Pharmacology Mind Maps for Medical Students and Allied Health Professionals

Pharmacology Mind Maps for Medical Students and Allied Health Professionals

Dr. Prasan Bhandari
Associate Professor, Department of Pharmacology
SDM College of Medical Sciences and Hospital, Sattur, Dharwad, Karnataka, India

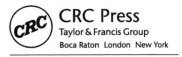

CRC Press
Taylor & Francis Group
Boca Raton London New York

CRC Press is an imprint of the
Taylor & Francis Group, an **informa** business

CRC Press
Taylor & Francis Group
6000 Broken Sound Parkway NW, Suite 300
Boca Raton, FL 33487-2742

Printed on acid-free paper

International Standard Book Number-13: 978-1-138-35124-0 (Paperback)

Library of Congress Cataloging-in-Publication Data

Names: Bhandari, Prasan R., author.
Title: Pharmacology mind maps for medical students and allied health professionals / Prasan R Bhandari.
Description: Boca Raton, FL : CRC Press/Taylor & Francis, 2020. | Includes bibliographical references and index.
Identifiers: LCCN 2019020058| ISBN 9781138351240 (pbk. : alk. paper) | ISBN 9780429023859 (ebook)
Subjects: | MESH: Pharmacological Phenomena | Drug Therapy--methods |
Handbook | Study Guide
Classification: LCC RM301.13 | NLM QV 39 | DDC 615.1076--dc23
LC record available at https://lccn.loc.gov/2019020058

Visit the Taylor & Francis Web site at
http://www.taylorandfrancis.com

and the CRC Press Web site at
http://www.crcpress.com

Dedicated to:

ALMIGHTY CREATOR

My parents, Mr. Ramchandra G. Bhandari and Mrs. Asha R. Bhandari

My in-laws, Mr. Dayanand A. Kamath and Mrs. Sharada D. Kamath

My sister, Mrs. Veebha (Lochan) V. Prabhu and my brother-in-law, Mr. Vishnu R. Prabhu

My sister-in-law, Mrs. Savita V. Shanbhag and my co-brother, Mr. Vinayak P. Shanbhag

My nephews, Ramnath V. Prabhu and Siddhant V. Shanbhag

My guru, guide, and philosopher, Mr. Dileep Keskar

A special thanks to Mr. Narasimha Bhat and family
(Mahalasa Narayani Temple, Mardol, Goa) for their constant guidance

Lastly, but most importantly, my wife, Mrs. Sangeeta P. Bhandari and
my two lovely daughters, Purva P. Bhandari and Neha P. Bhandari

Contents

PART IV CENTRAL NERVOUS SYSTEM (CNS) PHARMACOLOGY 199

Acknowledgments

I thank the management of the SDM College of Medical Sciences and Hospital, Dharwad, Karnataka, India, especially Dr. Niranjan Kumar (Medical Director), Dr. S.K. Joshi (Principal), Dr. P. Satyashankar (Medical Superintendent), Dr. J.V. Chowti (former Principal), and Dr. K.R. Pravin Chandra (Student Welfare Officer) for their support.

Thanks to my family members, relatives, friends for their active support, suggestions, and solutions.

In addition, my sincere thanks to Shivangi Pramanik and Mouli Sharma of CRC Press/Taylor & Francis Group, New Delhi, India, for providing me the opportunity to author this book.

The efforts put forth by the editorial staff, Nitasha Devasar and Himani Dwivedi, the Project Editor, Kyle Meyer, the Project Manager, Narayani Govindrajan, and the production team from Nova Techset are greatly appreciated.

Preface

During my tenure of teaching pharmacology, I noticed that undergraduate students find it difficult to read, remember, revise, and reproduce their subject material from standard textbooks. Empathizing with them, I wanted to write a book to provide them with alternative/supplementary material in a different format.

This book is designed for medical, dental, physiotherapy, and pharmacy students and any other healthcare professionals whose careers involve drug therapy and related aspects.

The book presents condensed and succinct descriptions of relevant and current information pertaining to pharmacology. It is not meant to be a substitute for the comprehensive presentation of information and difficult concepts found in standard textbooks of pharmacology.

Students are expected to master large amounts of information. There are few learning strategies accessible to these students to memorize and recall essential information to succeed in their medical colleges. When medical students receive very large amounts of information, passive learning results. Students remember facts rather than understanding and applying concepts.

As the medical profession continues to change, so do the methods by which medical students are taught. Various authors have accepted the need for alternative teaching and learning approaches that will help medical students to remember huge amounts of information, assimilate critical thinking skills, and explain a range of complex clinical problems.

There is a substantial necessity for faculty to move away from the customary teacher-centered educational method and enhance implementation of an active, student-centered learning environment.

One learning strategy that has been underutilized in medical education is *mind mapping*. Mind maps are multisensory tools that help students to organize, integrate, and retain information. A mind map is a diagram that represents words, concepts, ideas, or other items related to a given topic. Recent work suggests that using mind mapping as a note-taking strategy facilitates critical thinking.

Although the mind map as a learning strategy has not been extensively used in medical education, the latest research recommends using mind mapping in learning, as it increases students' long-term memory.

Mind maps, systematized by Tony Buzan, is a visual technique where information and knowledge are converted to a hierarchical formatted and illustrated diagram, with structural key terms associated with a subject. Mind maps are sprawling network diagrams that radiate out from a central point. The central topic contains a label of a general topic. Lines radiate out from that center to subtopics representing related concepts. More subtopics may radiate from those subtopics.

Mind mapping, a form of visual outlining, may seem superficial, but once mastered it provides a powerful tool for managing information overload and enabling one to quickly capture and organize a massive amount of ideas.

Mind maps are effective and can amplify productivity.

ONE SMALL STEP CAN CHANGE YOUR LIFE.

A mind map is a powerful graphic technique that can be applied to improve learning and clarify thinking. Mind maps can be used as self-learning methods to facilitate understanding of difficult concepts.

Mind mapping uses visual orientation to assimilate information and subsequently help students recall information in an organized manner. It is ideally suited for a last-minute study guide before examinations. This convenient and portable distillation of knowledge aids in memorizing and can save many hours of note taking.

We want to hear what you think. What do you like about the book's format—*the first of its kind in the world for pharmacology*? What do you think could be improved? Please share your feedback by emailing us at prasangeeta2012@gmail.com.

We are grateful to our students and our other colleagues who have taught us most of what we know about teaching. Examinations are stressful, but if you want to succeed, you have to put the work in.

However you choose to study, I hope you find this resource helpful throughout your preparation for your examinations.

Wishing you all the best for your examinations.

God Bless All.

Prasan Bhandari

Author

Dr. Prasan Bhandari obtained his MBBS degree from one of the oldest institutes in India, Grant Medical College and Sir JJ Group of Hospitals, Mumbai, India. He received his MD in Pharmacology from the academically renowned institute Topiwala National Medical College, BYL Nair Charitable Hospital, Mumbai, India.

Dr. Bhandari has over 23 years of academic, teaching, research, administrative, and industry experience. He has published several articles in both national and international journals and has served as an examiner in several universities for both postgraduate and undergraduate medical, dental, physiotherapy, and other allied paramedical students. He has guided several postgraduate students in their research work and dissertations.

He is currently Associate Professor in the Department of Pharmacology at SDM College of Medical Sciences and Hospital, Dharwad, India.

General pharmacology

Definitions, drug nomenclature, and sources of drugs

1.1 DEFINITIONS

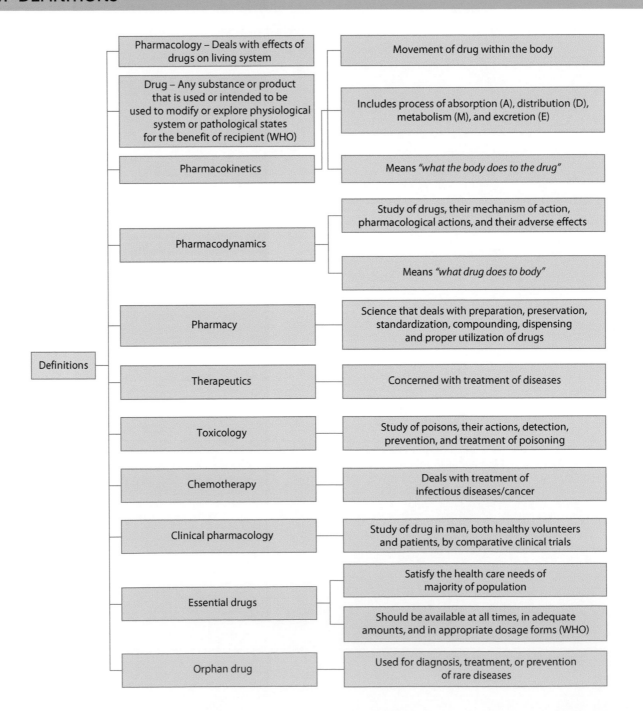

Definitions

- Pharmacology – Deals with effects of drugs on living system
- Drug – Any substance or product that is used or intended to be used to modify or explore physiological system or pathological states for the benefit of recipient (WHO)
- Pharmacokinetics
  - Movement of drug within the body
  - Includes process of absorption (A), distribution (D), metabolism (M), and excretion (E)
  - Means *"what the body does to the drug"*
- Pharmacodynamics
  - Study of drugs, their mechanism of action, pharmacological actions, and their adverse effects
  - Means *"what drug does to body"*
- Pharmacy
  - Science that deals with preparation, preservation, standardization, compounding, dispensing and proper utilization of drugs
- Therapeutics
  - Concerned with treatment of diseases
- Toxicology
  - Study of poisons, their actions, detection, prevention, and treatment of poisoning
- Chemotherapy
  - Deals with treatment of infectious diseases/cancer
- Clinical pharmacology
  - Study of drug in man, both healthy volunteers and patients, by comparative clinical trials
- Essential drugs
  - Satisfy the health care needs of majority of population
  - Should be available at all times, in adequate amounts, and in appropriate dosage forms (WHO)
- Orphan drug
  - Used for diagnosis, treatment, or prevention of rare diseases

1.2 DRUG NOMENCLATURE

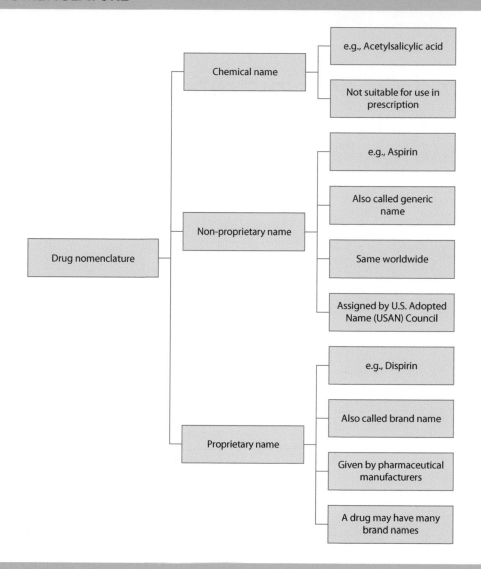

1.3 SOURCES OF DRUGS

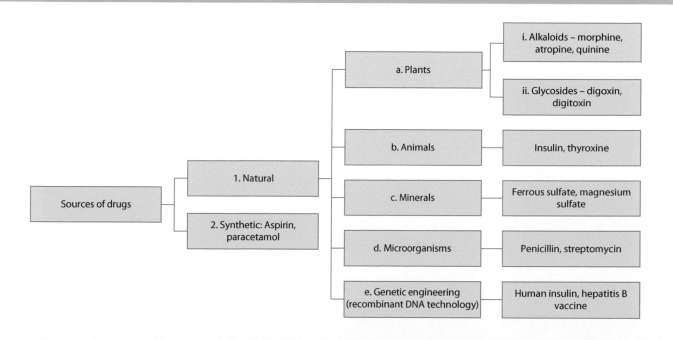

Routes of drug administration

2.1 FACTORS DETERMINING ROUTES OF DRUG ADMINISTRATION

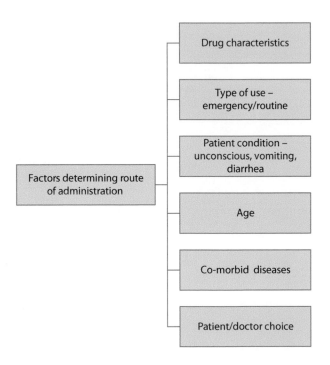

2.2 LOCAL ROUTE

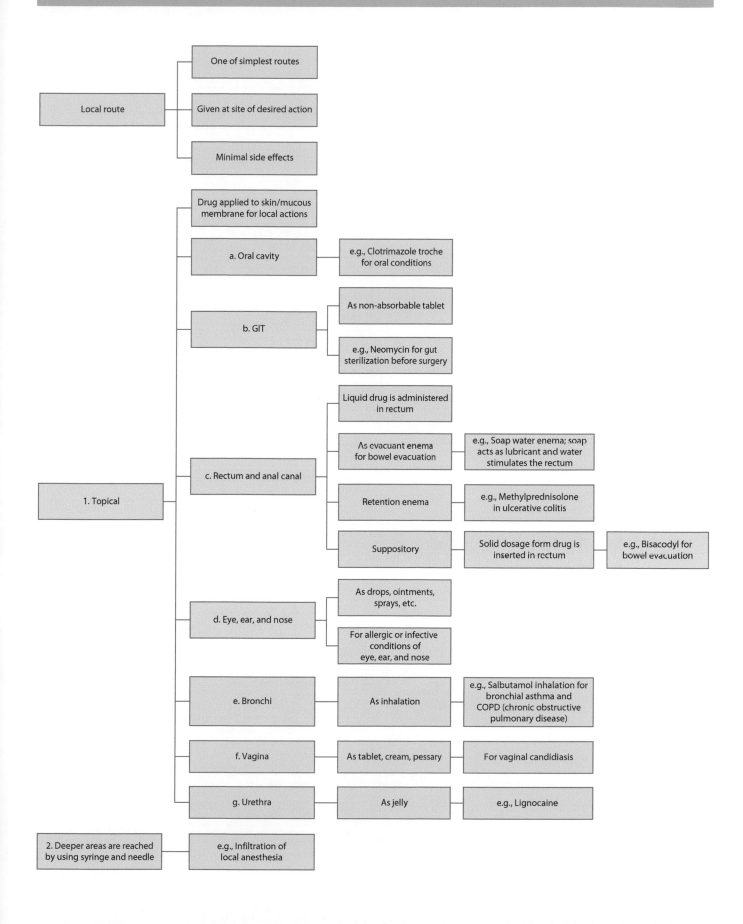

2.3 SYSTEMIC ROUTE

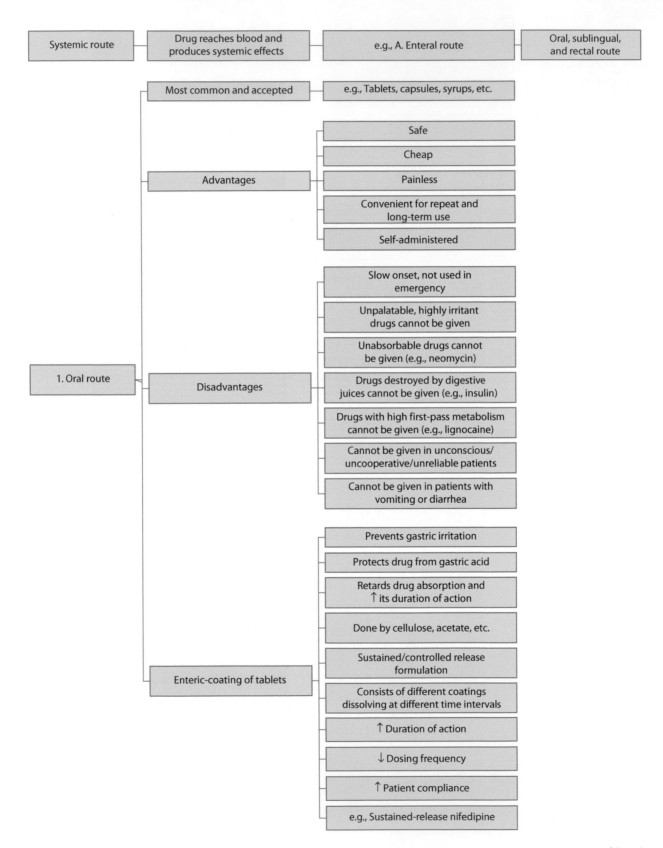

(Continued)

2.3 SYSTEMIC ROUTE (Continued)

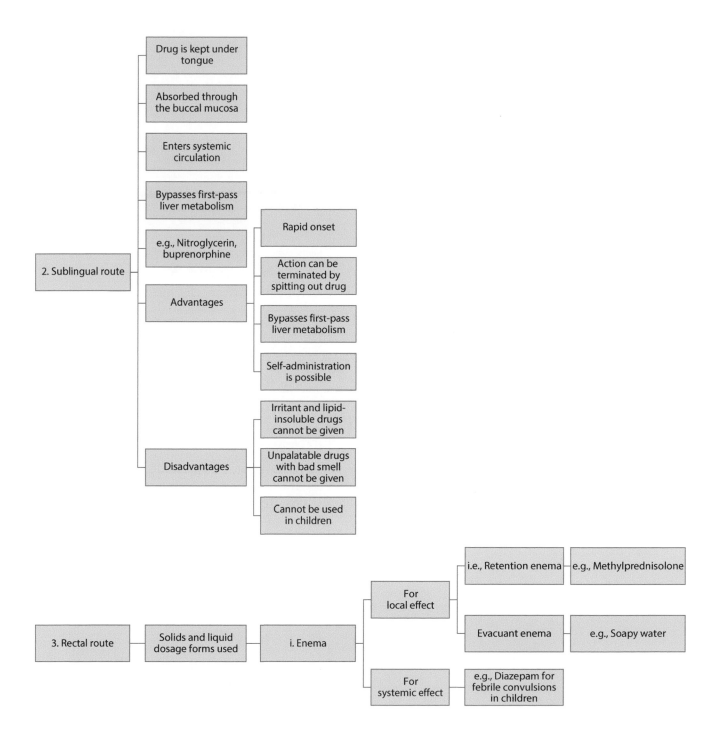

2.3 SYSTEMIC ROUTE (Continued)

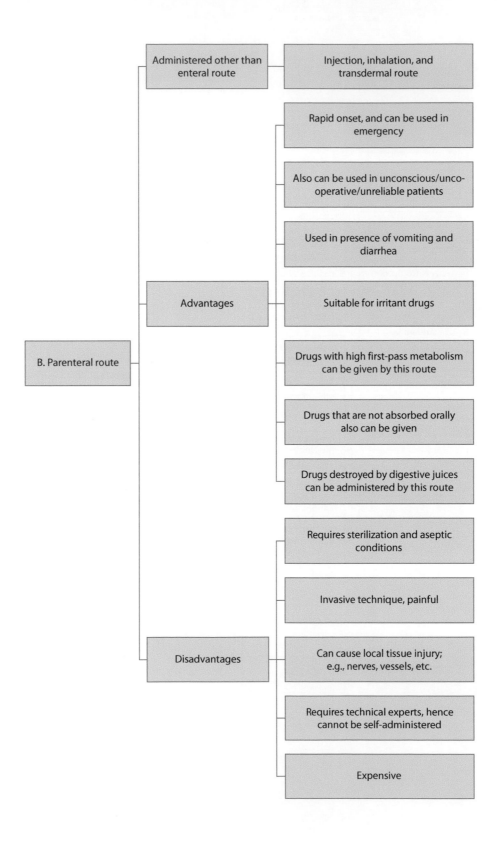

(Continued)

2.3 SYSTEMIC ROUTE (Continued)

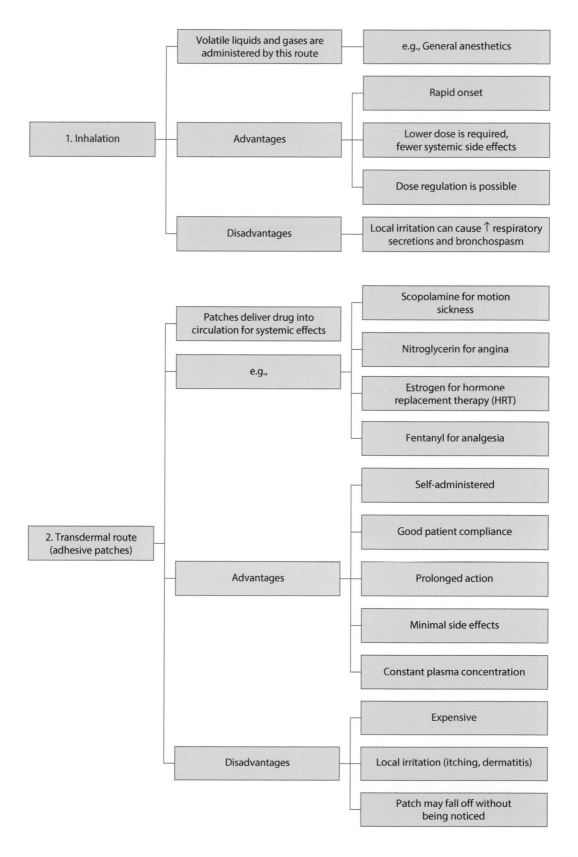

(Continued)

2.3 SYSTEMIC ROUTE (Continued)

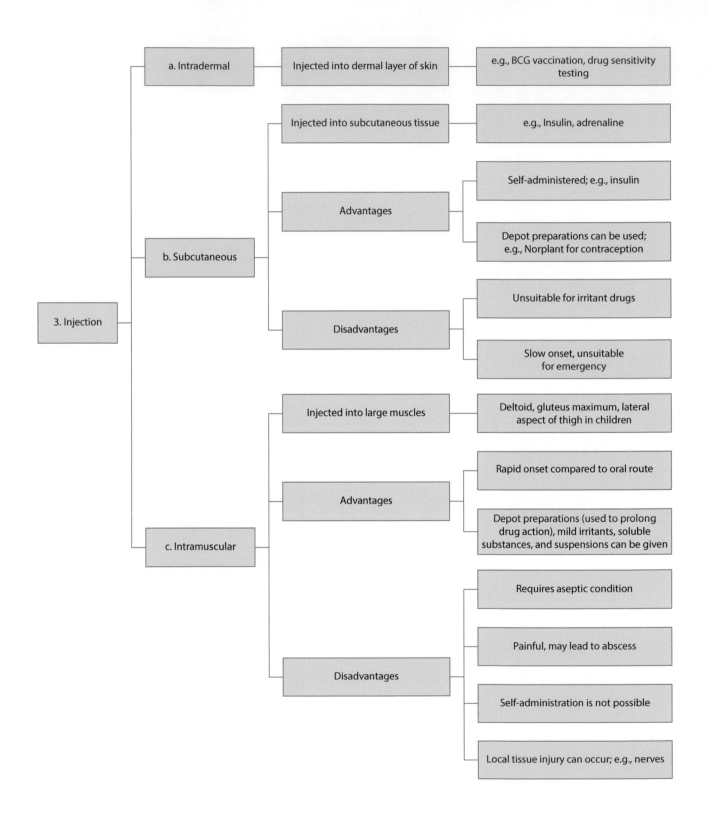

(Continued)

2.3 SYSTEMIC ROUTE (Continued)

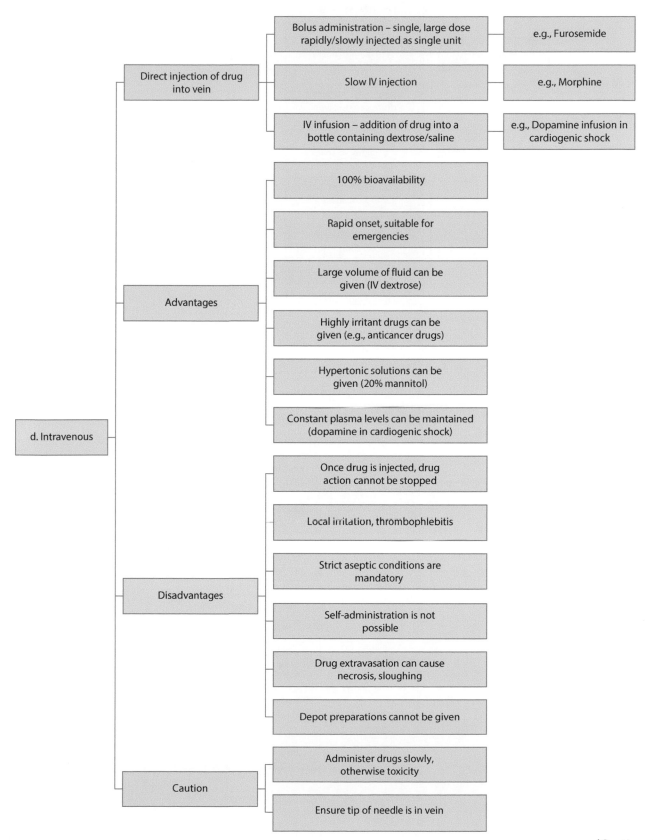

Direct injection of drug into vein
- Bolus administration – single, large dose rapidly/slowly injected as single unit → e.g., Furosemide
- Slow IV injection → e.g., Morphine
- IV infusion – addition of drug into a bottle containing dextrose/saline → e.g., Dopamine infusion in cardiogenic shock

d. Intravenous

Advantages
- 100% bioavailability
- Rapid onset, suitable for emergencies
- Large volume of fluid can be given (IV dextrose)
- Highly irritant drugs can be given (e.g., anticancer drugs)
- Hypertonic solutions can be given (20% mannitol)
- Constant plasma levels can be maintained (dopamine in cardiogenic shock)

Disadvantages
- Once drug is injected, drug action cannot be stopped
- Local irritation, thrombophlebitis
- Strict aseptic conditions are mandatory
- Self-administration is not possible
- Drug extravasation can cause necrosis, sloughing
- Depot preparations cannot be given

Caution
- Administer drugs slowly, otherwise toxicity
- Ensure tip of needle is in vein

(Continued)

2.3 SYSTEMIC ROUTE (Continued)

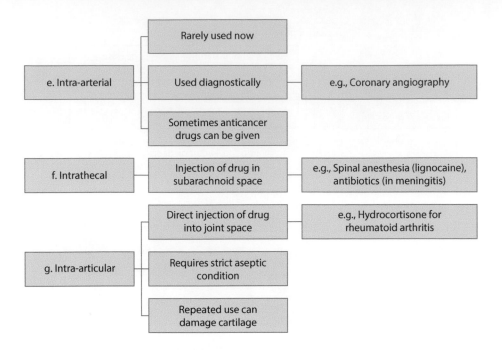

2.4 SPECIALIZED DRUG DELIVERY

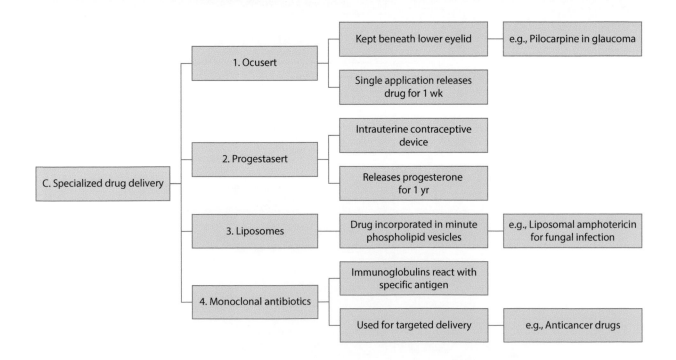

3

Pharmacokinetics and applied aspects

3.1 INTRODUCTION TO PHARMACOKINETICS

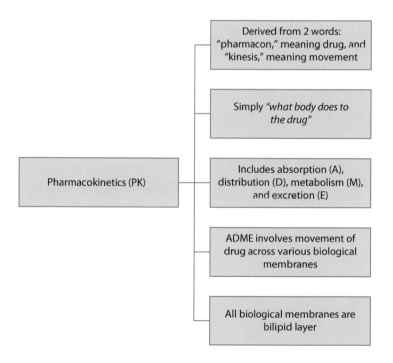

3.2 TRANSPORT OF DRUGS

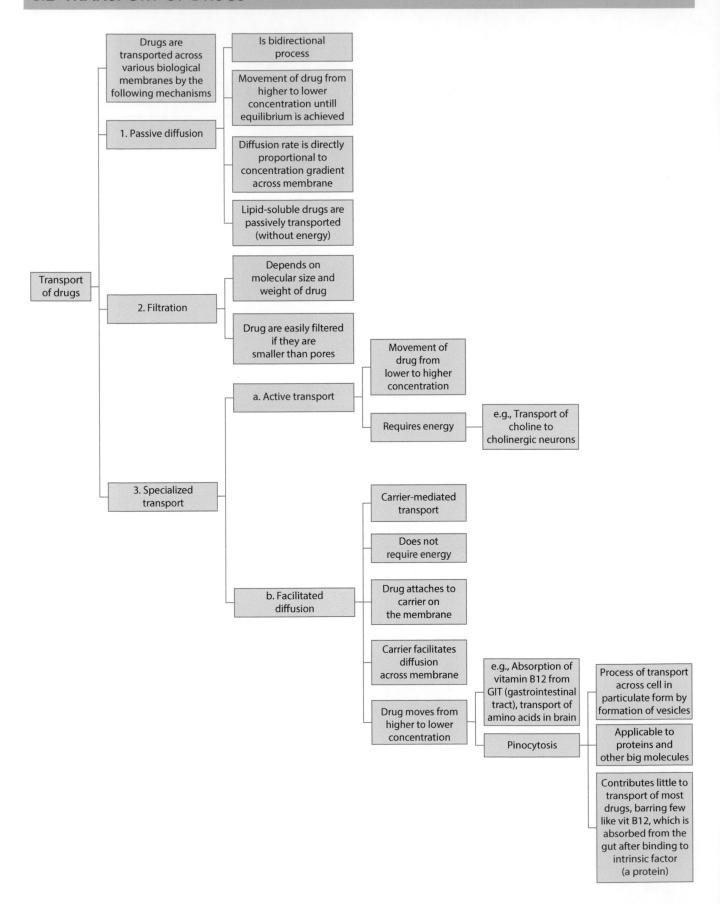

3.3 DRUG ABSORPTION

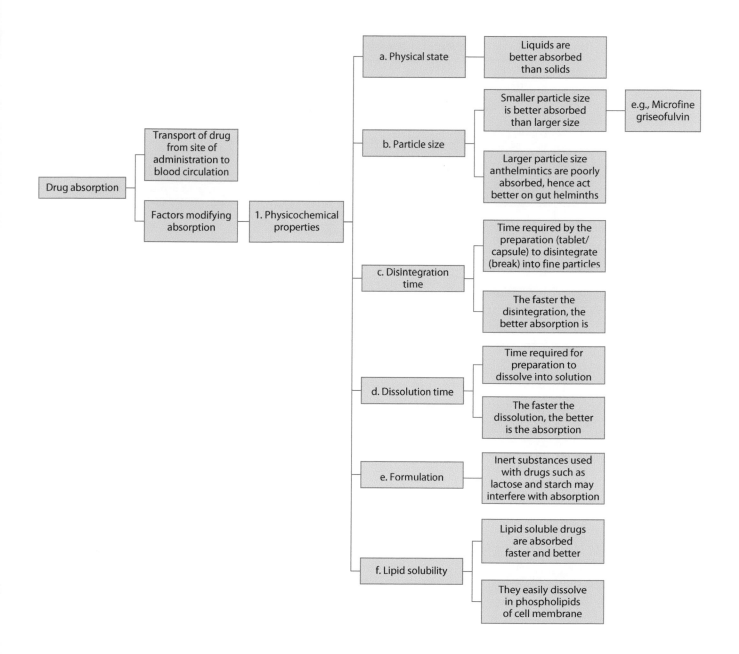

(*Continued*)

3.3 DRUG ABSORPTION (Continued)

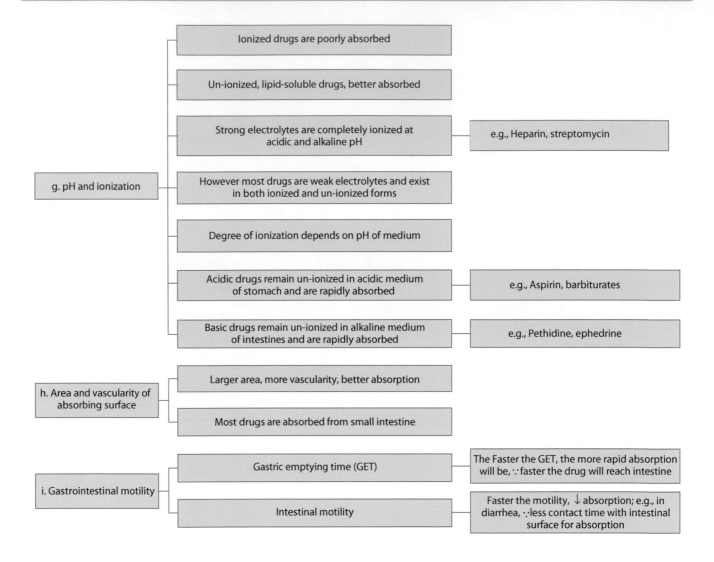

g. pH and ionization
- Ionized drugs are poorly absorbed
- Un-ionized, lipid-soluble drugs, better absorbed
- Strong electrolytes are completely ionized at acidic and alkaline pH — e.g., Heparin, streptomycin
- However most drugs are weak electrolytes and exist in both ionized and un-ionized forms
- Degree of ionization depends on pH of medium
- Acidic drugs remain un-ionized in acidic medium of stomach and are rapidly absorbed — e.g., Aspirin, barbiturates
- Basic drugs remain un-ionized in alkaline medium of intestines and are rapidly absorbed — e.g., Pethidine, ephedrine

h. Area and vascularity of absorbing surface
- Larger area, more vascularity, better absorption
- Most drugs are absorbed from small intestine

i. Gastrointestinal motility
- Gastric emptying time (GET) — The Faster the GET, the more rapid absorption will be, ∴ faster the drug will reach intestine
- Intestinal motility — Faster the motility, ↓ absorption; e.g., in diarrhea, ∴ less contact time with intestinal surface for absorption

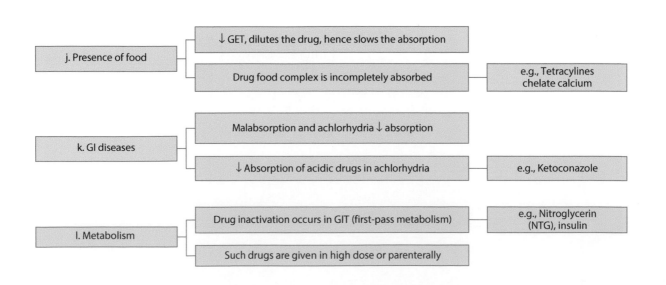

j. Presence of food
- ↓ GET, dilutes the drug, hence slows the absorption
- Drug food complex is incompletely absorbed — e.g., Tetracylines chelate calcium

k. GI diseases
- Malabsorption and achlorhydria ↓ absorption
- ↓ Absorption of acidic drugs in achlorhydria — e.g., Ketoconazole

l. Metabolism
- Drug inactivation occurs in GIT (first-pass metabolism) — e.g., Nitroglycerin (NTG), insulin
- Such drugs are given in high dose or parenterally

3.4 FIRST-PASS METABOLISM (PRESYSTEMIC METABOLISM)

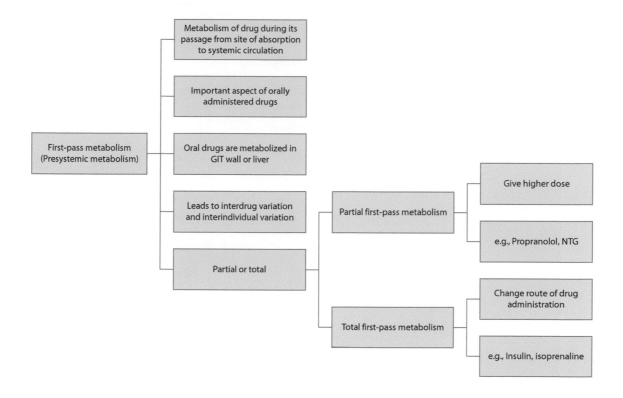

3.5 ABSORPTION FROM PARENTERAL ROUTE

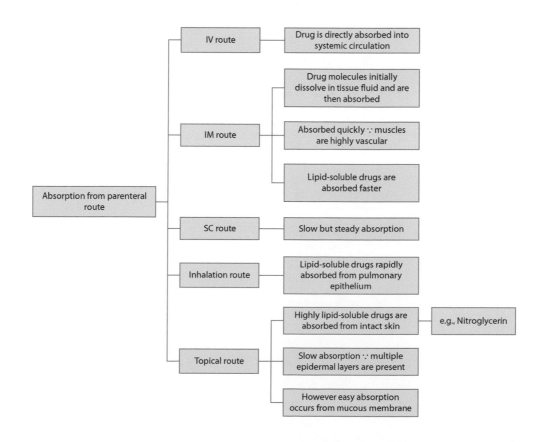

3.6 BIOAVAILABILITY AND BIOEQUIVALENCE

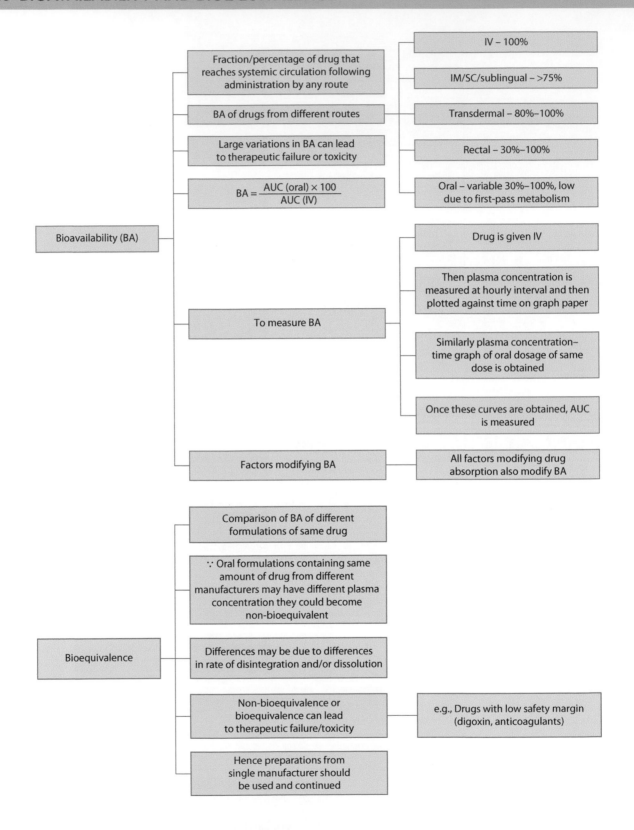

Bioavailability (BA)

- Fraction/percentage of drug that reaches systemic circulation following administration by any route
- BA of drugs from different routes
  - IV – 100%
  - IM/SC/sublingual – >75%
  - Transdermal – 80%–100%
  - Rectal – 30%–100%
  - Oral – variable 30%–100%, low due to first-pass metabolism
- Large variations in BA can lead to therapeutic failure or toxicity
- $BA = \dfrac{AUC\ (oral) \times 100}{AUC\ (IV)}$
- To measure BA
  - Drug is given IV
  - Then plasma concentration is measured at hourly interval and then plotted against time on graph paper
  - Similarly plasma concentration–time graph of oral dosage of same dose is obtained
  - Once these curves are obtained, AUC is measured
- Factors modifying BA
  - All factors modifying drug absorption also modify BA

Bioequivalence

- Comparison of BA of different formulations of same drug
- ∵ Oral formulations containing same amount of drug from different manufacturers may have different plasma concentration they could become non-bioequivalent
- Differences may be due to differences in rate of disintegration and/or dissolution
- Non-bioequivalence or bioequivalence can lead to therapeutic failure/toxicity
  - e.g., Drugs with low safety margin (digoxin, anticoagulants)
- Hence preparations from single manufacturer should be used and continued

3.7 DRUG DISTRIBUTION

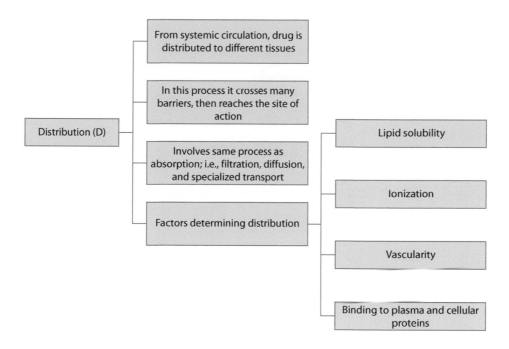

3.8 PLASMA PROTEIN BINDING

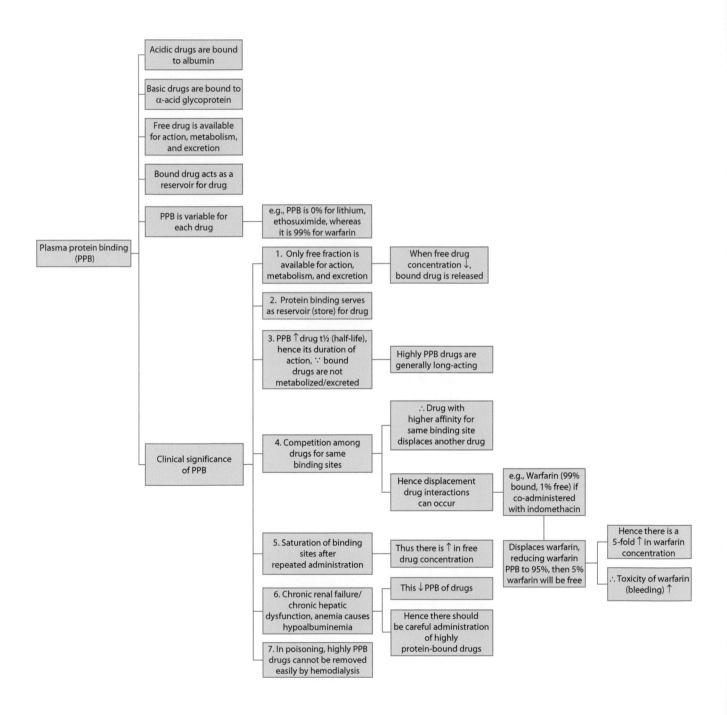

3.9 VOLUME OF DISTRIBUTION

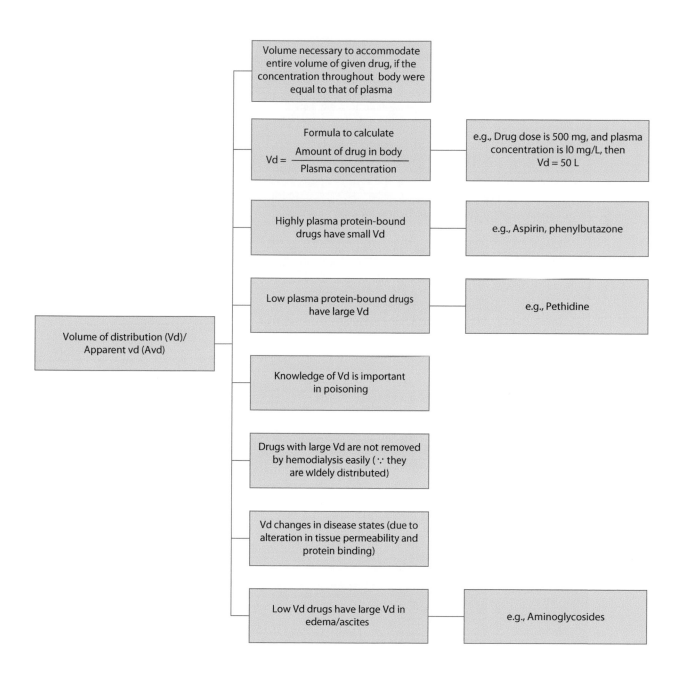

3.10 REDISTRIBUTION, BLOOD–BRAIN BARRIER, TISSUE BINDING, PLACENTAL BARRIER

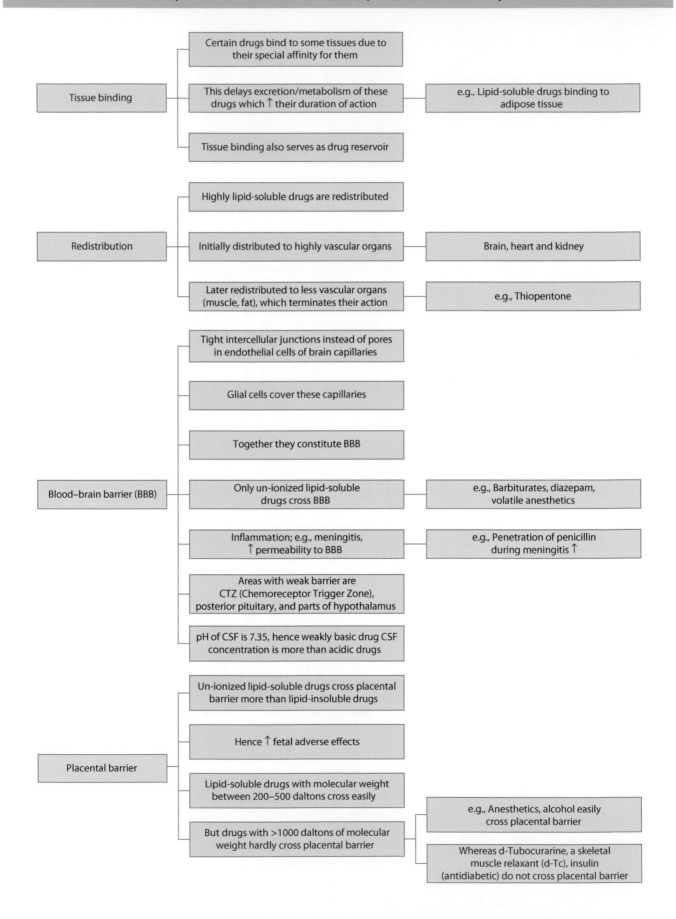

Tissue binding
- Certain drugs bind to some tissues due to their special affinity for them
- This delays excretion/metabolism of these drugs which ↑ their duration of action
  - e.g., Lipid-soluble drugs binding to adipose tissue
- Tissue binding also serves as drug reservoir

Redistribution
- Highly lipid-soluble drugs are redistributed
- Initially distributed to highly vascular organs
  - Brain, heart and kidney
- Later redistributed to less vascular organs (muscle, fat), which terminates their action
  - e.g., Thiopentone

Blood–brain barrier (BBB)
- Tight intercellular junctions instead of pores in endothelial cells of brain capillaries
- Glial cells cover these capillaries
- Together they constitute BBB
- Only un-ionized lipid-soluble drugs cross BBB
  - e.g., Barbiturates, diazepam, volatile anesthetics
- Inflammation; e.g., meningitis, ↑ permeability to BBB
  - e.g., Penetration of penicillin during meningitis ↑
- Areas with weak barrier are CTZ (Chemoreceptor Trigger Zone), posterior pituitary, and parts of hypothalamus
- pH of CSF is 7.35, hence weakly basic drug CSF concentration is more than acidic drugs

Placental barrier
- Un-ionized lipid-soluble drugs cross placental barrier more than lipid-insoluble drugs
- Hence ↑ fetal adverse effects
- Lipid-soluble drugs with molecular weight between 200–500 daltons cross easily
- But drugs with >1000 daltons of molecular weight hardly cross placental barrier
  - e.g., Anesthetics, alcohol easily cross placental barrier
  - Whereas d-Tubocurarine, a skeletal muscle relaxant (d-Tc), insulin (antidiabetic) do not cross placental barrier

3.11 FACTORS DETERMINING DISTRIBUTION

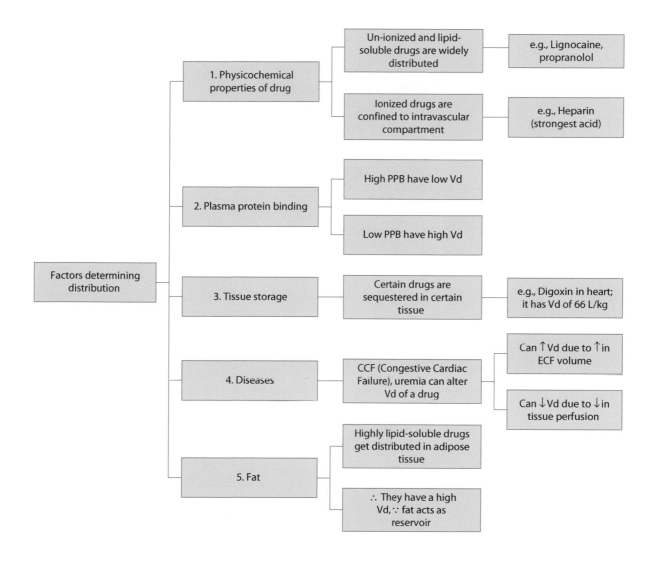

3.12 DRUG METABOLISM (BIOTRANSFORMATION)

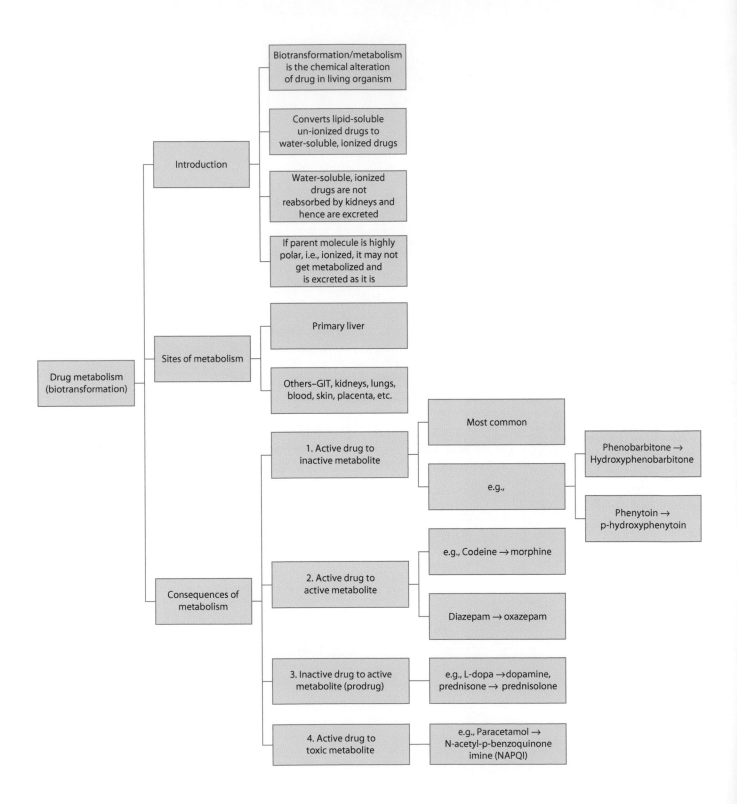

3.13 PATHWAYS OF METABOLISM AND PHASE I REACTIONS

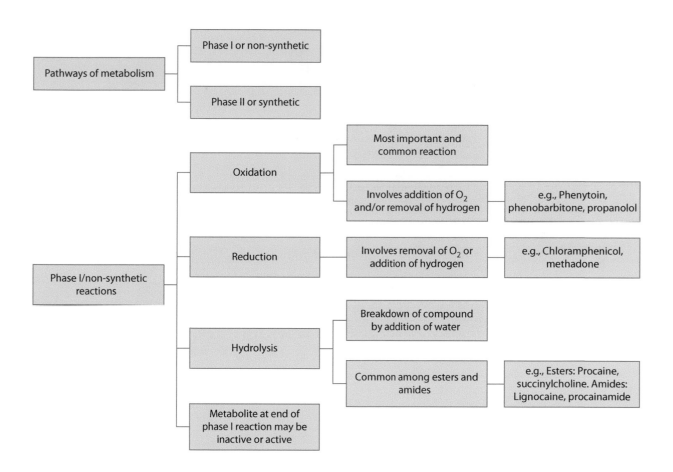

3.14 PHASE II/SYNTHETIC REACTIONS

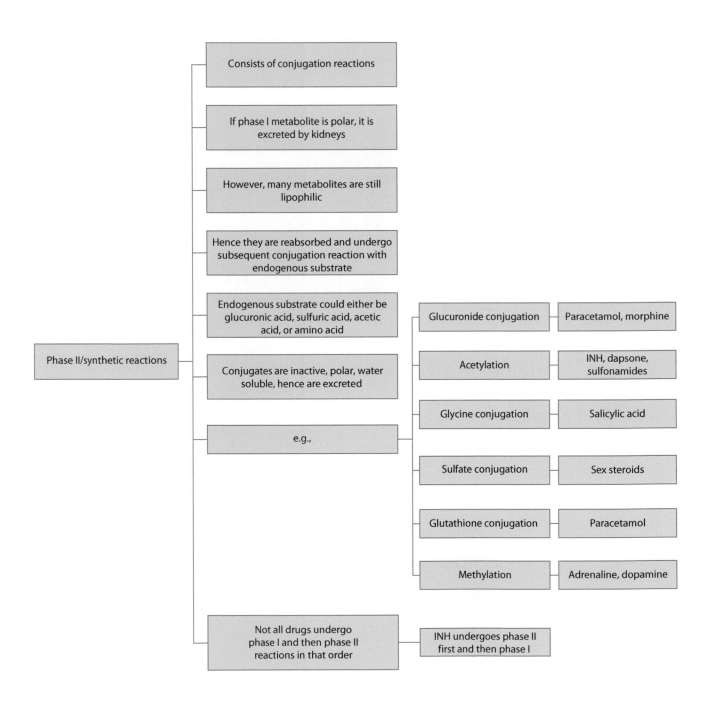

3.15 ENZYMES FOR METABOLISM

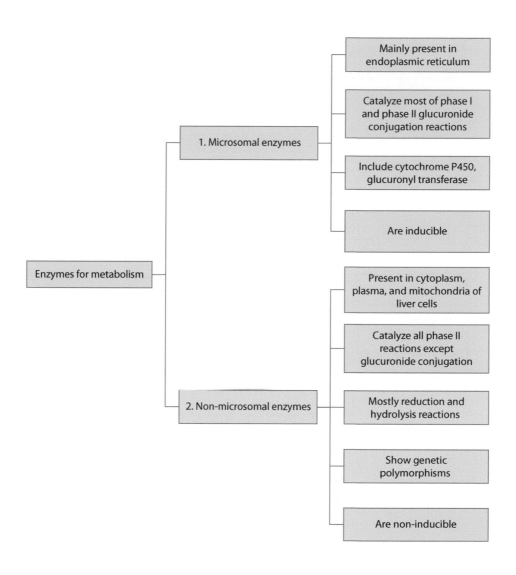

3.16 ENZYME INDUCTION

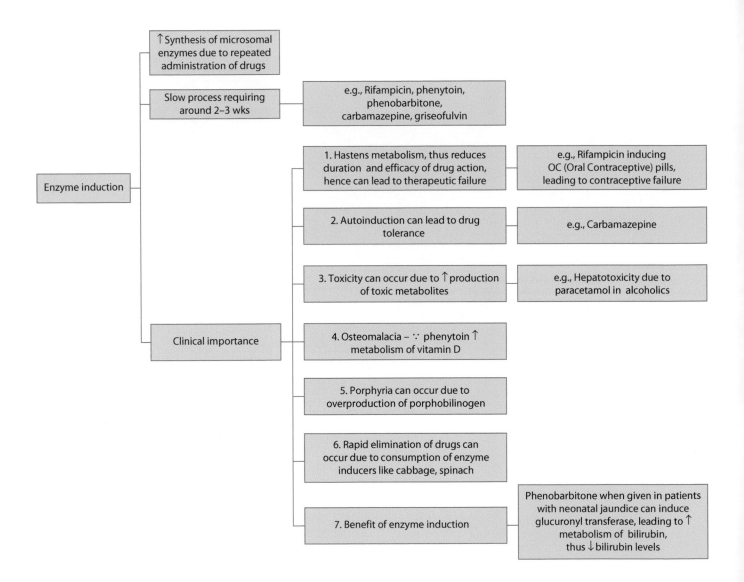

↑ Synthesis of microsomal enzymes due to repeated administration of drugs

Slow process requiring around 2–3 wks

e.g., Rifampicin, phenytoin, phenobarbitone, carbamazepine, griseofulvin

Enzyme induction

Clinical importance

1. Hastens metabolism, thus reduces duration and efficacy of drug action, hence can lead to therapeutic failure

e.g., Rifampicin inducing OC (Oral Contraceptive) pills, leading to contraceptive failure

2. Autoinduction can lead to drug tolerance

e.g., Carbamazepine

3. Toxicity can occur due to ↑ production of toxic metabolites

e.g., Hepatotoxicity due to paracetamol in alcoholics

4. Osteomalacia – ∵ phenytoin ↑ metabolism of vitamin D

5. Porphyria can occur due to overproduction of porphobilinogen

6. Rapid elimination of drugs can occur due to consumption of enzyme inducers like cabbage, spinach

7. Benefit of enzyme induction

Phenobarbitone when given in patients with neonatal jaundice can induce glucuronyl transferase, leading to ↑ metabolism of bilirubin, thus ↓ bilirubin levels

3.17 ENZYME INHIBITION

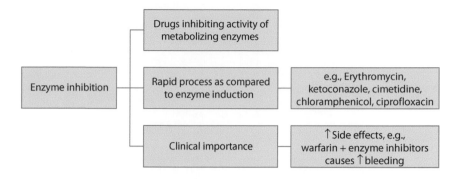

Enzyme inhibition
- Drugs inhibiting activity of metabolizing enzymes
- Rapid process as compared to enzyme induction — e.g., Erythromycin, ketoconazole, cimetidine, chloramphenicol, ciprofloxacin
- Clinical importance — ↑ Side effects, e.g., warfarin + enzyme inhibitors causes ↑ bleeding

3.18 FACTORS MODIFYING METABOLISM

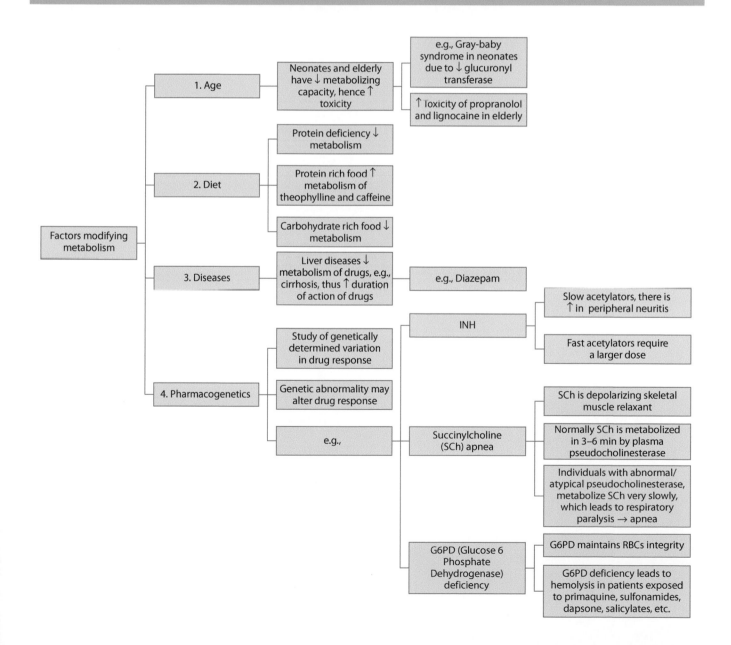

Factors modifying metabolism

1. Age — Neonates and elderly have ↓ metabolizing capacity, hence ↑ toxicity
   - e.g., Gray-baby syndrome in neonates due to ↓ glucuronyl transferase
   - ↑ Toxicity of propranolol and lignocaine in elderly

2. Diet
   - Protein deficiency ↓ metabolism
   - Protein rich food ↑ metabolism of theophylline and caffeine
   - Carbohydrate rich food ↓ metabolism

3. Diseases — Liver diseases ↓ metabolism of drugs, e.g., cirrhosis, thus ↑ duration of action of drugs — e.g., Diazepam

4. Pharmacogenetics
   - Study of genetically determined variation in drug response
   - Genetic abnormality may alter drug response
   - e.g.,
     - INH
       - Slow acetylators, there is ↑ in peripheral neuritis
       - Fast acetylators require a larger dose
     - Succinylcholine (SCh) apnea
       - SCh is depolarizing skeletal muscle relaxant
       - Normally SCh is metabolized in 3–6 min by plasma pseudocholinesterase
       - Individuals with abnormal/atypical pseudocholinesterase, metabolize SCh very slowly, which leads to respiratory paralysis → apnea
     - G6PD (Glucose 6 Phosphate Dehydrogenase) deficiency
       - G6PD maintains RBCs integrity
       - G6PD deficiency leads to hemolysis in patients exposed to primaquine, sulfonamides, dapsone, salicylates, etc.

3.19 PRODRUG

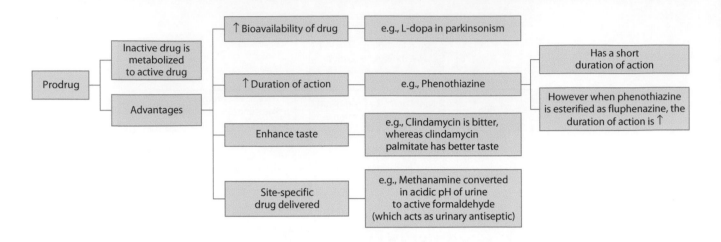

3.20 DRUG EXCRETION

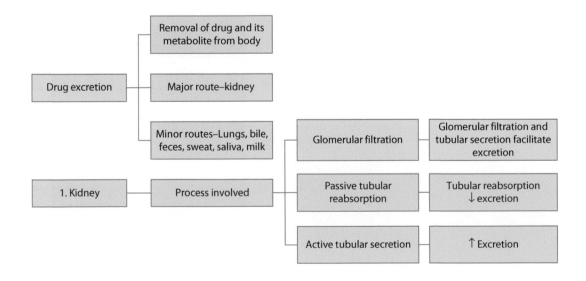

3.21 DRUG EXCRETION BY KIDNEYS

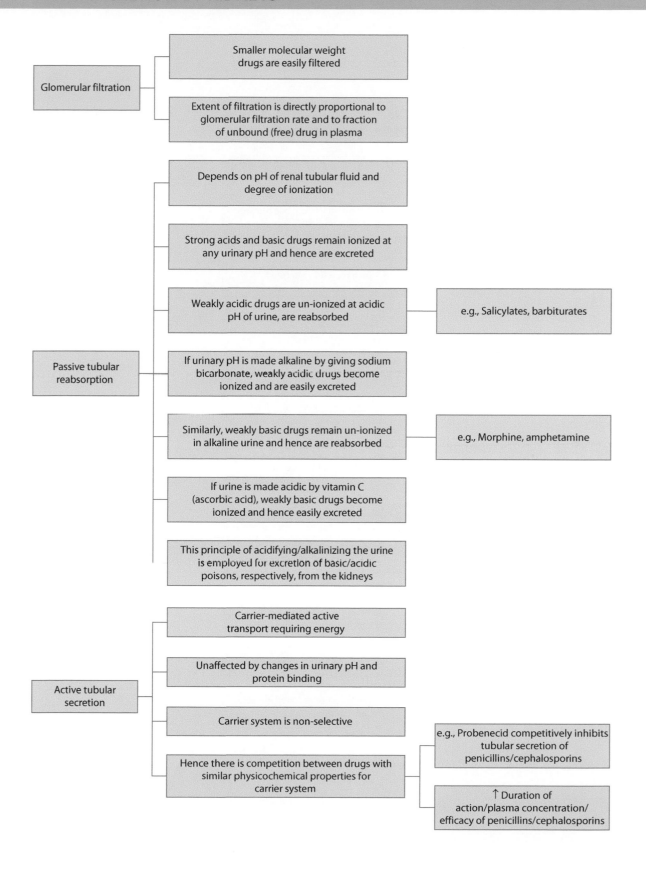

Glomerular filtration
- Smaller molecular weight drugs are easily filtered
- Extent of filtration is directly proportional to glomerular filtration rate and to fraction of unbound (free) drug in plasma

Passive tubular reabsorption
- Depends on pH of renal tubular fluid and degree of ionization
- Strong acids and basic drugs remain ionized at any urinary pH and hence are excreted
- Weakly acidic drugs are un-ionized at acidic pH of urine, are reabsorbed → e.g., Salicylates, barbiturates
- If urinary pH is made alkaline by giving sodium bicarbonate, weakly acidic drugs become ionized and are easily excreted
- Similarly, weakly basic drugs remain un-ionized in alkaline urine and hence are reabsorbed → e.g., Morphine, amphetamine
- If urine is made acidic by vitamin C (ascorbic acid), weakly basic drugs become ionized and hence easily excreted
- This principle of acidifying/alkalinizing the urine is employed for excretion of basic/acidic poisons, respectively, from the kidneys

Active tubular secretion
- Carrier-mediated active transport requiring energy
- Unaffected by changes in urinary pH and protein binding
- Carrier system is non-selective
- Hence there is competition between drugs with similar physicochemical properties for carrier system
  - e.g., Probenecid competitively inhibits tubular secretion of penicillins/cephalosporins
  - ↑ Duration of action/plasma concentration/efficacy of penicillins/cephalosporins

3.22 OTHER ROUTES OF DRUG EXCRETION

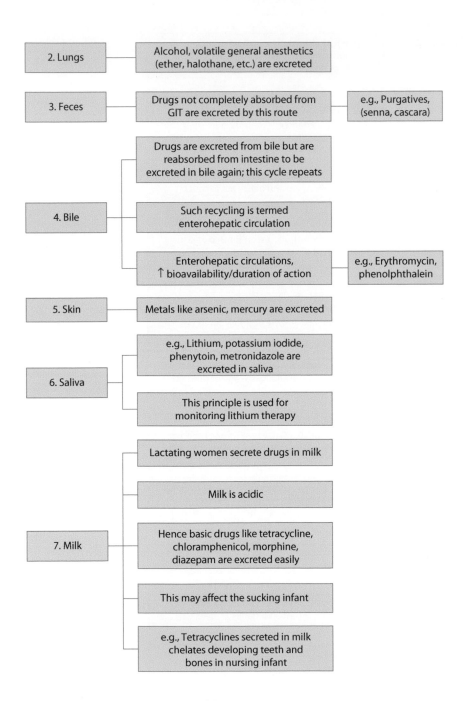

2. Lungs — Alcohol, volatile general anesthetics (ether, halothane, etc.) are excreted

3. Feces — Drugs not completely absorbed from GIT are excreted by this route — e.g., Purgatives, (senna, cascara)

4. Bile
- Drugs are excreted from bile but are reabsorbed from intestine to be excreted in bile again; this cycle repeats
- Such recycling is termed enterohepatic circulation
- Enterohepatic circulations, ↑ bioavailability/duration of action — e.g., Erythromycin, phenolphthalein

5. Skin — Metals like arsenic, mercury are excreted

6. Saliva
- e.g., Lithium, potassium iodide, phenytoin, metronidazole are excreted in saliva
- This principle is used for monitoring lithium therapy

7. Milk
- Lactating women secrete drugs in milk
- Milk is acidic
- Hence basic drugs like tetracycline, chloramphenicol, morphine, diazepam are excreted easily
- This may affect the sucking infant
- e.g., Tetracyclines secreted in milk chelates developing teeth and bones in nursing infant

3.23 APPLIED PHARMACOKINETICS

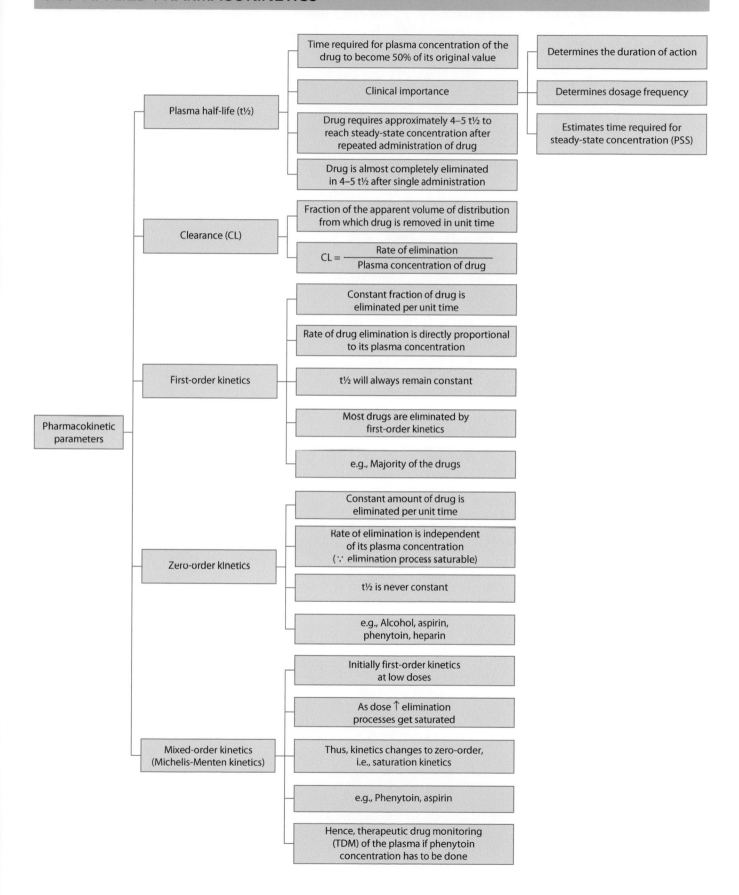

3.24 DRUG DOSING FACTORS

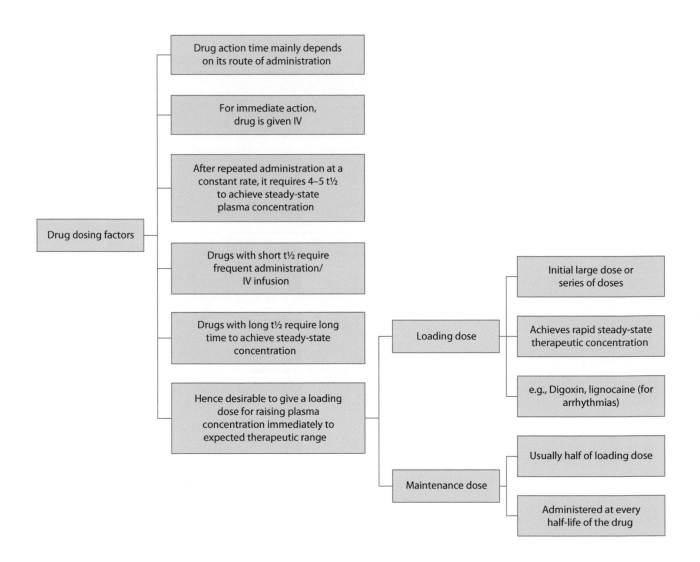

3.25 THERAPEUTIC DRUG MONITORING

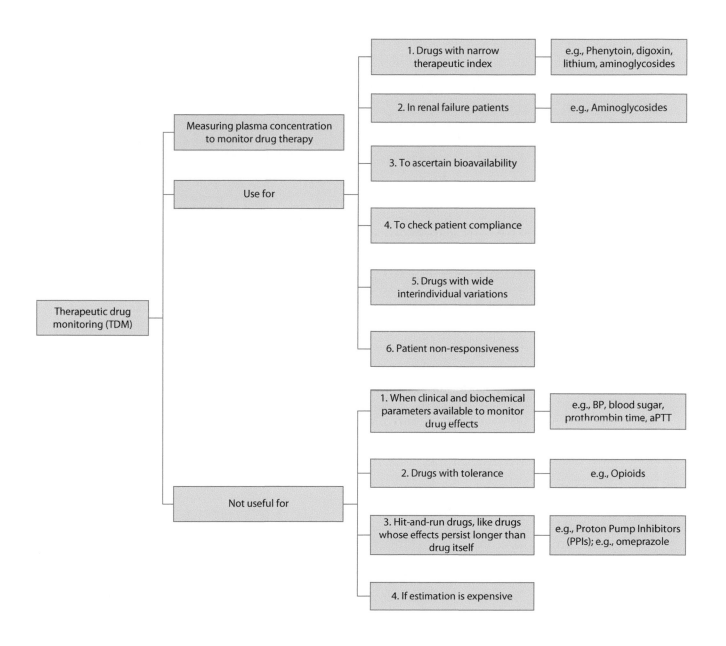

3.26 FIXED-DOSE COMBINATION

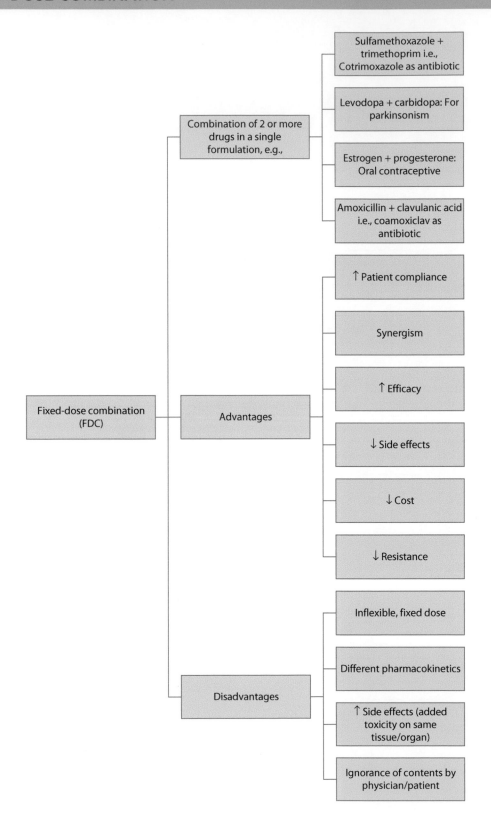

Fixed-dose combination (FDC)

Combination of 2 or more drugs in a single formulation, e.g.,
- Sulfamethoxazole + trimethoprim i.e., Cotrimoxazole as antibiotic
- Levodopa + carbidopa: For parkinsonism
- Estrogen + progesterone: Oral contraceptive
- Amoxicillin + clavulanic acid i.e., coamoxiclav as antibiotic

Advantages
- ↑ Patient compliance
- Synergism
- ↑ Efficacy
- ↓ Side effects
- ↓ Cost
- ↓ Resistance

Disadvantages
- Inflexible, fixed dose
- Different pharmacokinetics
- ↑ Side effects (added toxicity on same tissue/organ)
- Ignorance of contents by physician/patient

3.27 METHODS OF PROLONGING DRUG ACTION

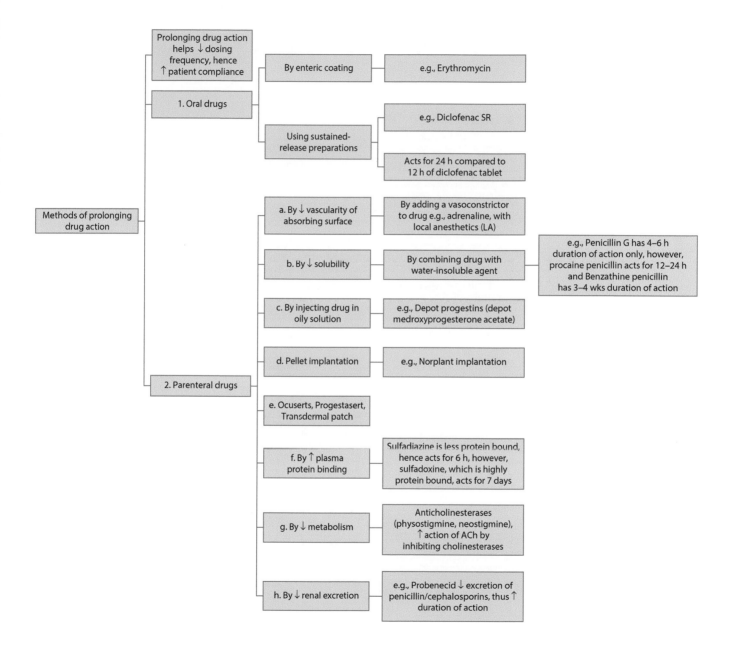

Pharmacodynamics

4.1 PHARMACODYNAMICS AND PRINCIPLES OF DRUG ACTION

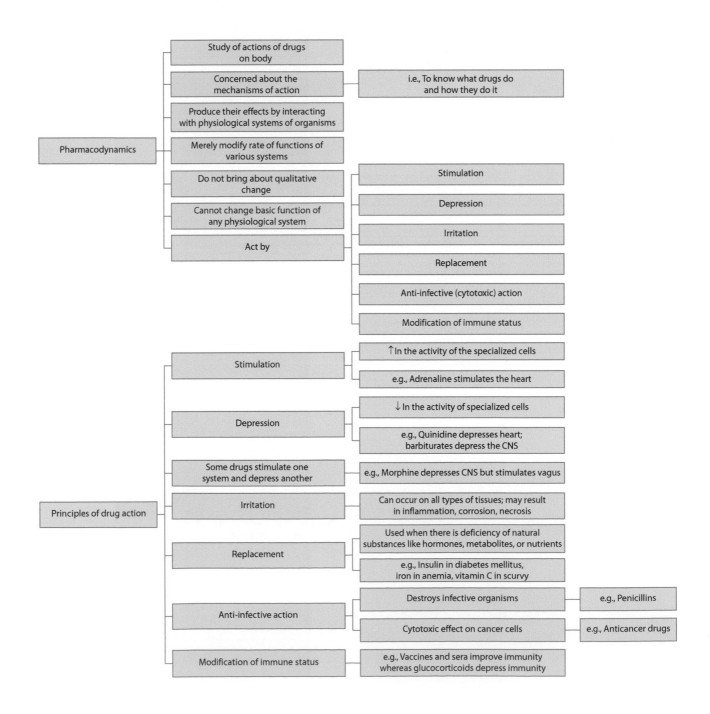

4.2 MECHANISMS OF DRUG ACTION

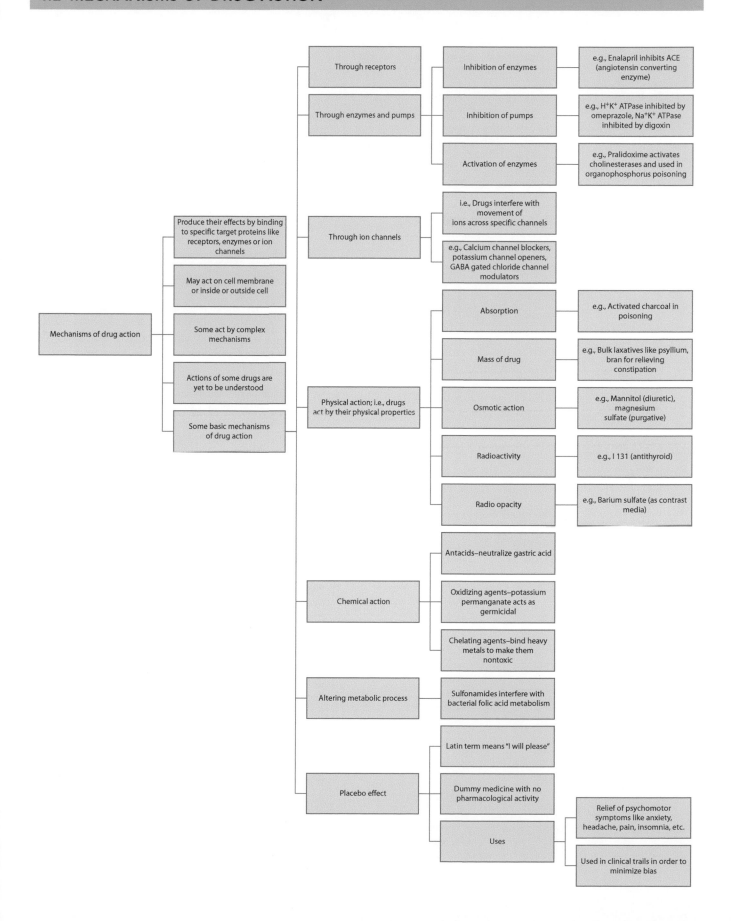

Mechanisms of drug action

- Produce their effects by binding to specific target proteins like receptors, enzymes or ion channels
- May act on cell membrane or inside or outside cell
- Some act by complex mechanisms
- Actions of some drugs are yet to be understood
- Some basic mechanisms of drug action

Through receptors

Through enzymes and pumps
- Inhibition of enzymes — e.g., Enalapril inhibits ACE (angiotensin converting enzyme)
- Inhibition of pumps — e.g., H^+K^+ ATPase inhibited by omeprazole, Na^+K^+ ATPase inhibited by digoxin
- Activation of enzymes — e.g., Pralidoxime activates cholinesterases and used in organophosphorus poisoning

Through ion channels
- i.e., Drugs interfere with movement of ions across specific channels
- e.g., Calcium channel blockers, potassium channel openers, GABA gated chloride channel modulators

Physical action; i.e., drugs act by their physical properties
- Absorption — e.g., Activated charcoal in poisoning
- Mass of drug — e.g., Bulk laxatives like psyllium, bran for relieving constipation
- Osmotic action — e.g., Mannitol (diuretic), magnesium sulfate (purgative)
- Radioactivity — e.g., I 131 (antithyroid)
- Radio opacity — e.g., Barium sulfate (as contrast media)

Chemical action
- Antacids–neutralize gastric acid
- Oxidizing agents–potassium permanganate acts as germicidal
- Chelating agents–bind heavy metals to make them nontoxic

Altering metabolic process
- Sulfonamides interfere with bacterial folic acid metabolism

Placebo effect
- Latin term means "I will please"
- Dummy medicine with no pharmacological activity
- Uses
  - Relief of psychomotor symptoms like anxiety, headache, pain, insomnia, etc.
  - Used in clinical trails in order to minimize bias

4.3 RECEPTOR

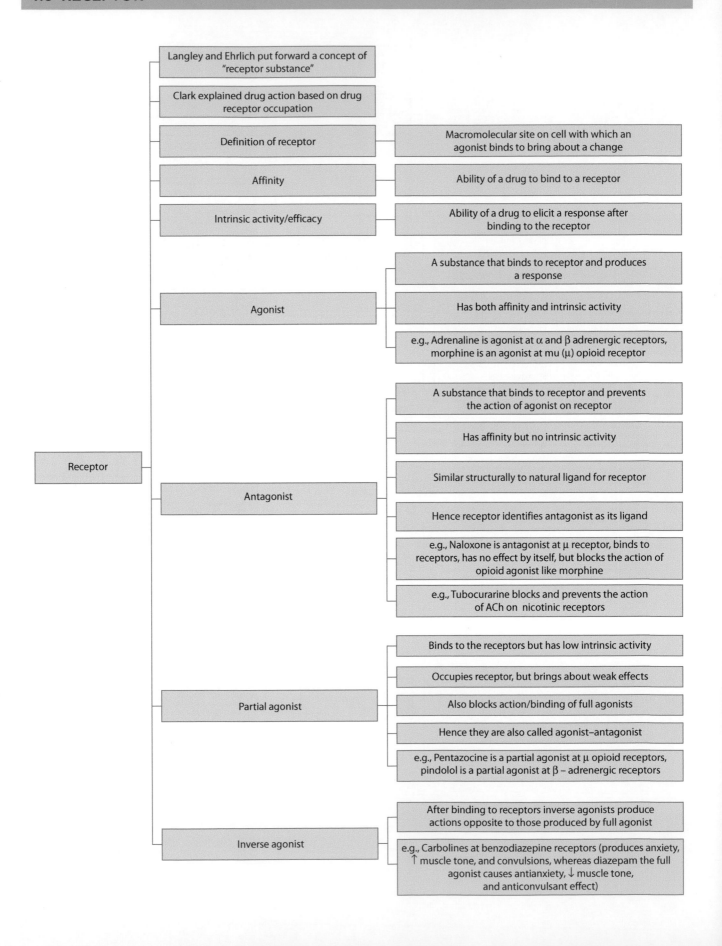

Langley and Ehrlich put forward a concept of "receptor substance"

Clark explained drug action based on drug receptor occupation

Definition of receptor — Macromolecular site on cell with which an agonist binds to bring about a change

Affinity — Ability of a drug to bind to a receptor

Intrinsic activity/efficacy — Ability of a drug to elicit a response after binding to the receptor

Agonist
- A substance that binds to receptor and produces a response
- Has both affinity and intrinsic activity
- e.g., Adrenaline is agonist at α and β adrenergic receptors, morphine is an agonist at mu (μ) opioid receptor

Antagonist
- A substance that binds to receptor and prevents the action of agonist on receptor
- Has affinity but no intrinsic activity
- Similar structurally to natural ligand for receptor
- Hence receptor identifies antagonist as its ligand
- e.g., Naloxone is antagonist at μ receptor, binds to receptors, has no effect by itself, but blocks the action of opioid agonist like morphine
- e.g., Tubocurarine blocks and prevents the action of ACh on nicotinic receptors

Partial agonist
- Binds to the receptors but has low intrinsic activity
- Occupies receptor, but brings about weak effects
- Also blocks action/binding of full agonists
- Hence they are also called agonist–antagonist
- e.g., Pentazocine is a partial agonist at μ opioid receptors, pindolol is a partial agonist at β – adrenergic receptors

Inverse agonist
- After binding to receptors inverse agonists produce actions opposite to those produced by full agonist
- e.g., Carbolines at benzodiazepine receptors (produces anxiety, ↑ muscle tone, and convulsions, whereas diazepam the full agonist causes antianxiety, ↓ muscle tone, and anticonvulsant effect)

Receptor

4.4 RECEPTOR – NATURE, SITES, AND FUNCTIONS

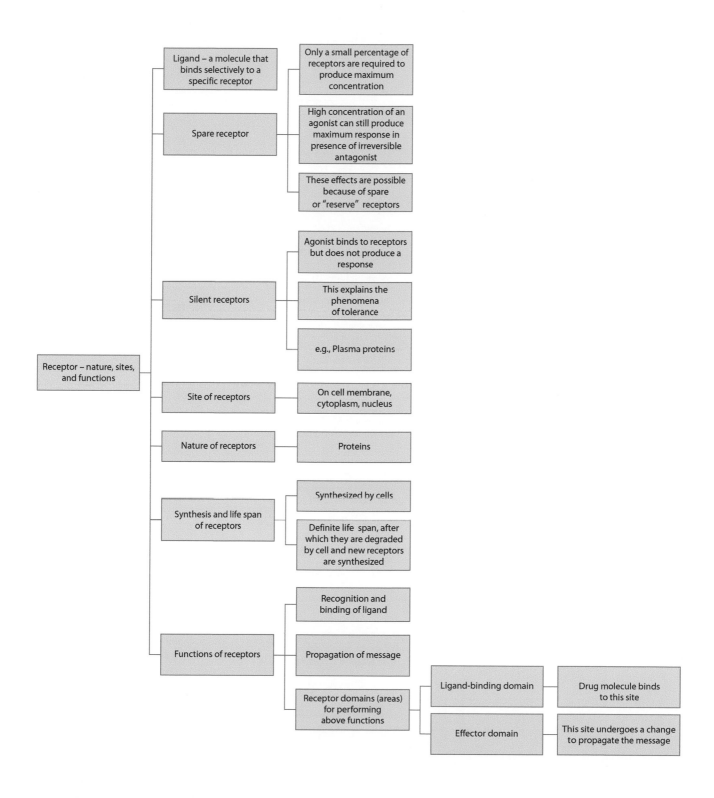

4.5 DRUG RECEPTOR INTERACTION THEORIES

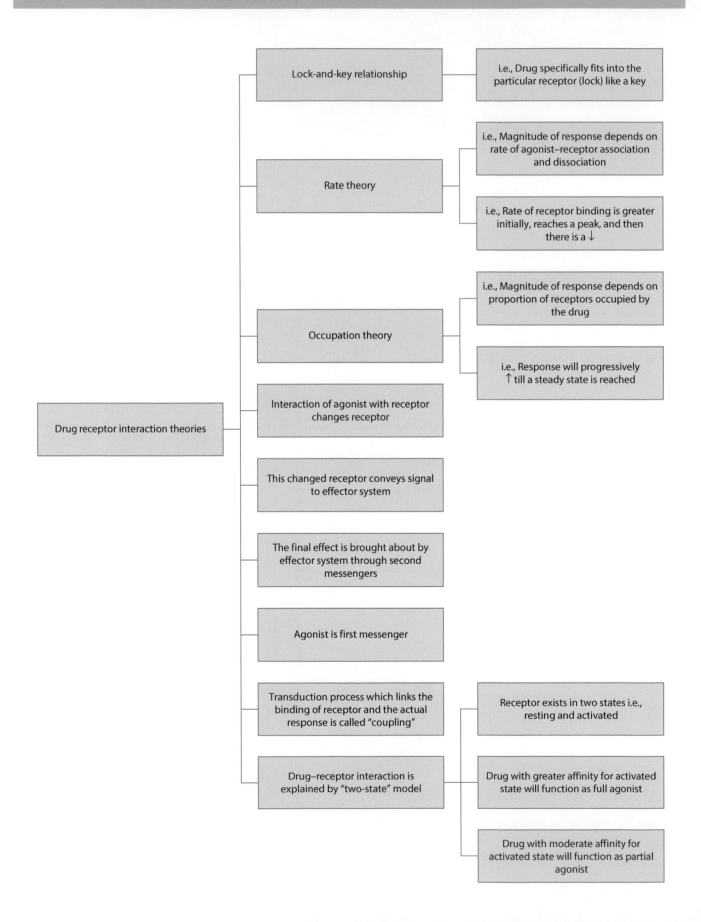

Drug receptor interaction theories

Lock-and-key relationship
— i.e., Drug specifically fits into the particular receptor (lock) like a key

Rate theory
— i.e., Magnitude of response depends on rate of agonist–receptor association and dissociation
— i.e., Rate of receptor binding is greater initially, reaches a peak, and then there is a ↓

Occupation theory
— i.e., Magnitude of response depends on proportion of receptors occupied by the drug
— i.e., Response will progressively ↑ till a steady state is reached

Interaction of agonist with receptor changes receptor

This changed receptor conveys signal to effector system

The final effect is brought about by effector system through second messengers

Agonist is first messenger

Transduction process which links the binding of receptor and the actual response is called "coupling"

Drug–receptor interaction is explained by "two-state" model
— Receptor exists in two states i.e., resting and activated
— Drug with greater affinity for activated state will function as full agonist
— Drug with moderate affinity for activated state will function as partial agonist

4.6 RECEPTOR FAMILIES

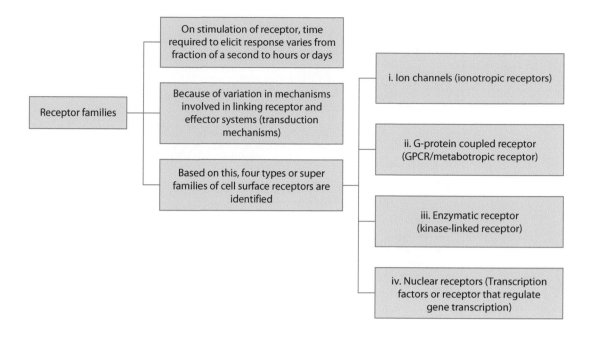

4.7 RECEPTOR FAMILIES AND THEIR TRANSDUCTION MECHANISMS – ION CHANNELS OR LIGAND-GATED ION CHANNELS

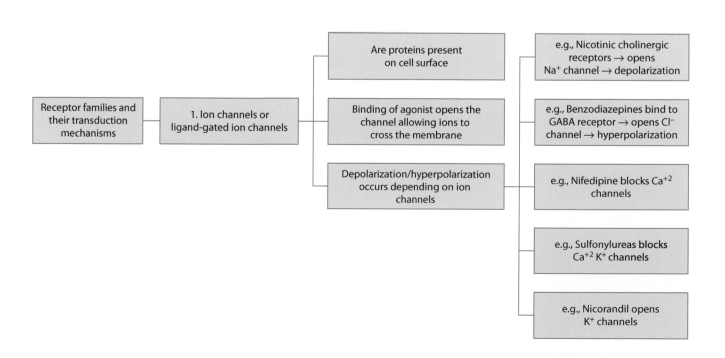

4.8 G-PROTEIN COUPLED RECEPTORS (GPCR)

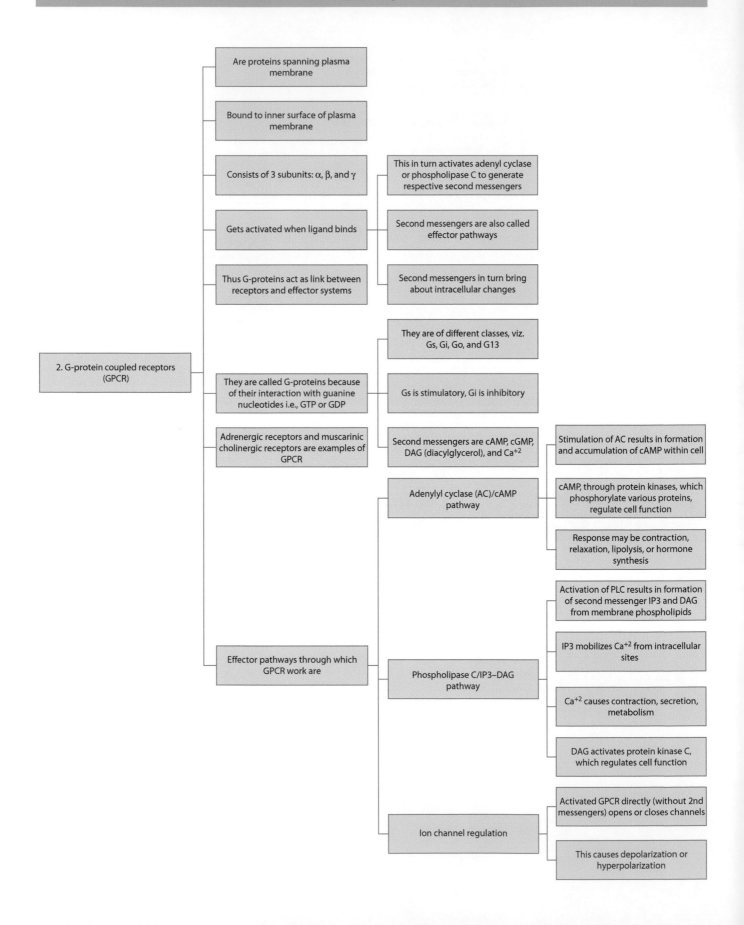

Are proteins spanning plasma membrane

Bound to inner surface of plasma membrane

Consists of 3 subunits: α, β, and γ

Gets activated when ligand binds

Thus G-proteins act as link between receptors and effector systems

2. G-protein coupled receptors (GPCR)

They are called G-proteins because of their interaction with guanine nucleotides i.e., GTP or GDP

Adrenergic receptors and muscarinic cholinergic receptors are examples of GPCR

Effector pathways through which GPCR work are

This in turn activates adenyl cyclase or phospholipase C to generate respective second messengers

Second messengers are also called effector pathways

Second messengers in turn bring about intracellular changes

They are of different classes, viz. Gs, Gi, Go, and G13

Gs is stimulatory, Gi is inhibitory

Second messengers are cAMP, cGMP, DAG (diacylglycerol), and Ca^{+2}

Adenylyl cyclase (AC)/cAMP pathway

Phospholipase C/IP3–DAG pathway

Ion channel regulation

Stimulation of AC results in formation and accumulation of cAMP within cell

cAMP, through protein kinases, which phosphorylate various proteins, regulate cell function

Response may be contraction, relaxation, lipolysis, or hormone synthesis

Activation of PLC results in formation of second messenger IP3 and DAG from membrane phospholipids

IP3 mobilizes Ca^{+2} from intracellular sites

Ca^{+2} causes contraction, secretion, metabolism

DAG activates protein kinase C, which regulates cell function

Activated GPCR directly (without 2nd messengers) opens or closes channels

This causes depolarization or hyperpolarization

4.9 ENZYMATIC RECEPTORS

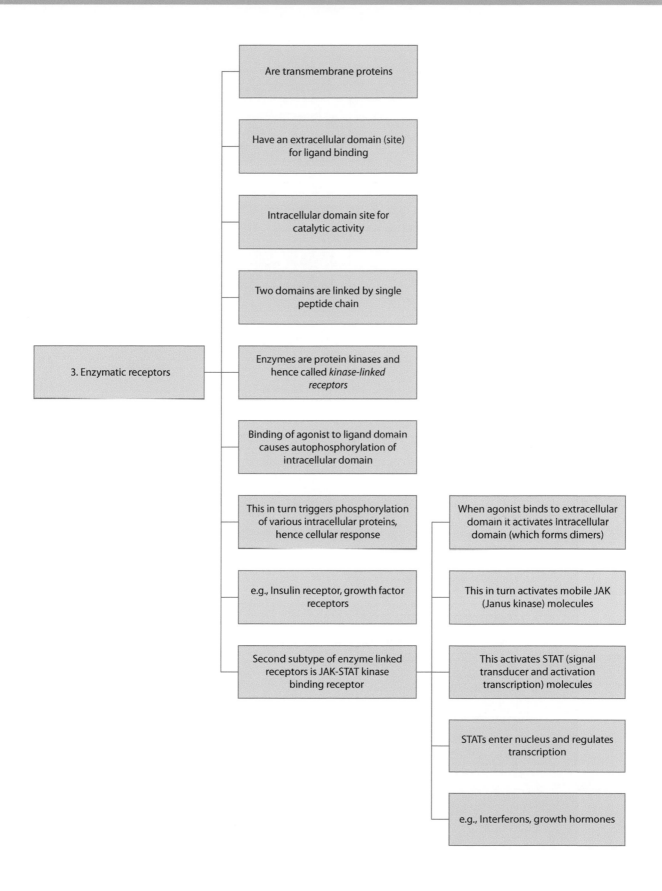

3. Enzymatic receptors

- Are transmembrane proteins
- Have an extracellular domain (site) for ligand binding
- Intracellular domain site for catalytic activity
- Two domains are linked by single peptide chain
- Enzymes are protein kinases and hence called *kinase-linked receptors*
- Binding of agonist to ligand domain causes autophosphorylation of intracellular domain
- This in turn triggers phosphorylation of various intracellular proteins, hence cellular response
- e.g., Insulin receptor, growth factor receptors
- Second subtype of enzyme linked receptors is JAK-STAT kinase binding receptor
  - When agonist binds to extracellular domain it activates intracellular domain (which forms dimers)
  - This in turn activates mobile JAK (Janus kinase) molecules
  - This activates STAT (signal transducer and activation transcription) molecules
  - STATs enter nucleus and regulates transcription
  - e.g., Interferons, growth hormones

4.10 NUCLEAR RECEPTOR

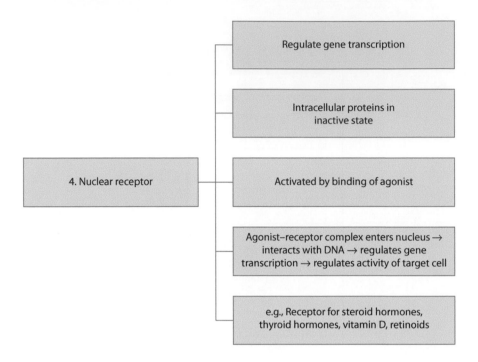

4. Nuclear receptor	Regulate gene transcription
	Intracellular proteins in inactive state
	Activated by binding of agonist
	Agonist–receptor complex enters nucleus → interacts with DNA → regulates gene transcription → regulates activity of target cell
	e.g., Receptor for steroid hormones, thyroid hormones, vitamin D, retinoids

4.11 RECEPTOR REGULATION

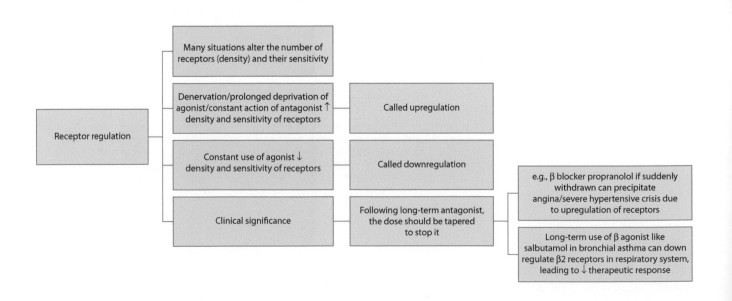

Receptor regulation

- Many situations alter the number of receptors (density) and their sensitivity
- Denervation/prolonged deprivation of agonist/constant action of antagonist ↑ density and sensitivity of receptors → Called upregulation
- Constant use of agonist ↓ density and sensitivity of receptors → Called downregulation
- Clinical significance → Following long-term antagonist, the dose should be tapered to stop it
  - e.g., β blocker propranolol if suddenly withdrawn can precipitate angina/severe hypertensive crisis due to upregulation of receptors
  - Long-term use of β agonist like salbutamol in bronchial asthma can down regulate β2 receptors in respiratory system, leading to ↓ therapeutic response

4.12 DOSE–RESPONSE RELATIONSHIP

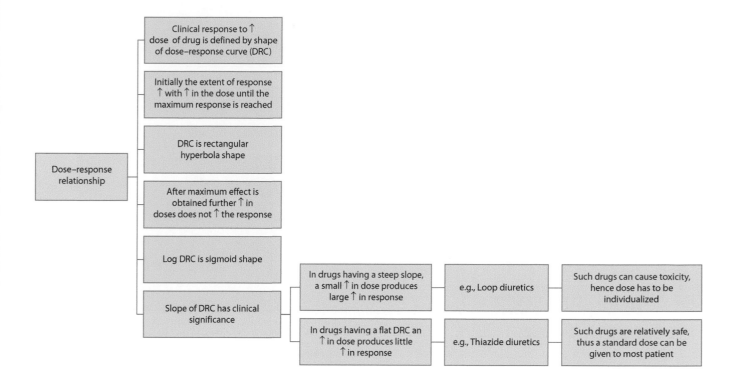

4.13 DRUG POTENCY

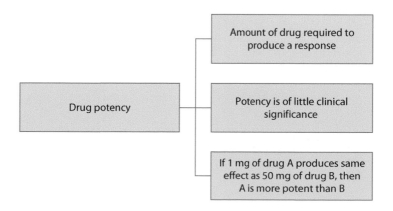

4.14 DRUG EFFICACY

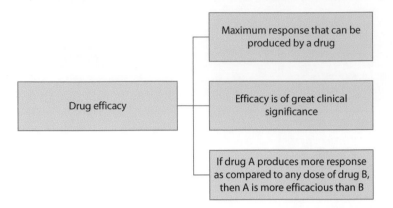

4.15 THERAPEUTIC INDEX (TI)

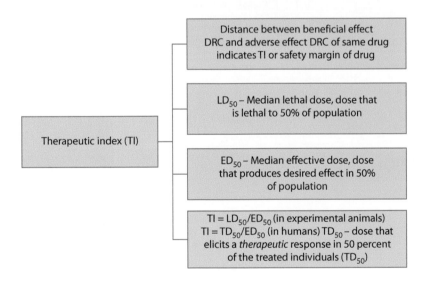

4.16 THERAPEUTIC WINDOW

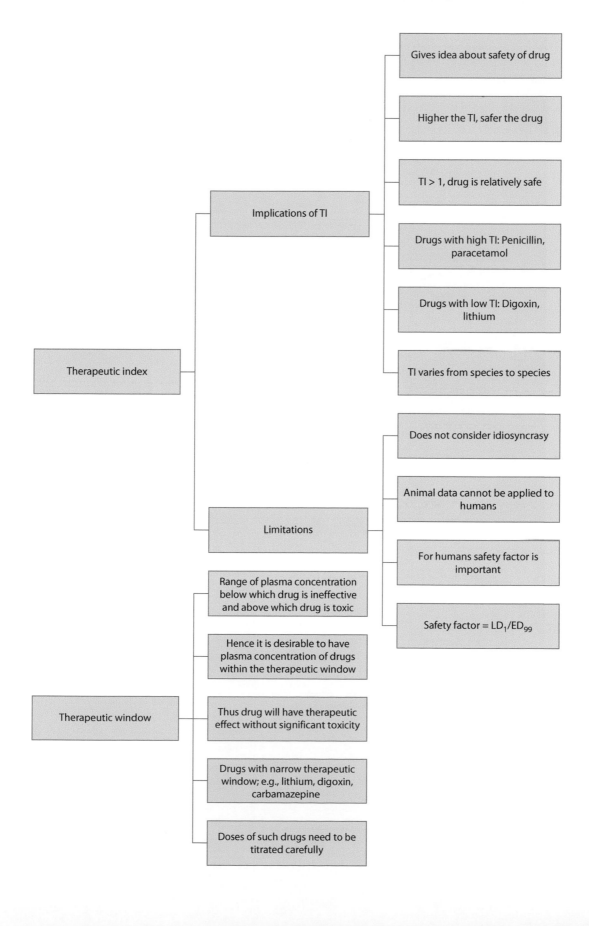

Therapeutic index

Implications of TI
- Gives idea about safety of drug
- Higher the TI, safer the drug
- TI > 1, drug is relatively safe
- Drugs with high TI: Penicillin, paracetamol
- Drugs with low TI: Digoxin, lithium
- TI varies from species to species

Limitations
- Does not consider idiosyncrasy
- Animal data cannot be applied to humans
- For humans safety factor is important
- Safety factor = LD_1/ED_{99}

Therapeutic window
- Range of plasma concentration below which drug is ineffective and above which drug is toxic
- Hence it is desirable to have plasma concentration of drugs within the therapeutic window
- Thus drug will have therapeutic effect without significant toxicity
- Drugs with narrow therapeutic window; e.g., lithium, digoxin, carbamazepine
- Doses of such drugs need to be titrated carefully

4.17 DRUG SYNERGISM AND ANTAGONISM

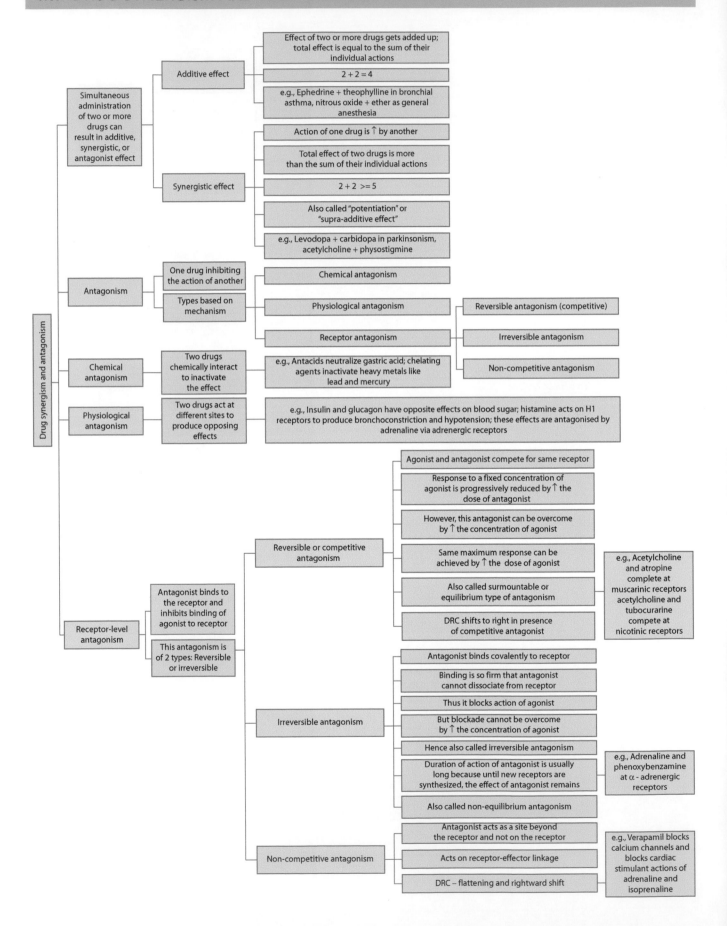

Drug synergism and antagonism

Simultaneous administration of two or more drugs can result in additive, synergistic, or antagonist effect

- **Additive effect**
  - Effect of two or more drugs gets added up; total effect is equal to the sum of their individual actions
  - 2 + 2 = 4
  - e.g., Ephedrine + theophylline in bronchial asthma, nitrous oxide + ether as general anesthesia
- **Synergistic effect**
  - Action of one drug is ↑ by another
  - Total effect of two drugs is more than the sum of their individual actions
  - 2 + 2 >= 5
  - Also called "potentiation" or "supra-additive effect"
  - e.g., Levodopa + carbidopa in parkinsonism, acetylcholine + physostigmine

Antagonism

- One drug inhibiting the action of another
- Types based on mechanism
  - Chemical antagonism
  - Physiological antagonism
  - Receptor antagonism
    - Reversible antagonism (competitive)
    - Irreversible antagonism
    - Non-competitive antagonism

Chemical antagonism

- Two drugs chemically interact to inactivate the effect
- e.g., Antacids neutralize gastric acid; chelating agents inactivate heavy metals like lead and mercury

Physiological antagonism

- Two drugs act at different sites to produce opposing effects
- e.g., Insulin and glucagon have opposite effects on blood sugar; histamine acts on H1 receptors to produce bronchoconstriction and hypotension; these effects are antagonised by adrenaline via adrenergic receptors

Receptor-level antagonism

- Antagonist binds to the receptor and inhibits binding of agonist to receptor
- This antagonism is of 2 types: Reversible or irreversible

- **Reversible or competitive antagonism**
  - Agonist and antagonist compete for same receptor
  - Response to a fixed concentration of agonist is progressively reduced by ↑ the dose of antagonist
  - However, this antagonist can be overcome by ↑ the concentration of agonist
  - Same maximum response can be achieved by ↑ the dose of agonist
  - Also called surmountable or equilibrium type of antagonism
  - DRC shifts to right in presence of competitive antagonist
  - e.g., Acetylcholine and atropine complete at muscarinic receptors acetylcholine and tubocurarine compete at nicotinic receptors

- **Irreversible antagonism**
  - Antagonist binds covalently to receptor
  - Binding is so firm that antagonist cannot dissociate from receptor
  - Thus it blocks action of agonist
  - But blockade cannot be overcome by ↑ the concentration of agonist
  - Hence also called irreversible antagonism
  - Duration of action of antagonist is usually long because until new receptors are synthesized, the effect of antagonist remains
  - Also called non-equilibrium antagonism
  - e.g., Adrenaline and phenoxybenzamine at α - adrenergic receptors

- **Non-competitive antagonism**
  - Antagonist acts as a site beyond the receptor and not on the receptor
  - Acts on receptor-effector linkage
  - DRC – flattening and rightward shift
  - e.g., Verapamil blocks calcium channels and blocks cardiac stimulant actions of adrenaline and isoprenaline

4.18 FACTORS THAT MODIFY EFFECTS OF DRUGS

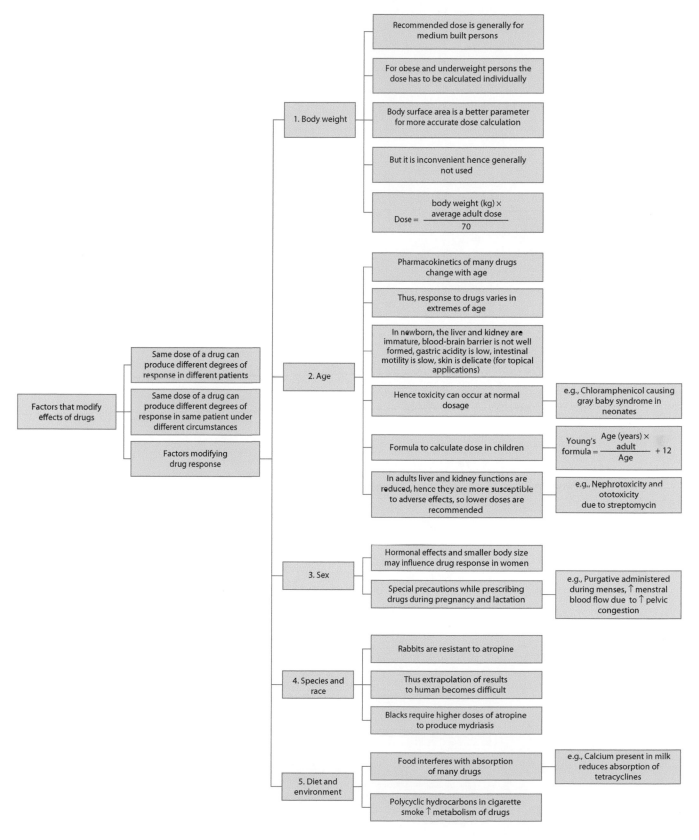

(Continued)

4.18 FACTORS THAT MODIFY EFFECTS OF DRUGS (Continued)

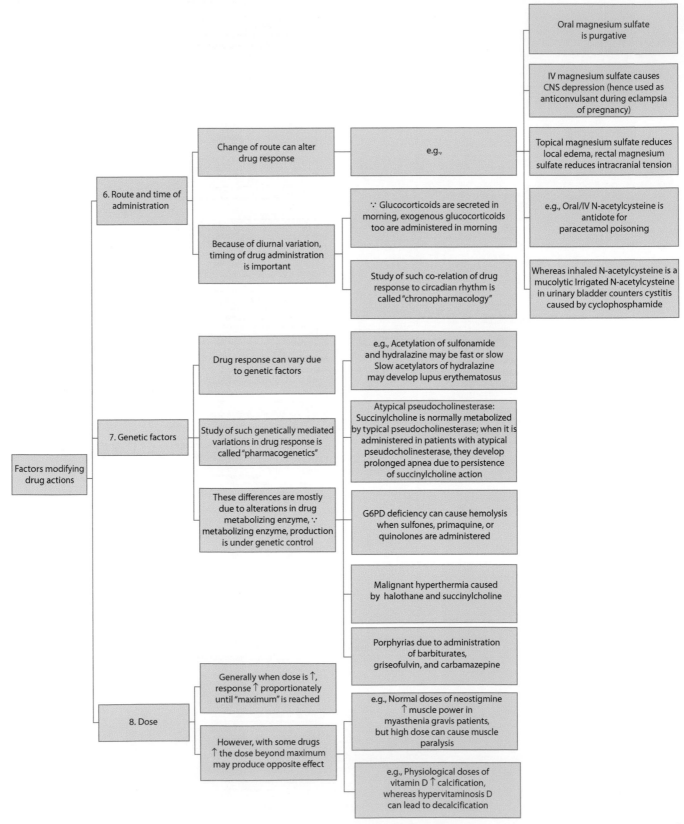

(Continued)

4.18 FACTORS THAT MODIFY EFFECTS OF DRUGS (Continued)

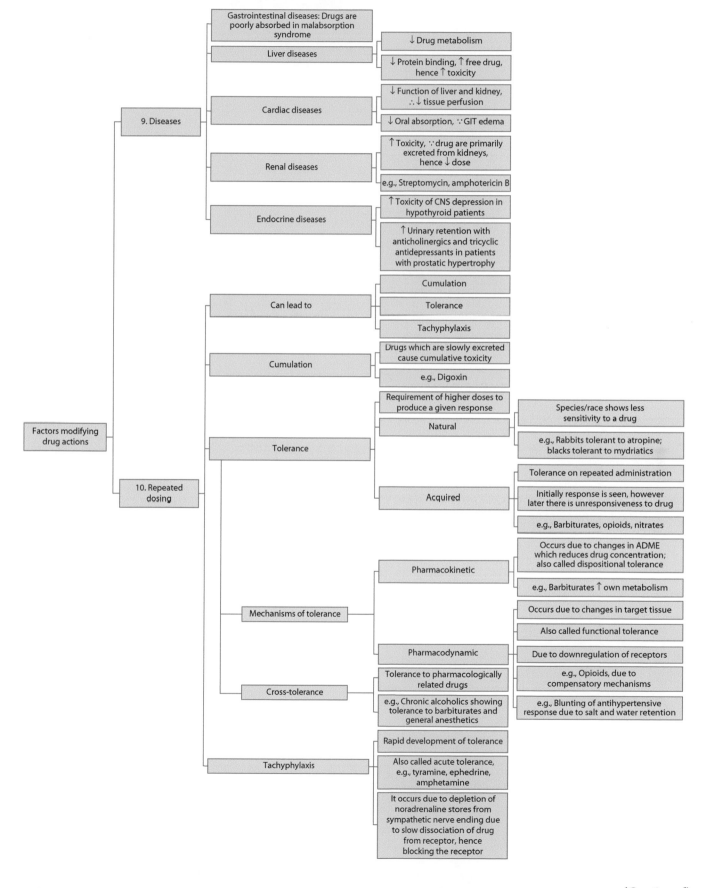

4.18 FACTORS THAT MODIFY EFFECTS OF DRUGS (Continued)

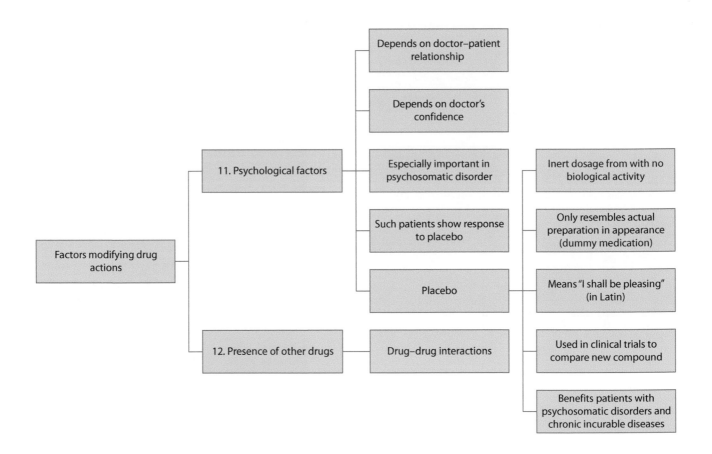

4.19 DRUG INTERACTIONS

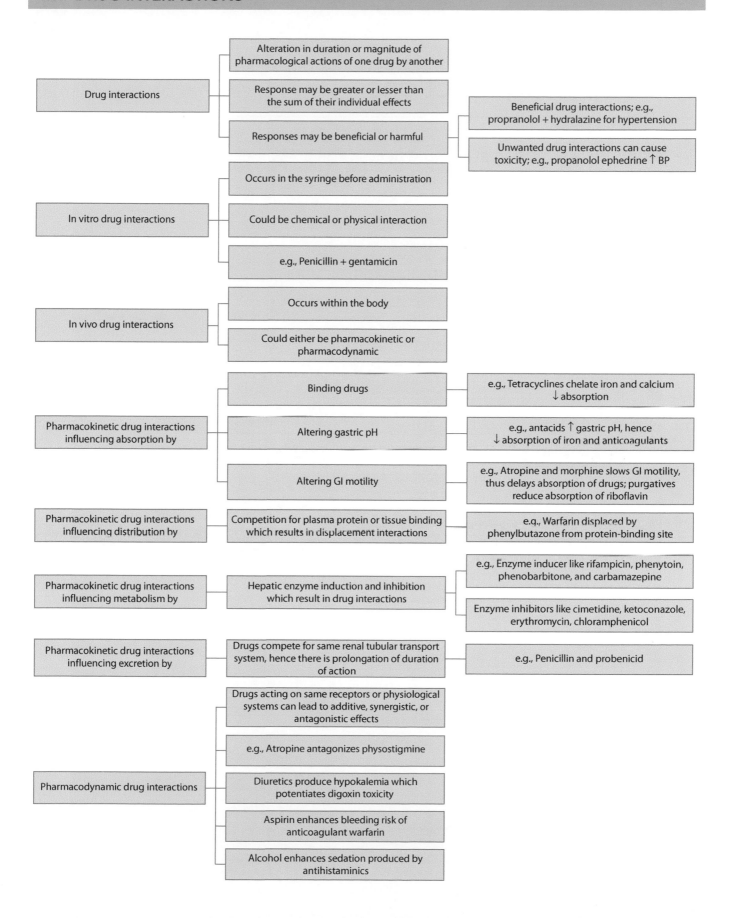

Drug interactions
- Alteration in duration or magnitude of pharmacological actions of one drug by another
- Response may be greater or lesser than the sum of their individual effects
- Responses may be beneficial or harmful
  - Beneficial drug interactions; e.g., propranolol + hydralazine for hypertension
  - Unwanted drug interactions can cause toxicity; e.g., propanolol ephedrine ↑ BP

In vitro drug interactions
- Occurs in the syringe before administration
- Could be chemical or physical interaction
- e.g., Penicillin + gentamicin

In vivo drug interactions
- Occurs within the body
- Could either be pharmacokinetic or pharmacodynamic

Pharmacokinetic drug interactions influencing absorption by
- Binding drugs
  - e.g., Tetracyclines chelate iron and calcium ↓ absorption
- Altering gastric pH
  - e.g., antacids ↑ gastric pH, hence ↓ absorption of iron and anticoagulants
- Altering GI motility
  - e.g., Atropine and morphine slows GI motility, thus delays absorption of drugs; purgatives reduce absorption of riboflavin

Pharmacokinetic drug interactions influencing distribution by
- Competition for plasma protein or tissue binding which results in displacement interactions
  - e.g., Warfarin displaced by phenylbutazone from protein-binding site

Pharmacokinetic drug interactions influencing metabolism by
- Hepatic enzyme induction and inhibition which result in drug interactions
  - e.g., Enzyme inducer like rifampicin, phenytoin, phenobarbitone, and carbamazepine
  - Enzyme inhibitors like cimetidine, ketoconazole, erythromycin, chloramphenicol

Pharmacokinetic drug interactions influencing excretion by
- Drugs compete for same renal tubular transport system, hence there is prolongation of duration of action
  - e.g., Penicillin and probenicid

Pharmacodynamic drug interactions
- Drugs acting on same receptors or physiological systems can lead to additive, synergistic, or antagonistic effects
- e.g., Atropine antagonizes physostigmine
- Diuretics produce hypokalemia which potentiates digoxin toxicity
- Aspirin enhances bleeding risk of anticoagulant warfarin
- Alcohol enhances sedation produced by antihistaminics

Adverse drug reactions

5.1 TYPES OF ADVERSE DRUG REACTIONS (ADRs)

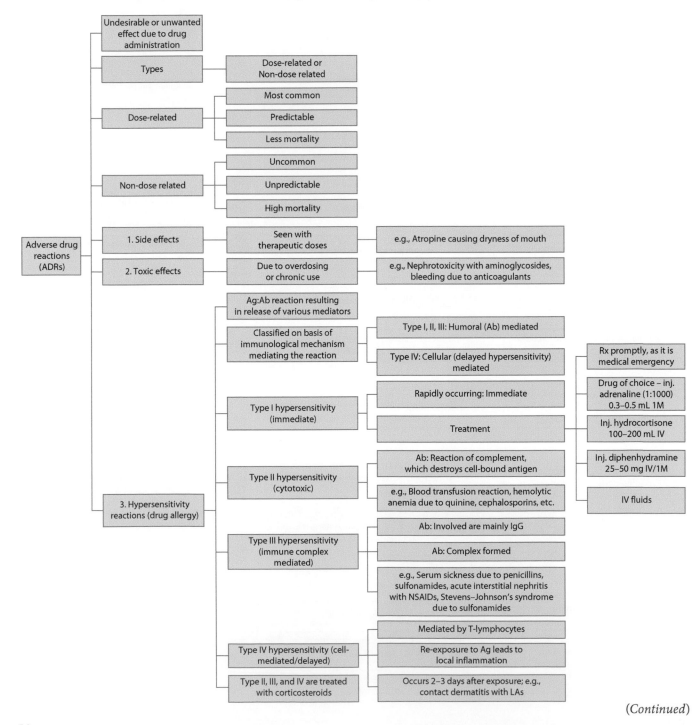

(Continued)

5.1 TYPES OF ADVERSE DRUG REACTIONS (ADRs) (Continued)

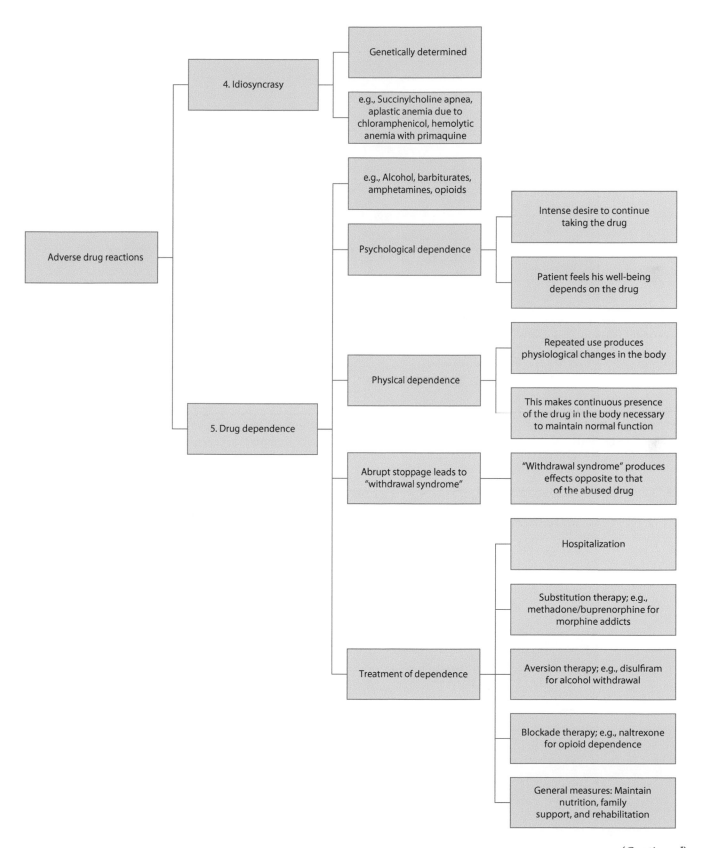

(Continued)

5.1 TYPES OF ADVERSE DRUG REACTIONS (ADRs) (Continued)

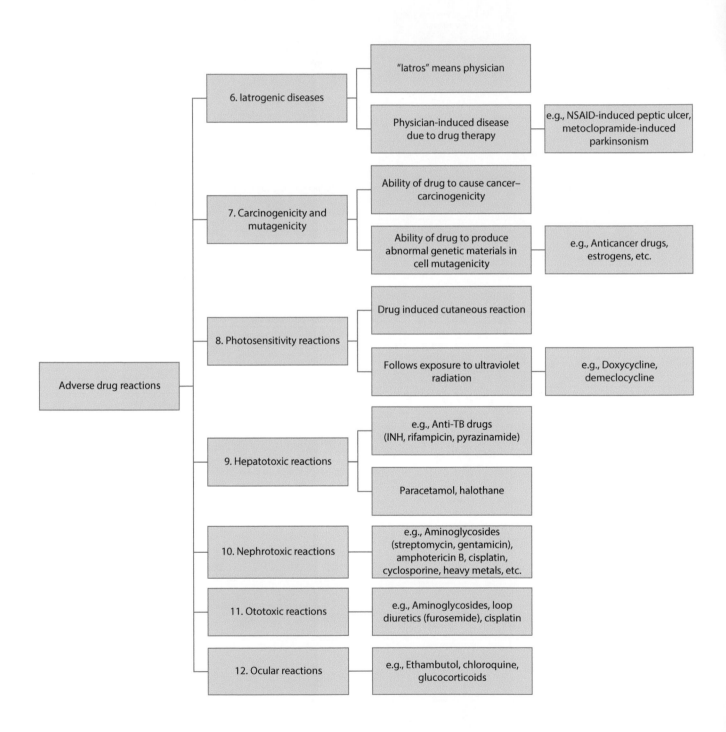

(Continued)

5.1 TYPES OF ADVERSE DRUG REACTIONS (ADRs) (Continued)

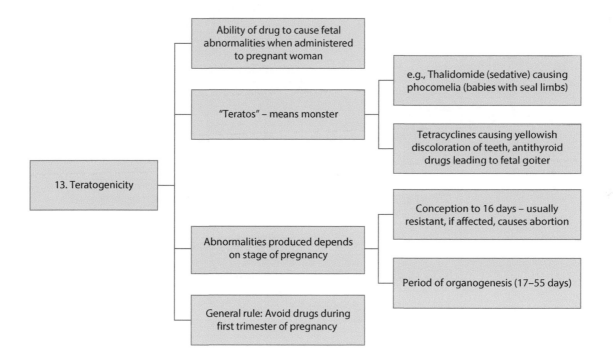

5.2 GENERAL PRINCIPLES OF TREATMENT OF POISONING (MNEMONICS [ABCDEFGHI])

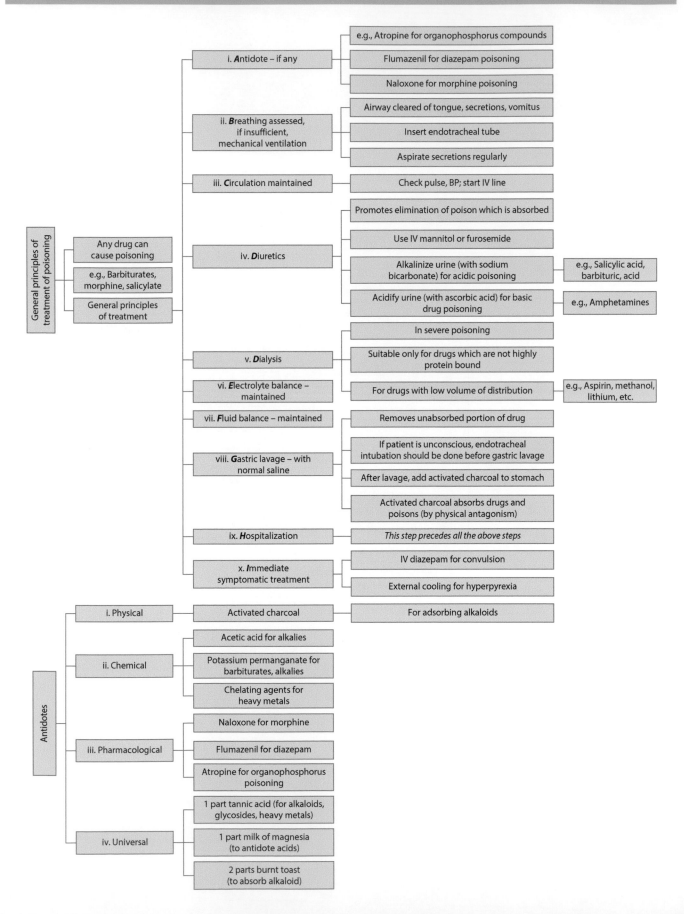

5.3 PHARMACOVIGILANCE

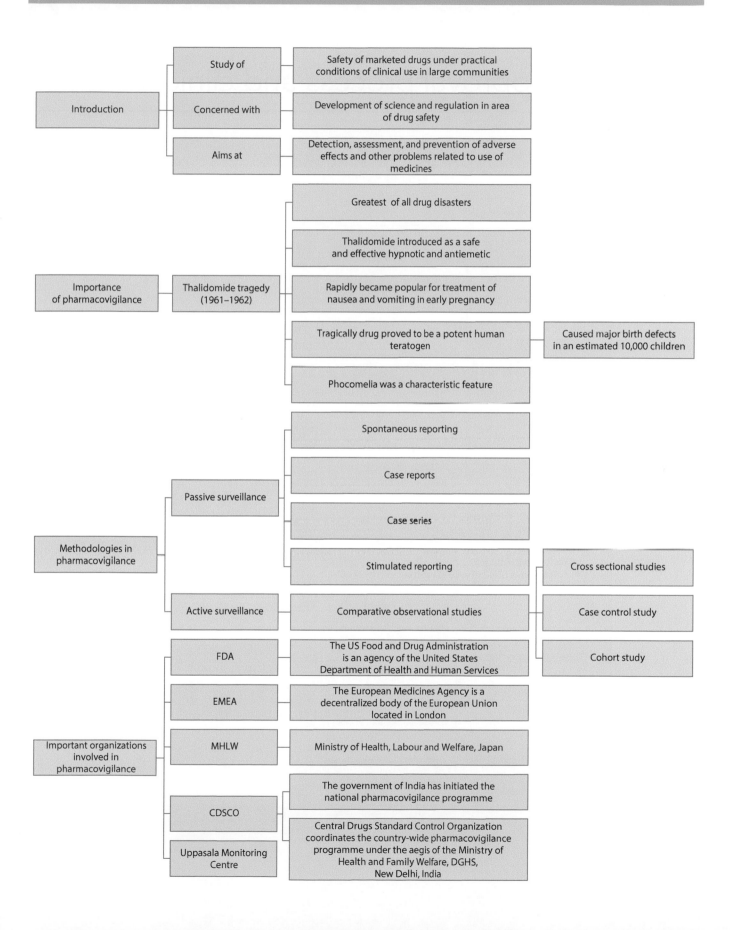

New drug approval process and clinical trials

6.1 NEW DRUG APPROVAL PROCESS

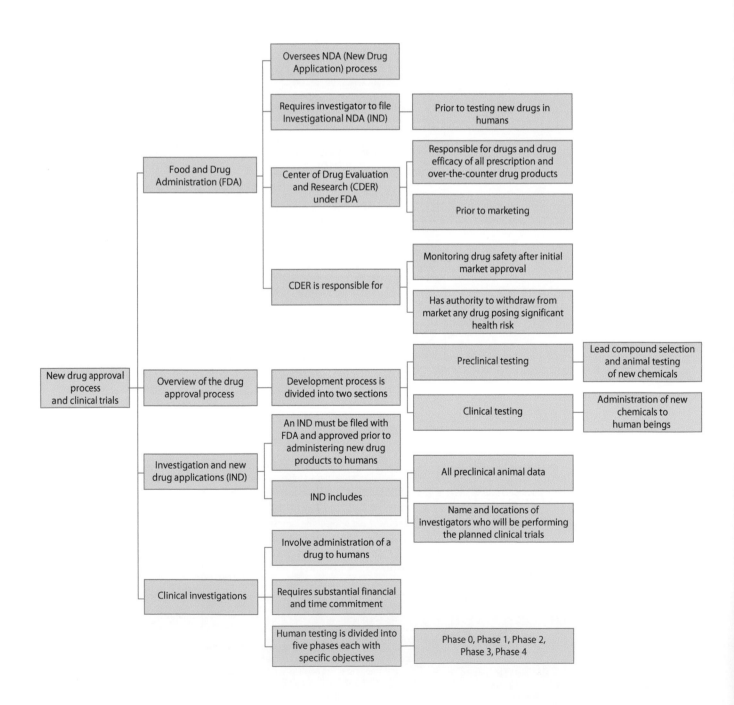

6.2 PHASES OF CLINICAL TRIALS (0, 1 AND 2)

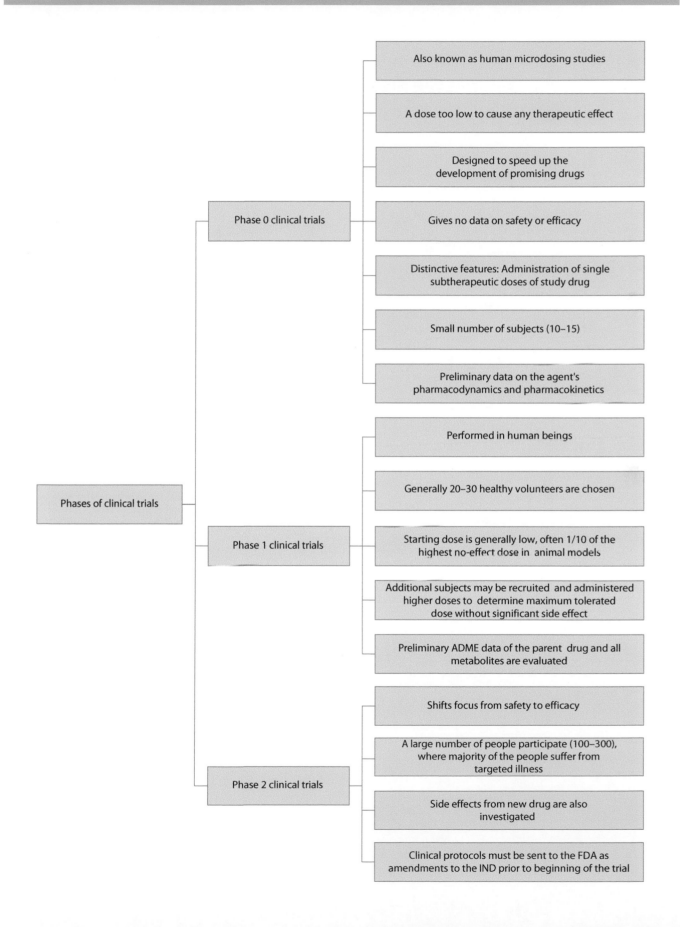

Phases of clinical trials

Phase 0 clinical trials
- Also known as human microdosing studies
- A dose too low to cause any therapeutic effect
- Designed to speed up the development of promising drugs
- Gives no data on safety or efficacy
- Distinctive features: Administration of single subtherapeutic doses of study drug
- Small number of subjects (10–15)
- Preliminary data on the agent's pharmacodynamics and pharmacokinetics

Phase 1 clinical trials
- Performed in human beings
- Generally 20–30 healthy volunteers are chosen
- Starting dose is generally low, often 1/10 of the highest no-effect dose in animal models
- Additional subjects may be recruited and administered higher doses to determine maximum tolerated dose without significant side effect
- Preliminary ADME data of the parent drug and all metabolites are evaluated

Phase 2 clinical trials
- Shifts focus from safety to efficacy
- A large number of people participate (100–300), where majority of the people suffer from targeted illness
- Side effects from new drug are also investigated
- Clinical protocols must be sent to the FDA as amendments to the IND prior to beginning of the trial

6.3 PHASES OF CLINICAL TRIALS (3 AND 4)

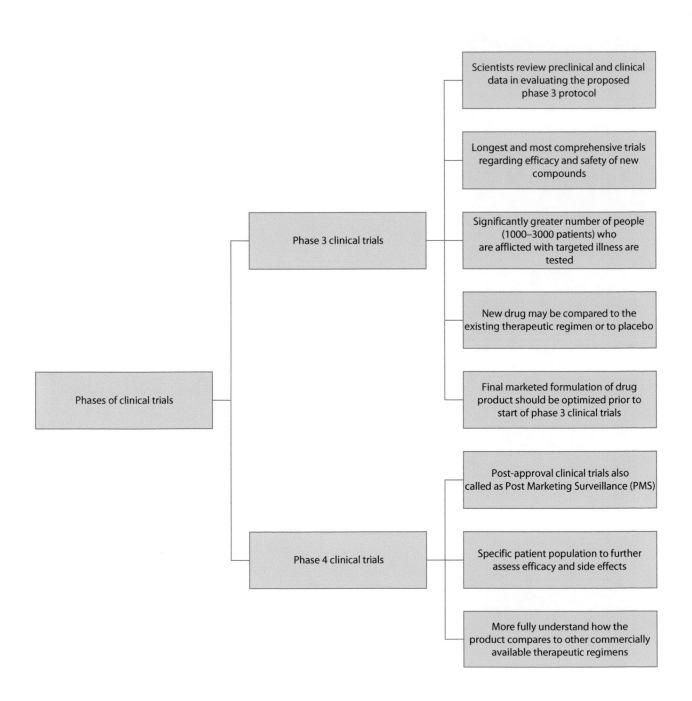

Phases of clinical trials

Phase 3 clinical trials

Scientists review preclinical and clinical data in evaluating the proposed phase 3 protocol

Longest and most comprehensive trials regarding efficacy and safety of new compounds

Significantly greater number of people (1000–3000 patients) who are afflicted with targeted illness are tested

New drug may be compared to the existing therapeutic regimen or to placebo

Final marketed formulation of drug product should be optimized prior to start of phase 3 clinical trials

Phase 4 clinical trials

Post-approval clinical trials also called as Post Marketing Surveillance (PMS)

Specific patient population to further assess efficacy and side effects

More fully understand how the product compares to other commercially available therapeutic regimens

PART II

Autonomic nervous system (ANS) pharmacology

Introduction to ANS

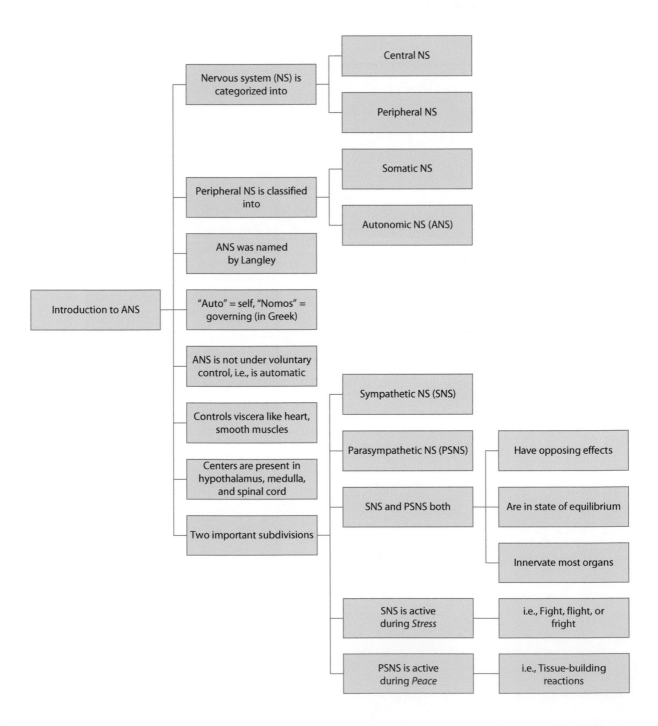

7.2 INNERVATIONS OF ANS

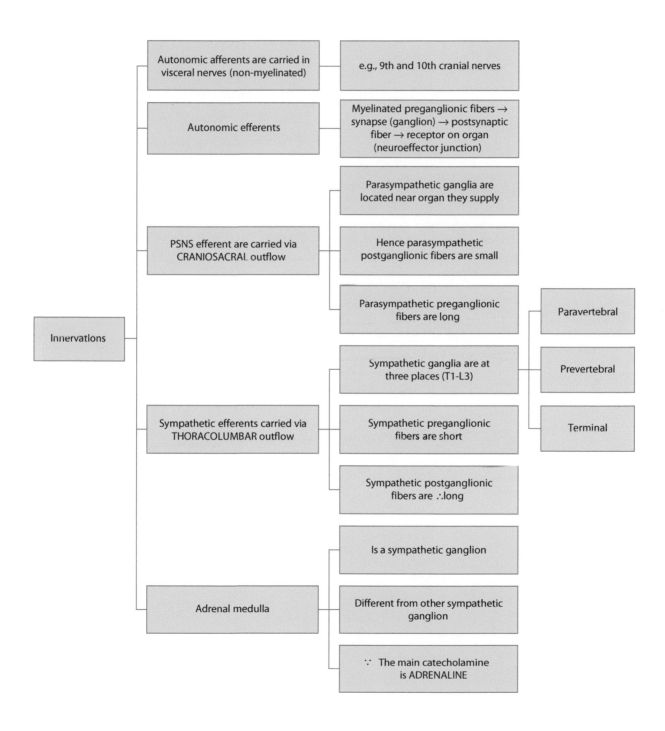

7.3 NEUROTRANSMITTERS

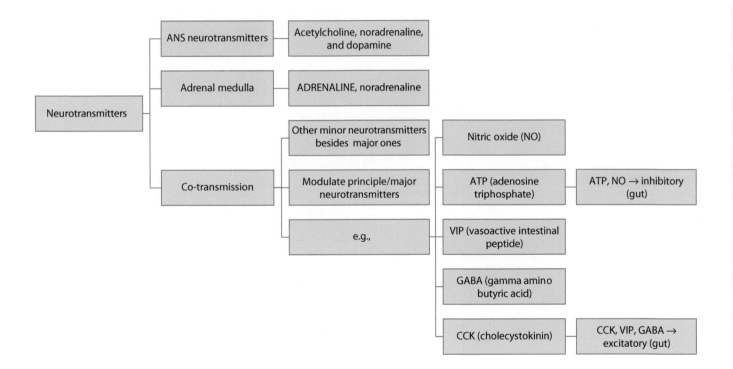

Cholinergic system and drugs

8.1 CHOLINERGIC SYSTEM

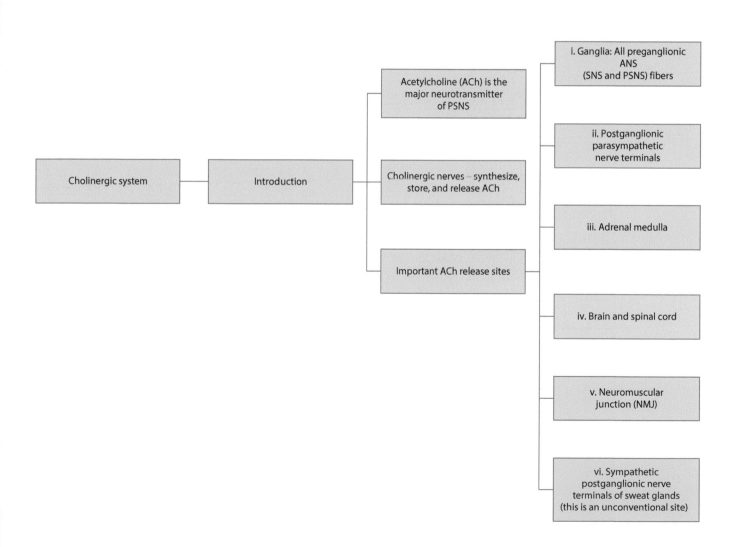

8.2 SYNTHESIS/TRANSMISSION/METABOLISM OF ACh

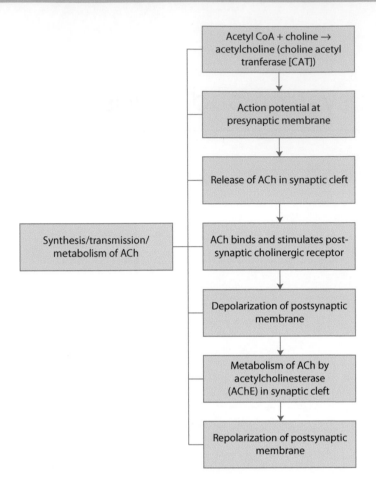

8.3 CHOLINESTERASES

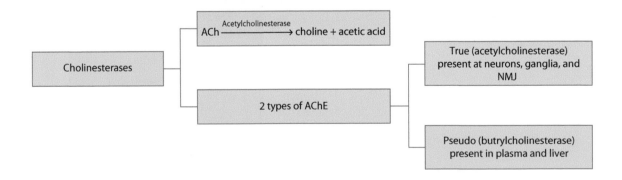

8.4 CHOLINERGIC RECEPTORS

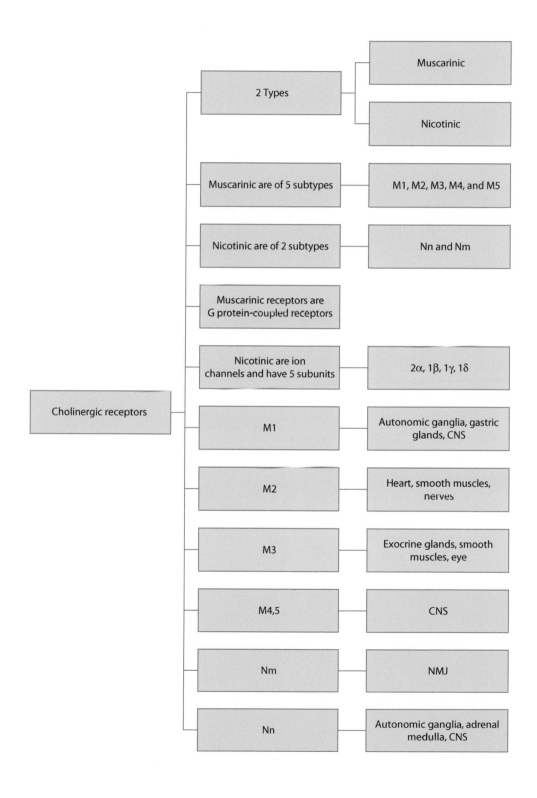

8.5 CHOLINERGIC DRUGS

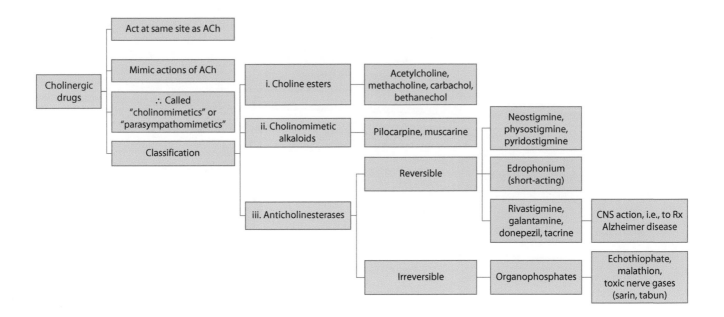

8.6 ACTIONS OF ACh

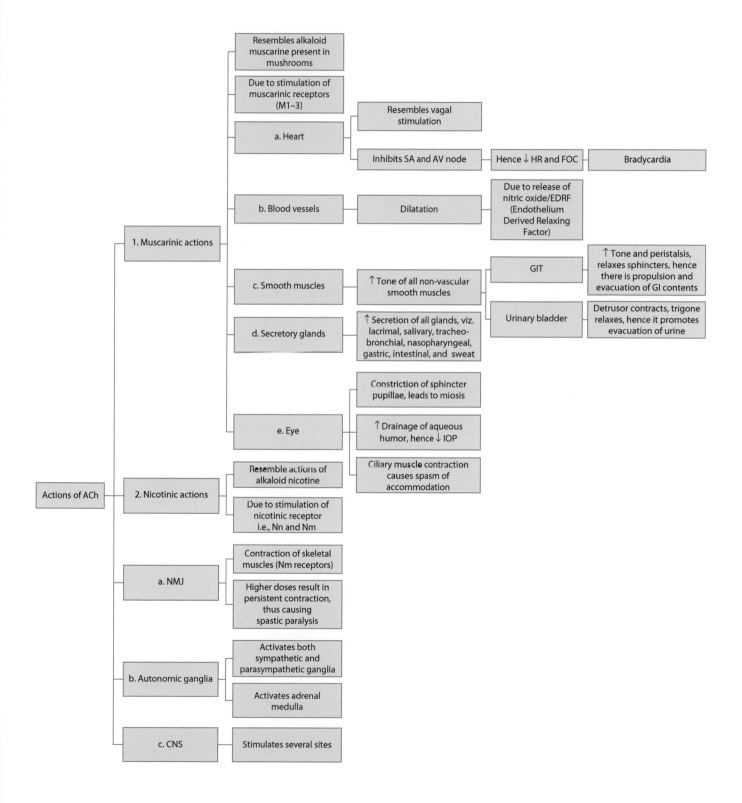

8.7 USES OF ACh AND CHOLINOMIMETICS

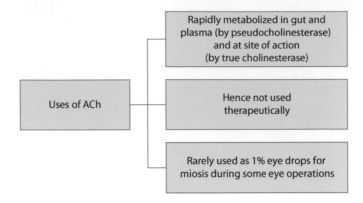

8.8 ADVERSE REACTIONS OF CHOLINOMIMETICS

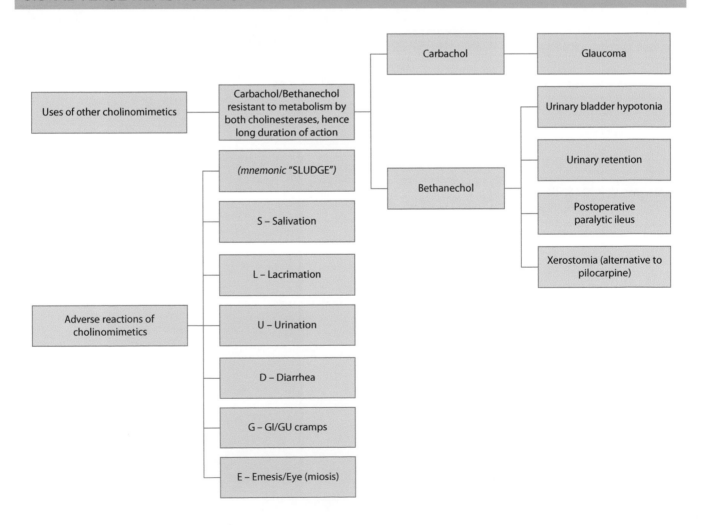

8.9 CHOLINOMIMETIC ALKALOIDS

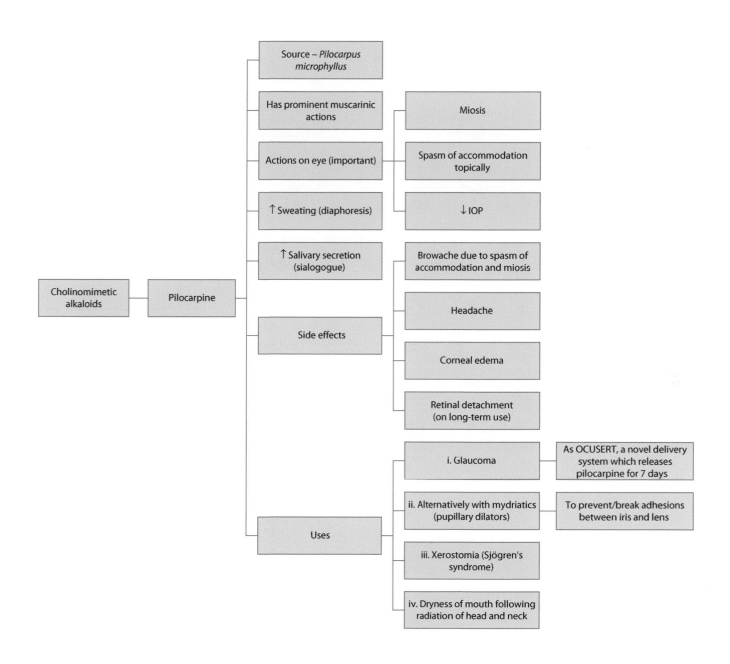

8.10 GLAUCOMA

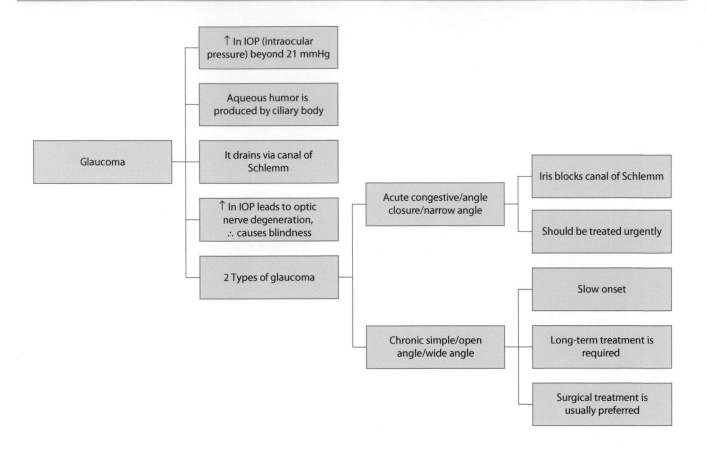

8.11 DRUGS FOR GLAUCOMA

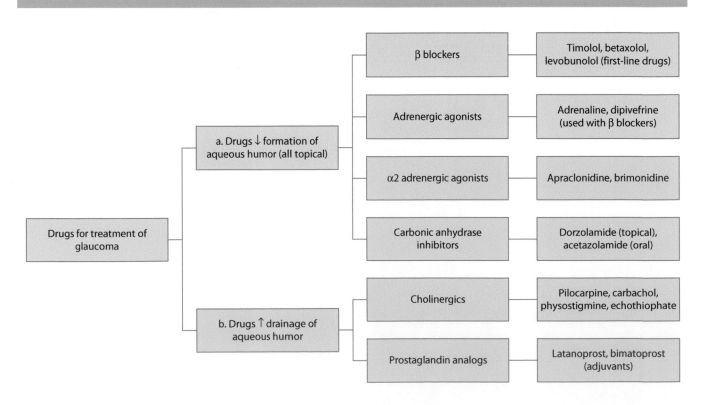

8.12 β BLOCKERS IN GLAUCOMA

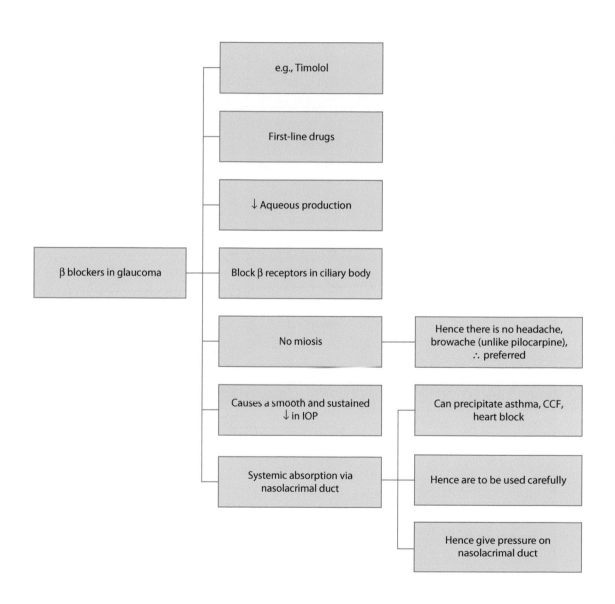

8.13 ADRENERGIC AGONISTS, MIOTICS, AND PROSTAGLANDIN ANALOGS IN GLAUCOMA

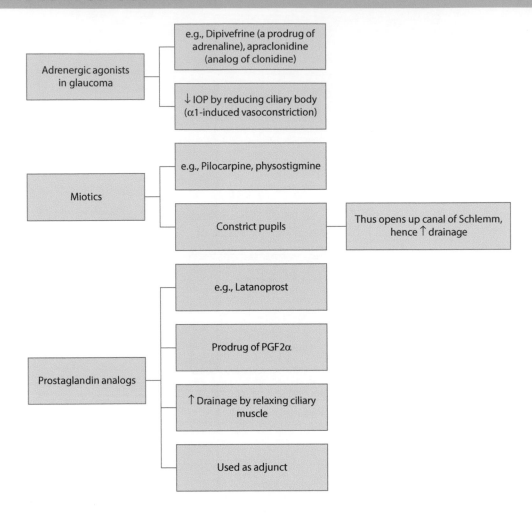

Adrenergic agonists in glaucoma
- e.g., Dipivefrine (a prodrug of adrenaline), apraclonidine (analog of clonidine)
- ↓ IOP by reducing ciliary body (α1-induced vasoconstriction)

Miotics
- e.g., Pilocarpine, physostigmine
- Constrict pupils → Thus opens up canal of Schlemm, hence ↑ drainage

Prostaglandin analogs
- e.g., Latanoprost
- Prodrug of PGF2α
- ↑ Drainage by relaxing ciliary muscle
- Used as adjunct

8.14 CARBONIC ANHYDRASE INHIBITORS (CAIs)

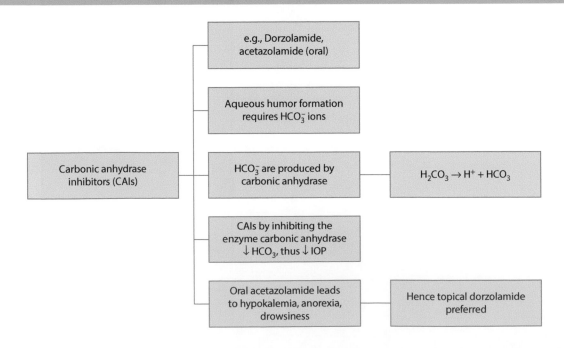

Carbonic anhydrase inhibitors (CAIs)
- e.g., Dorzolamide, acetazolamide (oral)
- Aqueous humor formation requires HCO_3^- ions
- HCO_3^- are produced by carbonic anhydrase → $H_2CO_3 \rightarrow H^+ + HCO_3$
- CAIs by inhibiting the enzyme carbonic anhydrase ↓ HCO_3, thus ↓ IOP
- Oral acetazolamide leads to hypokalemia, anorexia, drowsiness → Hence topical dorzolamide preferred

8.15 ANTICHOLINESTERASES (ANTIChE)

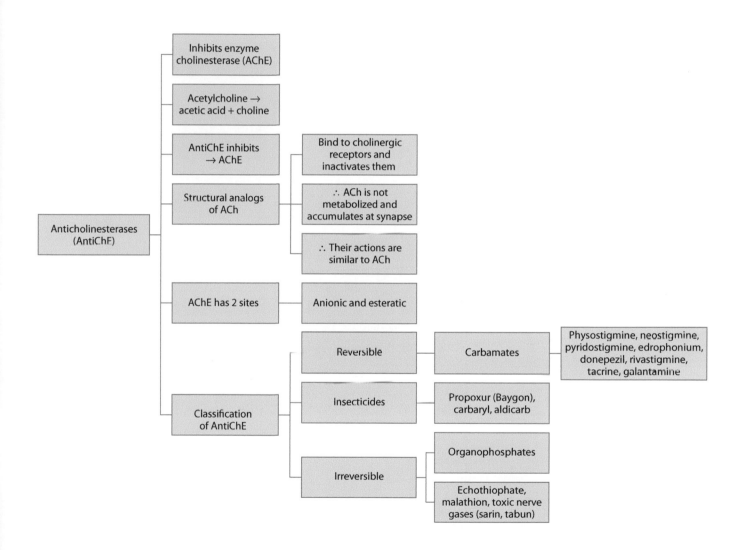

8.16 PHYSOSTIGMINE

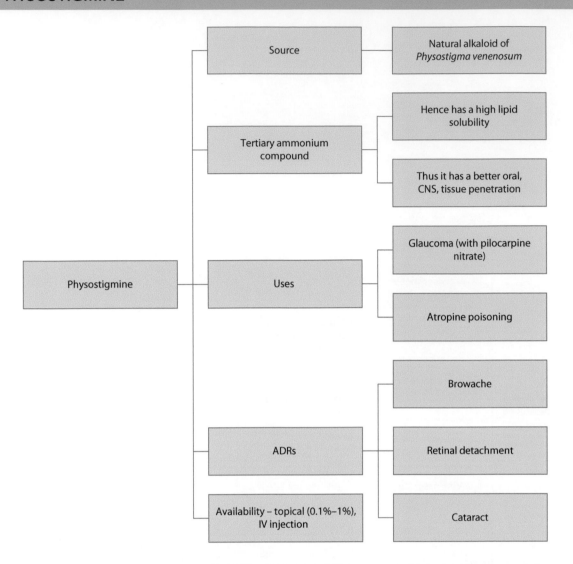

- Physostigmine
  - Source
    - Natural alkaloid of *Physostigma venenosum*
  - Tertiary ammonium compound
    - Hence has a high lipid solubility
    - Thus it has a better oral, CNS, tissue penetration
  - Uses
    - Glaucoma (with pilocarpine nitrate)
    - Atropine poisoning
  - ADRs
    - Browache
    - Retinal detachment
    - Cataract
  - Availability – topical (0.1%–1%), IV injection

8.17 NEOSTIGMINE

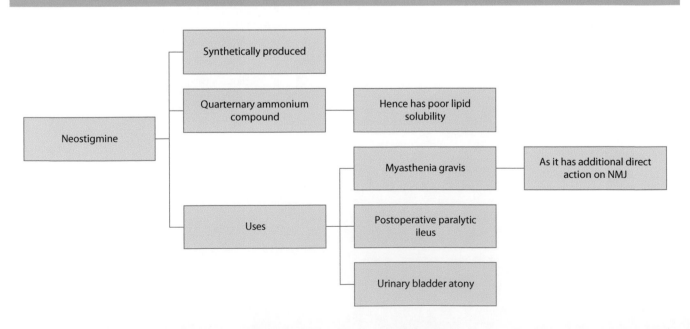

- Neostigmine
  - Synthetically produced
  - Quarternary ammonium compound
    - Hence has poor lipid solubility
  - Uses
    - Myasthenia gravis
      - As it has additional direct action on NMJ
    - Postoperative paralytic ileus
    - Urinary bladder atony

8.18 EDROPHONIUM

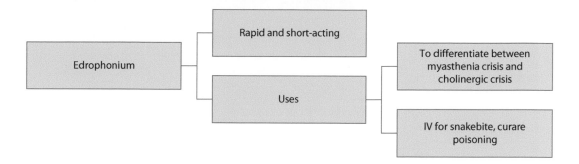

8.19 RIVASTIGMINE, DONEPEZIL, GALANTAMINE, TACRINE

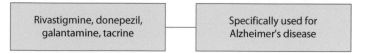

8.20 USES OF REVERSIBLE ANTIChE

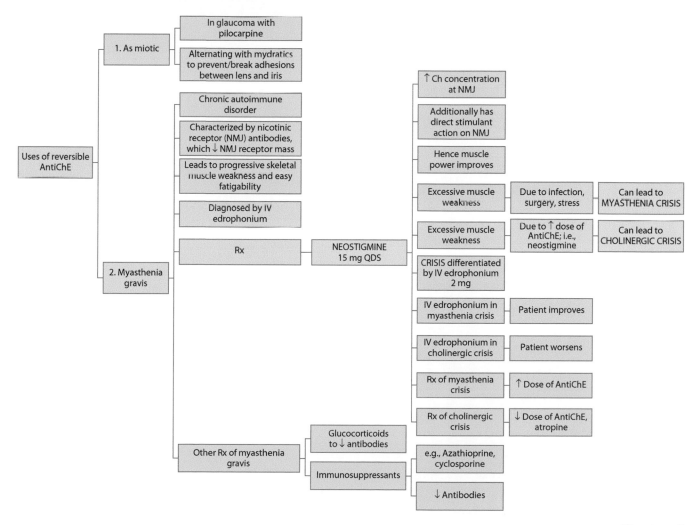

(Continued)

8.20 USES OF REVERSIBLE ANTIChE (Continued)

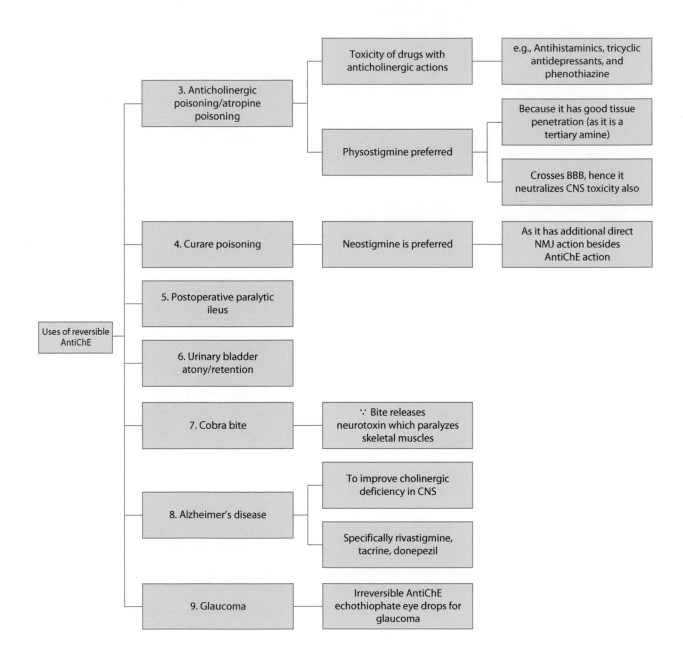

Uses of reversible AntiChE

3. Anticholinergic poisoning/atropine poisoning
- Toxicity of drugs with anticholinergic actions
  - e.g., Antihistaminics, tricyclic antidepressants, and phenothiazine
- Physostigmine preferred
  - Because it has good tissue penetration (as it is a tertiary amine)
  - Crosses BBB, hence it neutralizes CNS toxicity also

4. Curare poisoning
- Neostigmine is preferred
  - As it has additional direct NMJ action besides AntiChE action

5. Postoperative paralytic ileus

6. Urinary bladder atony/retention

7. Cobra bite
- ∵ Bite releases neurotoxin which paralyzes skeletal muscles

8. Alzheimer's disease
- To improve cholinergic deficiency in CNS
- Specifically rivastigmine, tacrine, donepezil

9. Glaucoma
- Irreversible AntiChE echothiophate eye drops for glaucoma

8.21 IRREVERSIBLE ANTIChE (ORGANOPHOSPHORUS COMPOUNDS)

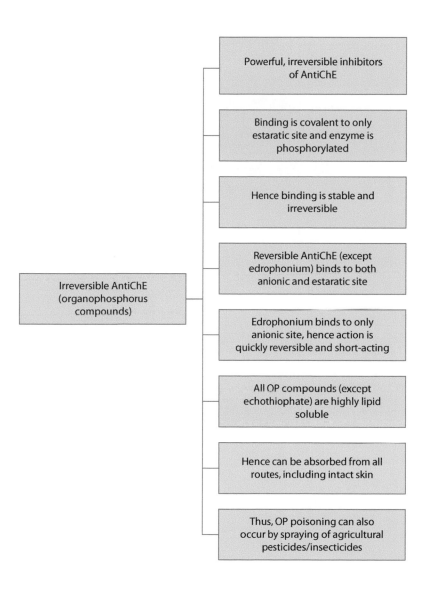

8.22 ORGANOPHOSPHORUS POISONING

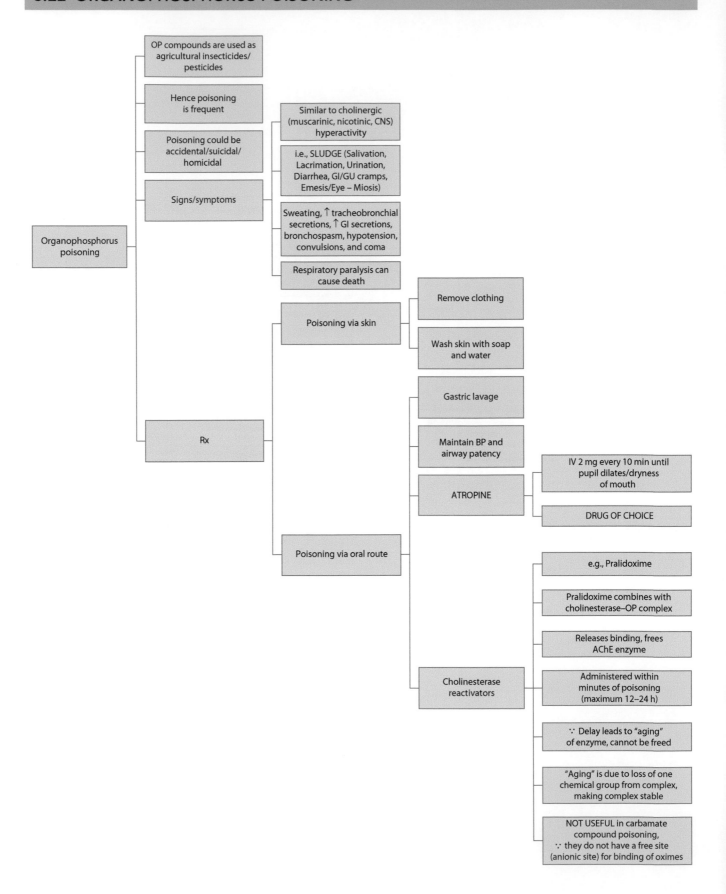

Organophosphorus poisoning

- OP compounds are used as agricultural insecticides/pesticides
- Hence poisoning is frequent
- Poisoning could be accidental/suicidal/homicidal
- Signs/symptoms
  - Similar to cholinergic (muscarinic, nicotinic, CNS) hyperactivity
  - i.e., SLUDGE (Salivation, Lacrimation, Urination, Diarrhea, GI/GU cramps, Emesis/Eye – Miosis)
  - Sweating, ↑ tracheobronchial secretions, ↑ GI secretions, bronchospasm, hypotension, convulsions, and coma
  - Respiratory paralysis can cause death
- Rx
  - Poisoning via skin
    - Remove clothing
    - Wash skin with soap and water
  - Poisoning via oral route
    - Gastric lavage
    - Maintain BP and airway patency
    - ATROPINE
      - IV 2 mg every 10 min until pupil dilates/dryness of mouth
      - DRUG OF CHOICE
    - Cholinesterase reactivators
      - e.g., Pralidoxime
      - Pralidoxime combines with cholinesterase–OP complex
      - Releases binding, frees AChE enzyme
      - Administered within minutes of poisoning (maximum 12–24 h)
      - ∵ Delay leads to "aging" of enzyme, cannot be freed
      - "Aging" is due to loss of one chemical group from complex, making complex stable
      - NOT USEFUL in carbamate compound poisoning, ∴ they do not have a free site (anionic site) for binding of oximes

8.23 DIFFERENCES BETWEEN PHYSOSTIGMINE AND NEOSTIGMINE

Physostigmine	Neostigmine
1. Natural (*Physostigma venenosum*)	Synthetic
2. Tertiary amine	Quarternary amine
3. Good oral absorption	Poor oral absorption
4. Good tissue penetration	Poor tissue penetration
5. Crosses BBB: CNS effects	Does not cross BBB, no CNS effects
6. Main indication – glaucoma	Myasthenia gravis
7. Used in atropine poisoning	Used in curare poisoning

Anticholinergics

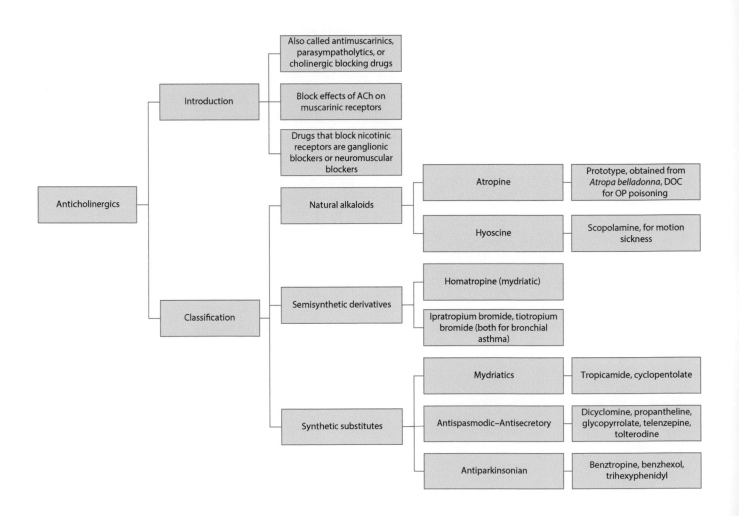

9.2 ACTIONS

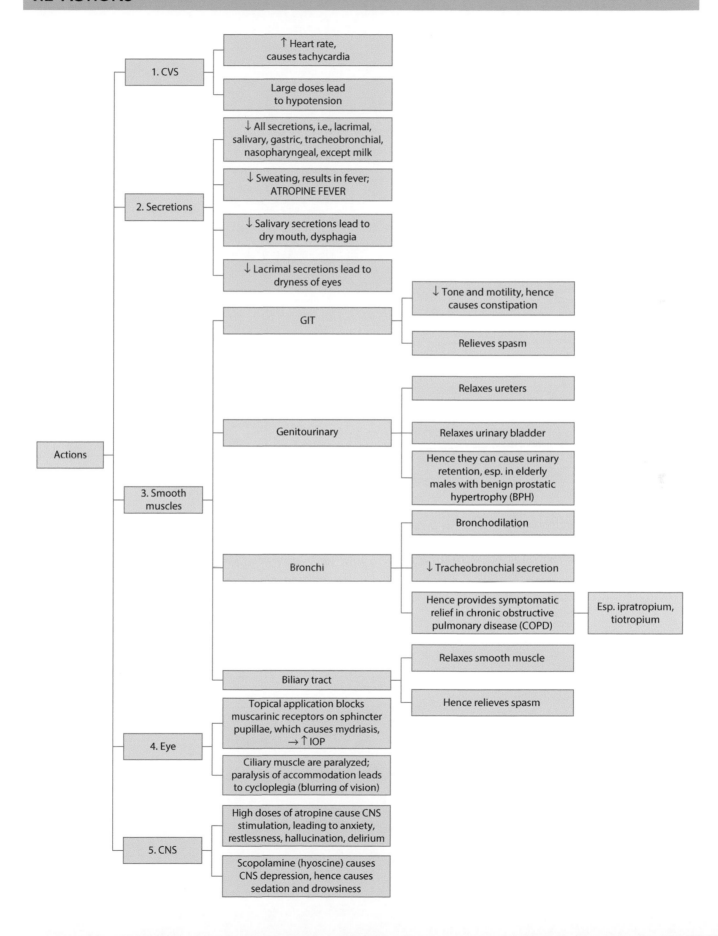

9.3 ADVERSE EFFECTS

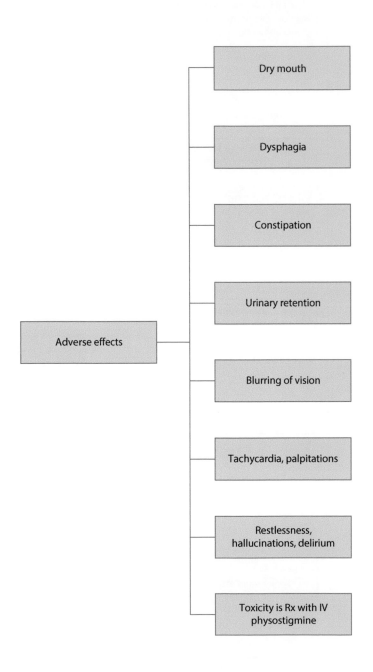

9.4 USES

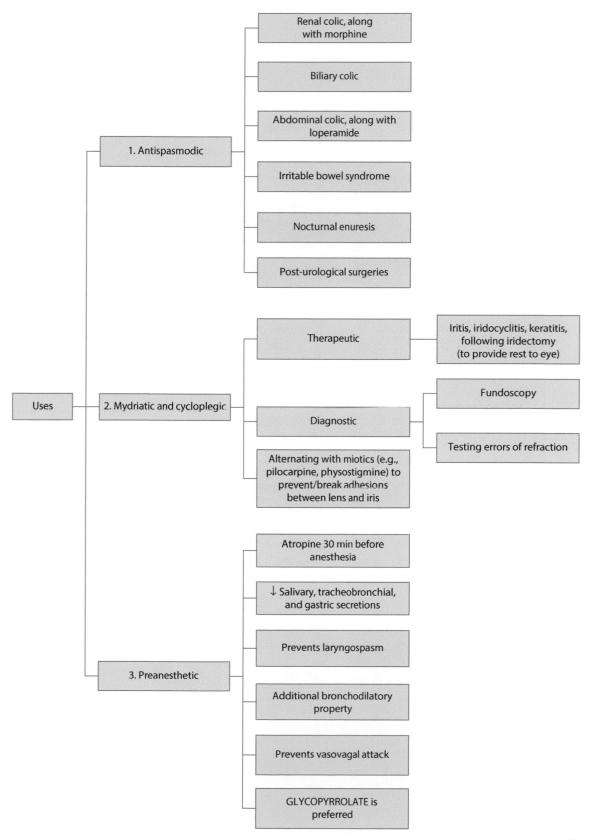

(Continued)

9.4 USES (Continued)

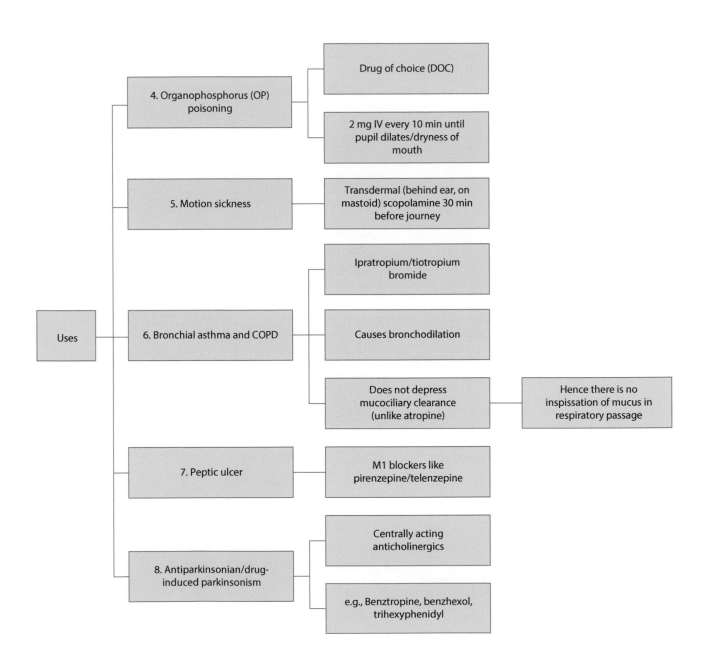

10

Skeletal muscle relaxants

10.1 INTRODUCTION

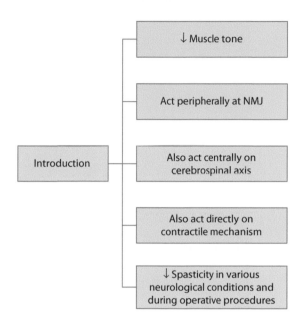

10.2 CLASSIFICATION

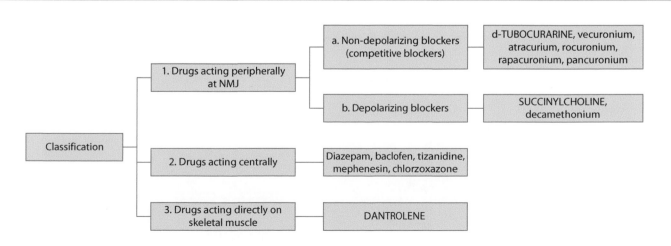

10.3 PERIPHERAL SMRs

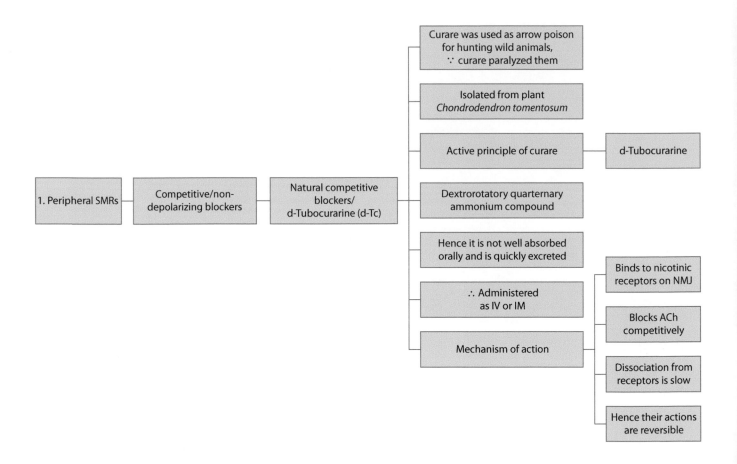

10.4 PHARMACOLOGICAL ACTIONS

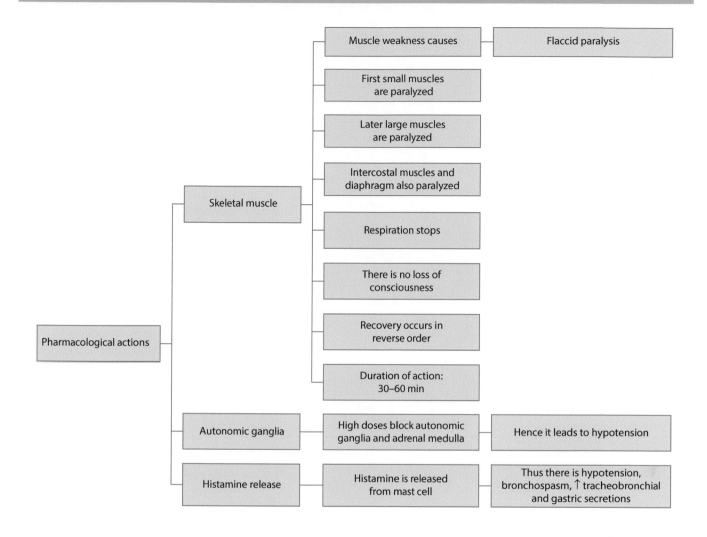

10.5 ADVERSE REACTIONS

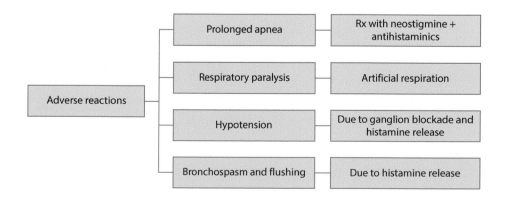

10.6 SYNTHETIC COMPETITIVE BLOCKERS

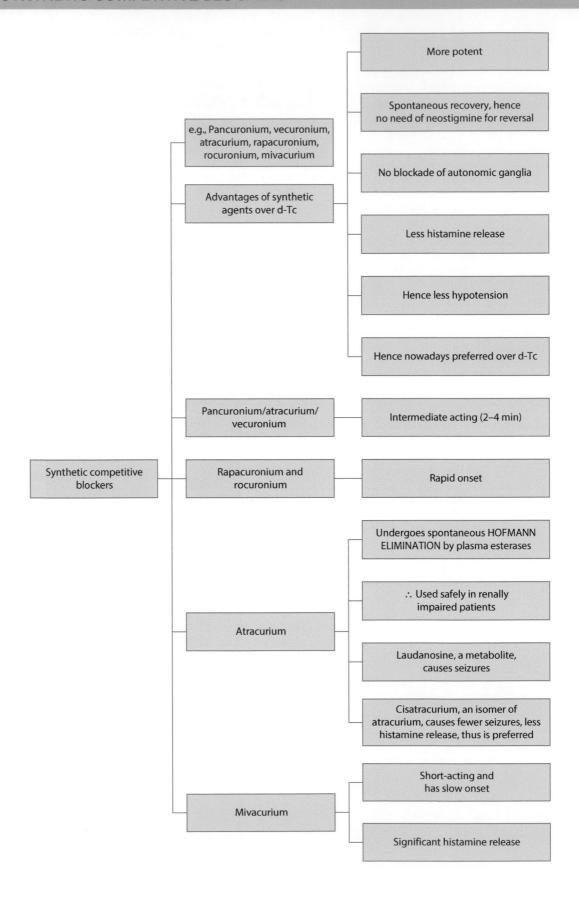

10.7 DEPOLARIZING BLOCKERS – SUCCINYLCHOLINE (SCh)

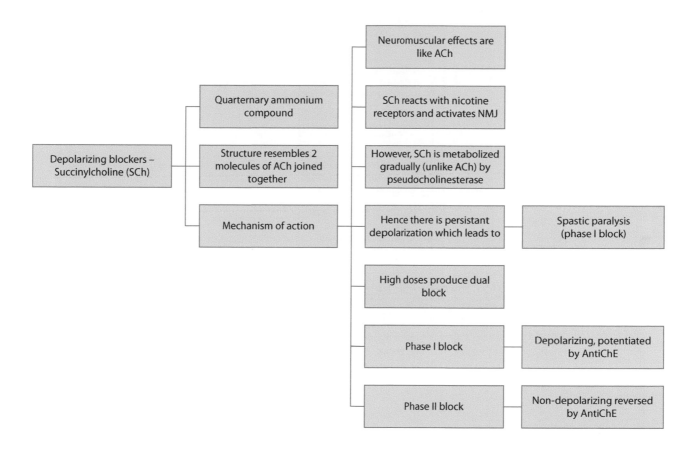

10.8 PHARMACOLOGICAL ACTIONS

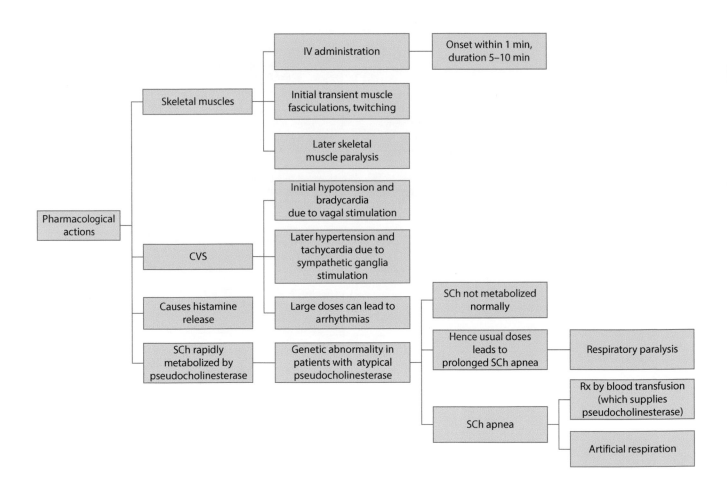

10.9 ADVERSE REACTIONS

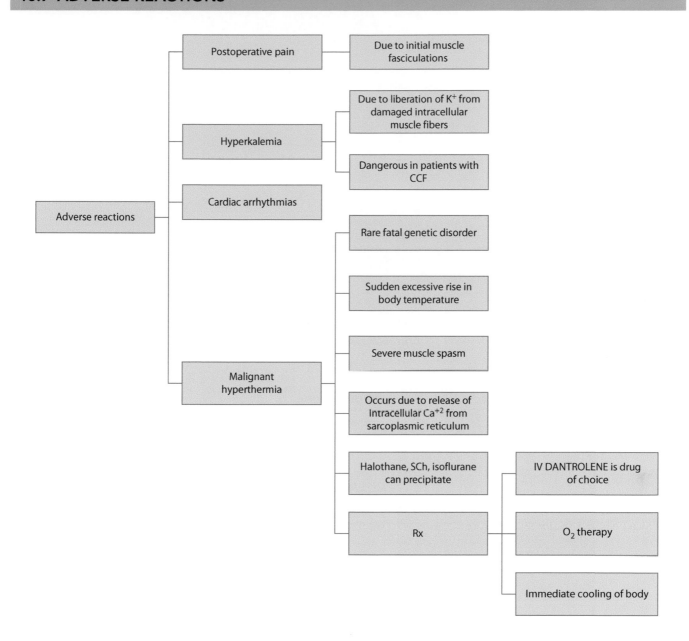

- Adverse reactions
  - Postoperative pain
    - Due to initial muscle fasciculations
  - Hyperkalemia
    - Due to liberation of K+ from damaged intracellular muscle fibers
    - Dangerous in patients with CCF
  - Cardiac arrhythmias
  - Malignant hyperthermia
    - Rare fatal genetic disorder
    - Sudden excessive rise in body temperature
    - Severe muscle spasm
    - Occurs due to release of Intracellular Ca^{+2} from sarcoplasmic reticulum
    - Halothane, SCh, isoflurane can precipitate
    - Rx
      - IV DANTROLENE is drug of choice
      - O$_2$ therapy
      - Immediate cooling of body

10.10 DRUG INTERACTIONS

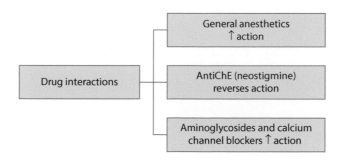

- Drug interactions
  - General anesthetics ↑ action
  - AntiChE (neostigmine) reverses action
  - Aminoglycosides and calcium channel blockers ↑ action

10.11 USES OF SMRs

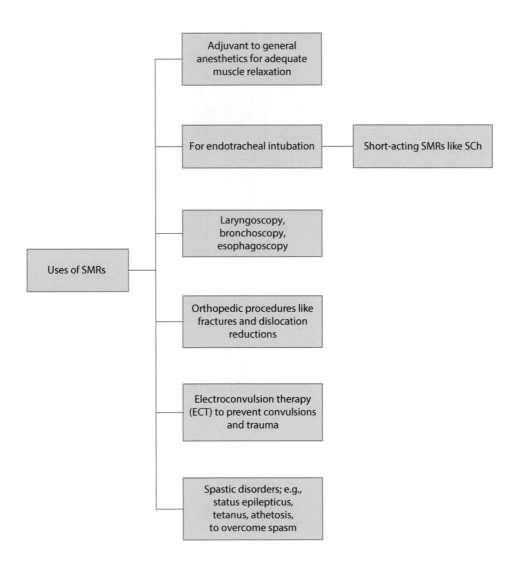

10.12 CENTRAL SMRs

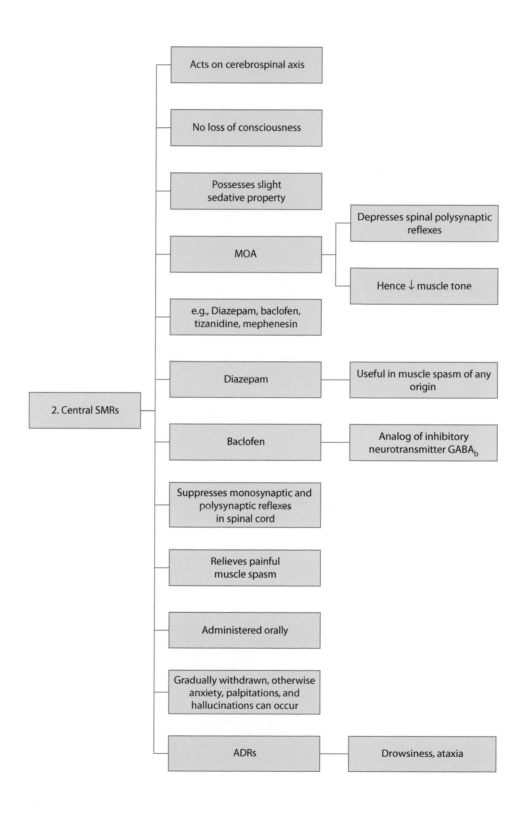

10.13 TIZANIDINE

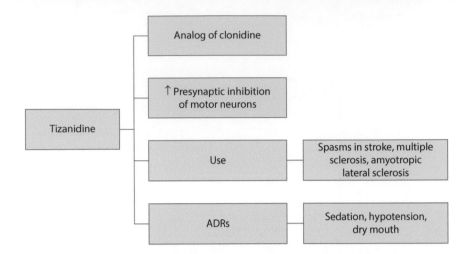

Tizanidine
- Analog of clonidine
- ↑ Presynaptic inhibition of motor neurons
- Use — Spasms in stroke, multiple sclerosis, amyotropic lateral sclerosis
- ADRs — Sedation, hypotension, dry mouth

10.14 MEPHENESIN, METHOCARBAMOL, CHLORZOXAZONE, CHLORMEZANONE

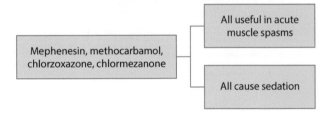

Mephenesin, methocarbamol, chlorzoxazone, chlormezanone
- All useful in acute muscle spasms
- All cause sedation

10.15 USES

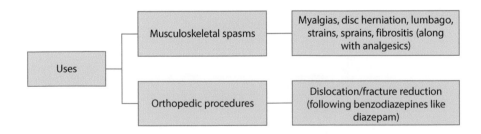

Uses
- Musculoskeletal spasms — Myalgias, disc herniation, lumbago, strains, sprains, fibrositis (along with analgesics)
- Orthopedic procedures — Dislocation/fracture reduction (following benzodiazepines like diazepam)

10.16 DIRECTLY ACTING SMRs

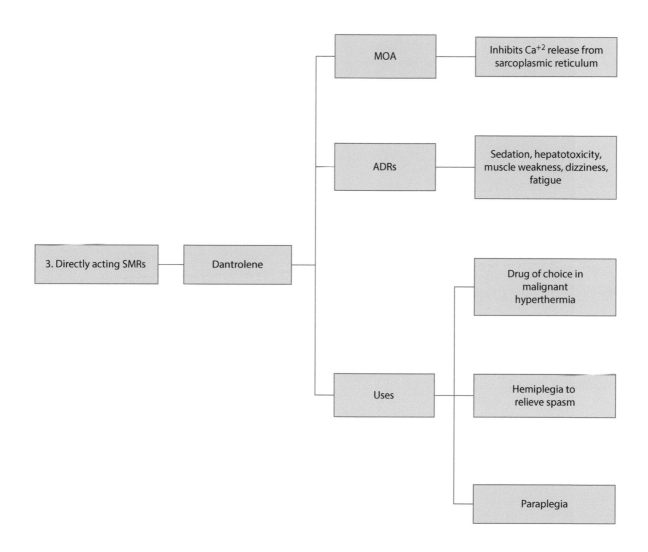

Adrenergic system and drugs

11.1 INTRODUCTION, DISTRIBUTION OF SNS, NEUROTRANSMITTERS

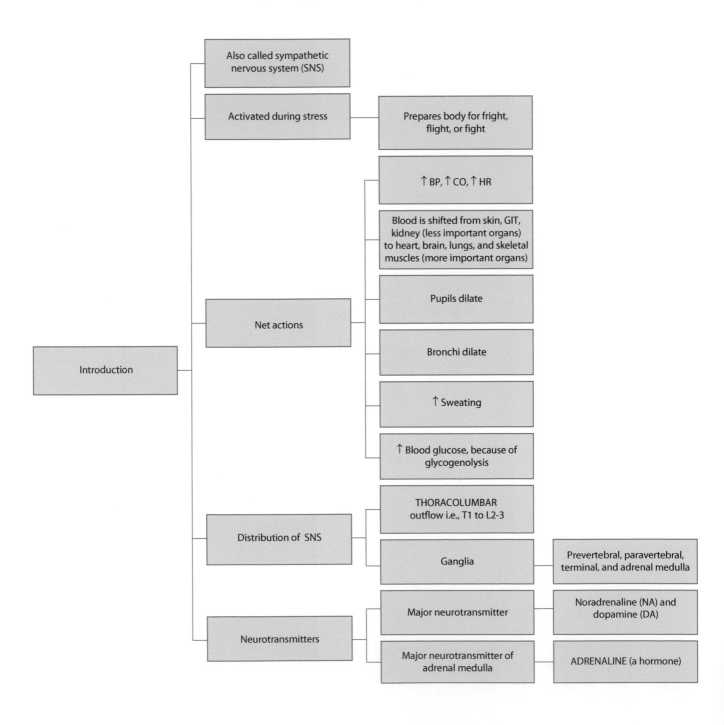

- Introduction
  - Also called sympathetic nervous system (SNS)
  - Activated during stress
    - Prepares body for fright, flight, or fight
  - Net actions
    - ↑ BP, ↑ CO, ↑ HR
    - Blood is shifted from skin, GIT, kidney (less important organs) to heart, brain, lungs, and skeletal muscles (more important organs)
    - Pupils dilate
    - Bronchi dilate
    - ↑ Sweating
    - ↑ Blood glucose, because of glycogenolysis
  - Distribution of SNS
    - THORACOLUMBAR outflow i.e., T1 to L2-3
    - Ganglia
      - Prevertebral, paravertebral, terminal, and adrenal medulla
  - Neurotransmitters
    - Major neurotransmitter
      - Noradrenaline (NA) and dopamine (DA)
    - Major neurotransmitter of adrenal medulla
      - ADRENALINE (a hormone)

11.2 BIOSYNTHESIS OF CATECHOLAMINES

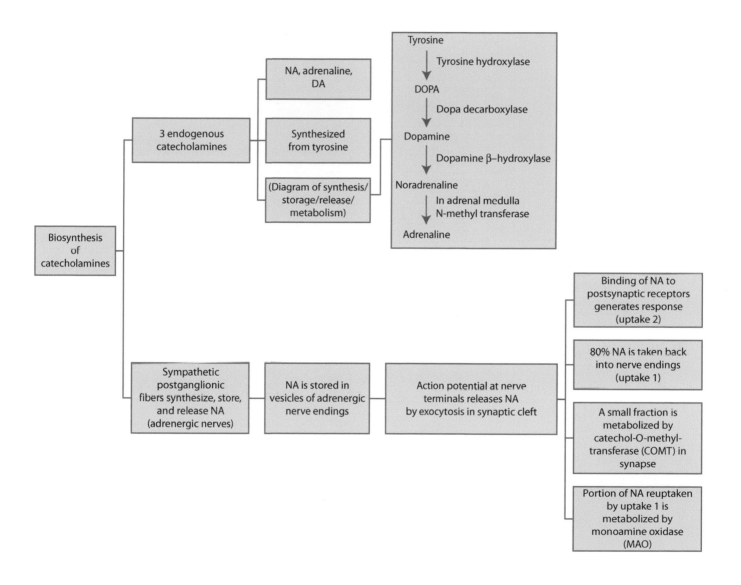

11.3 ADRENERGIC RECEPTORS

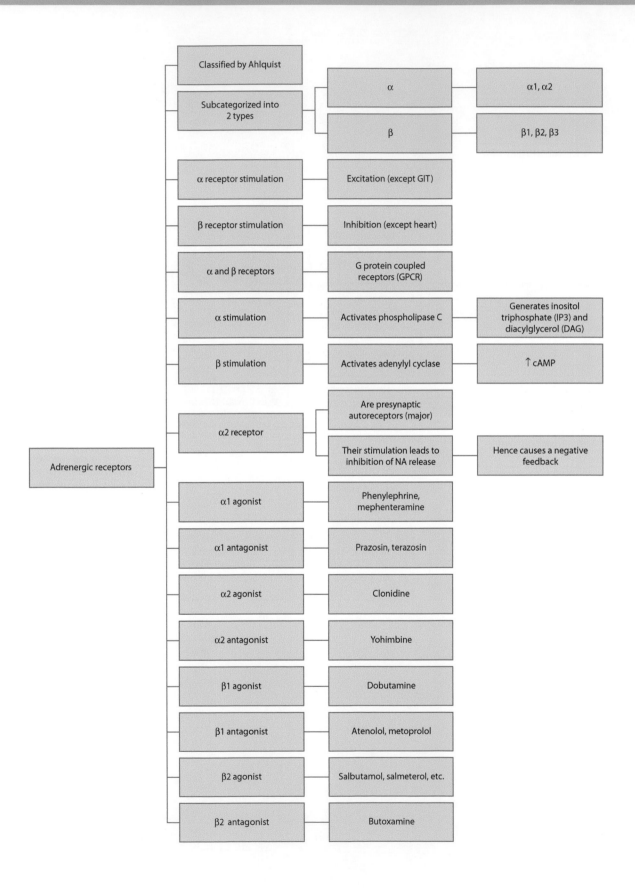

11.4 ADRENERGIC DRUGS (SYMPATHOMIMETICS) – CLASSIFICATION

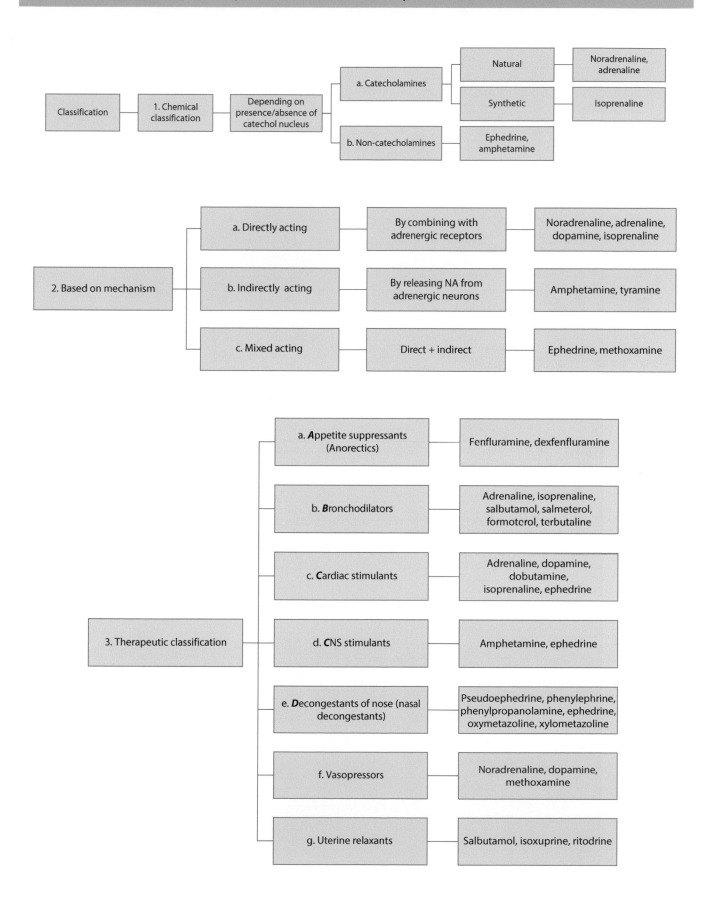

11.5 CATECHOLAMINES – ADRENALINE – PHARMACOLOGICAL ACTIONS

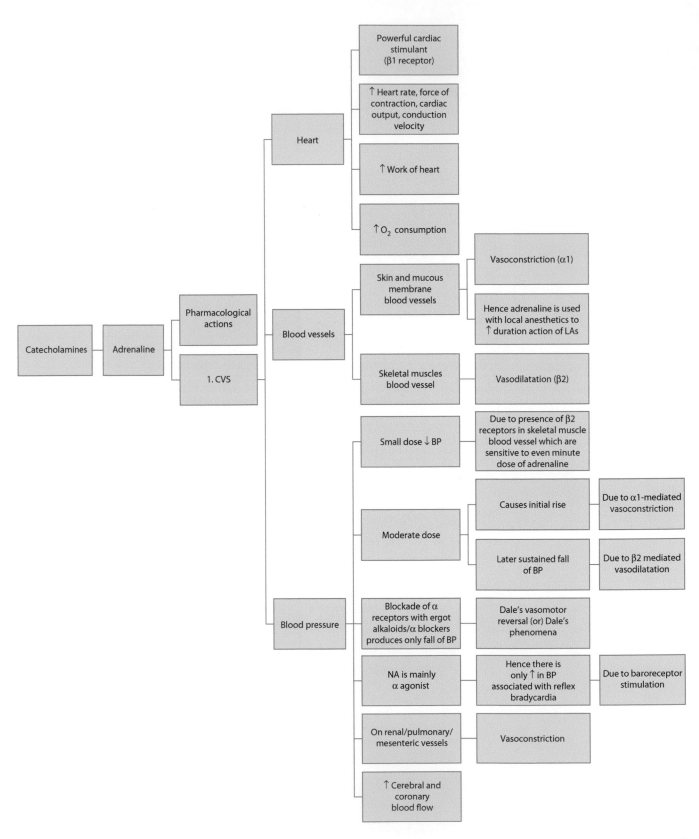

(Continued)

11.5 CATECHOLAMINES – ADRENALINE – PHARMACOLOGICAL ACTIONS (Continued)

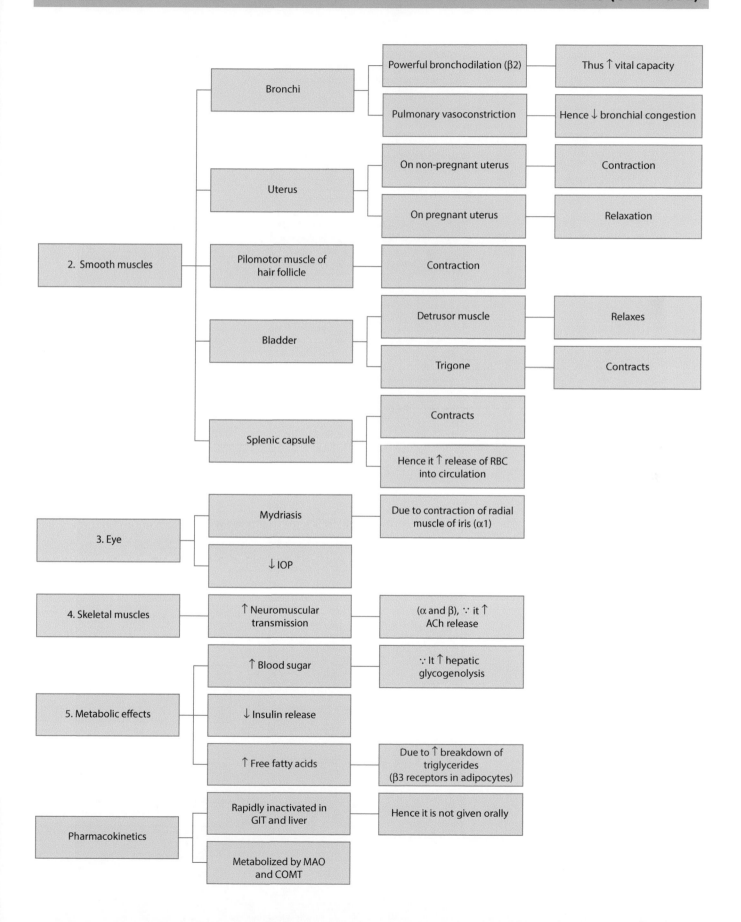

2. Smooth muscles

- **Bronchi**
  - Powerful bronchodilation (β2) → Thus ↑ vital capacity
  - Pulmonary vasoconstriction → Hence ↓ bronchial congestion
- **Uterus**
  - On non-pregnant uterus → Contraction
  - On pregnant uterus → Relaxation
- **Pilomotor muscle of hair follicle** → Contraction
- **Bladder**
  - Detrusor muscle → Relaxes
  - Trigone → Contracts
- **Splenic capsule**
  - Contracts
  - Hence it ↑ release of RBC into circulation

3. Eye
- Mydriasis → Due to contraction of radial muscle of iris (α1)
- ↓ IOP

4. Skeletal muscles
- ↑ Neuromuscular transmission → (α and β), ∵ it ↑ ACh release

5. Metabolic effects
- ↑ Blood sugar → ∵ It ↑ hepatic glycogenolysis
- ↓ Insulin release
- ↑ Free fatty acids → Due to ↑ breakdown of triglycerides (β3 receptors in adipocytes)

Pharmacokinetics
- Rapidly inactivated in GIT and liver → Hence it is not given orally
- Metabolized by MAO and COMT

11.6 ADVERSE REACTIONS, CONTRAINDICATIONS, PREPARATIONS

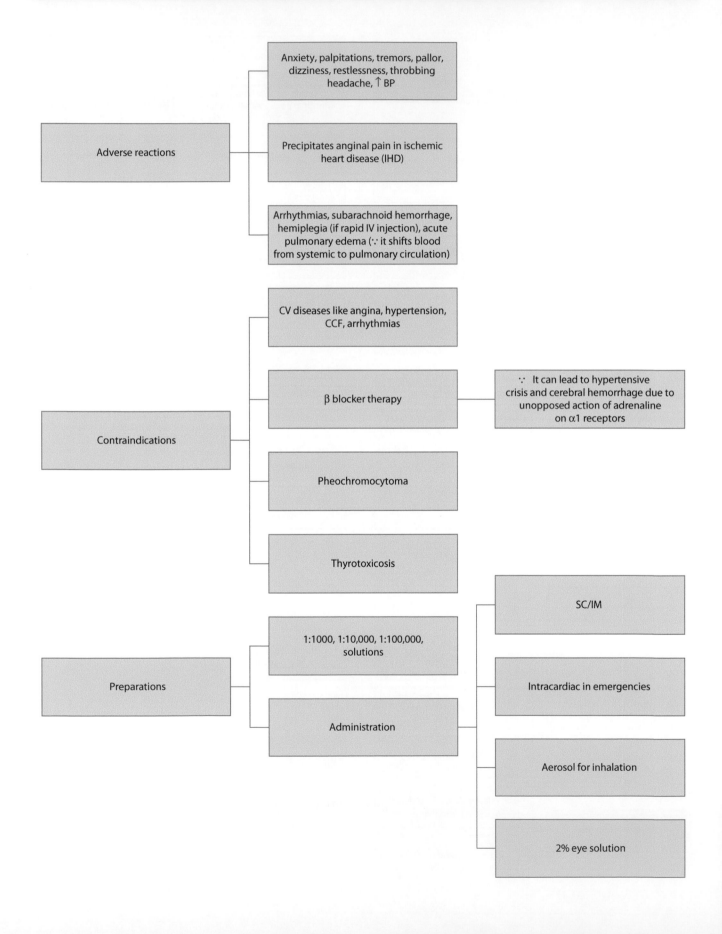

Adverse reactions

- Anxiety, palpitations, tremors, pallor, dizziness, restlessness, throbbing headache, ↑ BP
- Precipitates anginal pain in ischemic heart disease (IHD)
- Arrhythmias, subarachnoid hemorrhage, hemiplegia (if rapid IV injection), acute pulmonary edema (∵ it shifts blood from systemic to pulmonary circulation)

Contraindications

- CV diseases like angina, hypertension, CCF, arrhythmias
- β blocker therapy — ∵ It can lead to hypertensive crisis and cerebral hemorrhage due to unopposed action of adrenaline on α1 receptors
- Pheochromocytoma
- Thyrotoxicosis

Preparations

- 1:1000, 1:10,000, 1:100,000, solutions
- Administration
  - SC/IM
  - Intracardiac in emergencies
  - Aerosol for inhalation
  - 2% eye solution

11.7 USES OF ADRENALINE

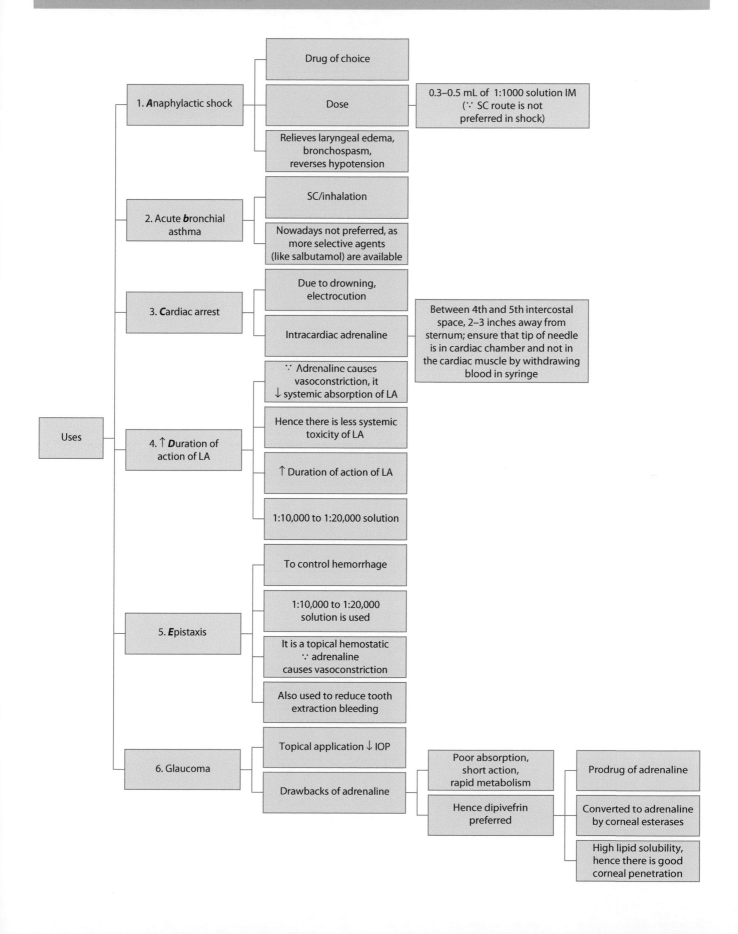

11.8 NORADRENALINE

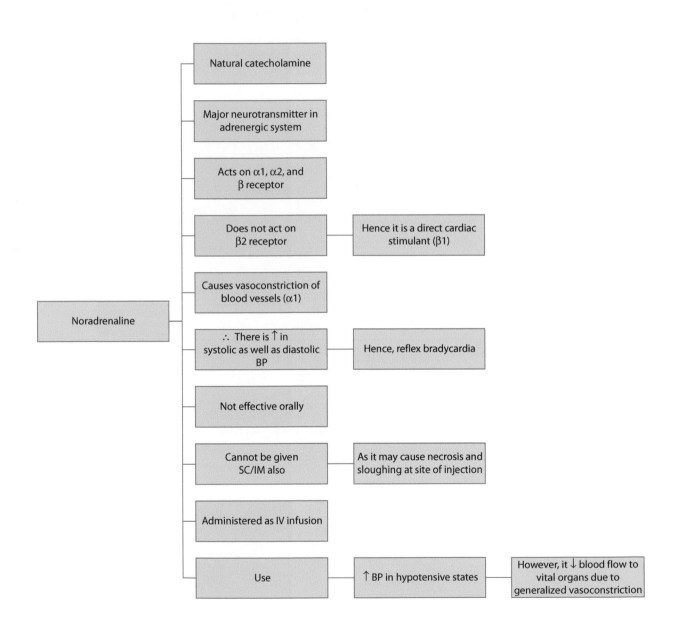

Noradrenaline

- Natural catecholamine
- Major neurotransmitter in adrenergic system
- Acts on α1, α2, and β receptor
- Does not act on β2 receptor → Hence it is a direct cardiac stimulant (β1)
- Causes vasoconstriction of blood vessels (α1)
- ∴ There is ↑ in systolic as well as diastolic BP → Hence, reflex bradycardia
- Not effective orally
- Cannot be given SC/IM also → As it may cause necrosis and sloughing at site of injection
- Administered as IV infusion
- Use → ↑ BP in hypotensive states → However, it ↓ blood flow to vital organs due to generalized vasoconstriction

11.9 ISOPRENALINE

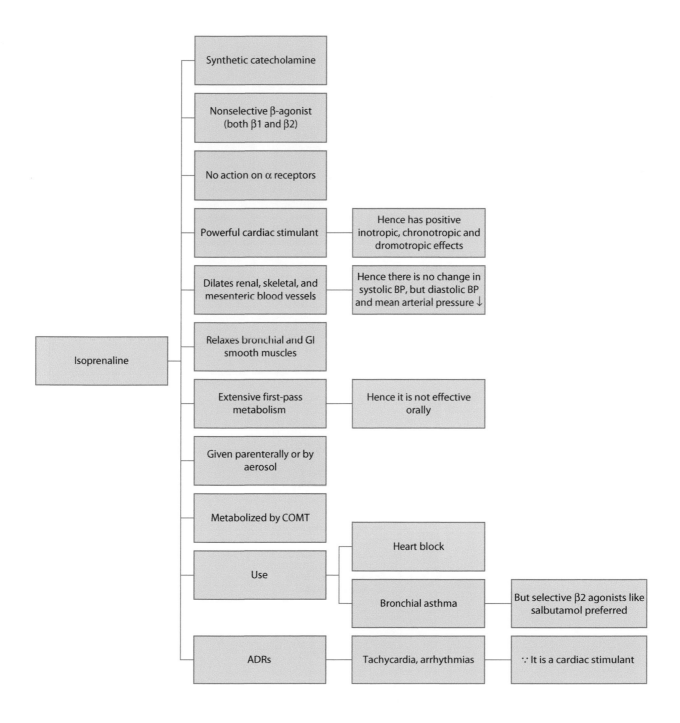

11.10 DOPAMINE

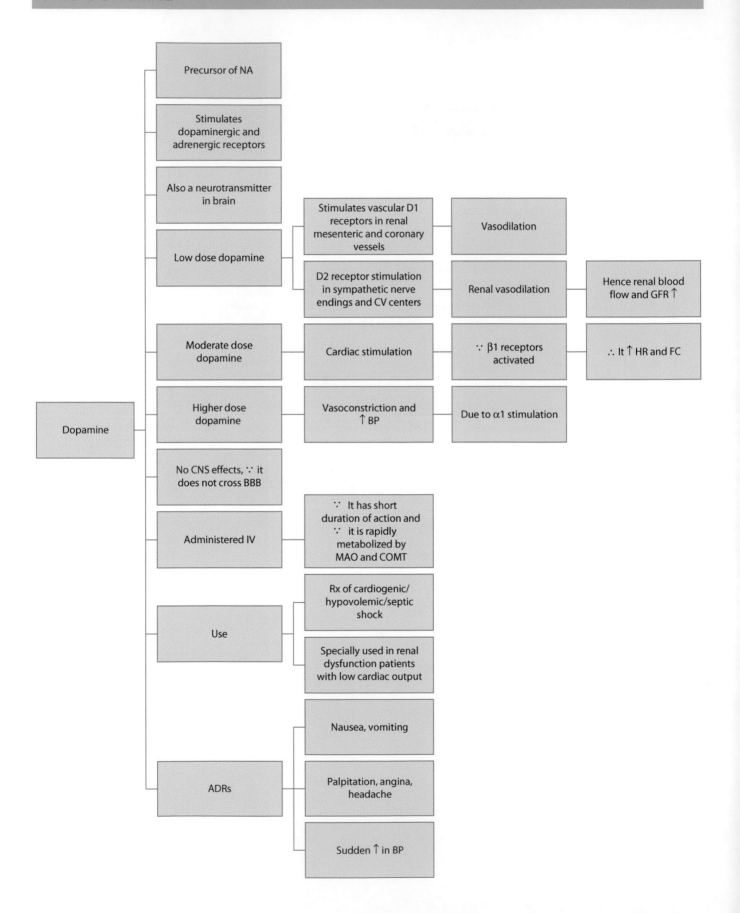

Dopamine

- Precursor of NA
- Stimulates dopaminergic and adrenergic receptors
- Also a neurotransmitter in brain
- Low dose dopamine
  - Stimulates vascular D1 receptors in renal mesenteric and coronary vessels → Vasodilation
  - D2 receptor stimulation in sympathetic nerve endings and CV centers → Renal vasodilation → Hence renal blood flow and GFR ↑
- Moderate dose dopamine → Cardiac stimulation → ∵ β1 receptors activated → ∴ It ↑ HR and FC
- Higher dose dopamine → Vasoconstriction and ↑ BP → Due to α1 stimulation
- No CNS effects, ∵ it does not cross BBB
- Administered IV → ∵ It has short duration of action and ∵ it is rapidly metabolized by MAO and COMT
- Use
  - Rx of cardiogenic/hypovolemic/septic shock
  - Specially used in renal dysfunction patients with low cardiac output
- ADRs
  - Nausea, vomiting
  - Palpitation, angina, headache
  - Sudden ↑ in BP

11.11 DOBUTAMINE, FENOLDOPAM

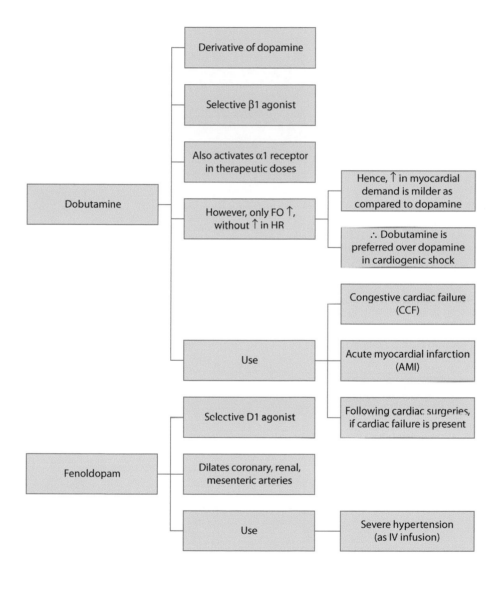

11.12 NONCATECHOLAMINES – INTRODUCTION AND EPHEDRINE

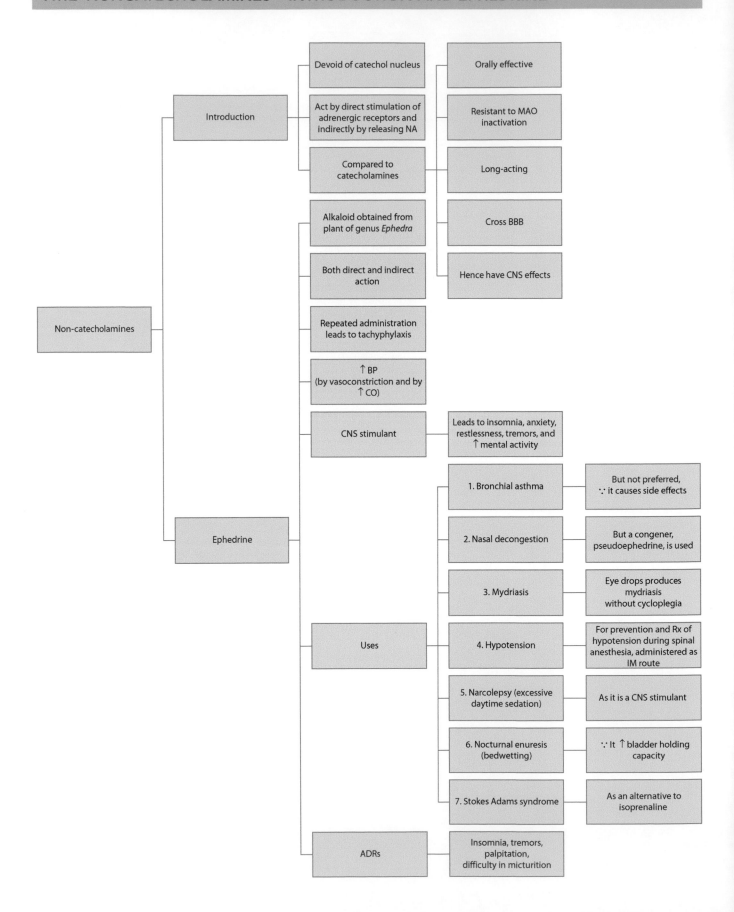

Non-catecholamines

Introduction
- Devoid of catechol nucleus
- Act by direct stimulation of adrenergic receptors and indirectly by releasing NA
- Compared to catecholamines
  - Orally effective
  - Resistant to MAO inactivation
  - Long-acting
  - Cross BBB
  - Hence have CNS effects

Ephedrine
- Alkaloid obtained from plant of genus *Ephedra*
- Both direct and indirect action
- Repeated administration leads to tachyphylaxis
- ↑ BP (by vasoconstriction and by ↑ CO)
- CNS stimulant
  - Leads to insomnia, anxiety, restlessness, tremors, and ↑ mental activity

Uses
1. Bronchial asthma — But not preferred, ∵ it causes side effects
2. Nasal decongestion — But a congener, pseudoephedrine, is used
3. Mydriasis — Eye drops produces mydriasis without cycloplegia
4. Hypotension — For prevention and Rx of hypotension during spinal anesthesia, administered as IM route
5. Narcolepsy (excessive daytime sedation) — As it is a CNS stimulant
6. Nocturnal enuresis (bedwetting) — ∵ It ↑ bladder holding capacity
7. Stokes Adams syndrome — As an alternative to isoprenaline

ADRs
- Insomnia, tremors, palpitation, difficulty in micturition

11.13 AMPHETAMINE

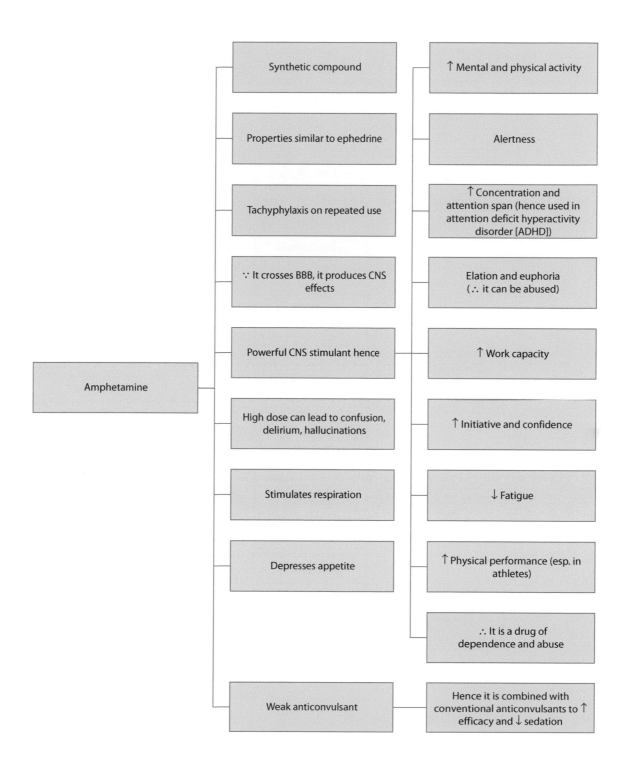

Amphetamine

- Synthetic compound
- Properties similar to ephedrine
- Tachyphylaxis on repeated use
- ∵ It crosses BBB, it produces CNS effects
- Powerful CNS stimulant hence
  - ↑ Mental and physical activity
  - Alertness
  - ↑ Concentration and attention span (hence used in attention deficit hyperactivity disorder [ADHD])
  - Elation and euphoria (∴ it can be abused)
  - ↑ Work capacity
  - ↑ Initiative and confidence
  - ↓ Fatigue
  - ↑ Physical performance (esp. in athletes)
  - ∴ It is a drug of dependence and abuse
- High dose can lead to confusion, delirium, hallucinations
- Stimulates respiration
- Depresses appetite
- Weak anticonvulsant
  - Hence it is combined with conventional anticonvulsants to ↑ efficacy and ↓ sedation

11.14 ADRs, USES

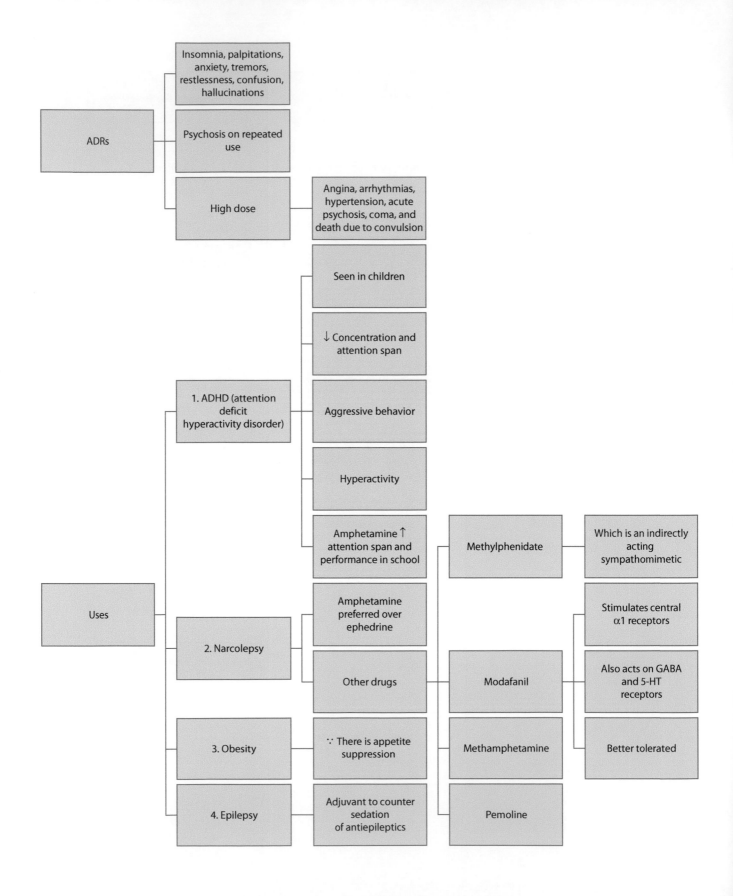

11.15 VASOPRESSORS

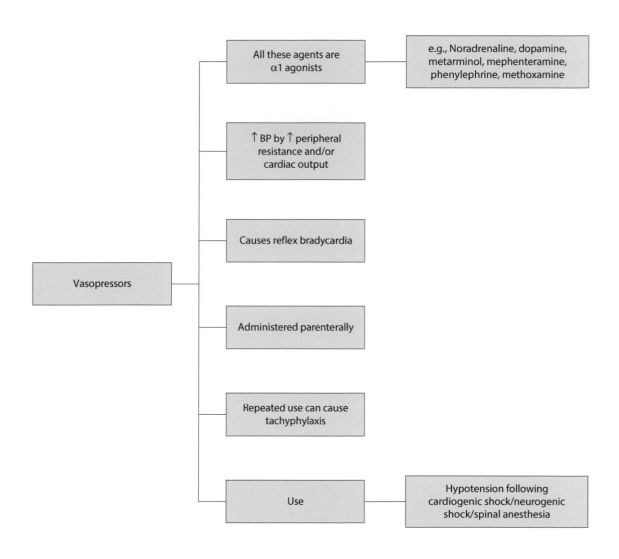

Vasopressors

- All these agents are α1 agonists — e.g., Noradrenaline, dopamine, metarminol, mephenteramine, phenylephrine, methoxamine
- ↑ BP by ↑ peripheral resistance and/or cardiac output
- Causes reflex bradycardia
- Administered parenterally
- Repeated use can cause tachyphylaxis
- Use — Hypotension following cardiogenic shock/neurogenic shock/spinal anesthesia

11.16 NASAL DECONGESTANTS

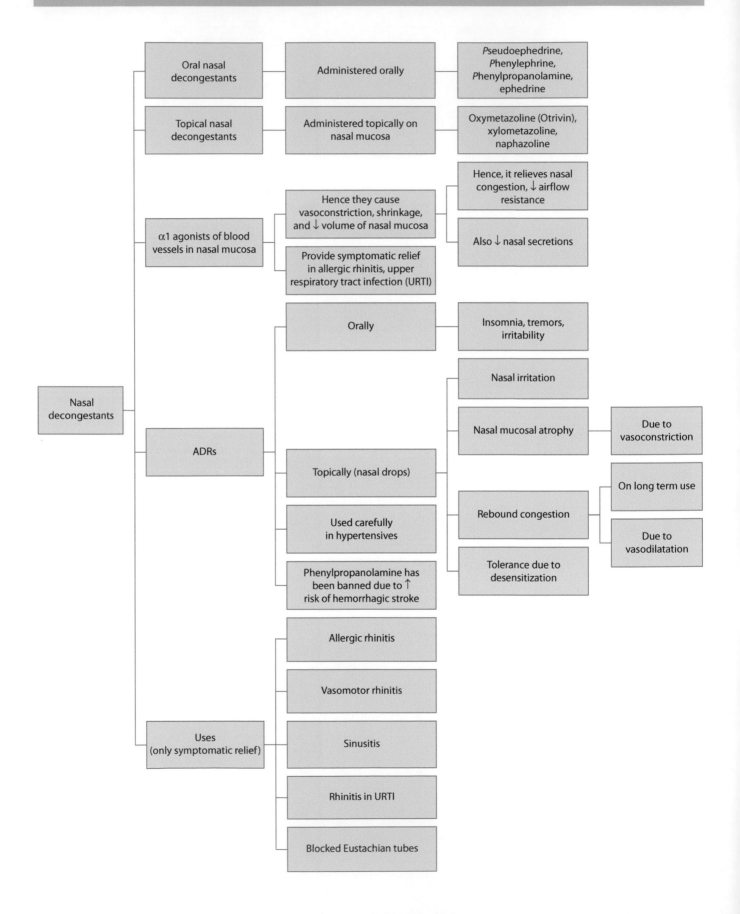

11.17 SELECTIVE β2-STIMULANTS, ANORECTICS (APPETITE SUPPRESSANTS)

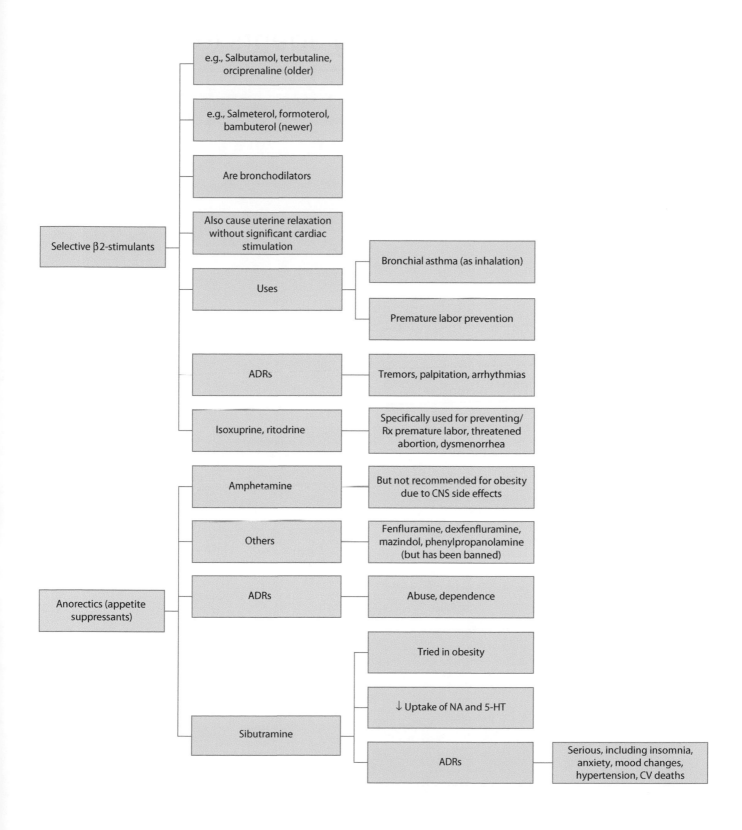

Alpha-adrenergic blocking agents (α blockers)

12

12.1 CLASSIFICATION

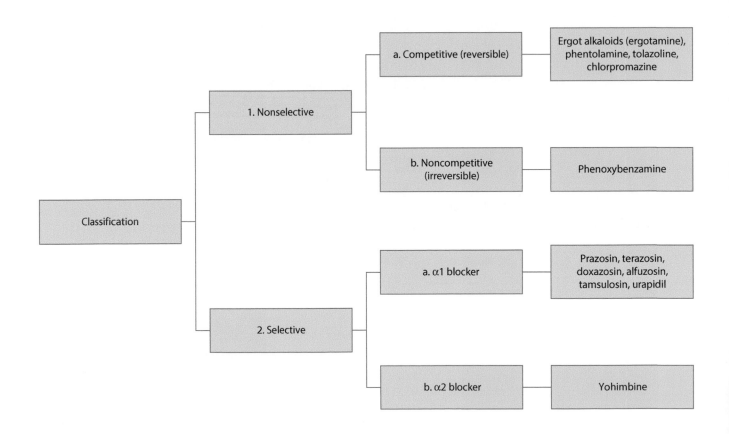

12.2 PHARMACOLOGICAL ACTIONS

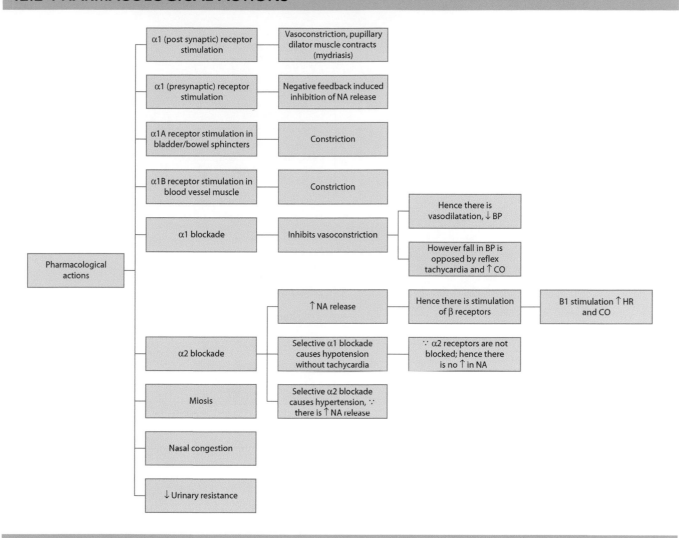

12.3 ADRs

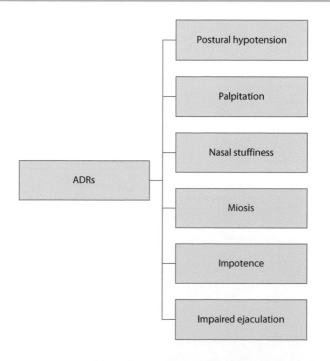

12.4 NONSELECTIVE α BLOCKERS

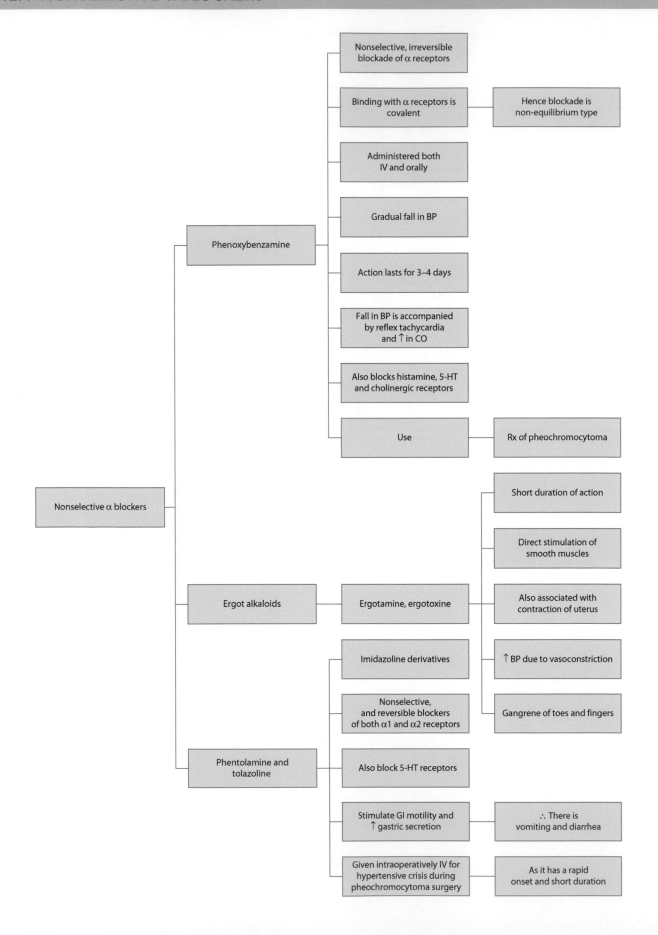

Nonselective α blockers

Phenoxybenzamine
- Nonselective, irreversible blockade of α receptors
- Binding with α receptors is covalent → Hence blockade is non-equilibrium type
- Administered both IV and orally
- Gradual fall in BP
- Action lasts for 3–4 days
- Fall in BP is accompanied by reflex tachycardia and ↑ in CO
- Also blocks histamine, 5-HT and cholinergic receptors
- Use → Rx of pheochromocytoma

Ergot alkaloids → Ergotamine, ergotoxine
- Short duration of action
- Direct stimulation of smooth muscles
- Also associated with contraction of uterus
- ↑ BP due to vasoconstriction
- Gangrene of toes and fingers

Phentolamine and tolazoline
- Imidazoline derivatives
- Nonselective, and reversible blockers of both α1 and α2 receptors
- Also block 5-HT receptors
- Stimulate GI motility and ↑ gastric secretion → ∴ There is vomiting and diarrhea
- Given intraoperatively IV for hypertensive crisis during pheochromocytoma surgery → As it has a rapid onset and short duration

12.5 SELECTIVE α1 BLOCKERS

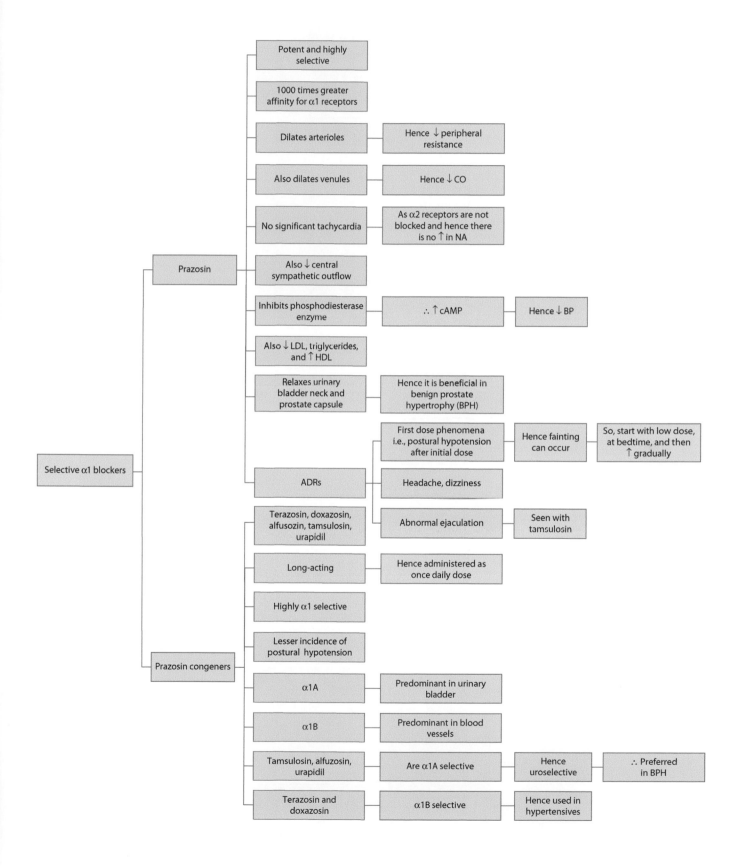

12.6 SELECTIVE α2 BLOCKERS

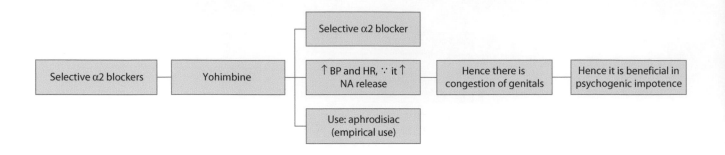

Selective α2 blockers → Yohimbine →

- Selective α2 blocker
- ↑ BP and HR, ∵ it ↑ NA release → Hence there is congestion of genitals → Hence it is beneficial in psychogenic impotence
- Use: aphrodisiac (empirical use)

12.7 USES OF α BLOCKERS

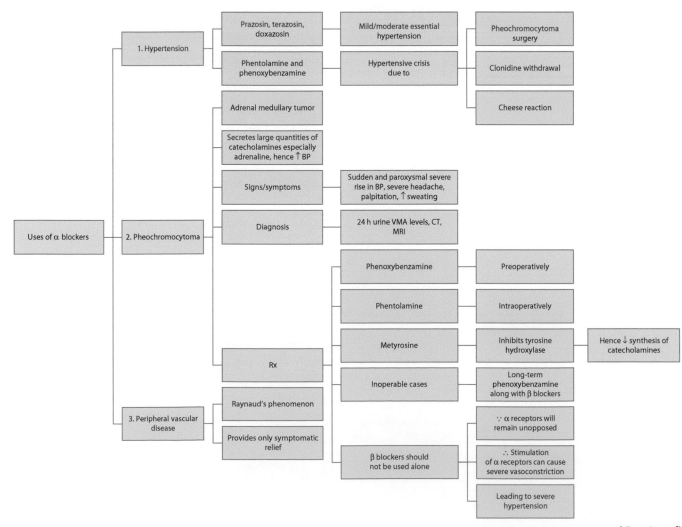

Uses of α blockers

1. Hypertension
   - Prazosin, terazosin, doxazosin → Mild/moderate essential hypertension
   - Phentolamine and phenoxybenzamine → Hypertensive crisis due to → Pheochromocytoma surgery / Clonidine withdrawal / Cheese reaction

2. Pheochromocytoma
   - Adrenal medullary tumor
   - Secretes large quantities of catecholamines especially adrenaline, hence ↑ BP
   - Signs/symptoms → Sudden and paroxysmal severe rise in BP, severe headache, palpitation, ↑ sweating
   - Diagnosis → 24 h urine VMA levels, CT, MRI
   - Rx
     - Phenoxybenzamine → Preoperatively
     - Phentolamine → Intraoperatively
     - Metyrosine → Inhibits tyrosine hydroxylase → Hence ↓ synthesis of catecholamines
     - Inoperable cases → Long-term phenoxybenzamine along with β blockers

3. Peripheral vascular disease
   - Raynaud's phenomenon
   - Provides only symptomatic relief
   - β blockers should not be used alone → ∵ α receptors will remain unopposed / ∴ Stimulation of α receptors can cause severe vasoconstriction / Leading to severe hypertension

(Continued)

12.7 USES OF α BLOCKERS (Continued)

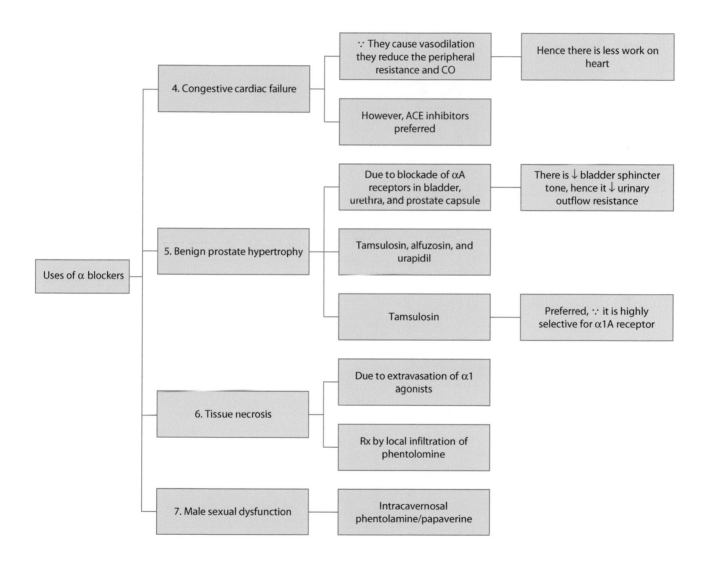

Beta-adrenergic blockers (β blockers)

13.1 CLASSIFICATION

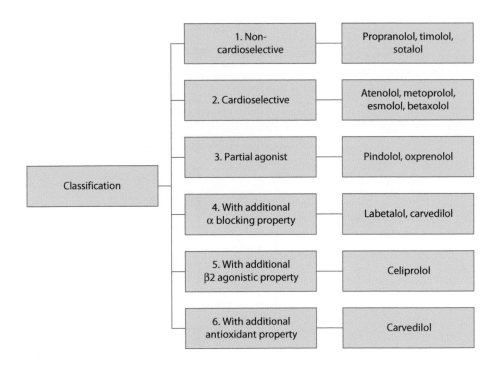

13.2 PHARMACOLOGICAL ACTIONS

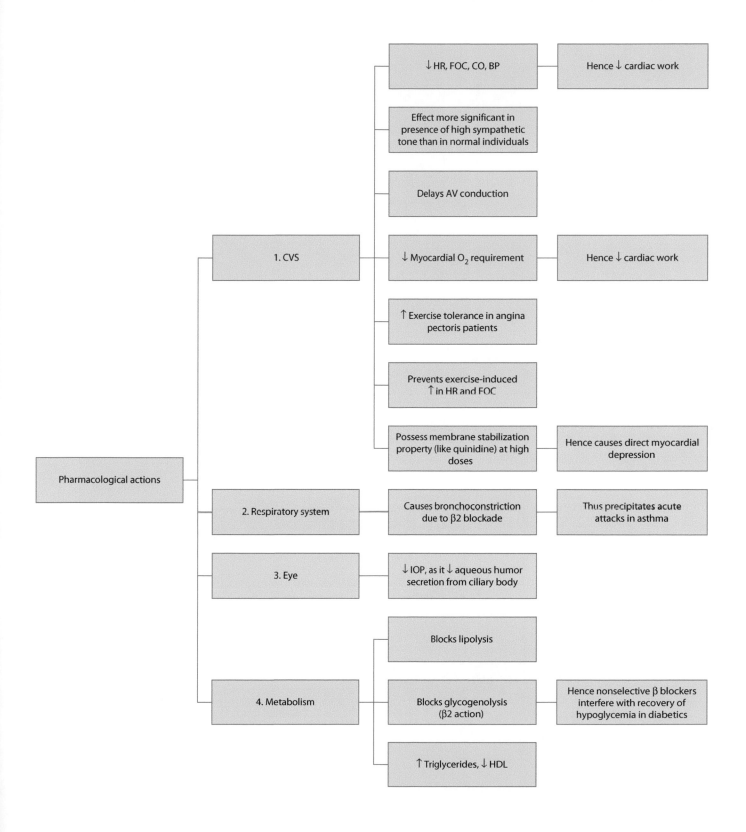

13.3 PHARMACOKINETICS

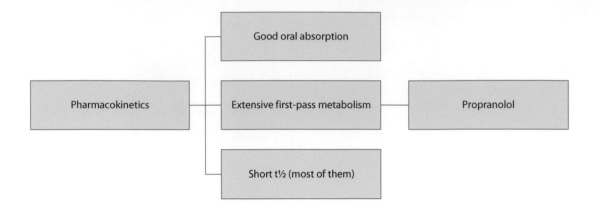

13.4 USES

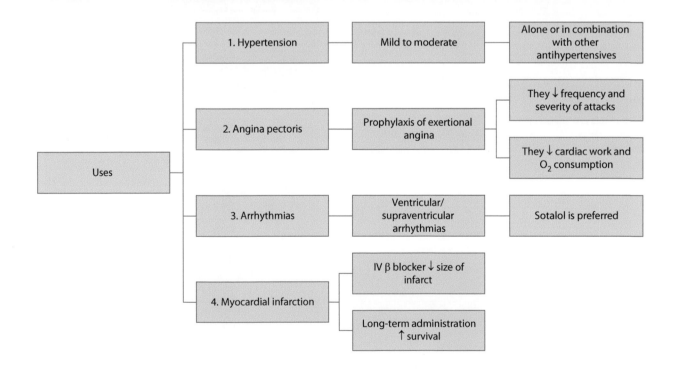

(Continued)

13.4 USES (Continued)

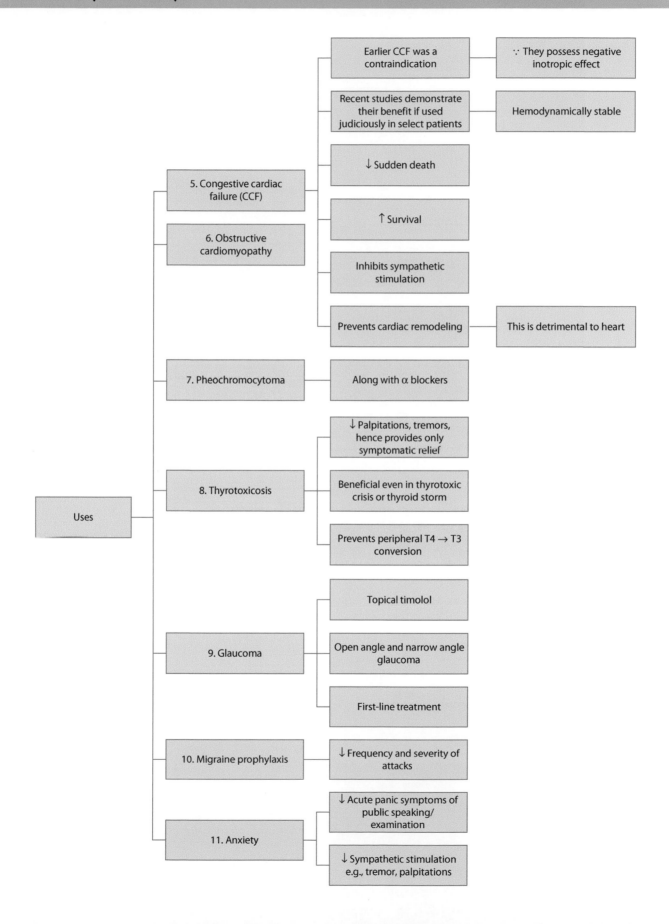

Uses

5. Congestive cardiac failure (CCF)
- Earlier CCF was a contraindication — ∵ They possess negative inotropic effect
- Recent studies demonstrate their benefit if used judiciously in select patients — Hemodynamically stable
- ↓ Sudden death
- ↑ Survival
- Inhibits sympathetic stimulation
- Prevents cardiac remodeling — This is detrimental to heart

6. Obstructive cardiomyopathy

7. Pheochromocytoma
- Along with α blockers

8. Thyrotoxicosis
- ↓ Palpitations, tremors, hence provides only symptomatic relief
- Beneficial even in thyrotoxic crisis or thyroid storm
- Prevents peripheral T4 → T3 conversion

9. Glaucoma
- Topical timolol
- Open angle and narrow angle glaucoma
- First-line treatment

10. Migraine prophylaxis
- ↓ Frequency and severity of attacks

11. Anxiety
- ↓ Acute panic symptoms of public speaking/ examination
- ↓ Sympathetic stimulation e.g., tremor, palpitations

13.5 ADVERSE REACTIONS

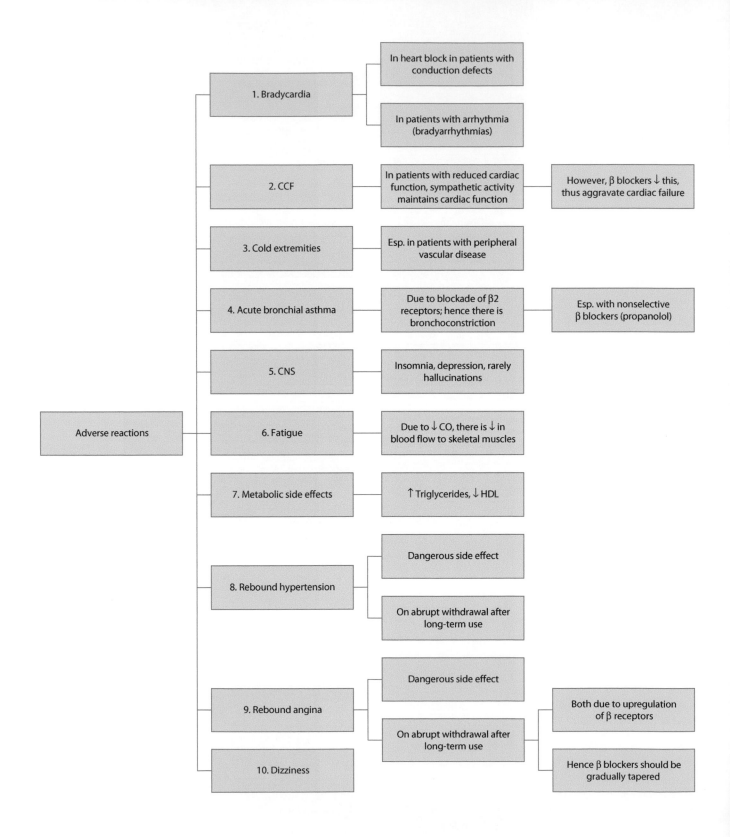

1. Bradycardia
- In heart block in patients with conduction defects
- In patients with arrhythmia (bradyarrhythmias)

2. CCF
- In patients with reduced cardiac function, sympathetic activity maintains cardiac function
  - However, β blockers ↓ this, thus aggravate cardiac failure

3. Cold extremities
- Esp. in patients with peripheral vascular disease

4. Acute bronchial asthma
- Due to blockade of β2 receptors; hence there is bronchoconstriction
  - Esp. with nonselective β blockers (propanolol)

5. CNS
- Insomnia, depression, rarely hallucinations

6. Fatigue
- Due to ↓ CO, there is ↓ in blood flow to skeletal muscles

7. Metabolic side effects
- ↑ Triglycerides, ↓ HDL

8. Rebound hypertension
- Dangerous side effect
- On abrupt withdrawal after long-term use

9. Rebound angina
- Dangerous side effect
- On abrupt withdrawal after long-term use
  - Both due to upregulation of β receptors
  - Hence β blockers should be gradually tapered

10. Dizziness

Adverse reactions

13.6 DRUG INTERACTIONS

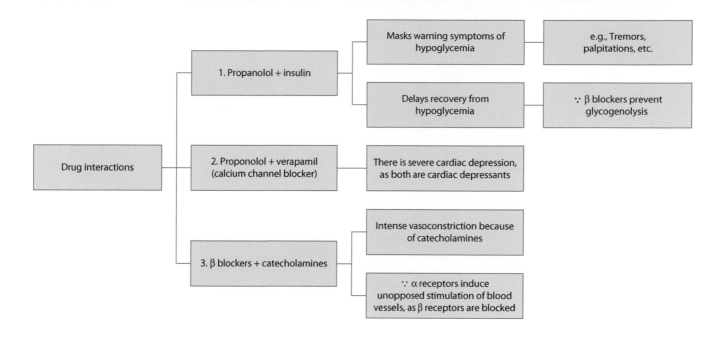

13.7 CONTRAINDICATIONS

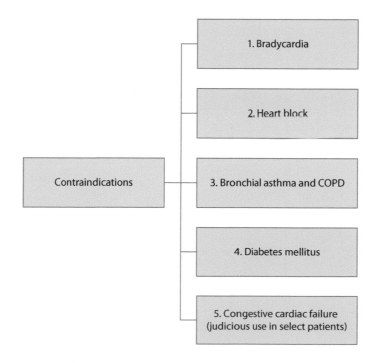

13.8 CARDIOSELECTIVE β BLOCKERS

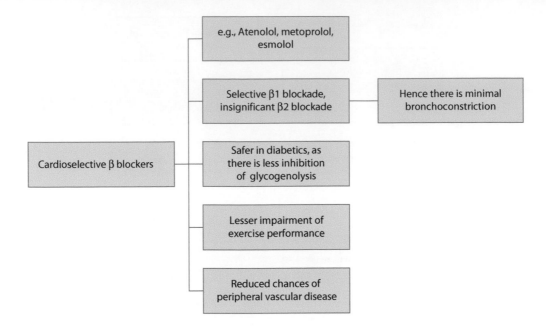

Cardioselective β blockers

- e.g., Atenolol, metoprolol, esmolol
- Selective β1 blockade, insignificant β2 blockade → Hence there is minimal bronchoconstriction
- Safer in diabetics, as there is less inhibition of glycogenolysis
- Lesser impairment of exercise performance
- Reduced chances of peripheral vascular disease

13.9 PARTIAL AGONISTS

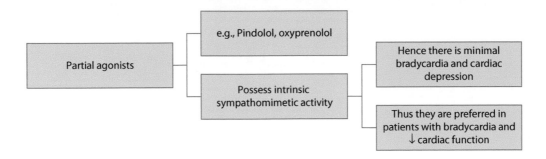

Partial agonists

- e.g., Pindolol, oxyprenolol
- Possess intrinsic sympathomimetic activity
  - Hence there is minimal bradycardia and cardiac depression
  - Thus they are preferred in patients with bradycardia and ↓ cardiac function

13.10 SOME INDIVIDUAL β BLOCKERS

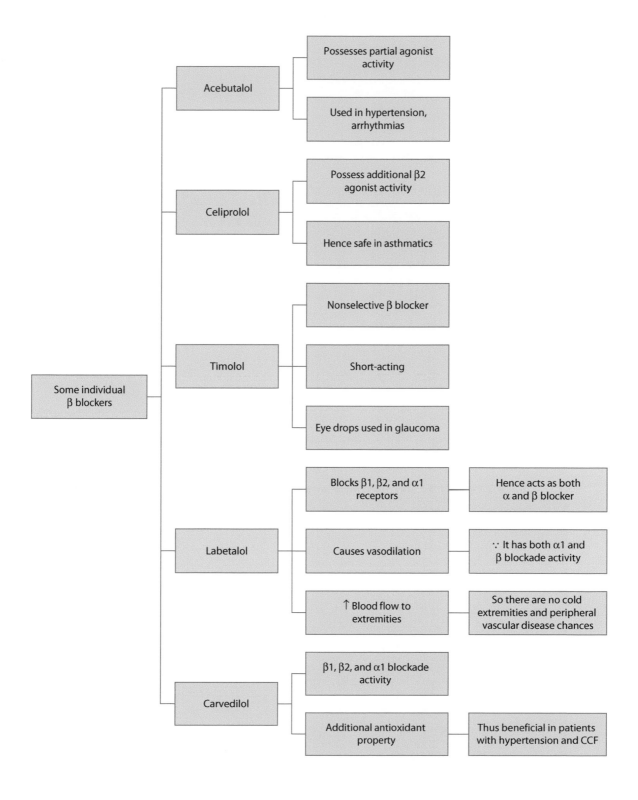

PART III

Cardiovascular pharmacology

Antihypertensives

14.1 INTRODUCTION

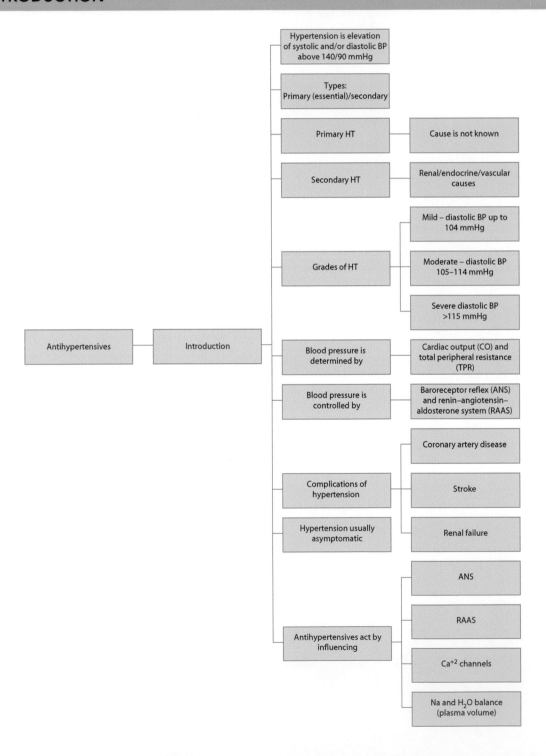

14.2 CLASSIFICATION

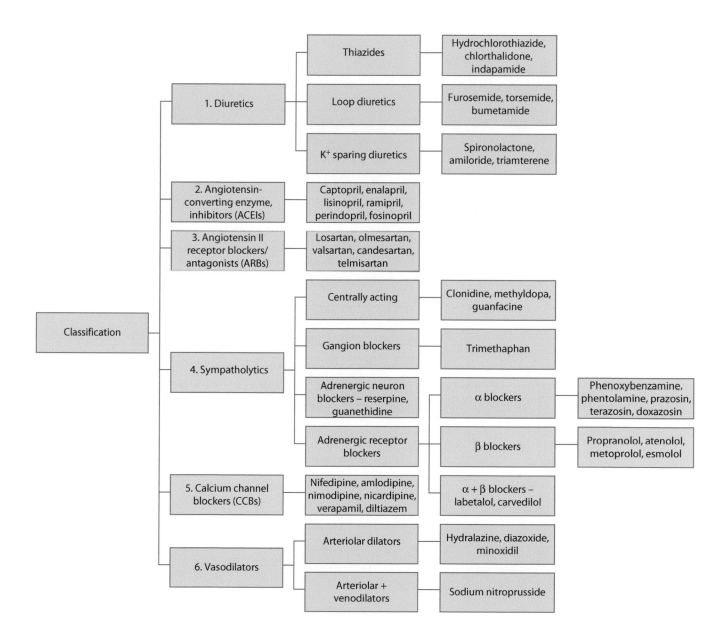

14.3 DIURETICS

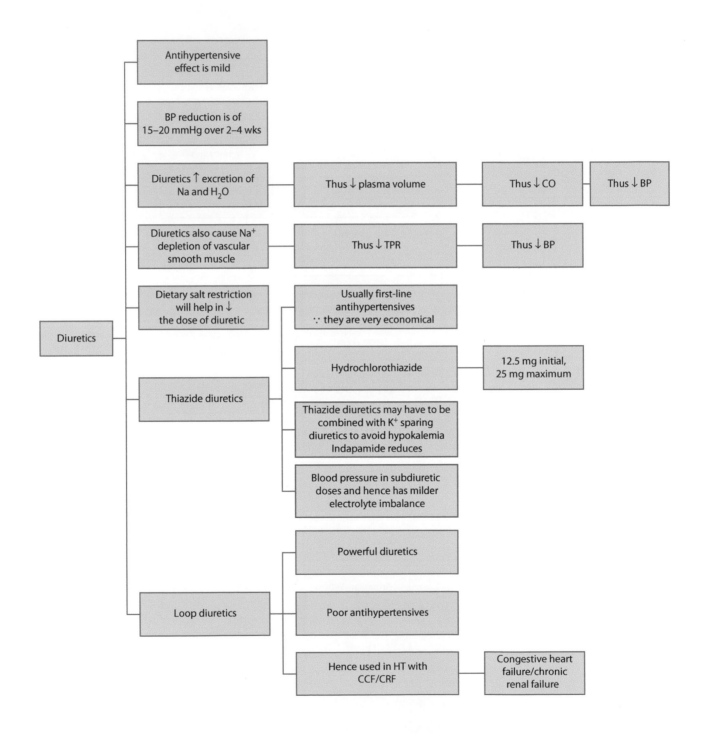

14.4 ANGIOTENSIN-CONVERTING ENZYME (ACE) INHIBITORS (ACEIs) AND ADRs

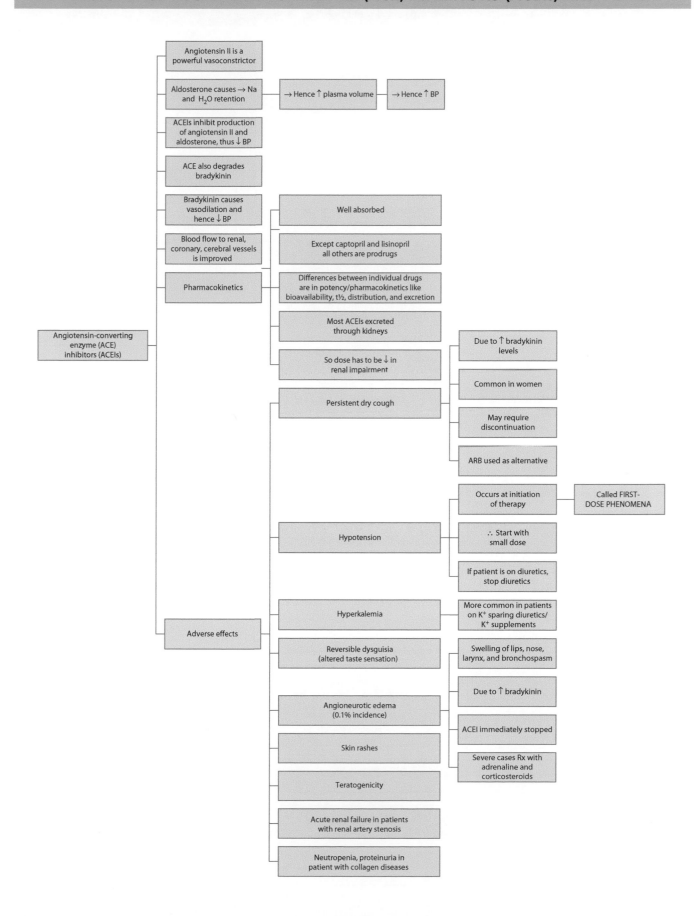

14.5 ANGIOTENSIN-CONVERTING ENZYME (ACE) INHIBITORS (ACEIs) – USES, PRECAUTIONS, AND CONTRAINDICATIONS

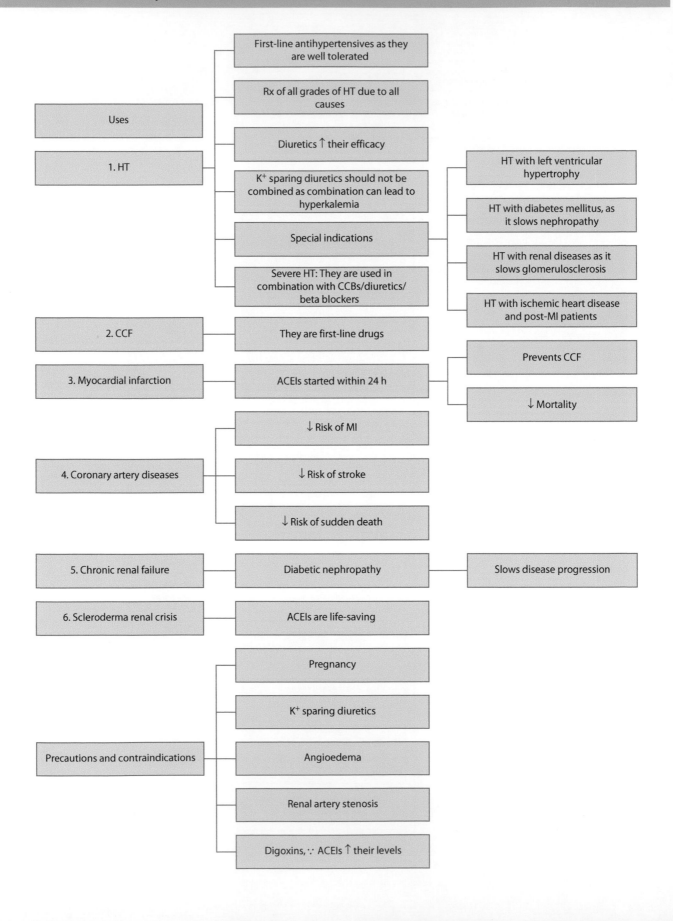

Uses

1. HT

First-line antihypertensives as they are well tolerated

Rx of all grades of HT due to all causes

Diuretics ↑ their efficacy

K⁺ sparing diuretics should not be combined as combination can lead to hyperkalemia

Special indications

Severe HT: They are used in combination with CCBs/diuretics/beta blockers

HT with left ventricular hypertrophy

HT with diabetes mellitus, as it slows nephropathy

HT with renal diseases as it slows glomerulosclerosis

HT with ischemic heart disease and post-MI patients

2. CCF — They are first-line drugs

3. Myocardial infarction — ACEIs started within 24 h

Prevents CCF

↓ Mortality

4. Coronary artery diseases

↓ Risk of MI

↓ Risk of stroke

↓ Risk of sudden death

5. Chronic renal failure — Diabetic nephropathy — Slows disease progression

6. Scleroderma renal crisis — ACEIs are life-saving

Precautions and contraindications

Pregnancy

K⁺ sparing diuretics

Angioedema

Renal artery stenosis

Digoxins, ∵ ACEIs ↑ their levels

14.6 ANGIOTENSIN II RECEPTOR BLOCKERS (ARBs)

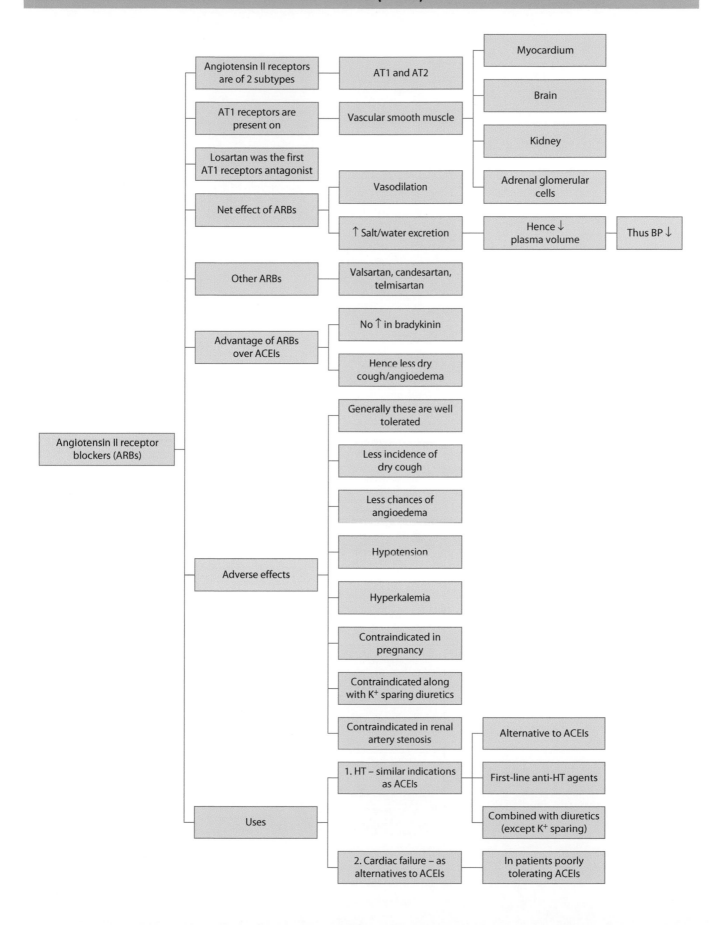

14.7 SYMPATHOLYTICS

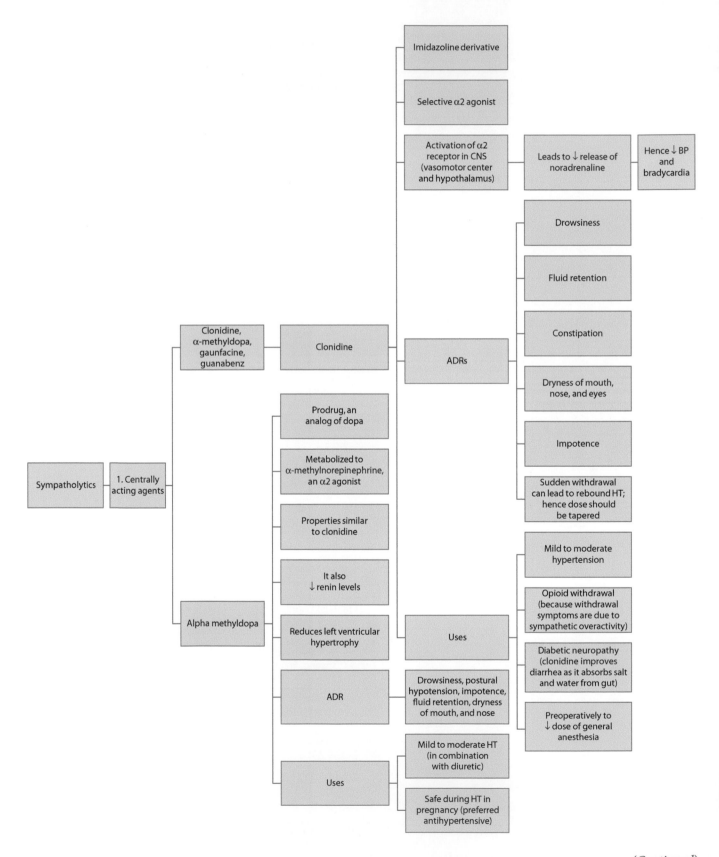

(Continued)

14.7 SYMPATHOLYTICS (Continued)

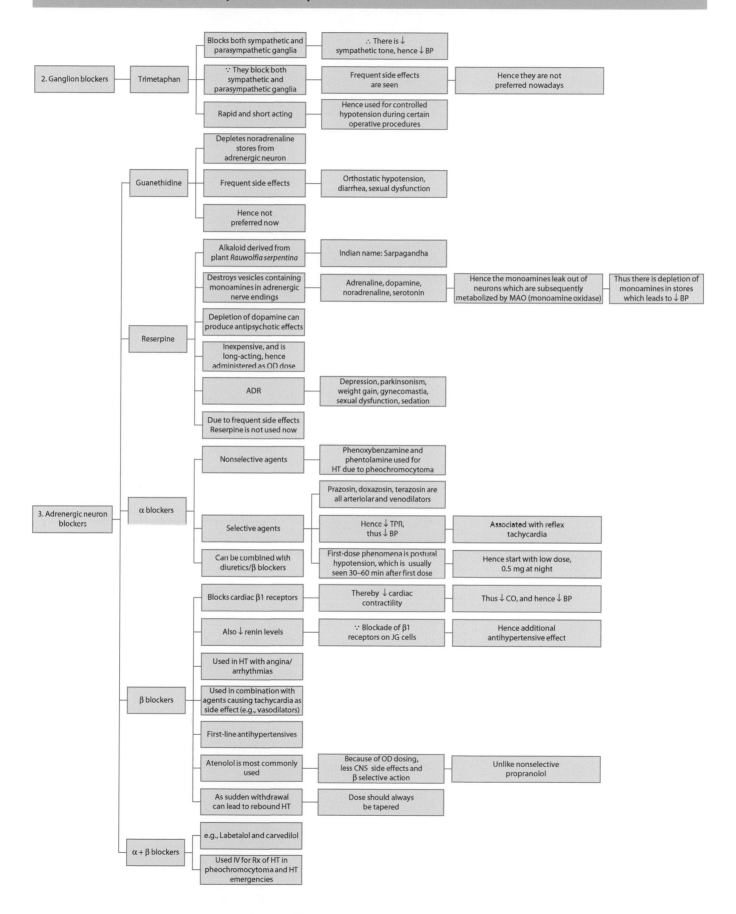

2. Ganglion blockers → **Trimetaphan**

- Blocks both sympathetic and parasympathetic ganglia → ∴ There is ↓ sympathetic tone, hence ↓ BP
- ∵ They block both sympathetic and parasympathetic ganglia → Frequent side effects are seen → Hence they are not preferred nowadays
- Rapid and short acting → Hence used for controlled hypotension during certain operative procedures

3. Adrenergic neuron blockers

Guanethidine
- Depletes noradrenaline stores from adrenergic neuron
- Frequent side effects → Orthostatic hypotension, diarrhea, sexual dysfunction
- Hence not preferred now

Reserpine
- Alkaloid derived from plant *Rauwolfia serpentina* → Indian name: Sarpagandha
- Destroys vesicles containing monoamines in adrenergic nerve endings → Adrenaline, dopamine, noradrenaline, serotonin → Hence the monoamines leak out of neurons which are subsequently metabolized by MAO (monoamine oxidase) → Thus there is depletion of monoamines in stores which leads to ↓ BP
- Depletion of dopamine can produce antipsychotic effects
- Inexpensive, and is long-acting, hence administered as OD dose
- ADR → Depression, parkinsonism, weight gain, gynecomastia, sexual dysfunction, sedation
- Due to frequent side effects Reserpine is not used now

α blockers
- Nonselective agents → Phenoxybenzamine and phentolamine used for HT due to pheochromocytoma
- Selective agents → Prazosin, doxazosin, terazosin are all arteriolar and venodilators
  - Hence ↓ TPR, thus ↓ BP → Associated with reflex tachycardia
  - First-dose phenomena is postural hypotension, which is usually seen 30–60 min after first dose → Hence start with low dose, 0.5 mg at night
- Can be combined with diuretics/β blockers

β blockers
- Blocks cardiac β1 receptors → Thereby ↓ cardiac contractility → Thus ↓ CO, and hence ↓ BP
- Also ↓ renin levels → ∵ Blockade of β1 receptors on JG cells → Hence additional antihypertensive effect
- Used in HT with angina/arrhythmias
- Used in combination with agents causing tachycardia as side effect (e.g., vasodilators)
- First-line antihypertensives
- Atenolol is most commonly used → Because of OD dosing, less CNS side effects and β selective action → Unlike nonselective propranolol
- As sudden withdrawal can lead to rebound HT → Dose should always be tapered

α + β blockers
- e.g., Labetalol and carvedilol
- Used IV for Rx of HT in pheochromocytoma and HT emergencies

14.8 CALCIUM CHANNEL BLOCKERS

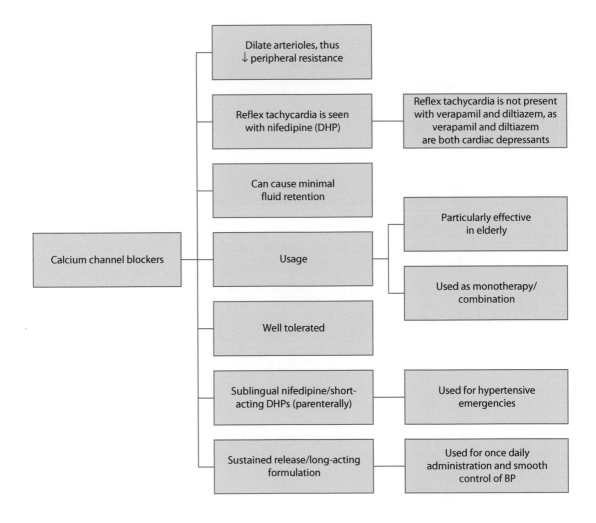

14.9 VASODILATORS

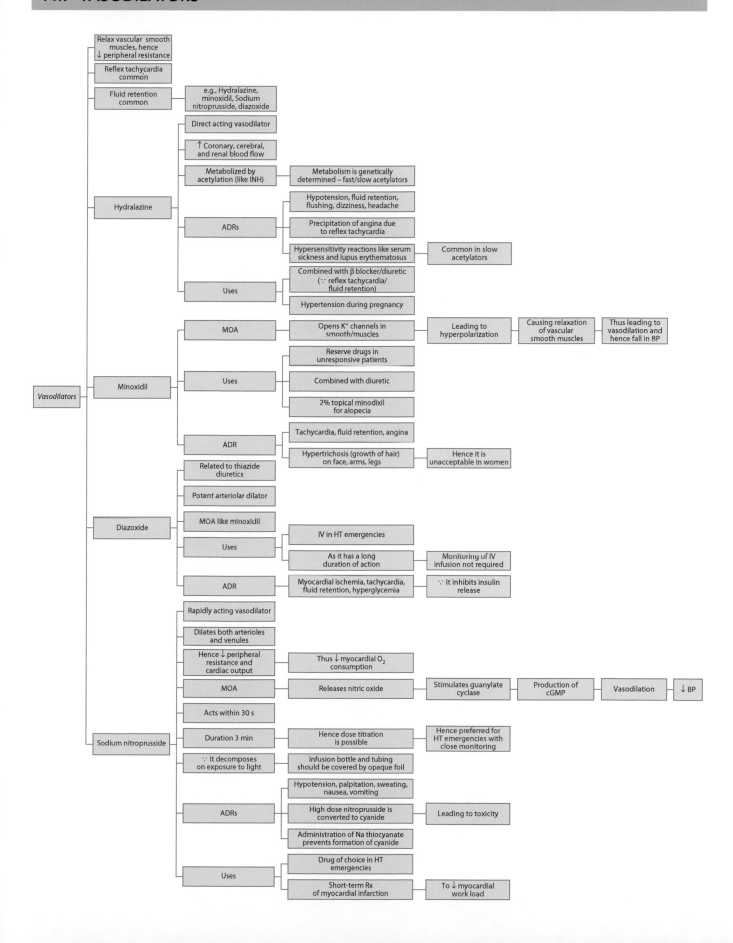

14.10 MANAGEMENT OF HT

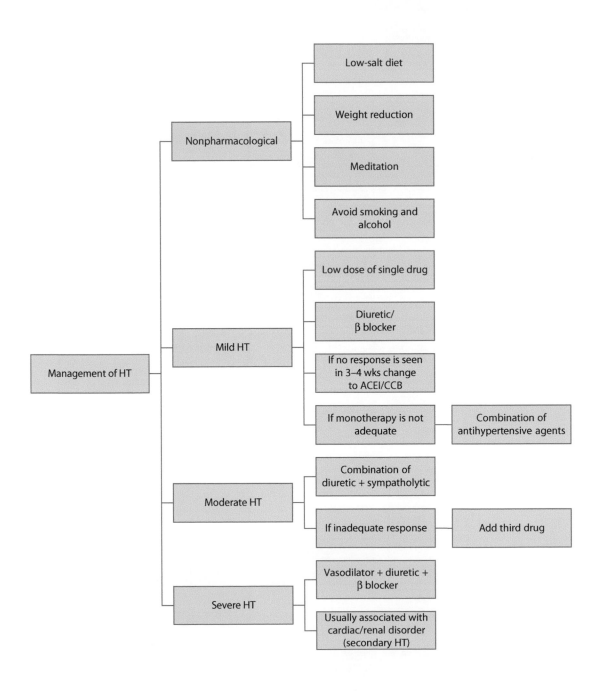

14.11 DRUG INTERACTIONS WITH ANTIHYPERTENSIVES, HYPERTENSIVE CRISIS, HT IN PREGNANCY, COMBINATION OF ANTIHYPERTENSIVES

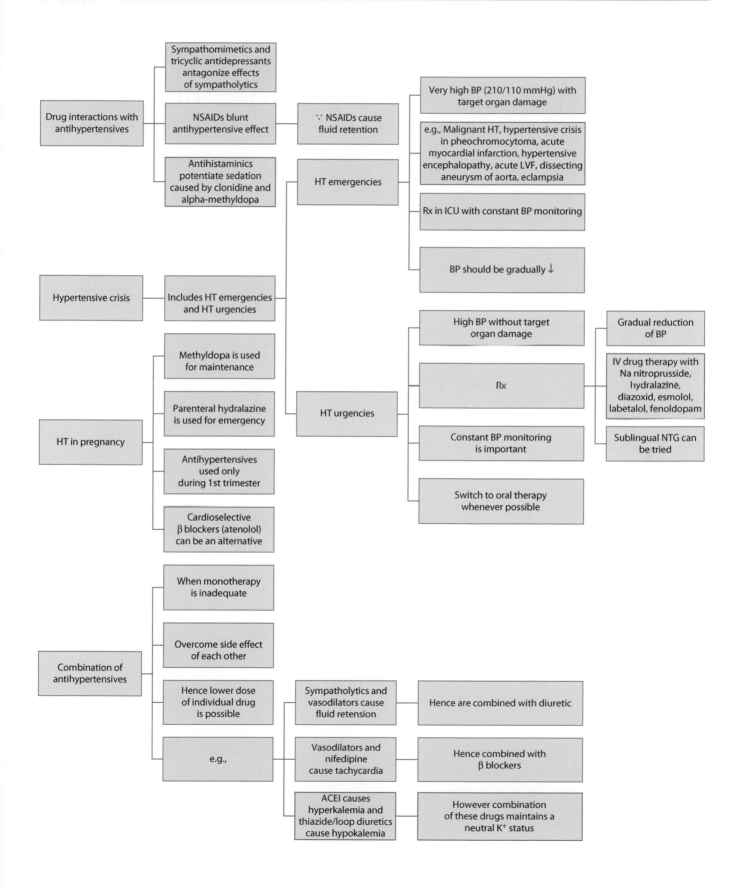

Calcium channel blockers, drug treatment of angina pectoris, and myocardial infarction

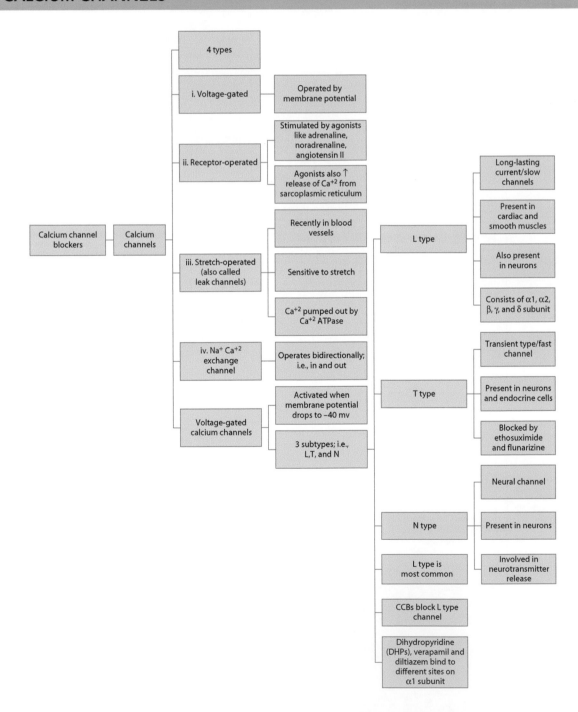

15.2 CLASSIFICATION OF CALCIUM CHANNEL BLOCKERS AND MECHANISM OF ACTION

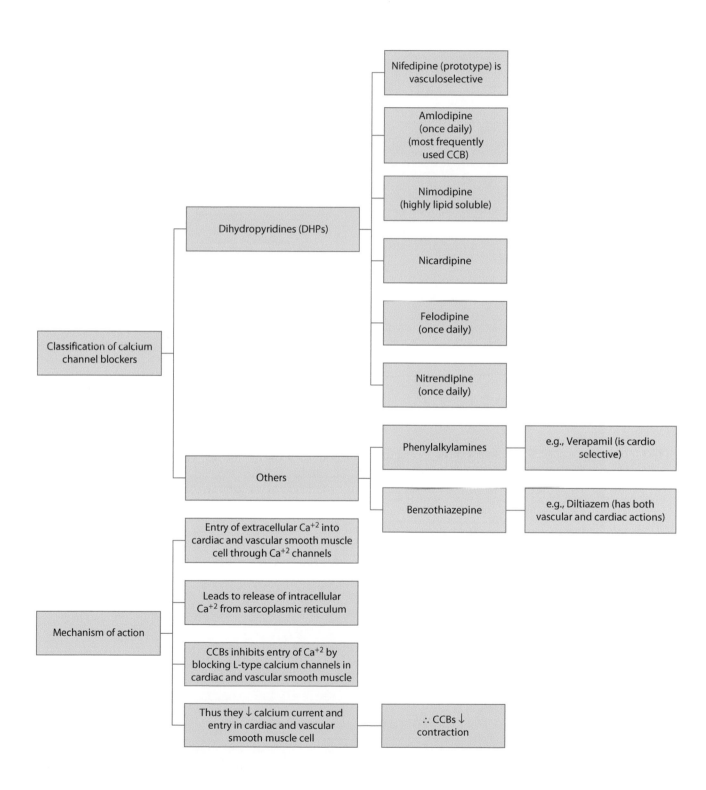

15.3 PHARMACOLOGICAL ACTIONS AND PHARMACOKINETICS

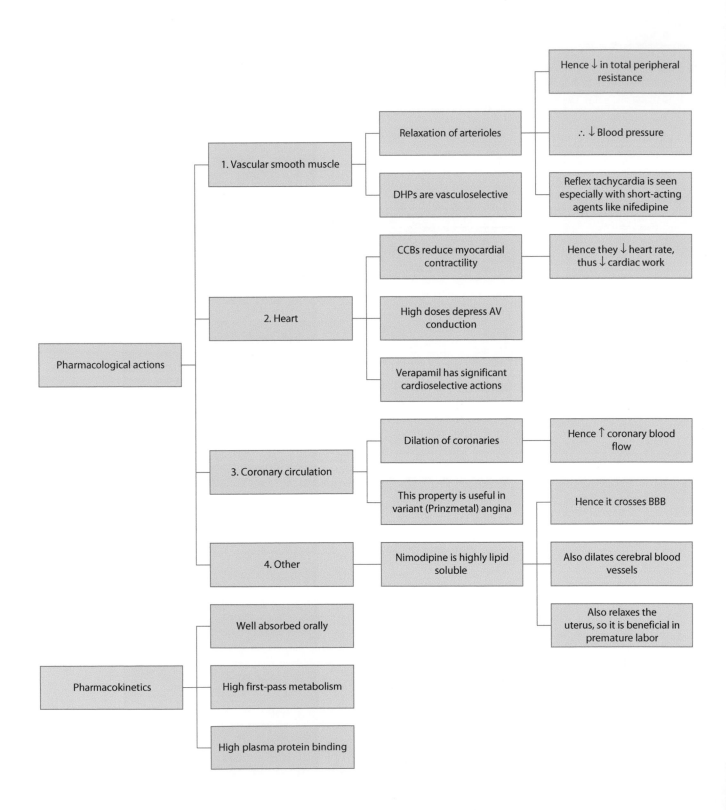

15.4 INDICATIONS

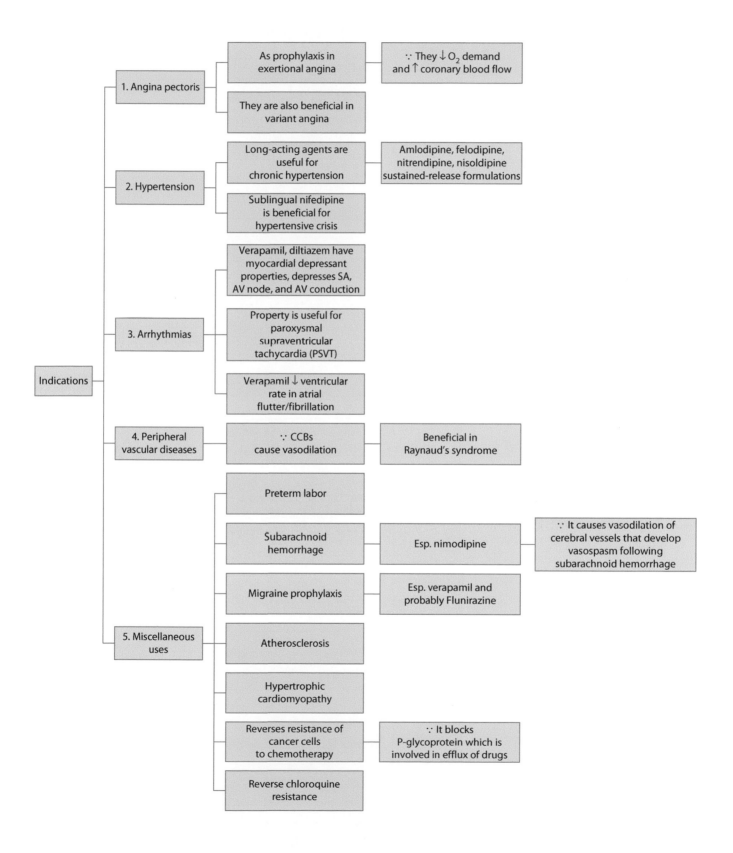

15.5 DRUG INTERACTIONS AND ADRs

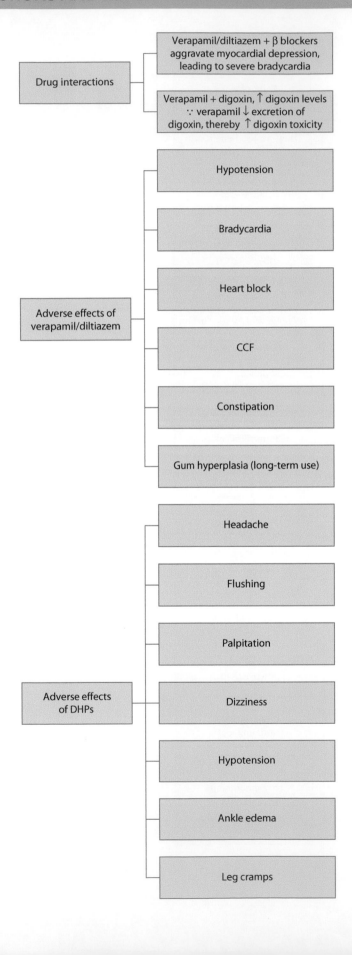

Drug interactions
- Verapamil/diltiazem + β blockers aggravate myocardial depression, leading to severe bradycardia
- Verapamil + digoxin, ↑ digoxin levels ∵ verapamil ↓ excretion of digoxin, thereby ↑ digoxin toxicity

Adverse effects of verapamil/diltiazem
- Hypotension
- Bradycardia
- Heart block
- CCF
- Constipation
- Gum hyperplasia (long-term use)

Adverse effects of DHPs
- Headache
- Flushing
- Palpitation
- Dizziness
- Hypotension
- Ankle edema
- Leg cramps

15.6 ANGINA PECTORIS

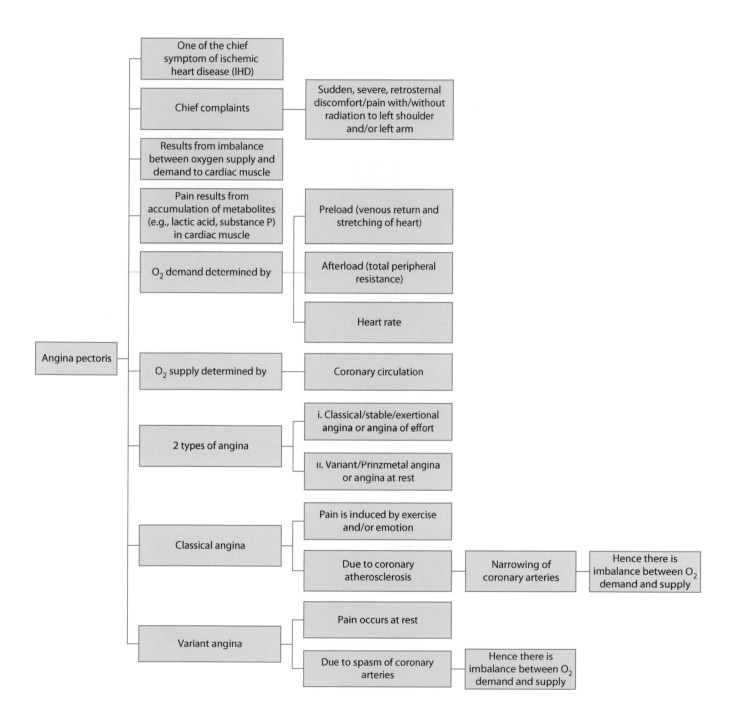

15.7 ANTIANGINALS – CLASSIFICATION

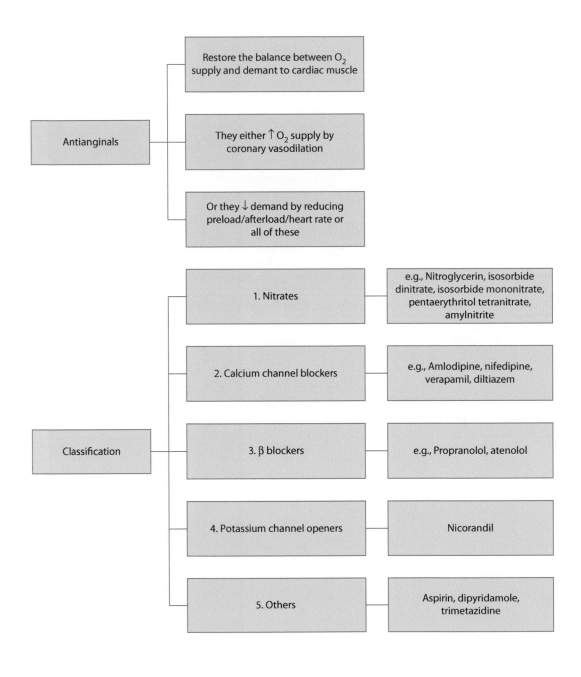

15.8 NITRATES – PHARMACOLOGICAL ACTIONS

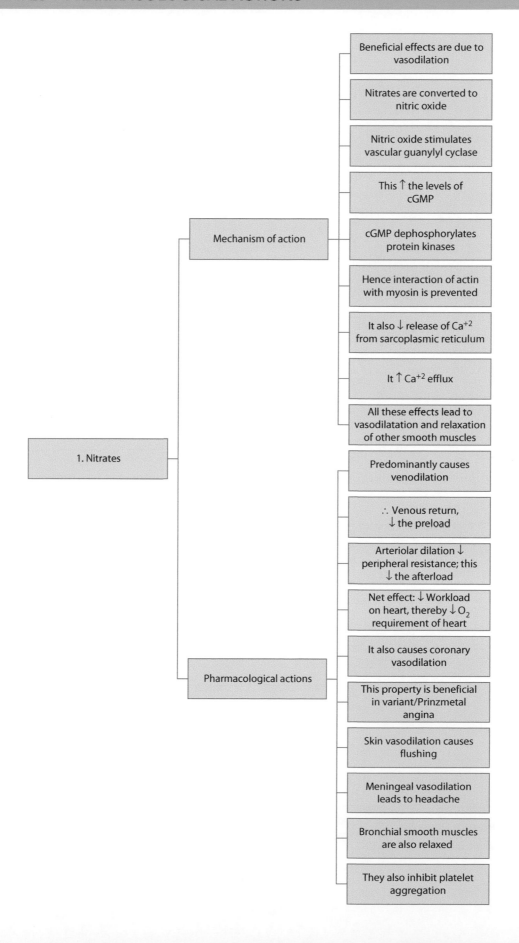

1. Nitrates

Mechanism of action
- Beneficial effects are due to vasodilation
- Nitrates are converted to nitric oxide
- Nitric oxide stimulates vascular guanylyl cyclase
- This ↑ the levels of cGMP
- cGMP dephosphorylates protein kinases
- Hence interaction of actin with myosin is prevented
- It also ↓ release of Ca^{+2} from sarcoplasmic reticulum
- It ↑ Ca^{+2} efflux
- All these effects lead to vasodilatation and relaxation of other smooth muscles

Pharmacological actions
- Predominantly causes venodilation
- ∴ Venous return, ↓ the preload
- Arteriolar dilation ↓ peripheral resistance; this ↓ the afterload
- Net effect: ↓ Workload on heart, thereby ↓ O_2 requirement of heart
- It also causes coronary vasodilation
- This property is beneficial in variant/Prinzmetal angina
- Skin vasodilation causes flushing
- Meningeal vasodilation leads to headache
- Bronchial smooth muscles are also relaxed
- They also inhibit platelet aggregation

15.9 PHARMACOKINETICS, ADRs, AND DRUG INTERACTIONS OF NITRATES

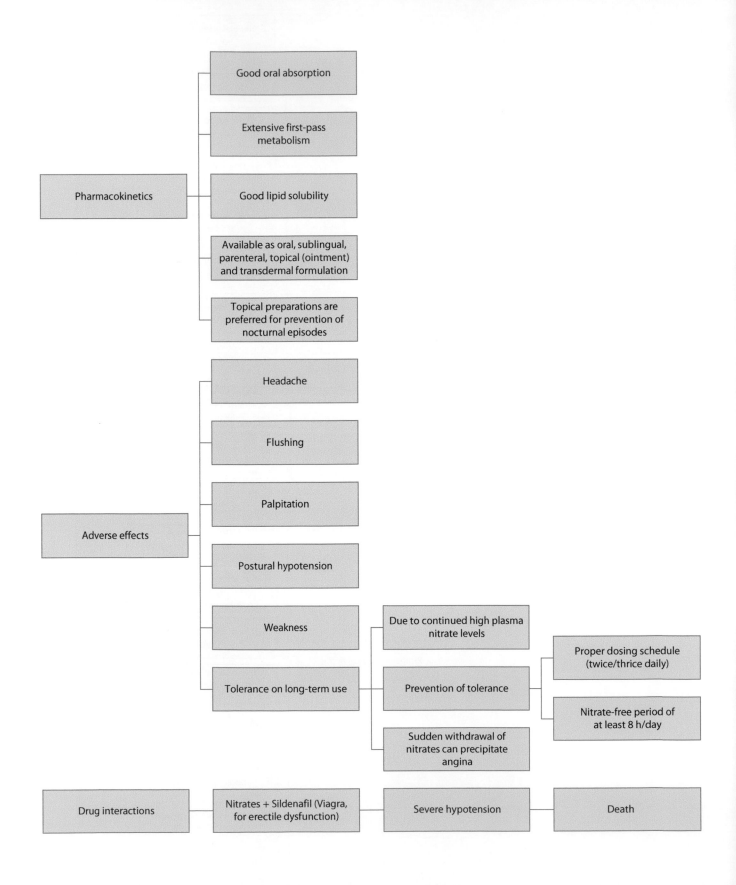

Pharmacokinetics
- Good oral absorption
- Extensive first-pass metabolism
- Good lipid solubility
- Available as oral, sublingual, parenteral, topical (ointment) and transdermal formulation
- Topical preparations are preferred for prevention of nocturnal episodes

Adverse effects
- Headache
- Flushing
- Palpitation
- Postural hypotension
- Weakness
- Tolerance on long-term use
  - Due to continued high plasma nitrate levels
  - Prevention of tolerance
    - Proper dosing schedule (twice/thrice daily)
    - Nitrate-free period of at least 8 h/day
  - Sudden withdrawal of nitrates can precipitate angina

Drug interactions — Nitrates + Sildenafil (Viagra, for erectile dysfunction) — Severe hypotension — Death

15.10 USES OF NITRATES

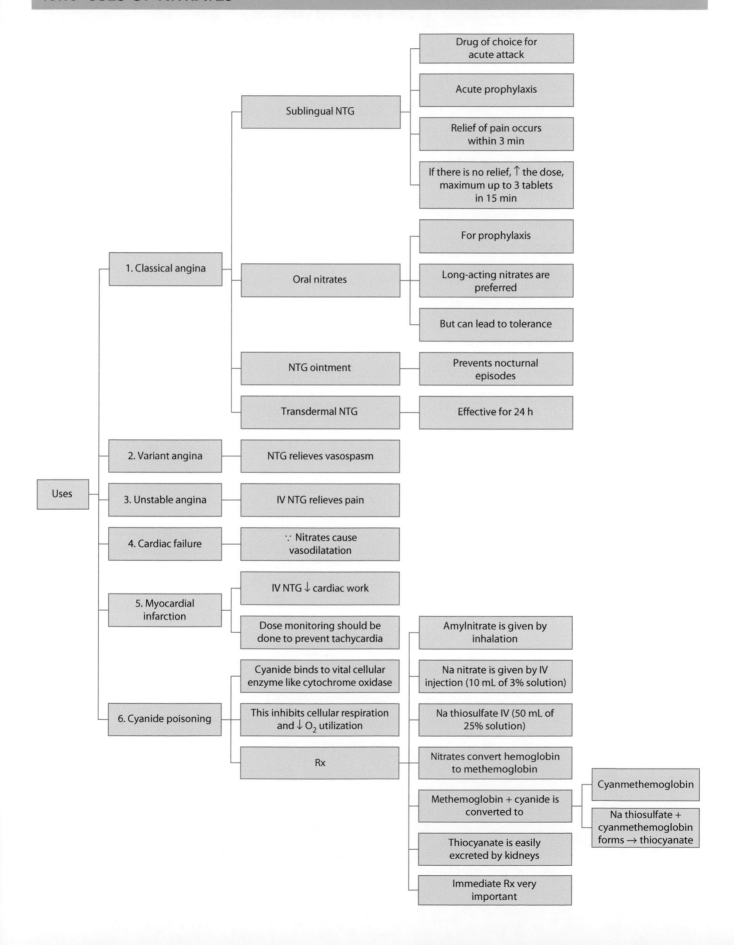

15.11 CALCIUM CHANNEL BLOCKERS (CCBs), BETA BLOCKERS (BBs), POTASSIUM CHANNEL OPENERS, AND OTHERS AS ANTIANGINALS

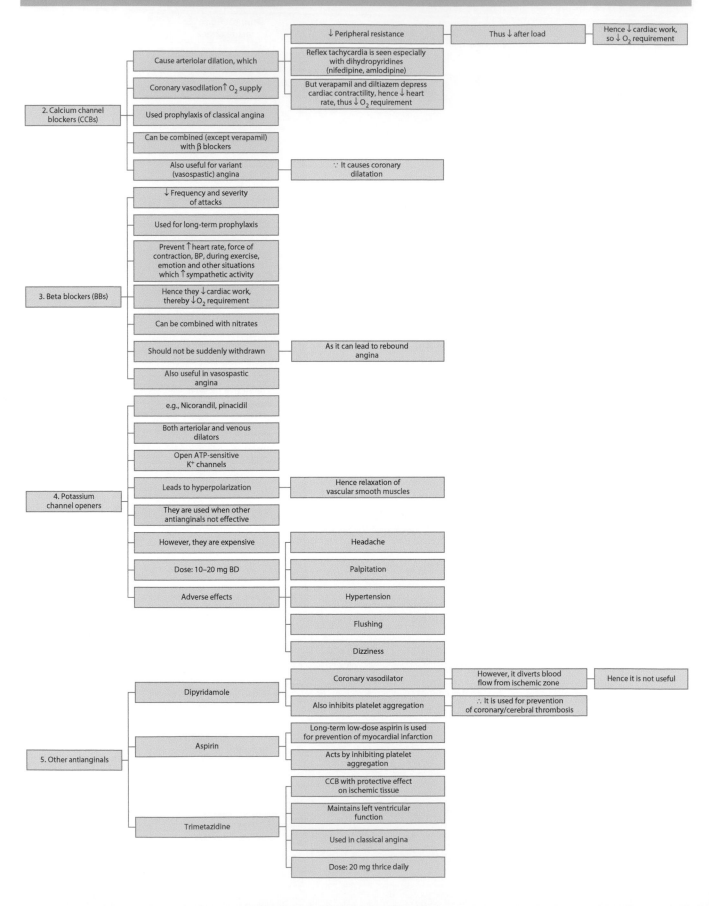

2. Calcium channel blockers (CCBs)

- Cause arteriolar dilation, which
  - ↓ Peripheral resistance → Thus ↓ after load → Hence ↓ cardiac work, so ↓ O_2 requirement
  - Reflex tachycardia is seen especially with dihydropyridines (nifedipine, amlodipine)
- Coronary vasodilation ↑ O_2 supply
  - But verapamil and diltiazem depress cardiac contractility, hence ↓ heart rate, thus ↓ O_2 requirement
- Used prophylaxis of classical angina
- Can be combined (except verapamil) with β blockers
- Also useful for variant (vasospastic) angina
  - ∵ It causes coronary dilatation

3. Beta blockers (BBs)

- ↓ Frequency and severity of attacks
- Used for long-term prophylaxis
- Prevent ↑ heart rate, force of contraction, BP, during exercise, emotion and other situations which ↑ sympathetic activity
- Hence they ↓ cardiac work, thereby ↓ O_2 requirement
- Can be combined with nitrates
- Should not be suddenly withdrawn
  - As it can lead to rebound angina
- Also useful in vasospastic angina

4. Potassium channel openers

- e.g., Nicorandil, pinacidil
- Both arteriolar and venous dilators
- Open ATP-sensitive K^+ channels
- Leads to hyperpolarization
  - Hence relaxation of vascular smooth muscles
- They are used when other antianginals not effective
- However, they are expensive
- Dose: 10–20 mg BD
- Adverse effects
  - Headache
  - Palpitation
  - Hypertension
  - Flushing
  - Dizziness

5. Other antianginals

- Dipyridamole
  - Coronary vasodilator → However, it diverts blood flow from ischemic zone → Hence it is not useful
  - Also inhibits platelet aggregation → ∴ It is used for prevention of coronary/cerebral thrombosis
- Aspirin
  - Long-term low-dose aspirin is used for prevention of myocardial infarction
  - Acts by inhibiting platelet aggregation
- Trimetazidine
  - CCB with protective effect on ischemic tissue
  - Maintains left ventricular function
  - Used in classical angina
  - Dose: 20 mg thrice daily

15.12 PHARMACOTHERAPY OF ANGINA

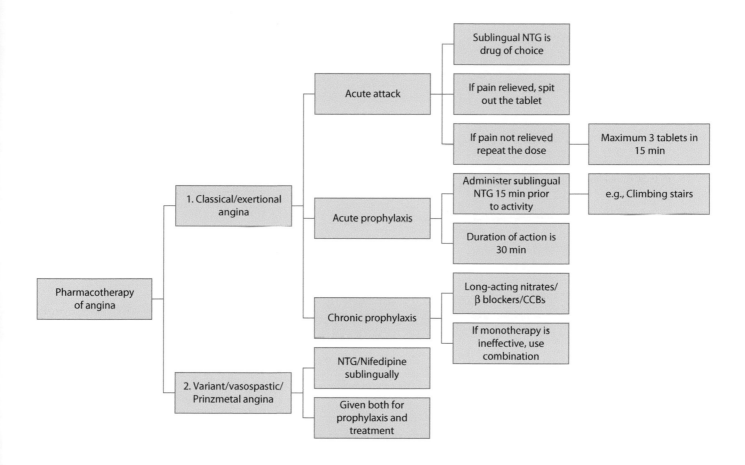

15.13 COMBINATION OF ANTIANGINALS

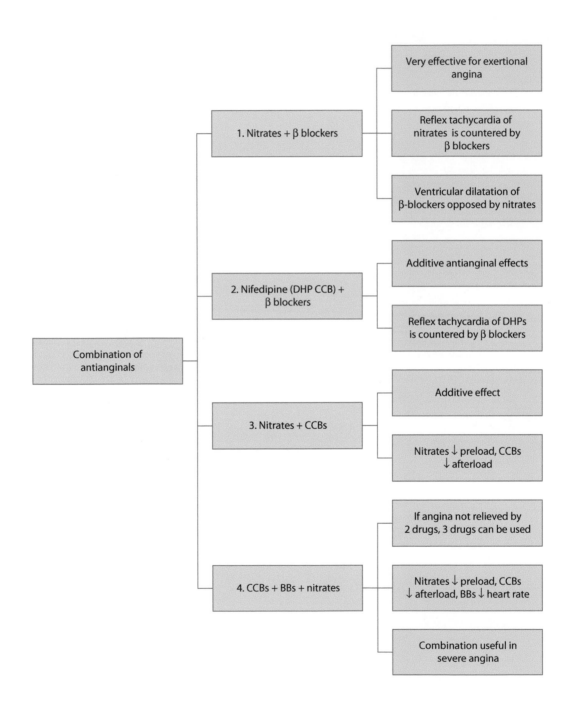

Combination of antianginals

1. Nitrates + β blockers
- Very effective for exertional angina
- Reflex tachycardia of nitrates is countered by β blockers
- Ventricular dilatation of β-blockers opposed by nitrates

2. Nifedipine (DHP CCB) + β blockers
- Additive antianginal effects
- Reflex tachycardia of DHPs is countered by β blockers

3. Nitrates + CCBs
- Additive effect
- Nitrates ↓ preload, CCBs ↓ afterload

4. CCBs + BBs + nitrates
- If angina not relieved by 2 drugs, 3 drugs can be used
- Nitrates ↓ preload, CCBs ↓ afterload, BBs ↓ heart rate
- Combination useful in severe angina

15.14 UNSTABLE ANGINA AND TREATMENT

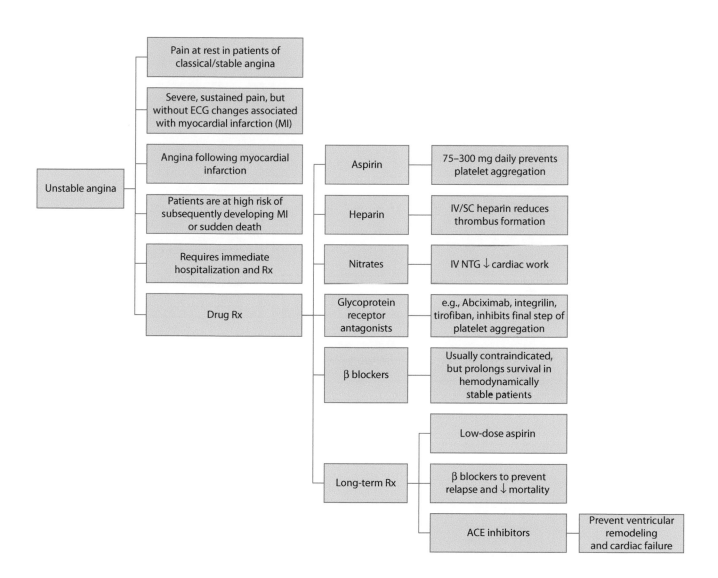

15.15 TREATMENT OF MYOCARDIAL INFARCTION

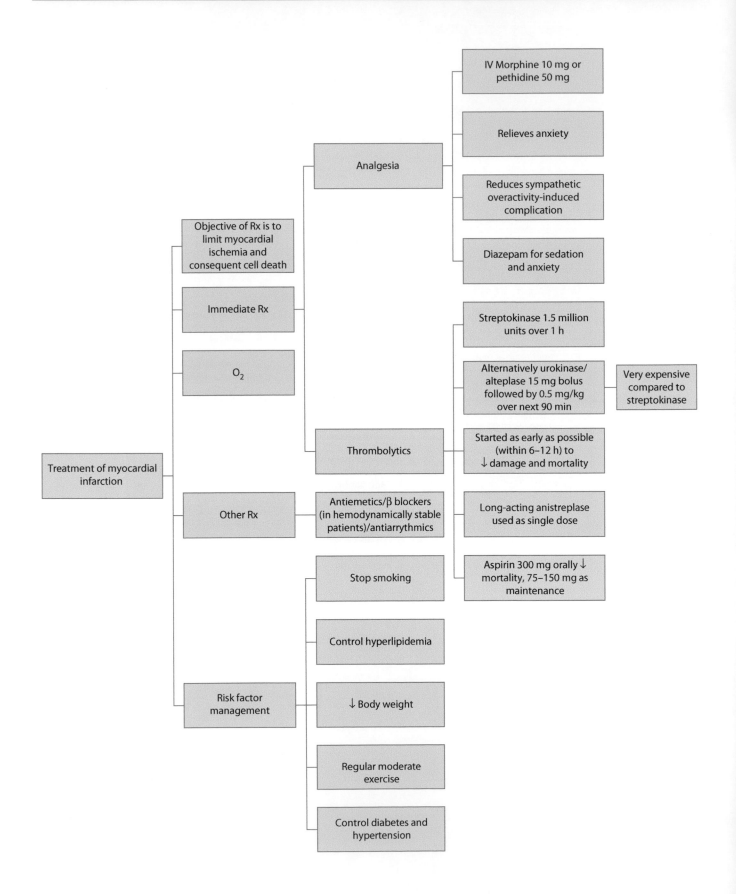

16

Cardiac glycosides and treatment of cardiac failure

16.1 INTRODUCTION

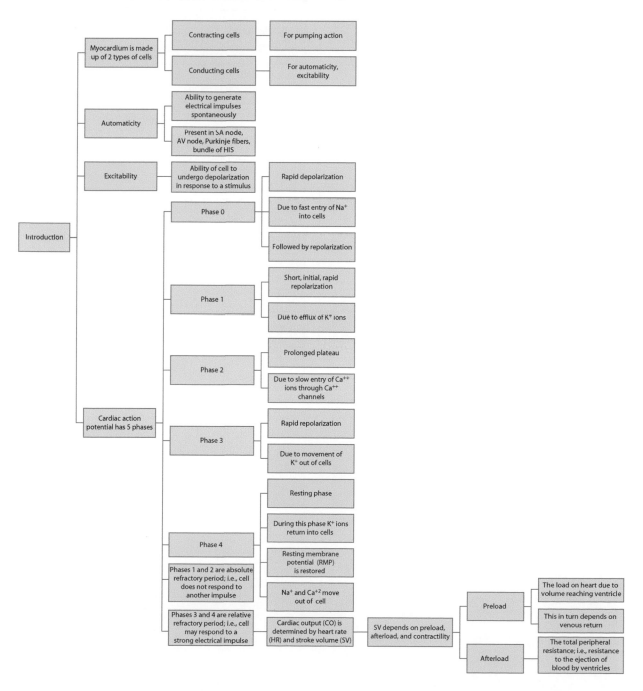

16.2 CONGESTIVE CARDIAC FAILURE (CCF)

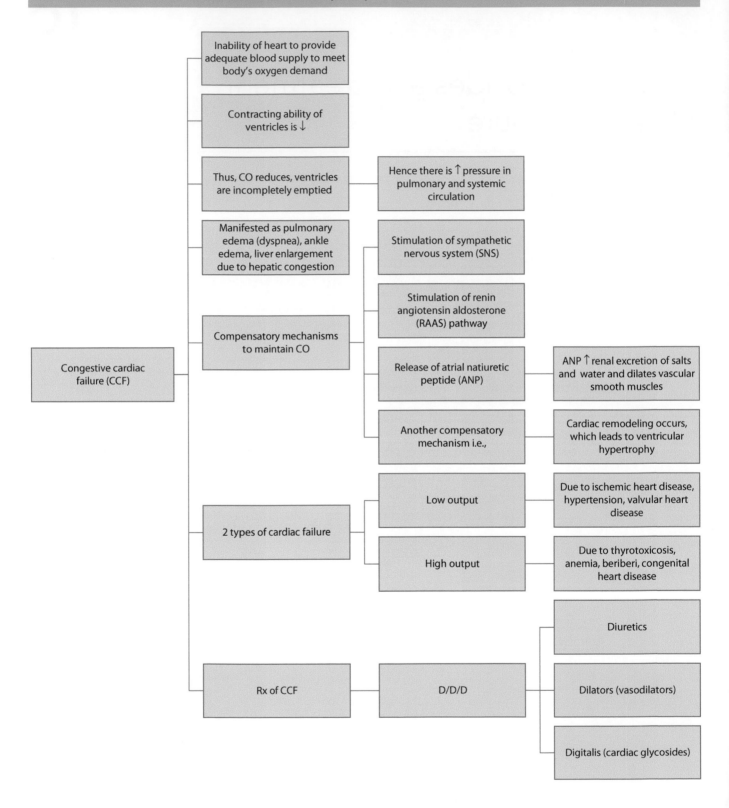

Inability of heart to provide adequate blood supply to meet body's oxygen demand

Contracting ability of ventricles is ↓

Thus, CO reduces, ventricles are incompletely emptied → Hence there is ↑ pressure in pulmonary and systemic circulation

Manifested as pulmonary edema (dyspnea), ankle edema, liver enlargement due to hepatic congestion

Congestive cardiac failure (CCF)

Compensatory mechanisms to maintain CO
- Stimulation of sympathetic nervous system (SNS)
- Stimulation of renin angiotensin aldosterone (RAAS) pathway
- Release of atrial natriuretic peptide (ANP) → ANP ↑ renal excretion of salts and water and dilates vascular smooth muscles
- Another compensatory mechanism i.e., → Cardiac remodeling occurs, which leads to ventricular hypertrophy

2 types of cardiac failure
- Low output → Due to ischemic heart disease, hypertension, valvular heart disease
- High output → Due to thyrotoxicosis, anemia, beriberi, congenital heart disease

Rx of CCF → D/D/D
- Diuretics
- Dilators (vasodilators)
- Digitalis (cardiac glycosides)

16.3 CARDIAC GLYCOSIDES

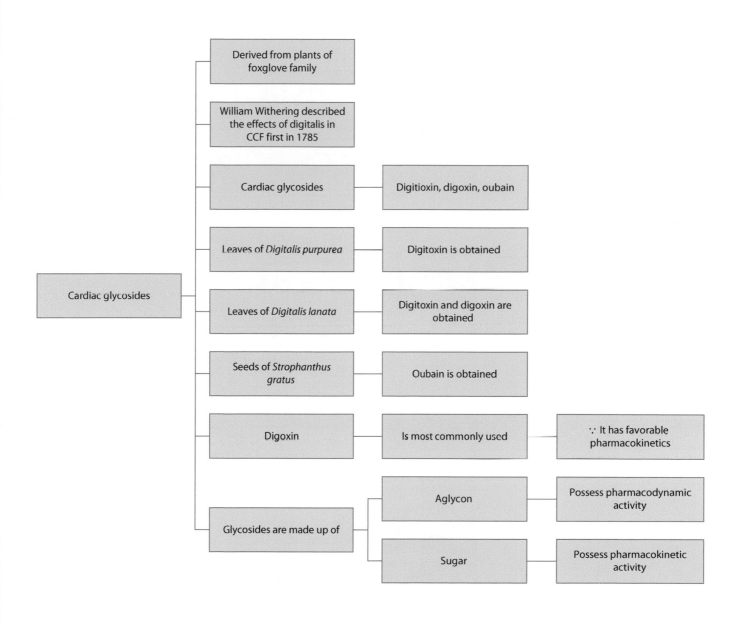

16.4 PHARMACOLOGICAL ACTIONS

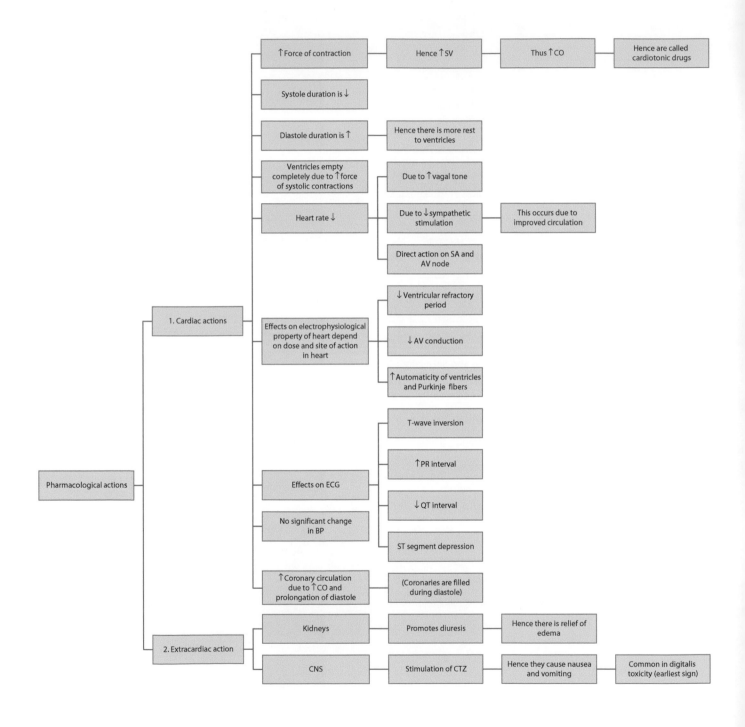

16.5 MECHANISM OF ACTION, PHARMACOKINETICS, DIGITALIZATION

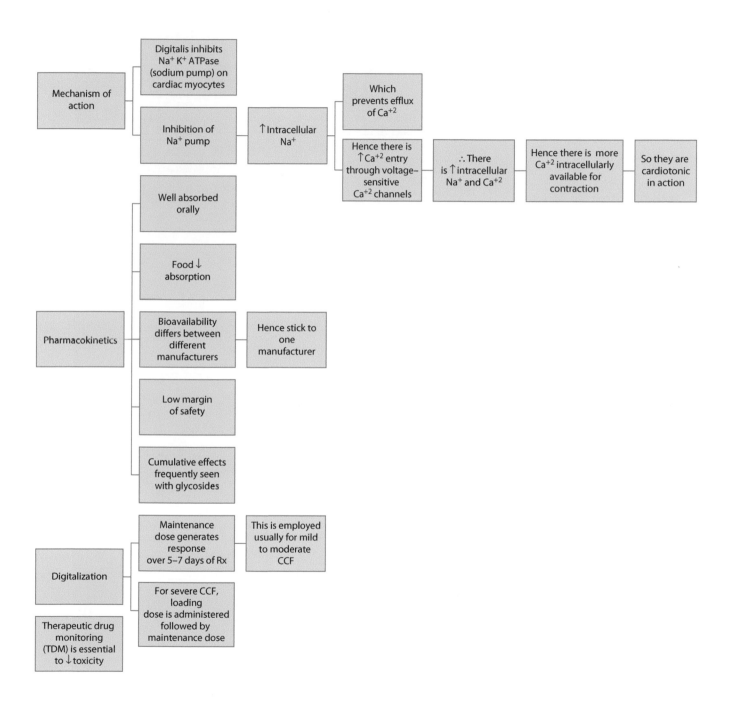

Mechanism of action

Digitalis inhibits Na⁺ K⁺ ATPase (sodium pump) on cardiac myocytes

Inhibition of Na⁺ pump → ↑Intracellular Na⁺

Which prevents efflux of Ca^{+2}

Hence there is ↑Ca^{+2} entry through voltage–sensitive Ca^{+2} channels

∴ There is ↑intracellular Na⁺ and Ca^{+2}

Hence there is more Ca^{+2} intracellularly available for contraction

So they are cardiotonic in action

Pharmacokinetics

Well absorbed orally

Food ↓ absorption

Bioavailability differs between different manufacturers → Hence stick to one manufacturer

Low margin of safety

Cumulative effects frequently seen with glycosides

Digitalization

Maintenance dose generates response over 5–7 days of Rx → This is employed usually for mild to moderate CCF

For severe CCF, loading dose is administered followed by maintenance dose

Therapeutic drug monitoring (TDM) is essential to ↓ toxicity

16.6 ADVERSE EFFECTS

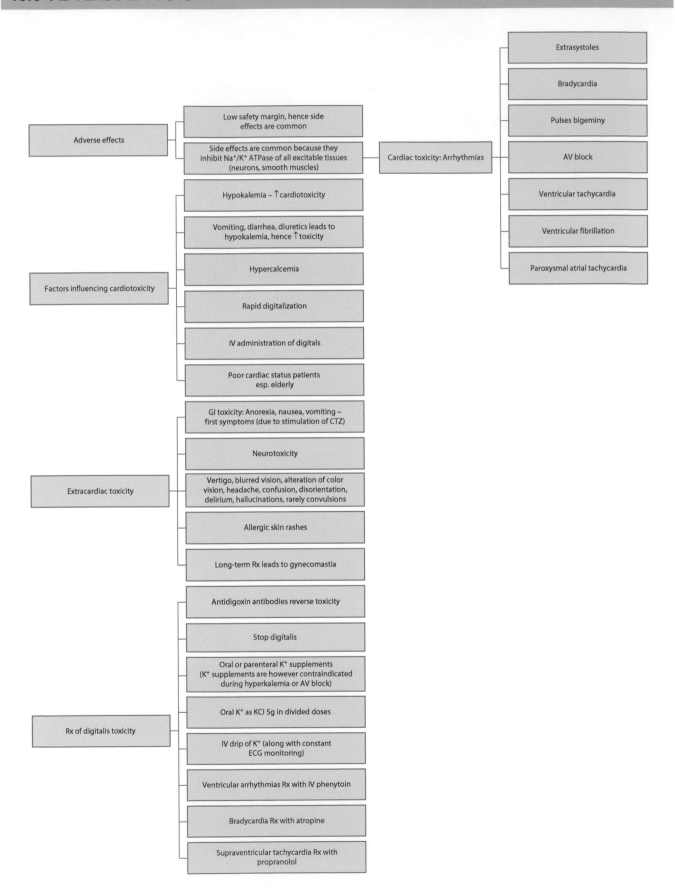

Adverse effects
- Low safety margin, hence side effects are common
- Side effects are common because they inhibit Na^+/K^+ ATPase of all excitable tissues (neurons, smooth muscles)
  - Cardiac toxicity: Arrhythmias
    - Extrasystoles
    - Bradycardia
    - Pulses bigeminy
    - AV block
    - Ventricular tachycardia
    - Ventricular fibrillation
    - Paroxysmal atrial tachycardia

Factors influencing cardiotoxicity
- Hypokalemia – ↑ cardiotoxicity
- Vomiting, diarrhea, diuretics leads to hypokalemia, hence ↑ toxicity
- Hypercalcemia
- Rapid digitalization
- IV administration of digitals
- Poor cardiac status patients esp. elderly

Extracardiac toxicity
- GI toxicity: Anorexia, nausea, vomiting – first symptoms (due to stimulation of CTZ)
- Neurotoxicity
- Vertigo, blurred vision, alteration of color vision, headache, confusion, disorientation, delirium, hallucinations, rarely convulsions
- Allergic skin rashes
- Long-term Rx leads to gynecomastia

Rx of digitalis toxicity
- Antidigoxin antibodies reverse toxicity
- Stop digitalis
- Oral or parenteral K^+ supplements (K^+ supplements are however contraindicated during hyperkalemia or AV block)
- Oral K^+ as KCl 5g in divided doses
- IV drip of K^+ (along with constant ECG monitoring)
- Ventricular arrhythmias Rx with IV phenytoin
- Bradycardia Rx with atropine
- Supraventricular tachycardia Rx with propranolol

16.7 DRUG INTERACTIONS, USES, PRECAUTIONS, AND CONTRAINDICATIONS

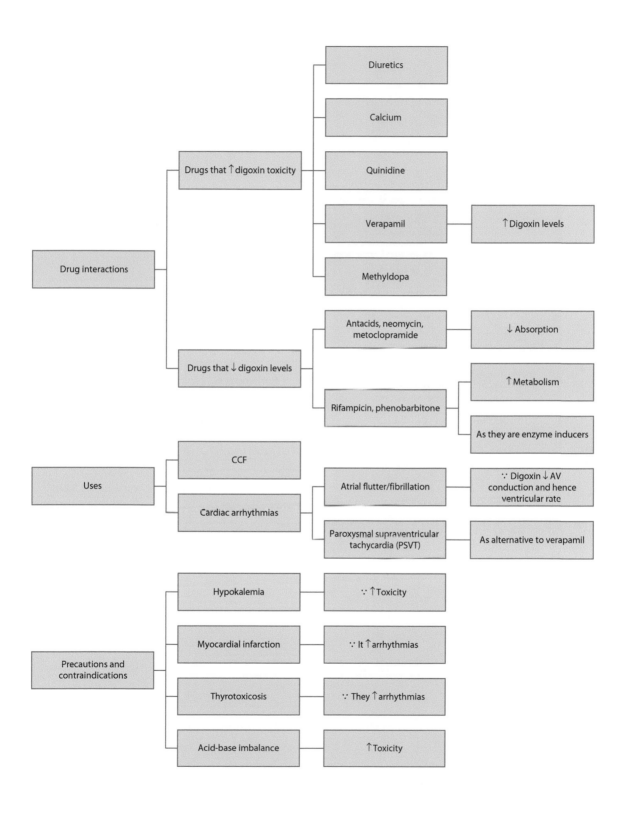

16.8 DRUGS FOR CCF, DIURETICS

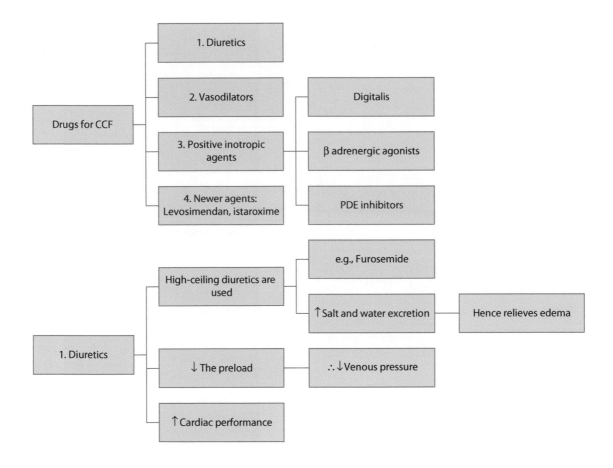

16.9 VASODILATORS

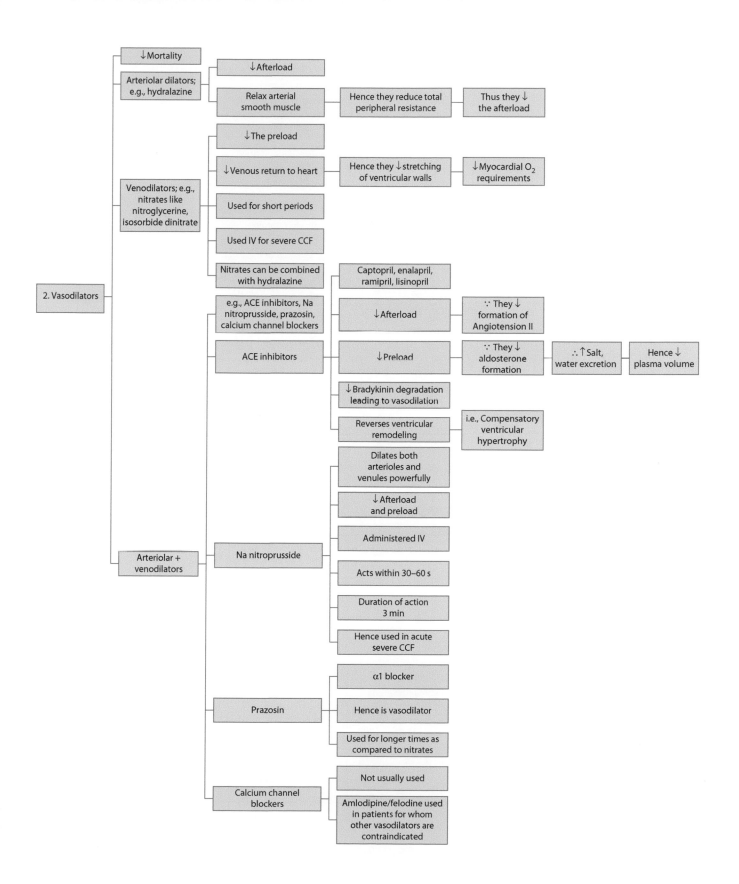

16.10 POSITIVE INOTROPIC AGENTS

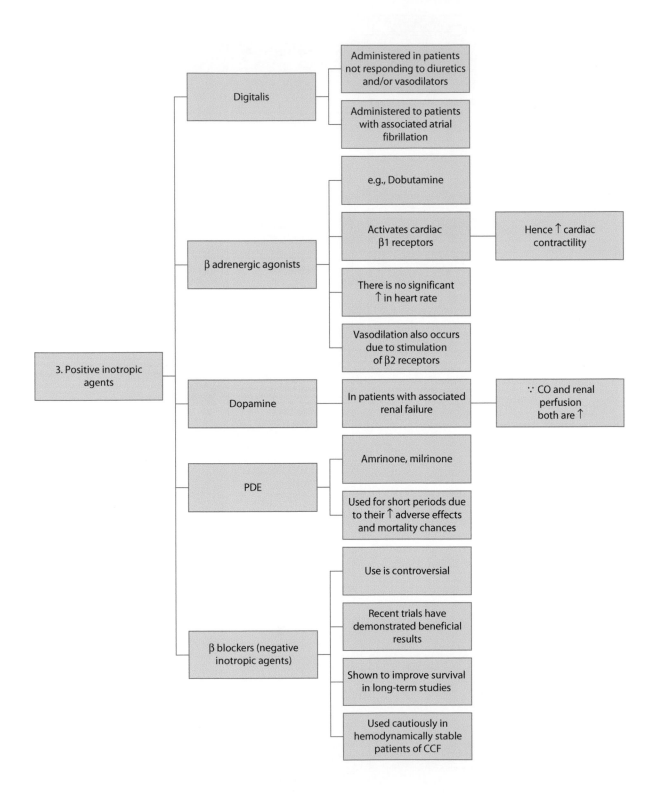

Digitalis
- Administered in patients not responding to diuretics and/or vasodilators
- Administered to patients with associated atrial fibrillation

β adrenergic agonists
- e.g., Dobutamine
- Activates cardiac β1 receptors — Hence ↑ cardiac contractility
- There is no significant ↑ in heart rate
- Vasodilation also occurs due to stimulation of β2 receptors

Dopamine
- In patients with associated renal failure — ∴ CO and renal perfusion both are ↑

PDE
- Amrinone, milrinone
- Used for short periods due to their ↑ adverse effects and mortality chances

β blockers (negative inotropic agents)
- Use is controversial
- Recent trials have demonstrated beneficial results
- Shown to improve survival in long-term studies
- Used cautiously in hemodynamically stable patients of CCF

3. Positive inotropic agents

Antiarrhythmics

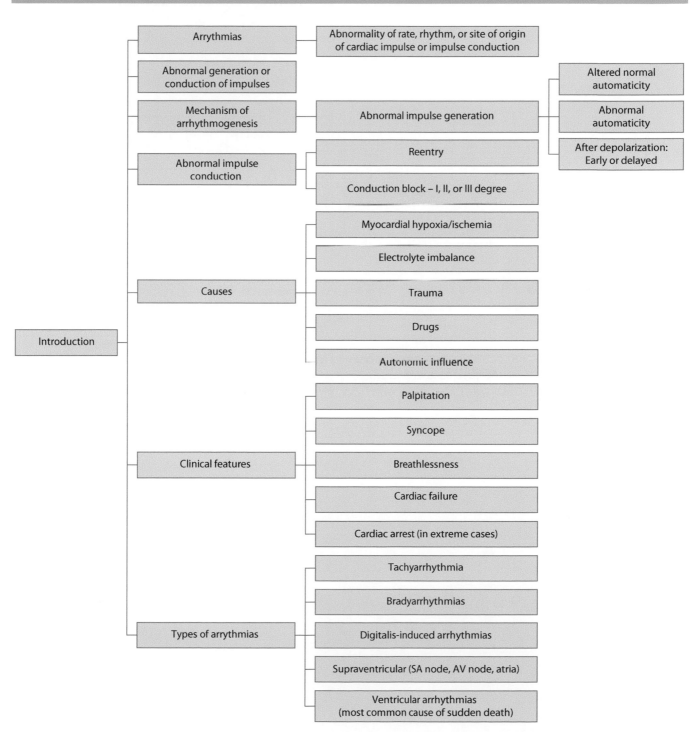

17.2 CLASSIFICATION OF ANTIARRYTHMICS

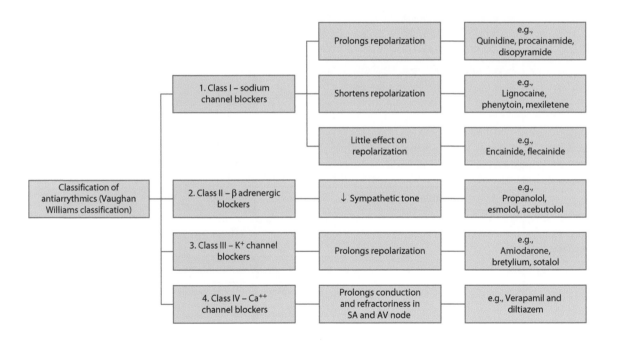

17.3 SODIUM CHANNEL BLOCKERS (CLASS IA) AND QUINIDINE

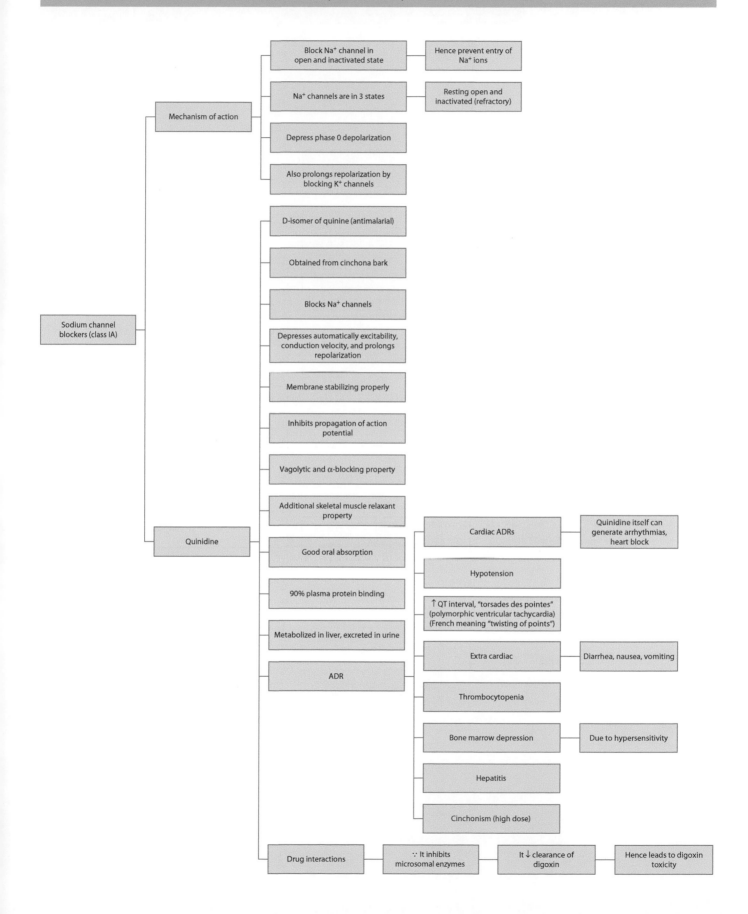

17.4 SODIUM CHANNEL BLOCKERS (CLASS IA) AND PROCAINAMIDE, DISOPYRAMIDE, AND USES OF CLASS 1A DRUGS

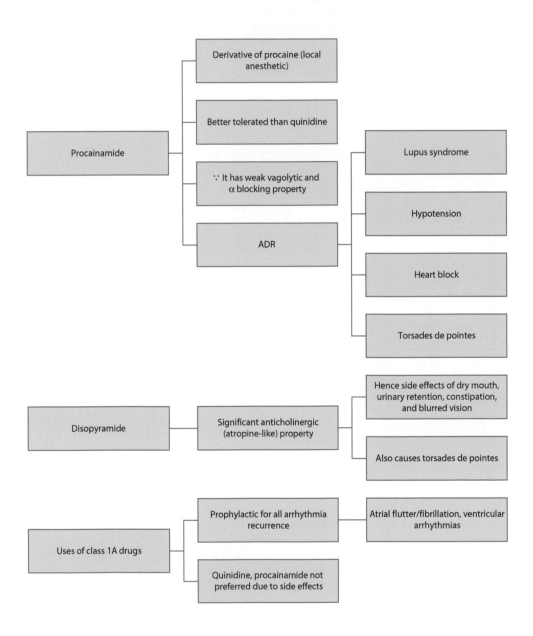

17.5 CLASS IB DRUGS – LIGNOCAINE, PHENYTOIN, AND MEXILETINE

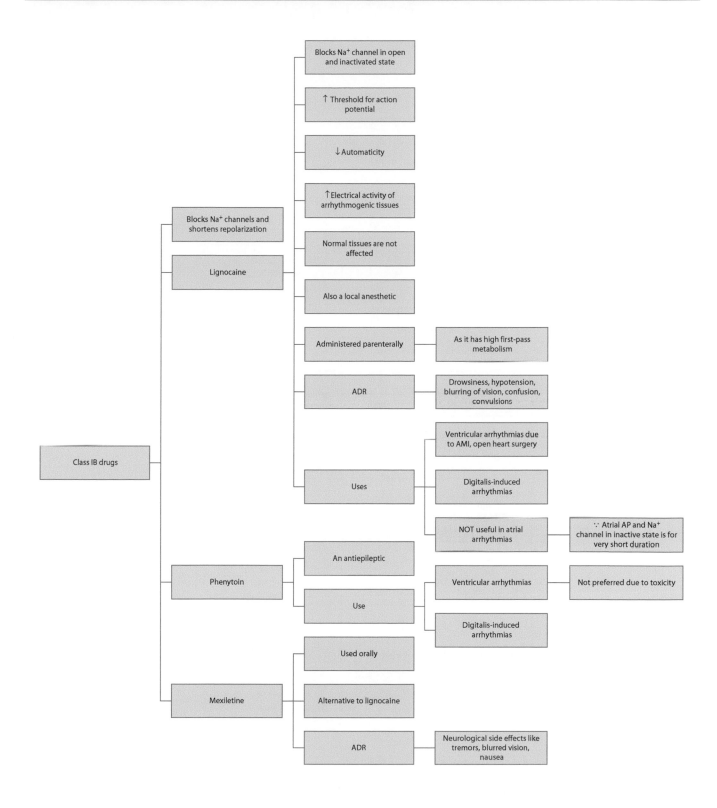

17.6 CLASS IC DRUGS AND CLASS II DRUGS

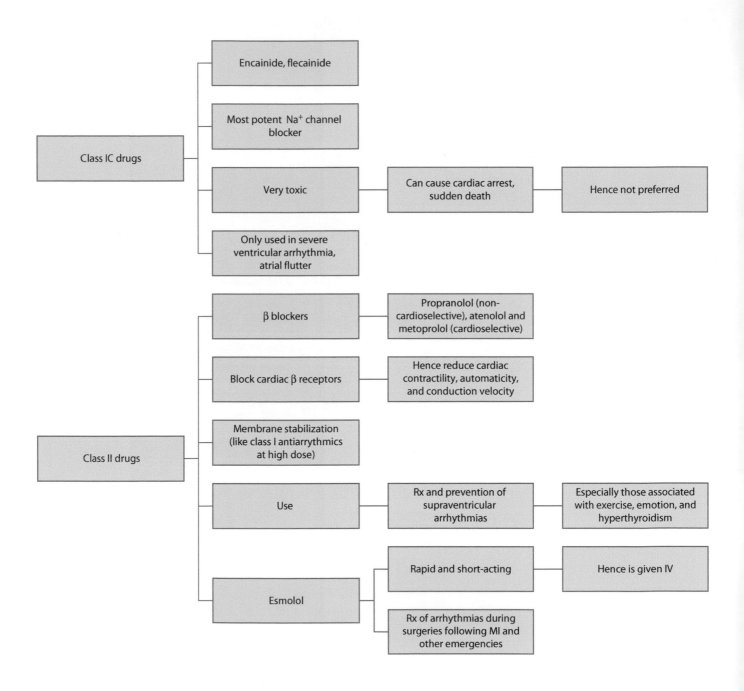

17.7 CLASS III DRUGS AND AMIODARONE

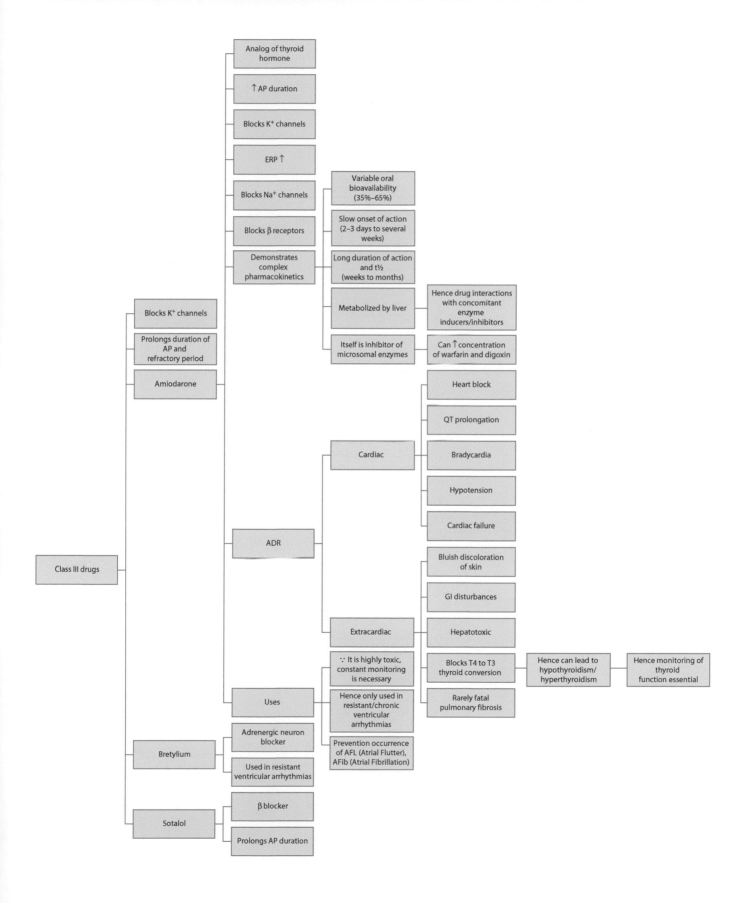

17.8 CLASS IV DRUGS AND MISCELLANEOUS AGENTS

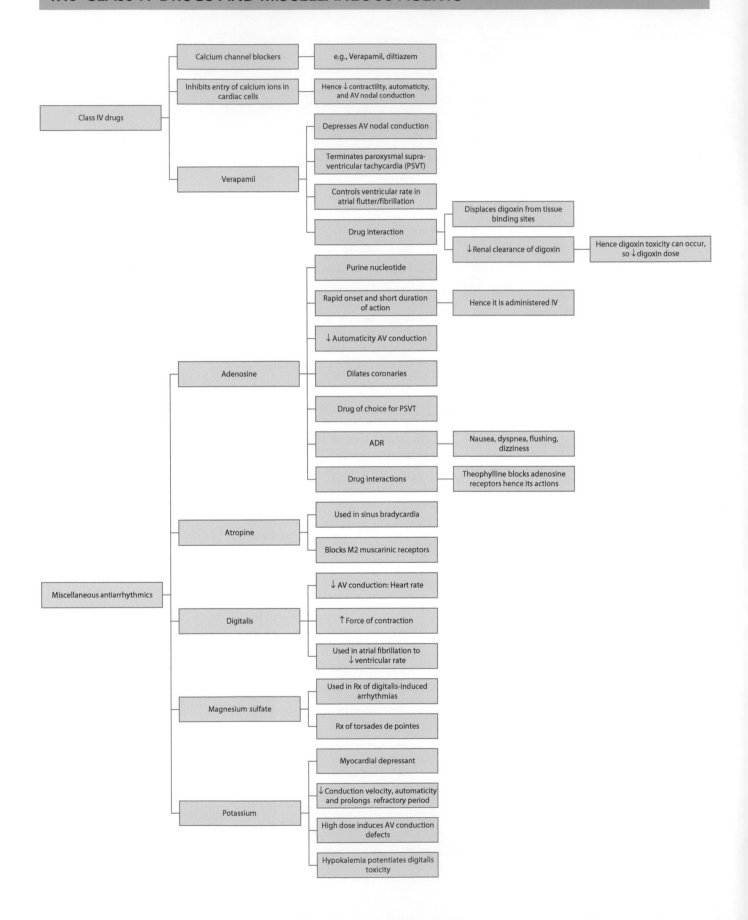

18

Diuretics and antidiuretics

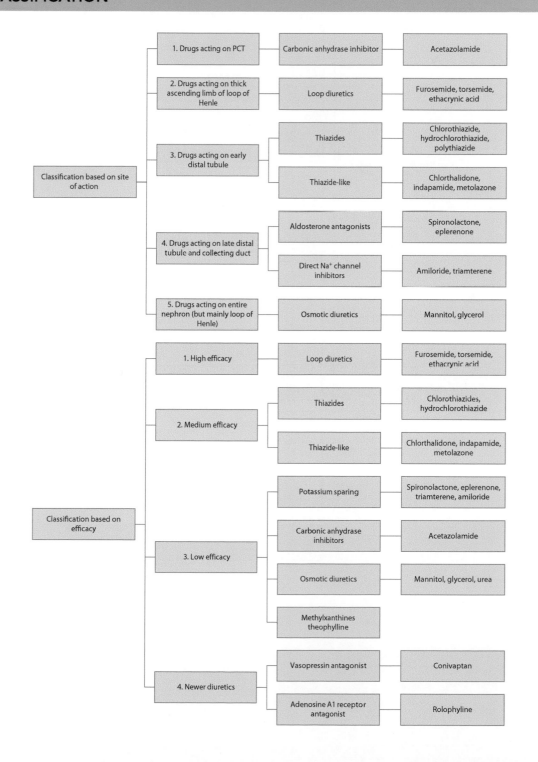

18.2 HIGH-EFFICACY/HIGH-CEILING/LOOP DIURETICS

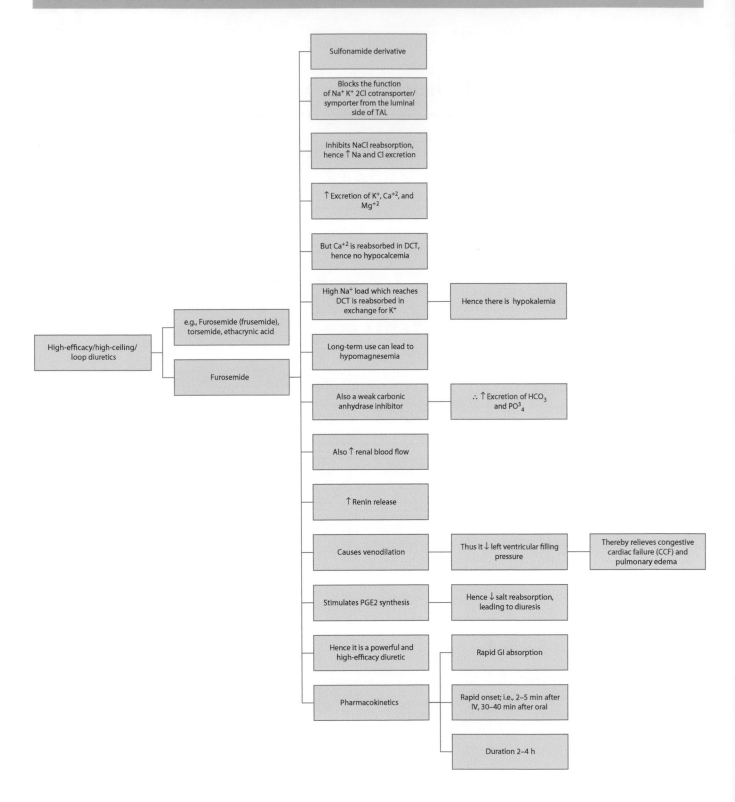

18.3 OTHER LOOP DIURETICS AND USES

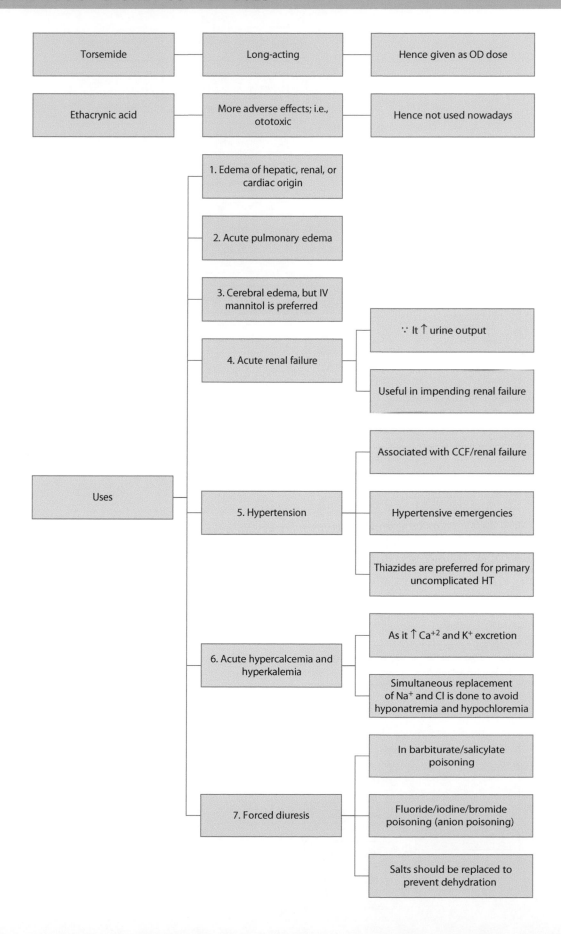

| Torsemide | Long-acting | Hence given as OD dose |

| Ethacrynic acid | More adverse effects; i.e., ototoxic | Hence not used nowadays |

Uses

1. Edema of hepatic, renal, or cardiac origin

2. Acute pulmonary edema

3. Cerebral edema, but IV mannitol is preferred

4. Acute renal failure
- ∵ It ↑ urine output
- Useful in impending renal failure

5. Hypertension
- Associated with CCF/renal failure
- Hypertensive emergencies
- Thiazides are preferred for primary uncomplicated HT

6. Acute hypercalcemia and hyperkalemia
- As it ↑ Ca^{+2} and K^+ excretion
- Simultaneous replacement of Na^+ and Cl is done to avoid hyponatremia and hypochloremia

7. Forced diuresis
- In barbiturate/salicylate poisoning
- Fluoride/iodine/bromide poisoning (anion poisoning)
- Salts should be replaced to prevent dehydration

18.4 ADRs

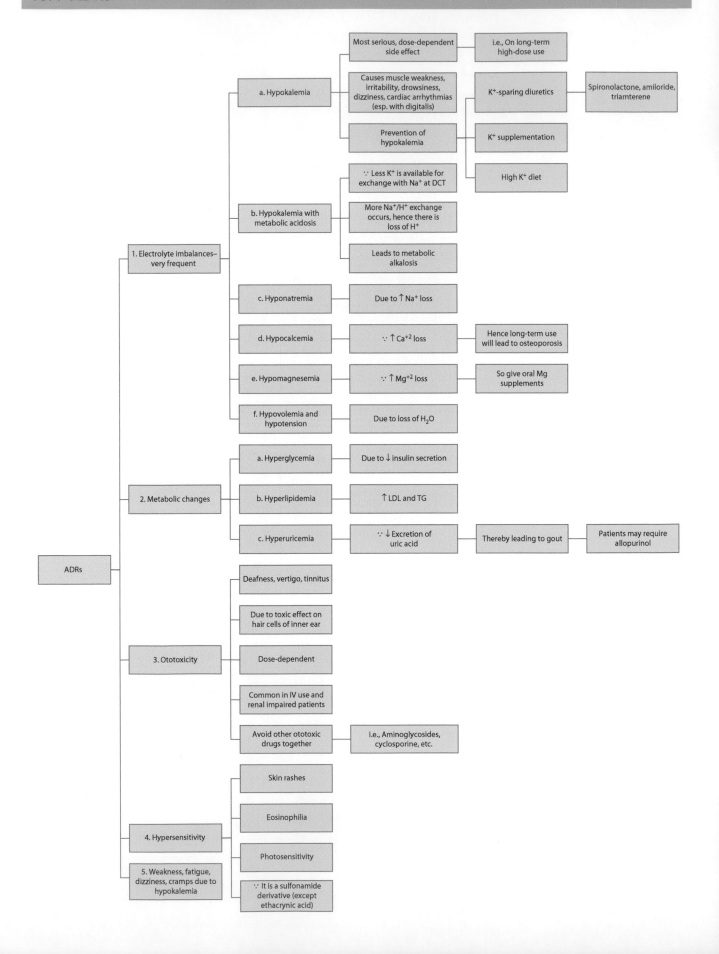

ADRs

1. Electrolyte imbalances–very frequent

a. Hypokalemia
- Most serious, dose-dependent side effect — i.e., On long-term high-dose use
- Causes muscle weakness, irritability, drowsiness, dizziness, cardiac arrhythmias (esp. with digitalis)
  - K^+-sparing diuretics — Spironolactone, amiloride, triamterene
- Prevention of hypokalemia
  - K^+ supplementation
  - High K^+ diet

b. Hypokalemia with metabolic acidosis
- ∵ Less K^+ is available for exchange with Na^+ at DCT
- More Na^+/H^+ exchange occurs, hence there is loss of H^+
- Leads to metabolic alkalosis

c. Hyponatremia
- Due to ↑ Na^+ loss

d. Hypocalcemia
- ∵ ↑ Ca^{+2} loss — Hence long-term use will lead to osteoporosis

e. Hypomagnesemia
- ∵ ↑ Mg^{+2} loss — So give oral Mg supplements

f. Hypovolemia and hypotension
- Due to loss of H_2O

2. Metabolic changes

a. Hyperglycemia
- Due to ↓ insulin secretion

b. Hyperlipidemia
- ↑ LDL and TG

c. Hyperuricemia
- ∵ ↓ Excretion of uric acid — Thereby leading to gout — Patients may require allopurinol

3. Ototoxicity
- Deafness, vertigo, tinnitus
- Due to toxic effect on hair cells of inner ear
- Dose-dependent
- Common in IV use and renal impaired patients
- Avoid other ototoxic drugs together — i.e., Aminoglycosides, cyclosporine, etc.

4. Hypersensitivity
- Skin rashes
- Eosinophilia
- Photosensitivity
- ∵ It is a sulfonamide derivative (except ethacrynic acid)

5. Weakness, fatigue, dizziness, cramps due to hypokalemia

18.5 DRUG INTERACTIONS AND CONTRAINDICATIONS

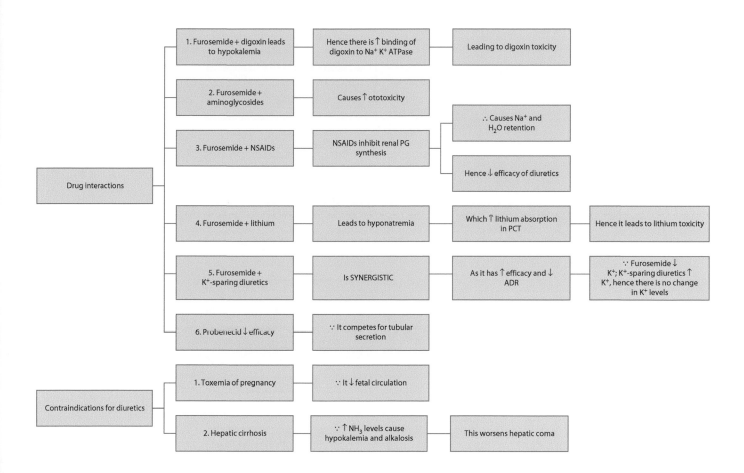

18.6 THIAZIDES AND THIAZIDE-LIKE DIURETICS

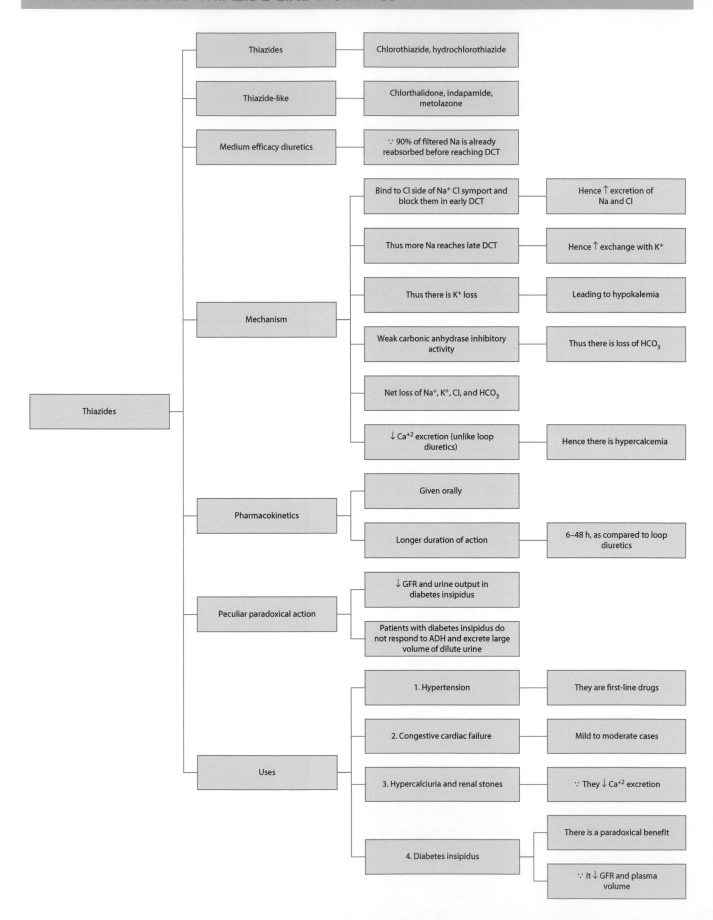

Thiazides

- Thiazides — Chlorothiazide, hydrochlorothiazide
- Thiazide-like — Chlorthalidone, indapamide, metolazone
- Medium efficacy diuretics — ∵ 90% of filtered Na is already reabsorbed before reaching DCT
- Mechanism
  - Bind to Cl side of Na$^+$ Cl symport and block them in early DCT — Hence ↑ excretion of Na and Cl
  - Thus more Na reaches late DCT — Hence ↑ exchange with K$^+$
  - Thus there is K$^+$ loss — Leading to hypokalemia
  - Weak carbonic anhydrase inhibitory activity — Thus there is loss of HCO$_3$
  - Net loss of Na$^+$, K$^+$, Cl, and HCO$_3$
  - ↓ Ca^{+2} excretion (unlike loop diuretics) — Hence there is hypercalcemia
- Pharmacokinetics
  - Given orally
  - Longer duration of action — 6–48 h, as compared to loop diuretics
- Peculiar paradoxical action
  - ↓ GFR and urine output in diabetes insipidus
  - Patients with diabetes insipidus do not respond to ADH and excrete large volume of dilute urine
- Uses
  - 1. Hypertension — They are first-line drugs
  - 2. Congestive cardiac failure — Mild to moderate cases
  - 3. Hypercalciuria and renal stones — ∵ They ↓ Ca^{+2} excretion
  - 4. Diabetes insipidus
    - There is a paradoxical benefit
    - ∵ It ↓ GFR and plasma volume

18.7 OTHER THIAZIDE DIURETICS AND ADRs

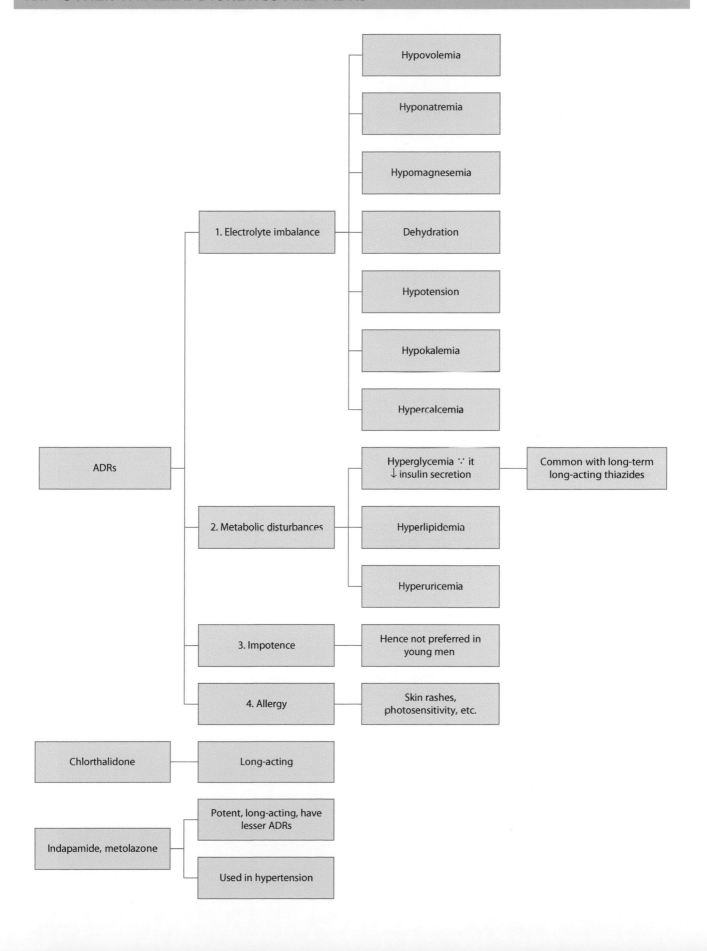

18.8 POTASSIUM-SPARING DIURETICS

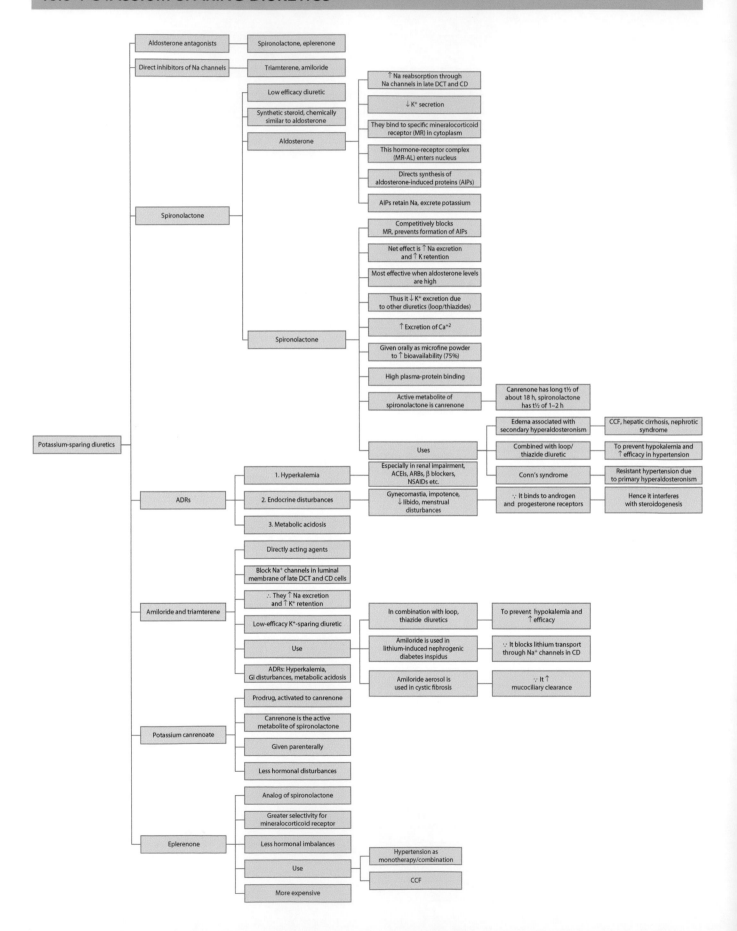

18.9 CARBONIC ANHYDRASE (CA) INHIBITORS (CAIs)

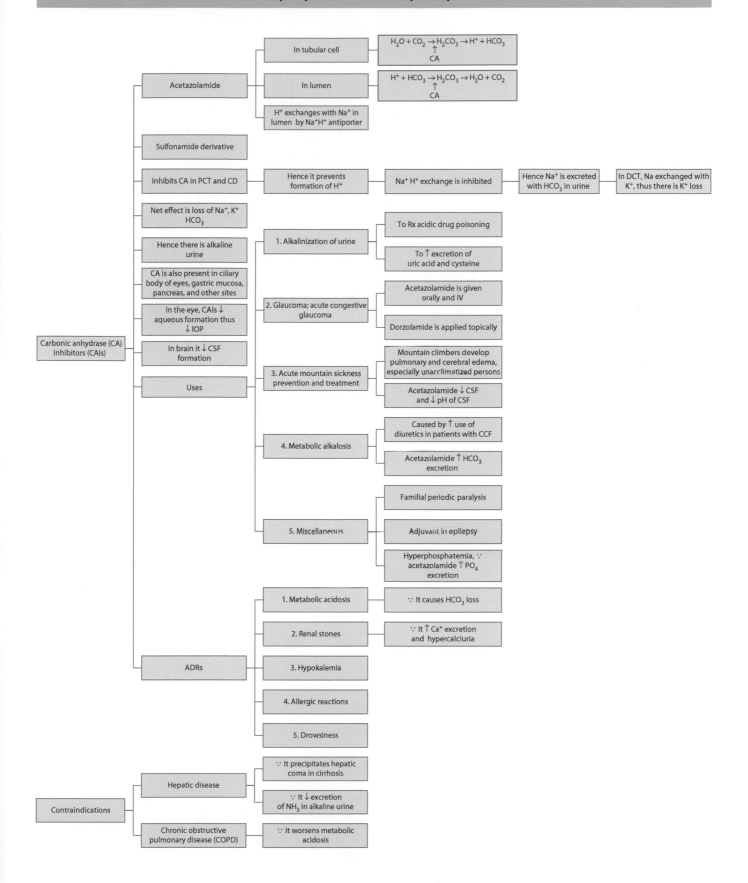

Carbonic anhydrase (CA) inhibitors (CAIs)

- **Acetazolamide**
  - In tubular cell
    $$H_2O + CO_2 \rightarrow H_2CO_3 \rightarrow H^+ + HCO_3$$
    $$\uparrow$$
    $$CA$$
  - In lumen
    $$H^+ + HCO_3 \rightarrow H_2CO_3 \rightarrow H_2O + CO_2$$
    $$\uparrow$$
    $$CA$$
  - H^+ exchanges with Na^+ in lumen by Na^+H^+ antiporter
- Sulfonamide derivative
- Inhibits CA in PCT and CD → Hence it prevents formation of H^+ → $Na^+ H^+$ exchange is inhibited → Hence Na^+ is excreted with HCO_3 in urine → In DCT, Na exchanged with K^+, thus there is K^+ loss
- Net effect is loss of Na^+, K^+ HCO_3
- Hence there is alkaline urine
- CA is also present in ciliary body of eyes, gastric mucosa, pancreas, and other sites
- In the eye, CAIs ↓ aqueous formation thus ↓ IOP
- In brain it ↓ CSF formation
- **Uses**
  - 1. Alkalinization of urine
    - To Rx acidic drug poisoning
    - To ↑ excretion of uric acid and cysteine
  - 2. Glaucoma; acute congestive glaucoma
    - Acetazolamide is given orally and IV
    - Dorzolamide is applied topically
  - 3. Acute mountain sickness prevention and treatment
    - Mountain climbers develop pulmonary and cerebral edema, especially unacclimatized persons
    - Acetazolamide ↓ CSF and ↓ pH of CSF
  - 4. Metabolic alkalosis
    - Caused by ↑ use of diuretics in patients with CCF
    - Acetazolamide ↑ HCO_3 excretion
  - 5. Miscellaneous
    - Familial periodic paralysis
    - Adjuvant in epilepsy
    - Hyperphosphatemia, ∵ acetazolamide ↑ PO_4 excretion
- **ADRs**
  - 1. Metabolic acidosis → ∵ It causes HCO_3 loss
  - 2. Renal stones → ∵ It ↑ Ca^+ excretion and hypercalciuria
  - 3. Hypokalemia
  - 4. Allergic reactions
  - 5. Drowsiness

Contraindications
- Hepatic disease
  - ∵ It precipitates hepatic coma in cirrhosis
  - ∵ It ↓ excretion of NH_3 in alkaline urine
- Chronic obstructive pulmonary disease (COPD)
  - ∵ It worsens metabolic acidosis

18.10 OSMOTIC DIURETICS

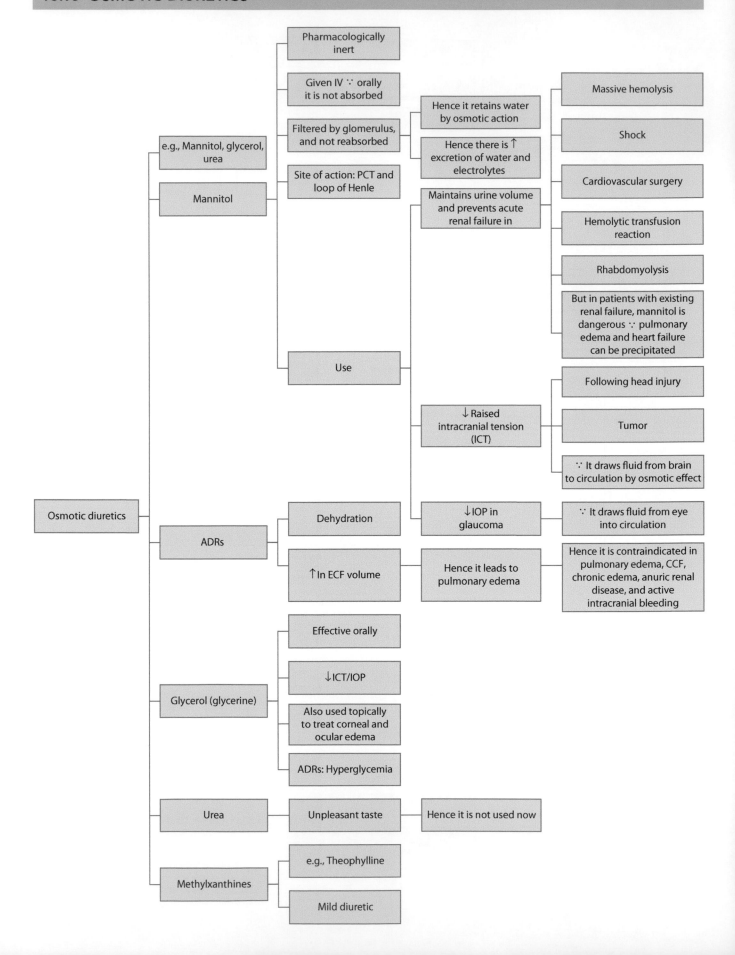

18.11 NEWER DIURETICS

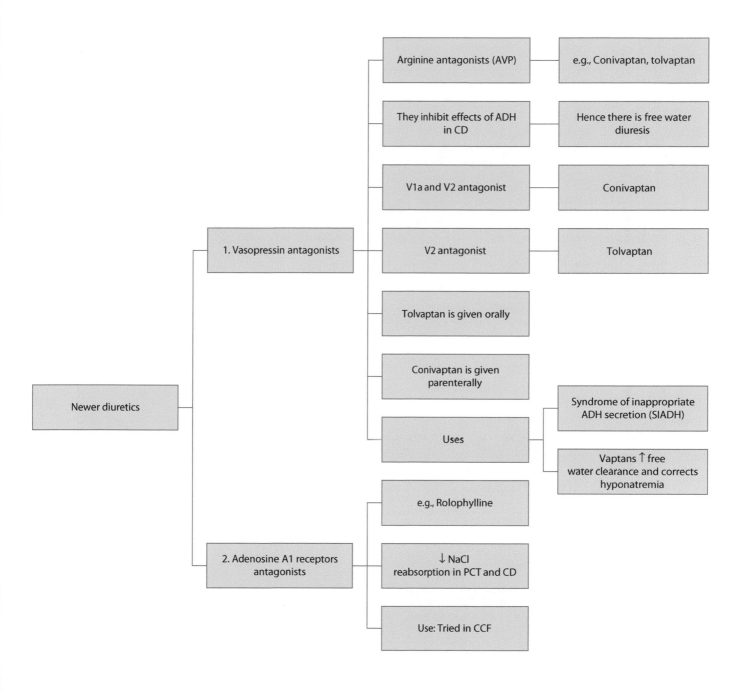

18.12 TABLE ON DIFFERENCES BETWEEN DIURETICS

Thiazide	Furosemide
Medium efficacy	High
Acts on early DCT	TALH
Inhibits Na^+ Cl symport	Na^+ K^+ 2Cl cotransport
Onset 1 h	20–40 min
Duration of action long: 8–12 h	8–6 h
No response on ↑ dose	Dose dependent ↑
Causes hyperuricemia	No change
↑ Blood sugar	No change
No ototoxicity	Ototoxic
Use: Hypertension	Edema

Furosemide	Spironolactone
Sulfonamide	Steroid
Acts on TALH	DCT and CD
Na^+ K^+ 2Cl cotransport blocked	Aldosterone blocker
High efficacy	Low efficacy
Quick onset (minutes)	Slow onset (days)
Hypokalemia	Hyperkalemia
Causes ototoxicity	Causes gynecomastia, hirsutism
Use – edema	Hyperaldosteronism, as adjuvant to diuretics
Caution: Allergy to sulfonamides	Caution: Peptic ulcer

18.13 ANTIDIURETICS

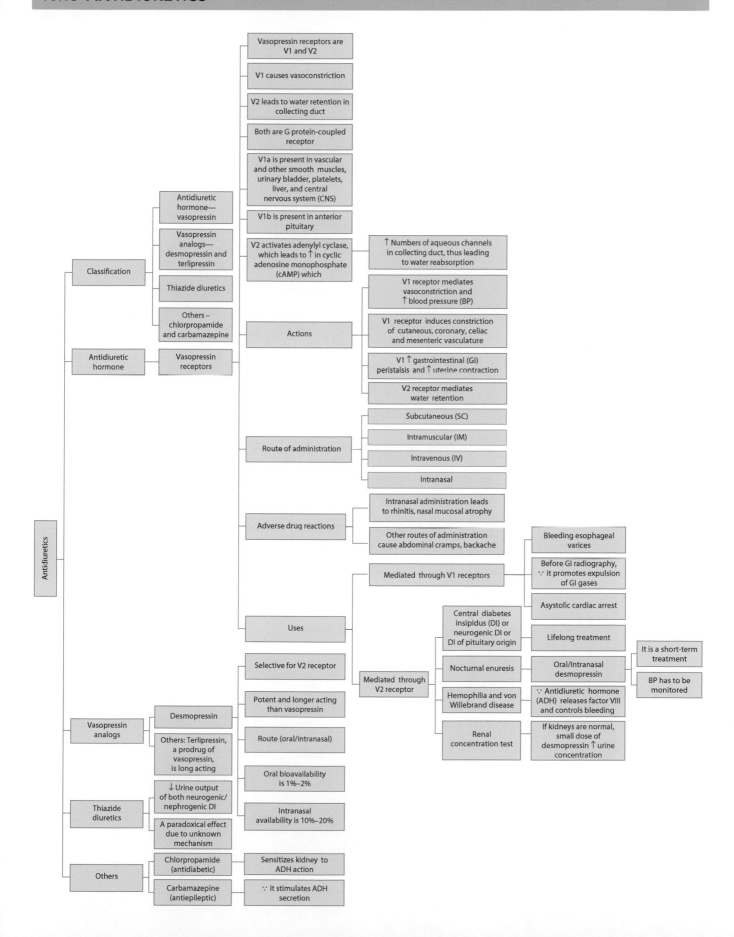

19

Pharmacotherapy of shock

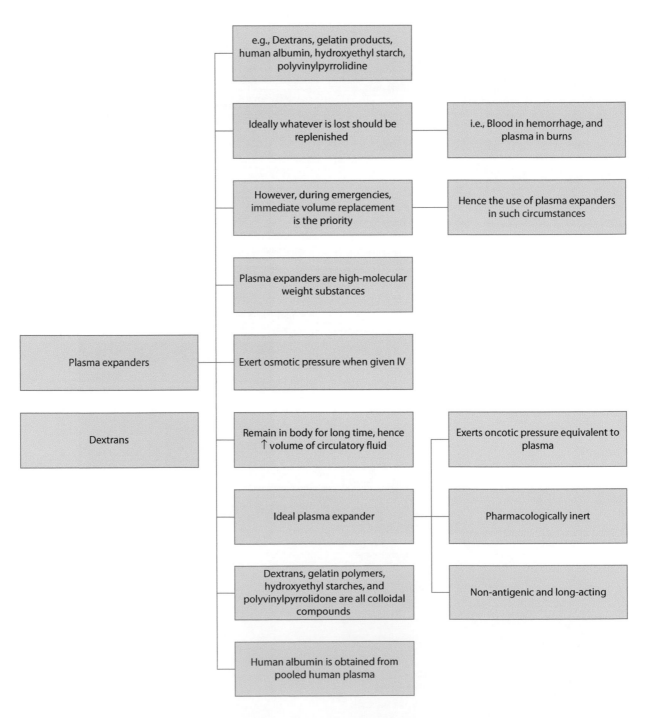

19.2 DEXTRANS

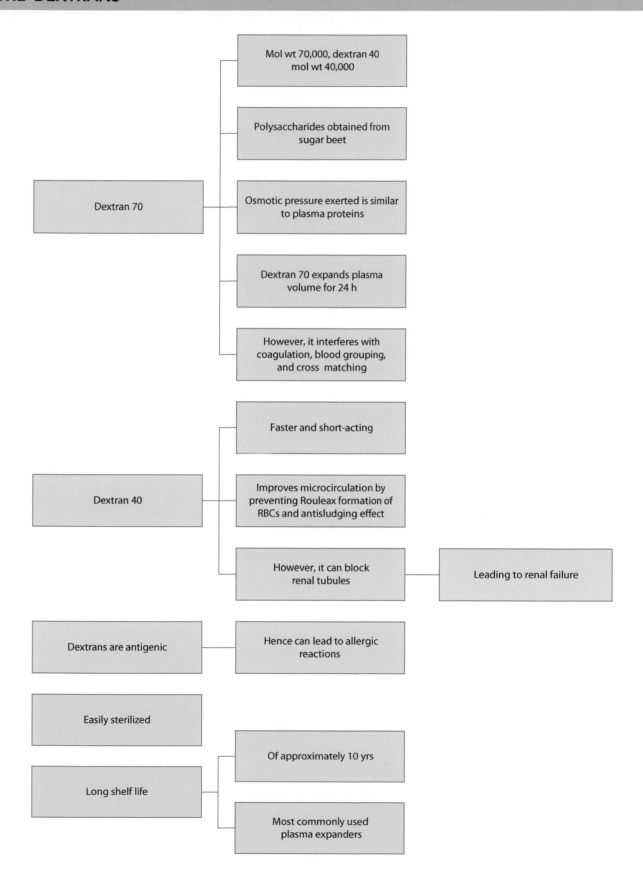

Dextran 70
- Mol wt 70,000, dextran 40 mol wt 40,000
- Polysaccharides obtained from sugar beet
- Osmotic pressure exerted is similar to plasma proteins
- Dextran 70 expands plasma volume for 24 h
- However, it interferes with coagulation, blood grouping, and cross matching

Dextran 40
- Faster and short-acting
- Improves microcirculation by preventing Rouleax formation of RBCs and antisludging effect
- However, it can block renal tubules → Leading to renal failure

Dextrans are antigenic → Hence can lead to allergic reactions

Easily sterilized

Long shelf life
- Of approximately 10 yrs
- Most commonly used plasma expanders

19.3 GELATIN PRODUCTS

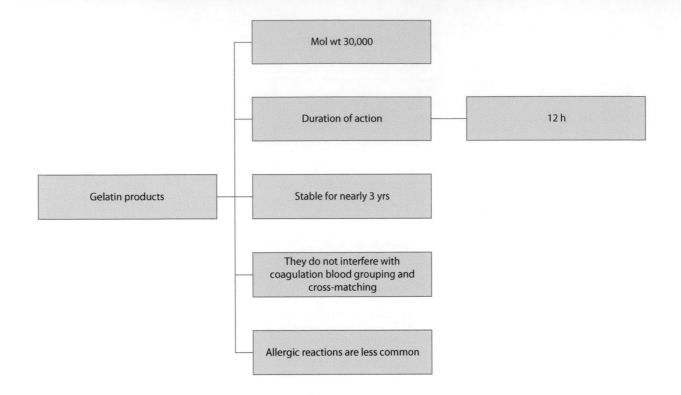

Gelatin products

Mol wt 30,000

Duration of action — 12 h

Stable for nearly 3 yrs

They do not interfere with coagulation blood grouping and cross-matching

Allergic reactions are less common

19.4 HYDROXYETHYL STARCH

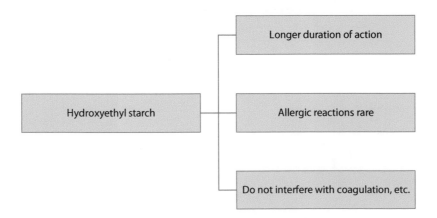

Hydroxyethyl starch

Longer duration of action

Allergic reactions rare

Do not interfere with coagulation, etc.

19.5 POLYVINYLPYRROLIDONE

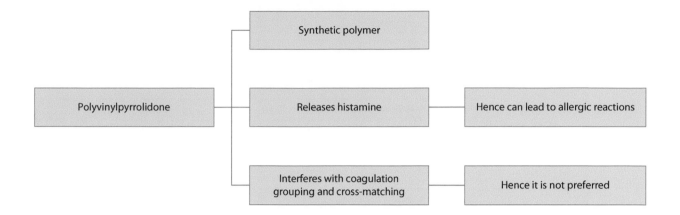

19.6 HUMAN ALBUMIN

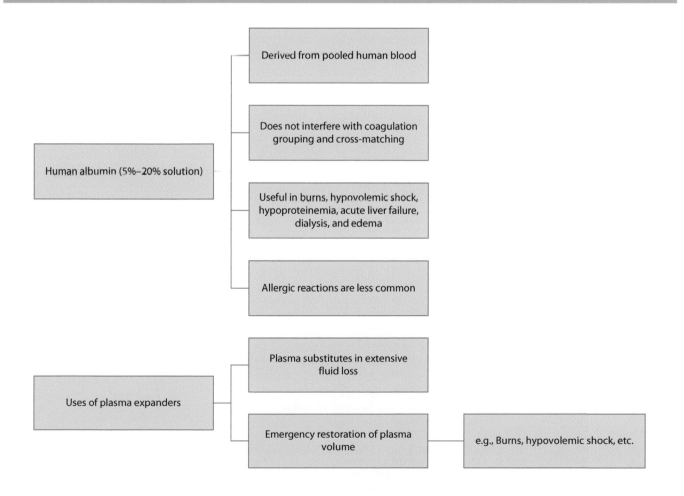

19.7 INTRAVENOUS FLUIDS

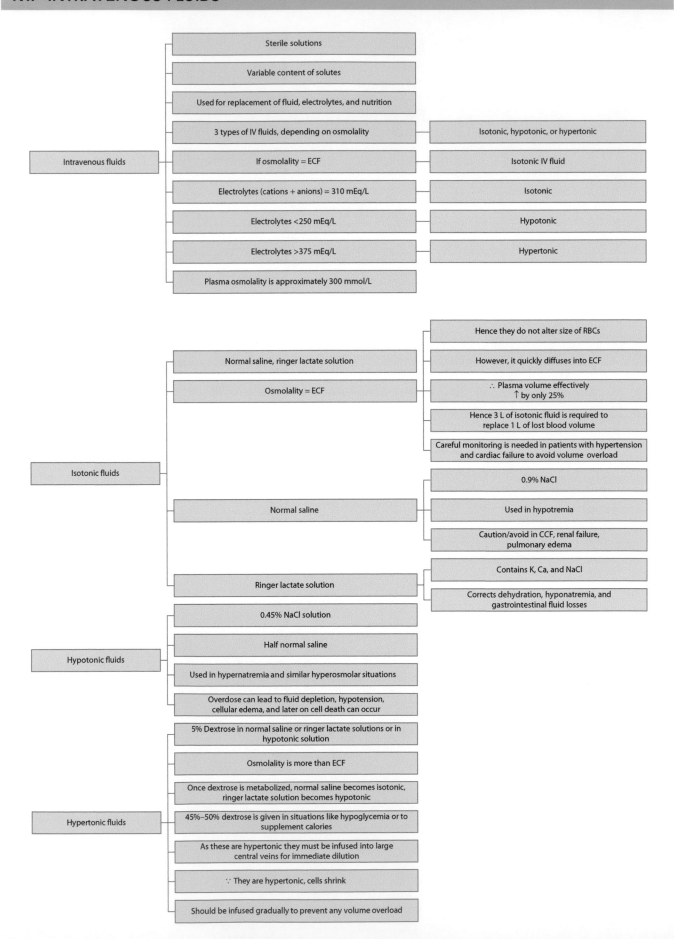

Intravenous fluids
- Sterile solutions
- Variable content of solutes
- Used for replacement of fluid, electrolytes, and nutrition
- 3 types of IV fluids, depending on osmolality — Isotonic, hypotonic, or hypertonic
- If osmolality = ECF — Isotonic IV fluid
- Electrolytes (cations + anions) = 310 mEq/L — Isotonic
- Electrolytes <250 mEq/L — Hypotonic
- Electrolytes >375 mEq/L — Hypertonic
- Plasma osmolality is approximately 300 mmol/L

Isotonic fluids
- Normal saline, ringer lactate solution
- Osmolality = ECF
  - Hence they do not alter size of RBCs
  - However, it quickly diffuses into ECF
  - ∴ Plasma volume effectively ↑ by only 25%
  - Hence 3 L of isotonic fluid is required to replace 1 L of lost blood volume
  - Careful monitoring is needed in patients with hypertension and cardiac failure to avoid volume overload
- Normal saline
  - 0.9% NaCl
  - Used in hypotremia
  - Caution/avoid in CCF, renal failure, pulmonary edema
- Ringer lactate solution
  - Contains K, Ca, and NaCl
  - Corrects dehydration, hyponatremia, and gastrointestinal fluid losses

Hypotonic fluids
- 0.45% NaCl solution
- Half normal saline
- Used in hypernatremia and similar hyperosmolar situations
- Overdose can lead to fluid depletion, hypotension, cellular edema, and later on cell death can occur

Hypertonic fluids
- 5% Dextrose in normal saline or ringer lactate solutions or in hypotonic solution
- Osmolality is more than ECF
- Once dextrose is metabolized, normal saline becomes isotonic, ringer lactate solution becomes hypotonic
- 45%–50% dextrose is given in situations like hypoglycemia or to supplement calories
- As these are hypertonic they must be infused into large central veins for immediate dilution
- ∵ They are hypertonic, cells shrink
- Should be infused gradually to prevent any volume overload

PART IV

Central nervous system (CNS) pharmacology

Introduction to CNS and alcohol

20.1 INTRODUCTION TO CNS, CNS NEUROTRANSMITTERS, EXCITATORY NEUROTRANSMITTERS, INHIBITORY NEUROTRANSMITTERS

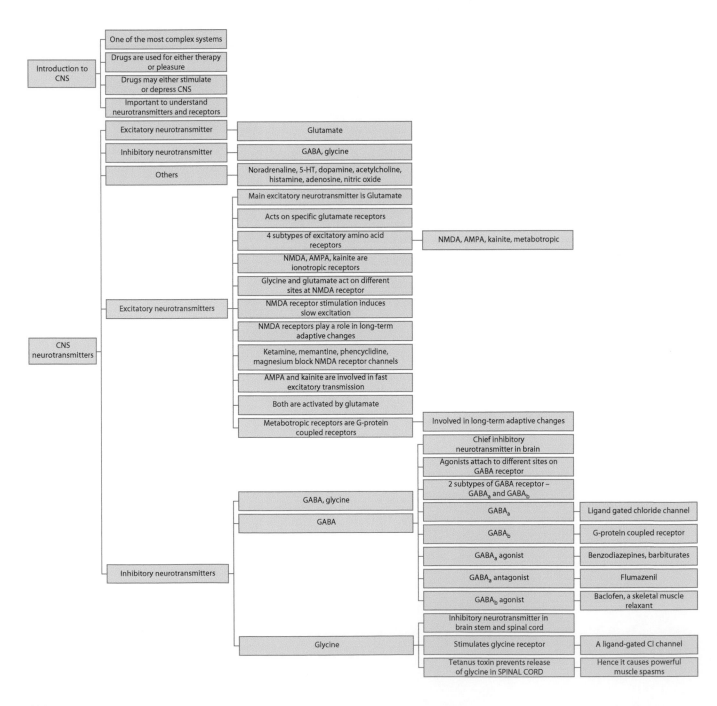

20.2 ALCOHOLS, ETHYL ALCOHOL – INTRODUCTION AND ACTIONS

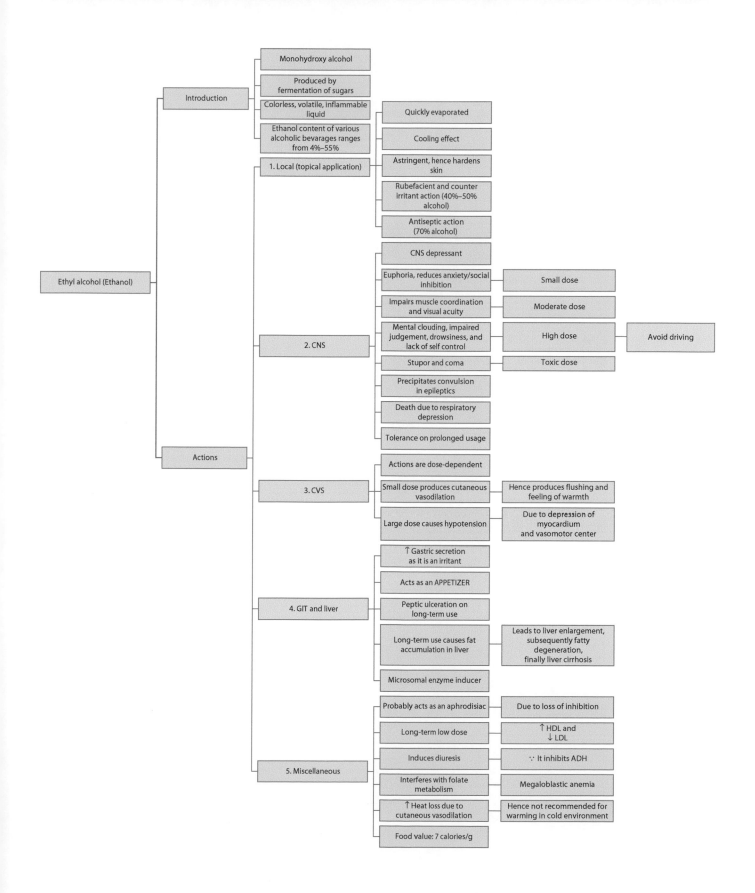

20.3 MECHANISM OF ACTION, PHARMACOKINETICS, DRUG INTERACTION, AND USES

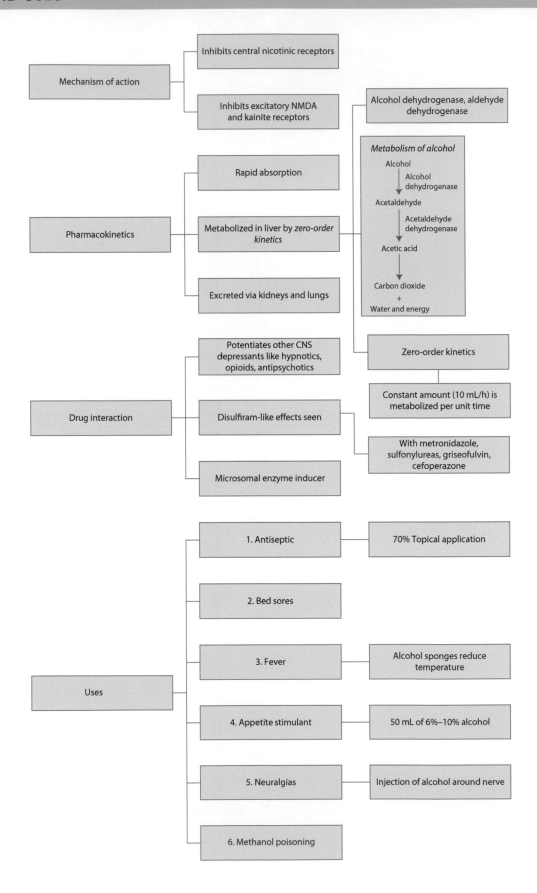

20.4 DISULFIRAM

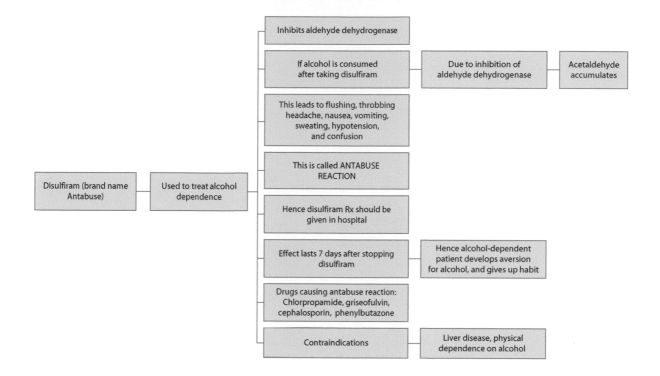

Disulfiram (brand name Antabuse) — Used to treat alcohol dependence

- Inhibits aldehyde dehydrogenase
- If alcohol is consumed after taking disulfiram → Due to inhibition of aldehyde dehydrogenase → Acetaldehyde accumulates
- This leads to flushing, throbbing headache, nausea, vomiting, sweating, hypotension, and confusion
- This is called ANTABUSE REACTION
- Hence disulfiram Rx should be given in hospital
- Effect lasts 7 days after stopping disulfiram → Hence alcohol-dependent patient develops aversion for alcohol, and gives up habit
- Drugs causing antabuse reaction: Chlorpropamide, griseofulvin, cephalosporin, phenylbutazone
- Contraindications → Liver disease, physical dependence on alcohol

20.5 DRUGS TO TREAT ALCOHOL DEPENDENCE

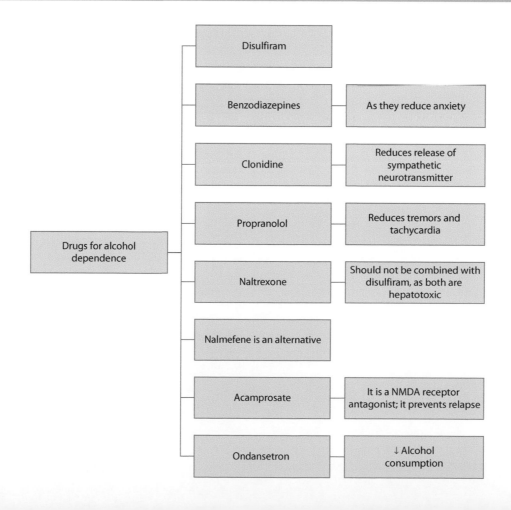

Drugs for alcohol dependence

- Disulfiram
- Benzodiazepines → As they reduce anxiety
- Clonidine → Reduces release of sympathetic neurotransmitter
- Propranolol → Reduces tremors and tachycardia
- Naltrexone → Should not be combined with disulfiram, as both are hepatotoxic
- Nalmefene is an alternative
- Acamprosate → It is a NMDA receptor antagonist; it prevents relapse
- Ondansetron → ↓ Alcohol consumption

20.6 METHYL ALCOHOL (METHANOL)

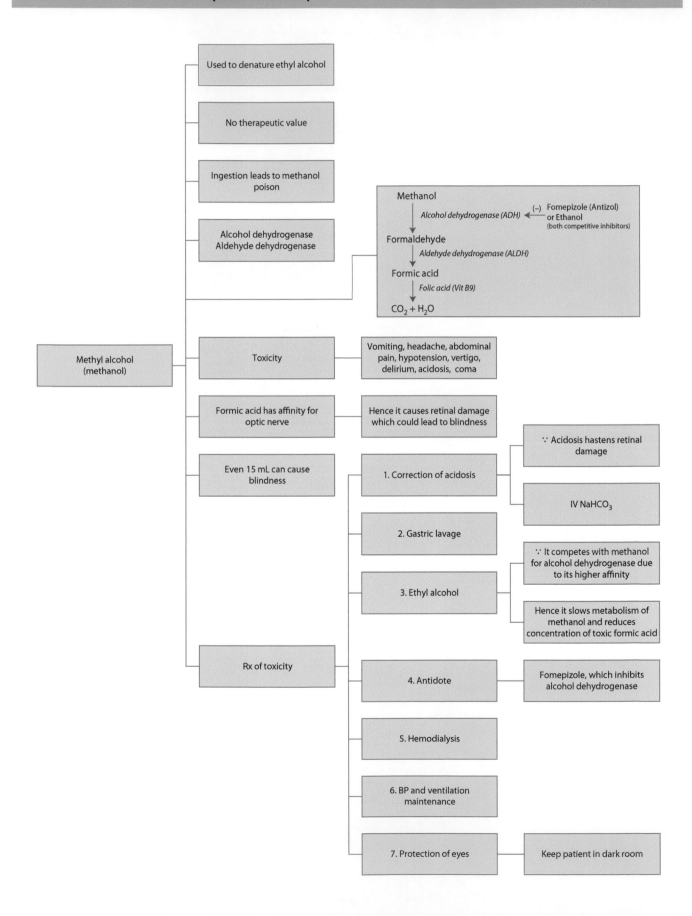

Sedative hypnotics

21.1 INTRODUCTION TO SEDATIVE HYPNOTICS

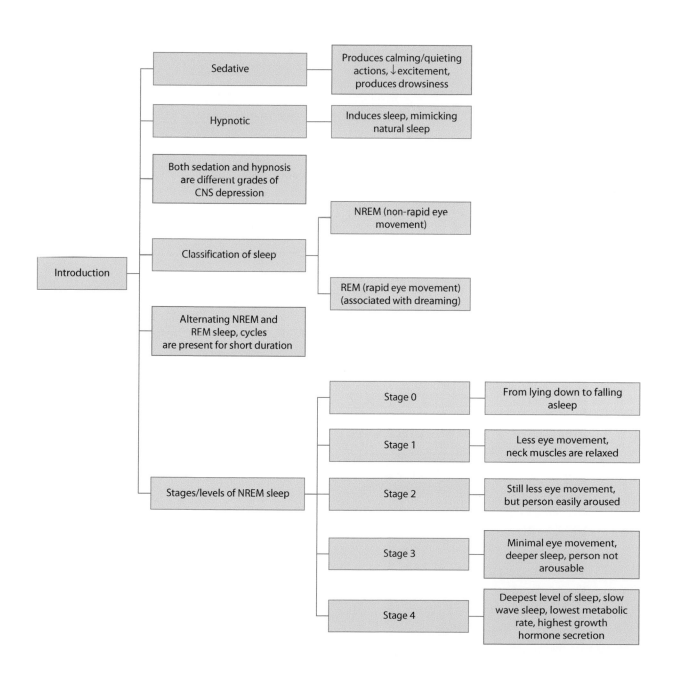

21.2 CLASSIFICATION

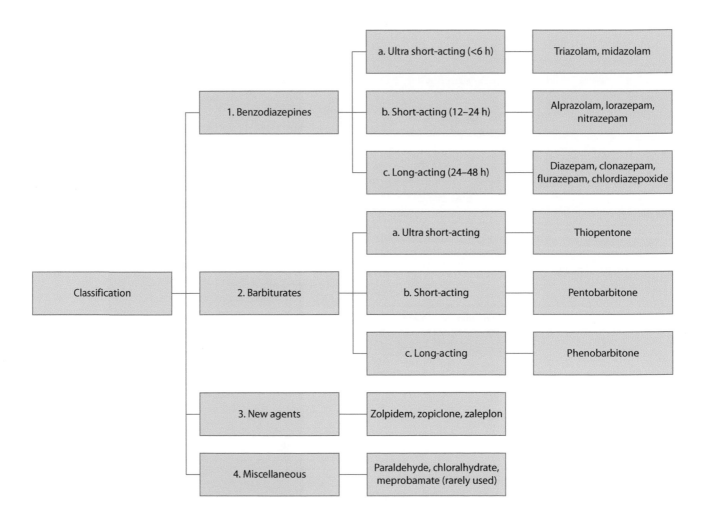

21.3 MECHANISM OF ACTION

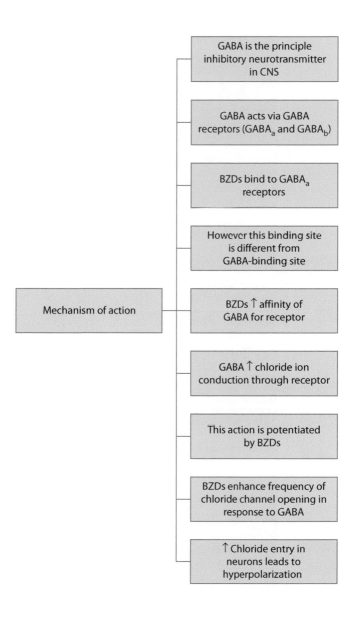

21.4 PHARMACOLOGICAL ACTIONS

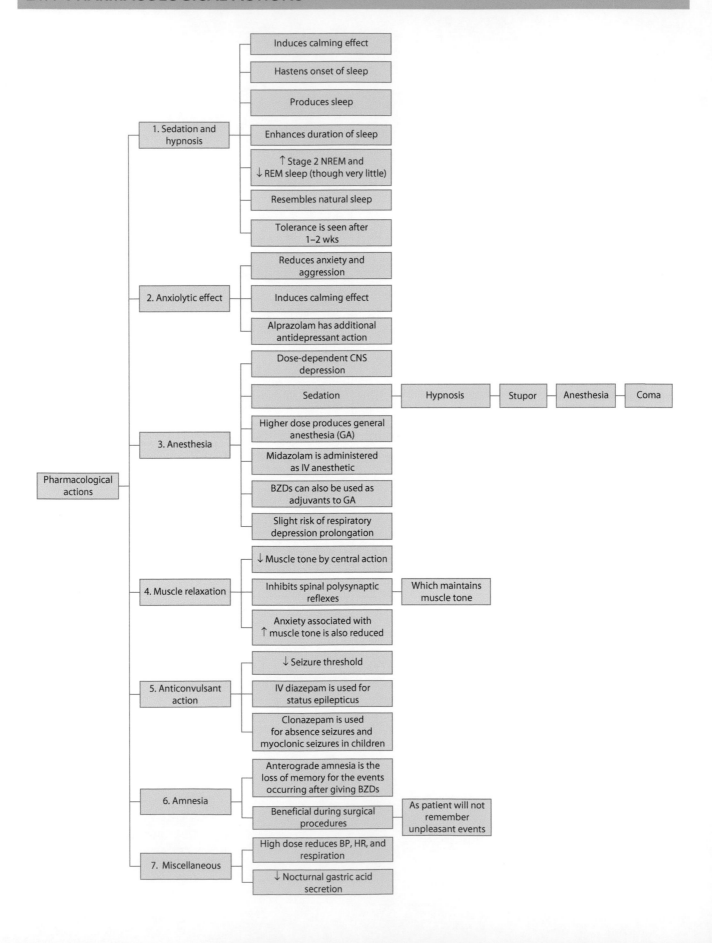

21.5 ADVANTAGES OF BZDs OVER BARBITURATES

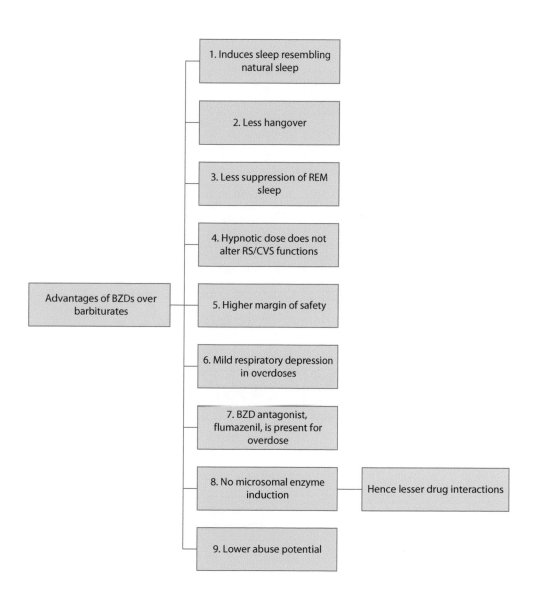

21.6 PHARMACOKINETICS AND ADRs

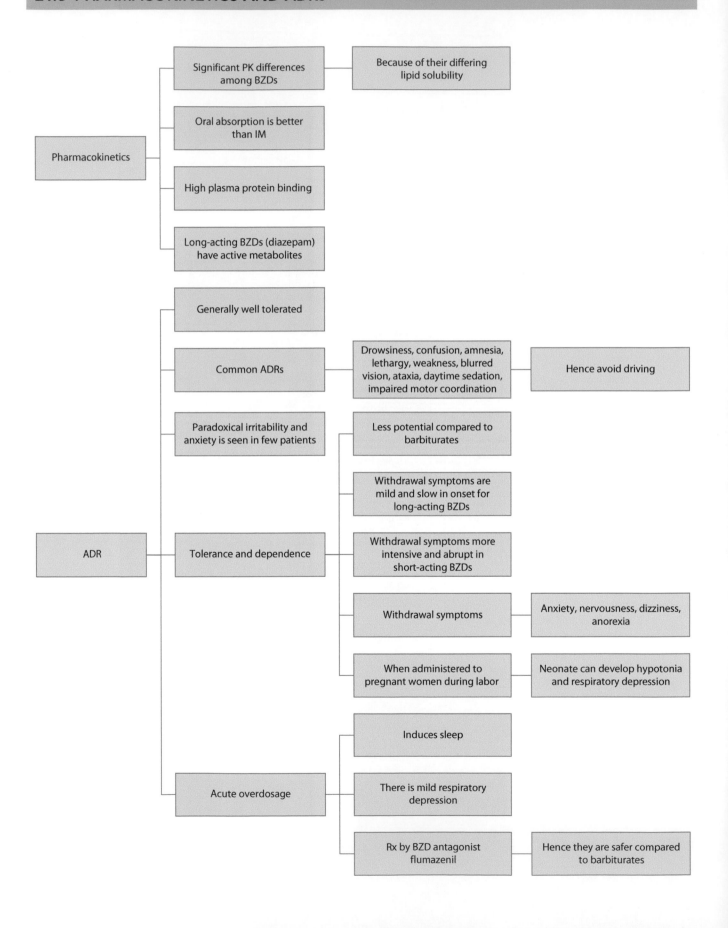

21.7 USES OF BZDs AND BZD ANTAGONIST

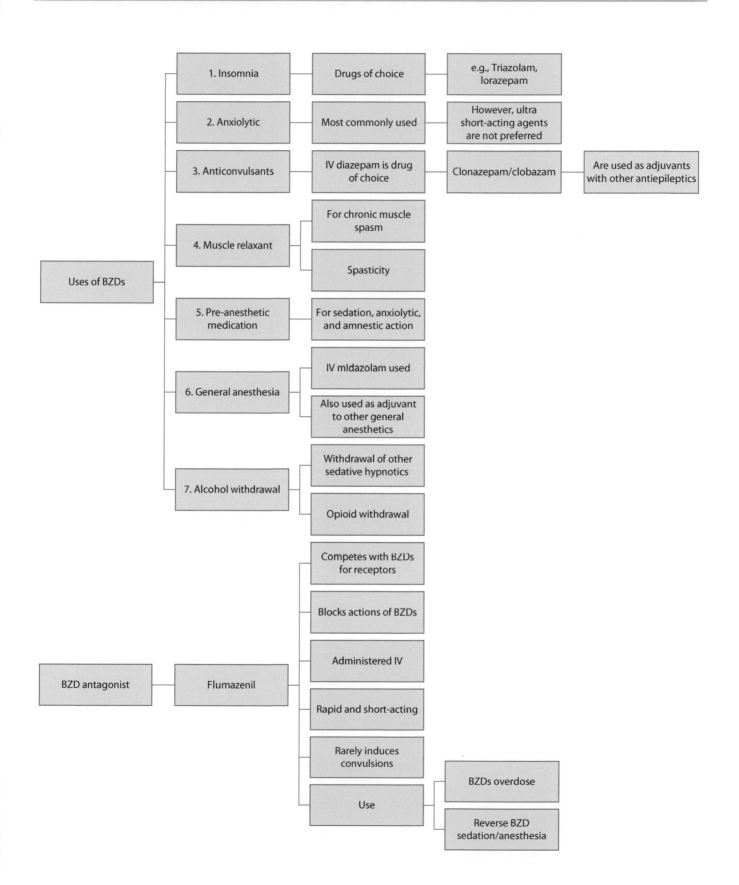

21.8 NEWER AGENTS

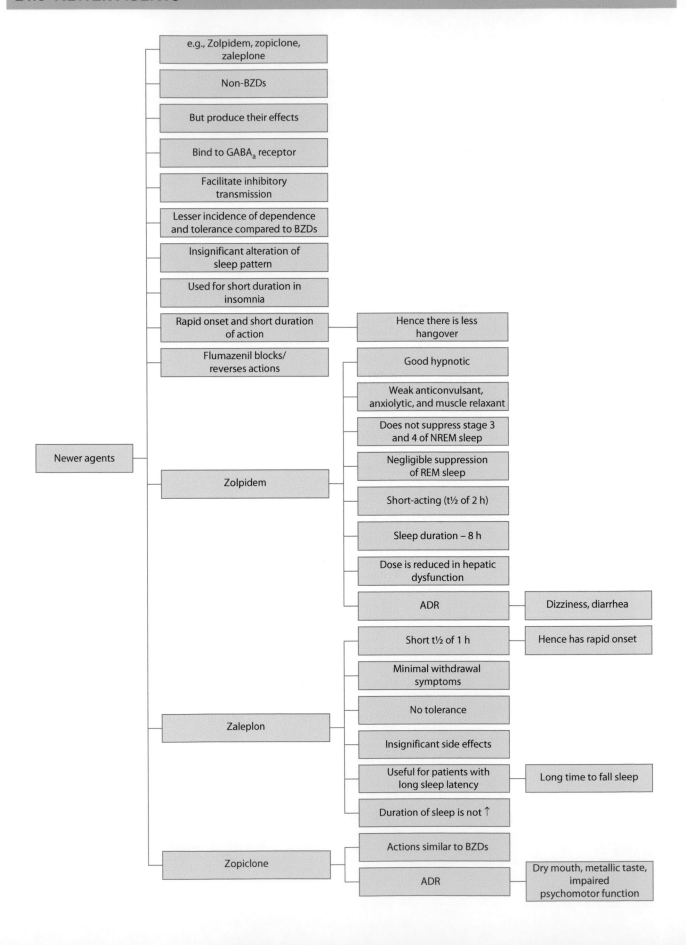

21.9 BARBITURATES CLASSIFICATION, MECHANISM OF ACTION, AND PHARMACOLOGICAL ACTION

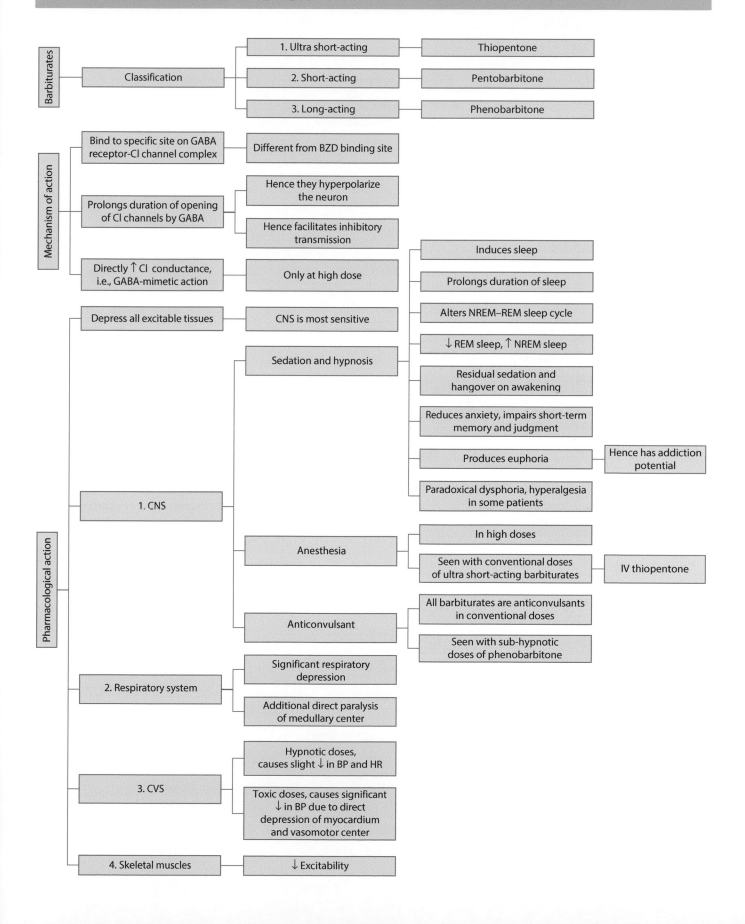

21.10 PHARMACOKINETICS, ADVERSE REACTIONS, AND USES

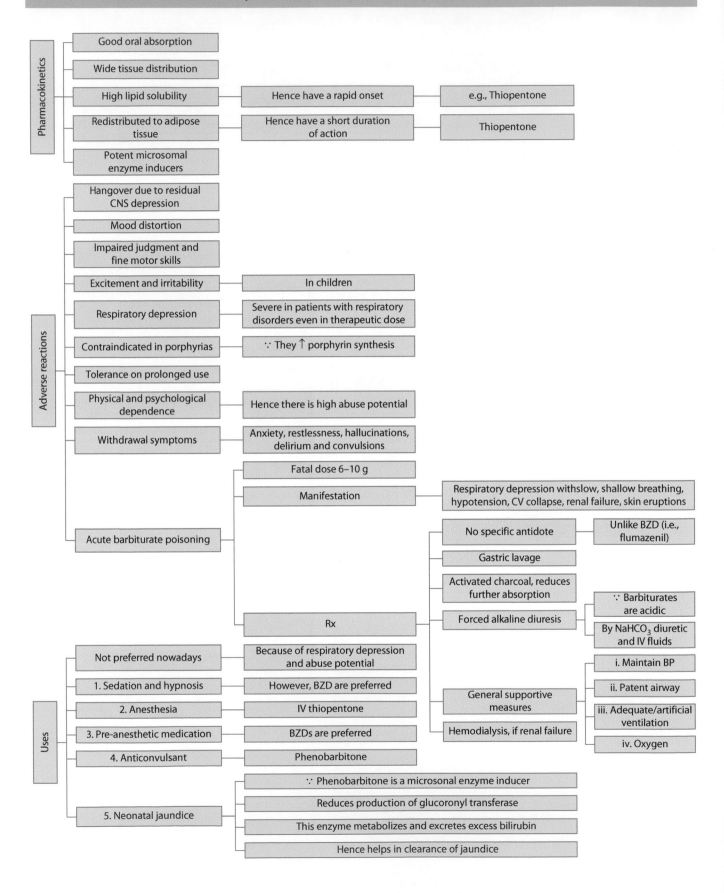

Pharmacokinetics
- Good oral absorption
- Wide tissue distribution
- High lipid solubility → Hence have a rapid onset → e.g., Thiopentone
- Redistributed to adipose tissue → Hence have a short duration of action → Thiopentone
- Potent microsomal enzyme inducers

Adverse reactions
- Hangover due to residual CNS depression
- Mood distortion
- Impaired judgment and fine motor skills
- Excitement and irritability → In children
- Respiratory depression → Severe in patients with respiratory disorders even in therapeutic dose
- Contraindicated in porphyrias → ∵ They ↑ porphyrin synthesis
- Tolerance on prolonged use
- Physical and psychological dependence → Hence there is high abuse potential
- Withdrawal symptoms → Anxiety, restlessness, hallucinations, delirium and convulsions
- Acute barbiturate poisoning
  - Fatal dose 6–10 g
  - Manifestation → Respiratory depression withslow, shallow breathing, hypotension, CV collapse, renal failure, skin eruptions
  - Rx
    - No specific antidote → Unlike BZD (i.e., flumazenil)
    - Gastric lavage
    - Activated charcoal, reduces further absorption
    - Forced alkaline diuresis → ∵ Barbiturates are acidic / By NaHCO₃ diuretic and IV fluids
    - General supportive measures → i. Maintain BP / ii. Patent airway / iii. Adequate/artificial ventilation / iv. Oxygen
    - Hemodialysis, if renal failure

Uses
- Not preferred nowadays → Because of respiratory depression and abuse potential
- 1. Sedation and hypnosis → However, BZD are preferred
- 2. Anesthesia → IV thiopentone
- 3. Pre-anesthetic medication → BZDs are preferred
- 4. Anticonvulsant → Phenobarbitone
- 5. Neonatal jaundice
  - ∵ Phenobarbitone is a microsonal enzyme inducer
  - Reduces production of glucoronyl transferase
  - This enzyme metabolizes and excretes excess bilirubin
  - Hence helps in clearance of jaundice

22

Antiepileptics

22.1 ANTIEPILEPTICS CLASSIFICATION AND MECHANISM OF ACTION

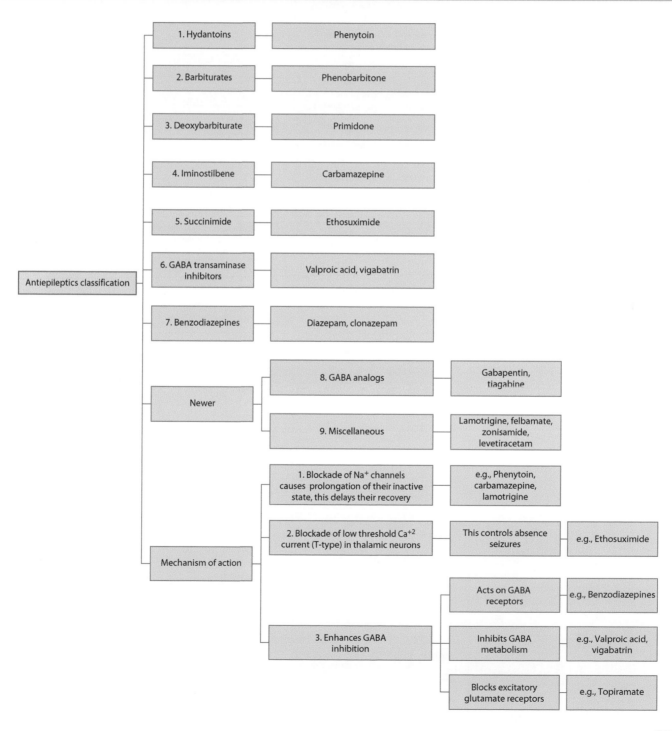

215

22.2 PHENYTOIN

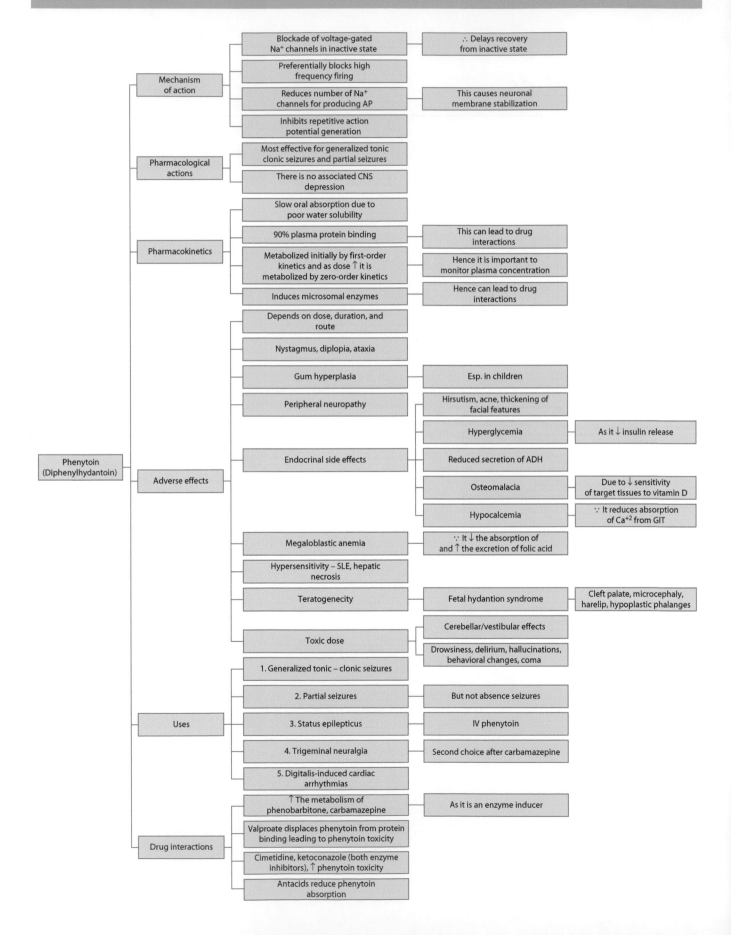

Phenytoin (Diphenylhydantoin)

Mechanism of action
- Blockade of voltage-gated Na+ channels in inactive state → ∴ Delays recovery from inactive state
- Preferentially blocks high frequency firing
- Reduces number of Na+ channels for producing AP → This causes neuronal membrane stabilization
- Inhibits repetitive action potential generation

Pharmacological actions
- Most effective for generalized tonic clonic seizures and partial seizures
- There is no associated CNS depression

Pharmacokinetics
- Slow oral absorption due to poor water solubility
- 90% plasma protein binding → This can lead to drug interactions
- Metabolized initially by first-order kinetics and as dose ↑ it is metabolized by zero-order kinetics → Hence it is important to monitor plasma concentration
- Induces microsomal enzymes → Hence can lead to drug interactions

Adverse effects
- Depends on dose, duration, and route
- Nystagmus, diplopia, ataxia
- Gum hyperplasia → Esp. in children
- Peripheral neuropathy
- Endocrinal side effects
  - Hirsutism, acne, thickening of facial features
  - Hyperglycemia → As it ↓ insulin release
  - Reduced secretion of ADH
  - Osteomalacia → Due to ↓ sensitivity of target tissues to vitamin D
  - Hypocalcemia → ∵ It reduces absorption of Ca+2 from GIT
- Megaloblastic anemia → ∵ It ↓ the absorption of and ↑ the excretion of folic acid
- Hypersensitivity – SLE, hepatic necrosis
- Teratogenecity → Fetal hydantion syndrome → Cleft palate, microcephaly, harelip, hypoplastic phalanges
- Toxic dose
  - Cerebellar/vestibular effects
  - Drowsiness, delirium, hallucinations, behavioral changes, coma

Uses
1. Generalized tonic – clonic seizures
2. Partial seizures → But not absence seizures
3. Status epilepticus → IV phenytoin
4. Trigeminal neuralgia → Second choice after carbamazepine
5. Digitalis-induced cardiac arrhythmias

Drug interactions
- ↑ The metabolism of phenobarbitone, carbamazepine → As it is an enzyme inducer
- Valproate displaces phenytoin from protein binding leading to phenytoin toxicity
- Cimetidine, ketoconazole (both enzyme inhibitors), ↑ phenytoin toxicity
- Antacids reduce phenytoin absorption

22.3 PHENOBARBITONE

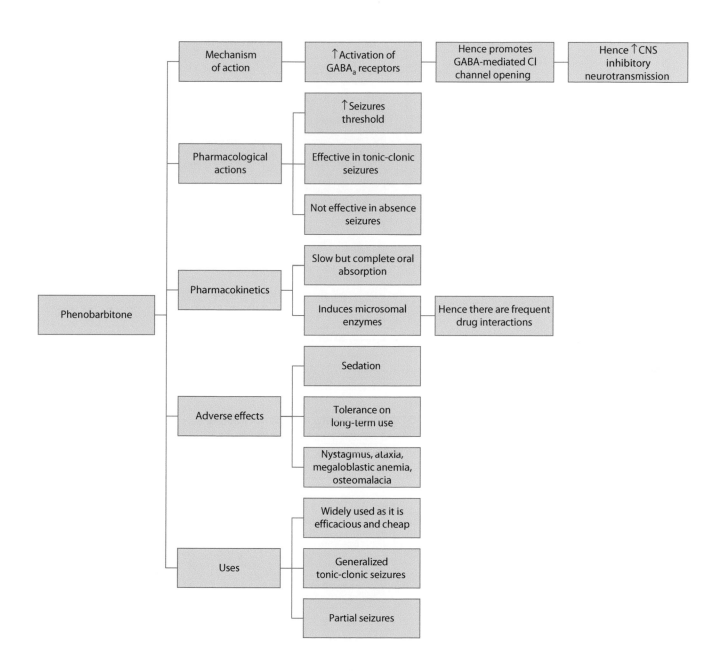

22.4 CARBAMAZEPINE AND ETHOSUXIMIDE

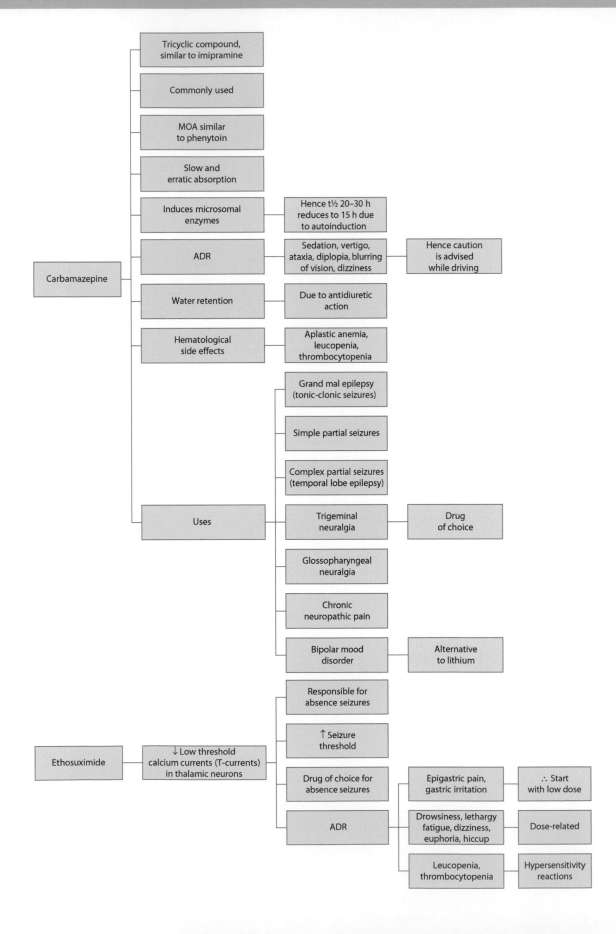

22.5 VALPROIC ACID

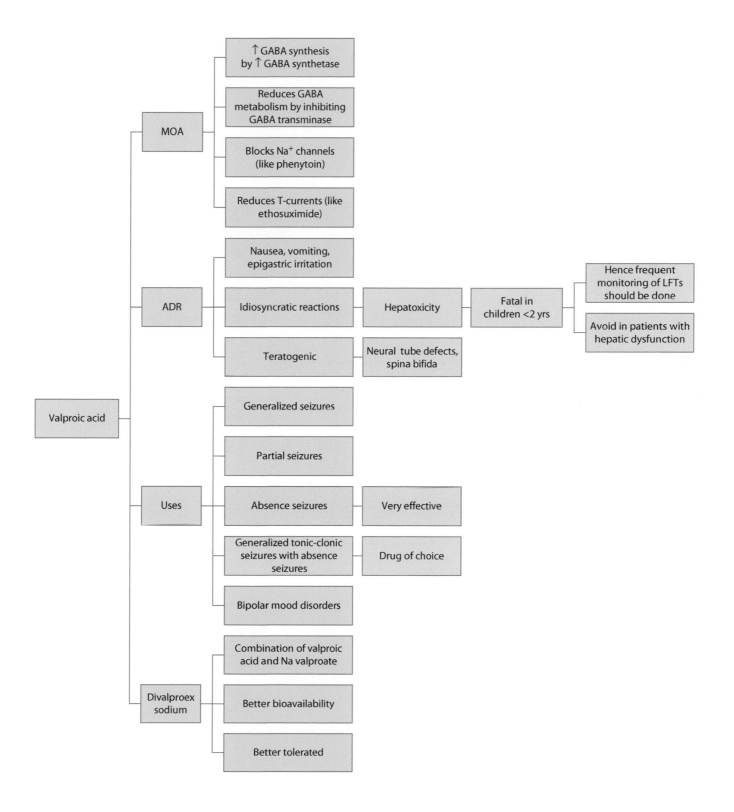

22.6 BENZODIAZEPINES

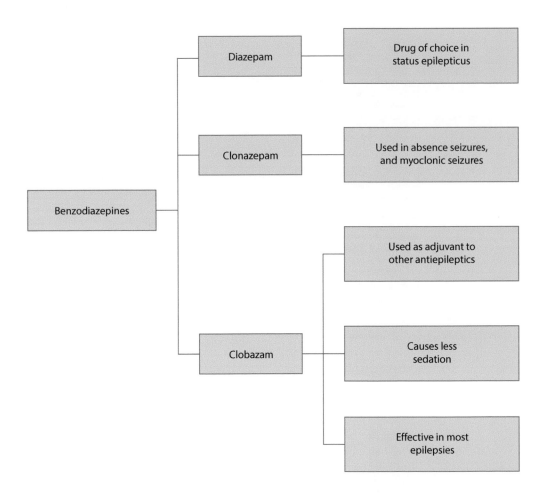

22.7 NEWER ANTIEPILEPTICS

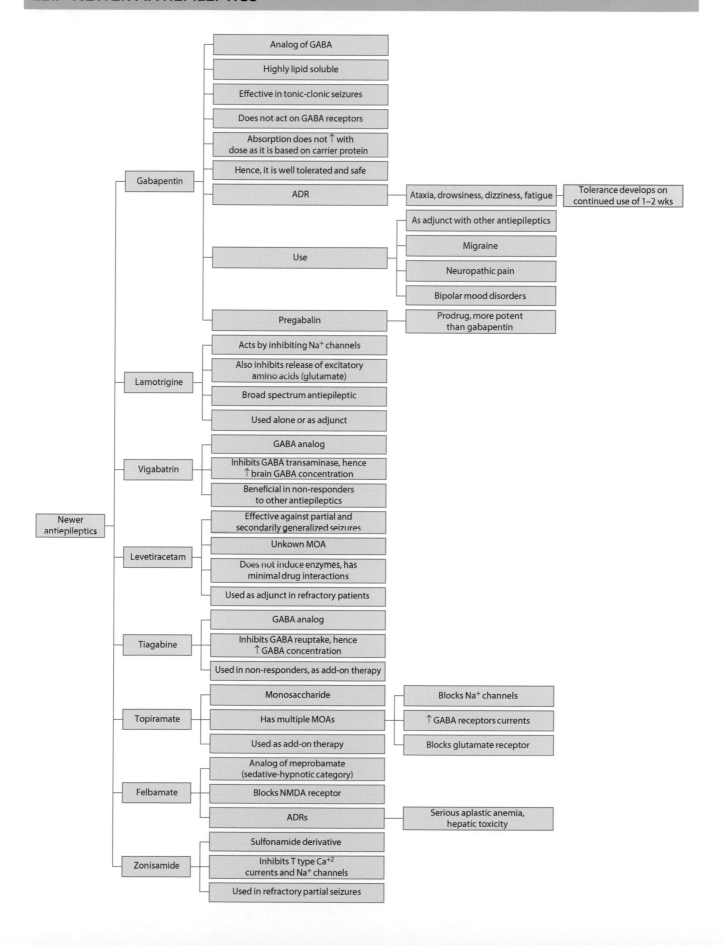

Newer antiepileptics

Gabapentin
- Analog of GABA
- Highly lipid soluble
- Effective in tonic-clonic seizures
- Does not act on GABA receptors
- Absorption does not ↑ with dose as it is based on carrier protein
- Hence, it is well tolerated and safe
- ADR → Ataxia, drowsiness, dizziness, fatigue → Tolerance develops on continued use of 1–2 wks
- Use →
  - As adjunct with other antiepileptics
  - Migraine
  - Neuropathic pain
  - Bipolar mood disorders
- Pregabalin → Prodrug, more potent than gabapentin

Lamotrigine
- Acts by inhibiting Na⁺ channels
- Also inhibits release of excitatory amino acids (glutamate)
- Broad spectrum antiepileptic
- Used alone or as adjunct

Vigabatrin
- GABA analog
- Inhibits GABA transaminase, hence ↑brain GABA concentration
- Beneficial in non-responders to other antiepileptics

Levetiracetam
- Effective against partial and secondarily generalized seizures
- Unkown MOA
- Does not induce enzymes, has minimal drug interactions
- Used as adjunct in refractory patients

Tiagabine
- GABA analog
- Inhibits GABA reuptake, hence ↑GABA concentration
- Used in non-responders, as add-on therapy

Topiramate
- Monosaccharide
- Has multiple MOAs →
  - Blocks Na⁺ channels
  - ↑GABA receptors currents
  - Blocks glutamate receptor
- Used as add-on therapy

Felbamate
- Analog of meprobamate (sedative-hypnotic category)
- Blocks NMDA receptor
- ADRs → Serious aplastic anemia, hepatic toxicity

Zonisamide
- Sulfonamide derivative
- Inhibits T type Ca⁺² currents and Na⁺ channels
- Used in refractory partial seizures

23

Antidepressants

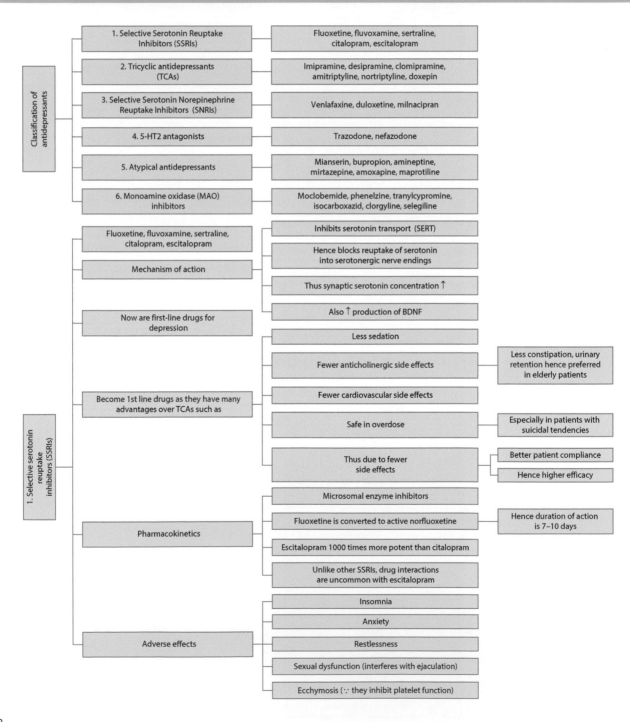

Classification of antidepressants

1. Selective Serotonin Reuptake Inhibitors (SSRIs) — Fluoxetine, fluvoxamine, sertraline, citalopram, escitalopram

2. Tricyclic antidepressants (TCAs) — Imipramine, desipramine, clomipramine, amitriptyline, nortriptyline, doxepin

3. Selective Serotonin Norepinephrine Reuptake Inhibitors (SNRIs) — Venlafaxine, duloxetine, milnacipran

4. 5-HT2 antagonists — Trazodone, nefazodone

5. Atypical antidepressants — Mianserin, bupropion, amineptine, mirtazepine, amoxapine, maprotiline

6. Monoamine oxidase (MAO) inhibitors — Moclobemide, phenelzine, tranylcypromine, isocarboxazid, clorgyline, selegiline

1. Selective serotonin reuptake inhibitors (SSRIs)

Fluoxetine, fluvoxamine, sertraline, citalopram, escitalopram

Mechanism of action
- Inhibits serotonin transport (SERT)
- Hence blocks reuptake of serotonin into serotonergic nerve endings
- Thus synaptic serotonin concentration ↑
- Also ↑ production of BDNF

Now are first-line drugs for depression

Become 1st line drugs as they have many advantages over TCAs such as
- Less sedation
- Fewer anticholinergic side effects → Less constipation, urinary retention hence preferred in elderly patients
- Fewer cardiovascular side effects
- Safe in overdose → Especially in patients with suicidal tendencies
- Thus due to fewer side effects → Better patient compliance / Hence higher efficacy

Pharmacokinetics
- Microsomal enzyme inhibitors
- Fluoxetine is converted to active norfluoxetine → Hence duration of action is 7–10 days
- Escitalopram 1000 times more potent than citalopram
- Unlike other SSRIs, drug interactions are uncommon with escitalopram

Adverse effects
- Insomnia
- Anxiety
- Restlessness
- Sexual dysfunction (interferes with ejaculation)
- Ecchymosis (∵ they inhibit platelet function)

23.2 TRICYCLIC ANTIDEPRESSANTS (TCAs)

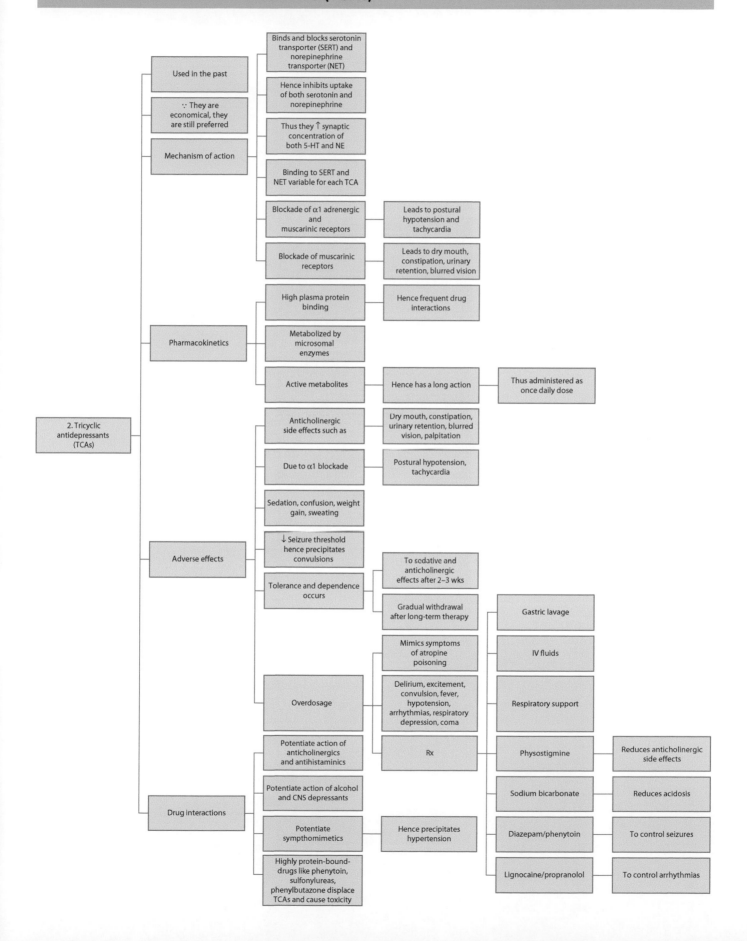

23.3 SELECTIVE SEROTONIN – NOREPINEPHRINE REUPTAKE INHIBITORS (SNRIs), 5-HT2 ANTAGONISTS, AND ATYPICAL ANTIDEPRESSANTS

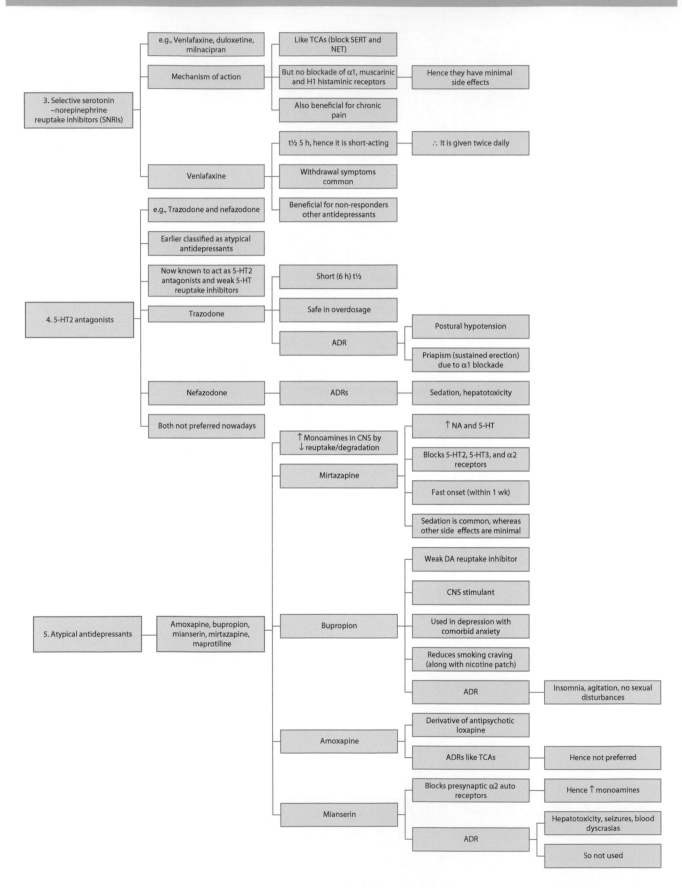

3. Selective serotonin –norepinephrine reuptake inhibitors (SNRIs)

- e.g., Venlafaxine, duloxetine, milnacipran
- Mechanism of action
  - Like TCAs (block SERT and NET)
  - But no blockade of α1, muscarinic and H1 histaminic receptors → Hence they have minimal side effects
  - Also beneficial for chronic pain
- Venlafaxine
  - t½ 5 h, hence it is short-acting → ∴ It is given twice daily
  - Withdrawal symptoms common
  - Beneficial for non-responders other antidepressants

4. 5-HT2 antagonists

- e.g., Trazodone and nefazodone
- Earlier classified as atypical antidepressants
- Now known to act as 5-HT2 antagonists and weak 5-HT reuptake inhibitors
- Trazodone
  - Short (6 h) t½
  - Safe in overdosage
  - ADR
    - Postural hypotension
    - Priapism (sustained erection) due to α1 blockade
- Nefazodone
  - ADRs → Sedation, hepatotoxicity
- Both not preferred nowadays

5. Atypical antidepressants

- Amoxapine, bupropion, mianserin, mirtazapine, maprotiline
  - Mirtazapine
    - ↑ Monoamines in CNS by ↓ reuptake/degradation → ↑ NA and 5-HT
    - Blocks 5-HT2, 5-HT3, and α2 receptors
    - Fast onset (within 1 wk)
    - Sedation is common, whereas other side effects are minimal
  - Bupropion
    - Weak DA reuptake inhibitor
    - CNS stimulant
    - Used in depression with comorbid anxiety
    - Reduces smoking craving (along with nicotine patch)
    - ADR → Insomnia, agitation, no sexual disturbances
  - Amoxapine
    - Derivative of antipsychotic loxapine
    - ADRs like TCAs → Hence not preferred
  - Mianserin
    - Blocks presynaptic α2 auto receptors → Hence ↑ monoamines
    - ADR
      - Hepatotoxicity, seizures, blood dyscrasias
      - So not used

23.4 MONOAMINE OXIDASE (MAO) INHIBITORS

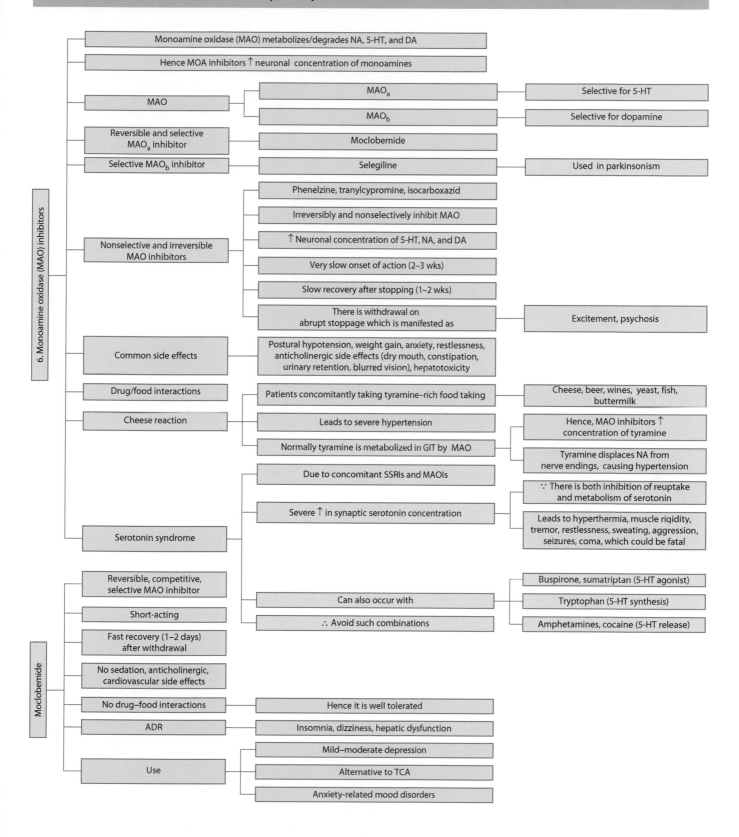

6. Monoamine oxidase (MAO) inhibitors

Monoamine oxidase (MAO) metabolizes/degrades NA, 5-HT, and DA

Hence MOA inhibitors ↑ neuronal concentration of monoamines

MAO
- MAO$_a$ — Selective for 5-HT
- MAO$_b$ — Selective for dopamine

Reversible and selective MAO$_a$ inhibitor — Moclobemide

Selective MAO$_b$ inhibitor — Selegiline — Used in parkinsonism

Nonselective and irreversible MAO inhibitors
- Phenelzine, tranylcypromine, isocarboxazid
- Irreversibly and nonselectively inhibit MAO
- ↑ Neuronal concentration of 5-HT, NA, and DA
- Very slow onset of action (2–3 wks)
- Slow recovery after stopping (1–2 wks)
- There is withdrawal on abrupt stoppage which is manifested as — Excitement, psychosis

Common side effects — Postural hypotension, weight gain, anxiety, restlessness, anticholinergic side effects (dry mouth, constipation, urinary retention, blurred vision), hepatotoxicity

Drug/food interactions

Cheese reaction
- Patients concomitantly taking tyramine–rich food taking — Cheese, beer, wines, yeast, fish, buttermilk
- Leads to severe hypertension — Hence, MAO inhibitors ↑ concentration of tyramine
- Normally tyramine is metabolized in GIT by MAO — Tyramine displaces NA from nerve endings, causing hypertension

Serotonin syndrome
- Due to concomitant SSRIs and MAOIs
- Severe ↑ in synaptic serotonin concentration
  - ∵ There is both inhibition of reuptake and metabolism of serotonin
  - Leads to hyperthermia, muscle rigidity, tremor, restlessness, sweating, aggression, seizures, coma, which could be fatal
- Can also occur with
  - Buspirone, sumatriptan (5-HT agonist)
  - Tryptophan (5-HT synthesis)
  - Amphetamines, cocaine (5-HT release)
- ∴ Avoid such combinations

Moclobemide

Reversible, competitive, selective MAO inhibitor

Short-acting

Fast recovery (1–2 days) after withdrawal

No sedation, anticholinergic, cardiovascular side effects

No drug–food interactions — Hence it is well tolerated

ADR — Insomnia, dizziness, hepatic dysfunction

Use
- Mild–moderate depression
- Alternative to TCA
- Anxiety-related mood disorders

23.5 USES OF ANTIDEPRESSANTS

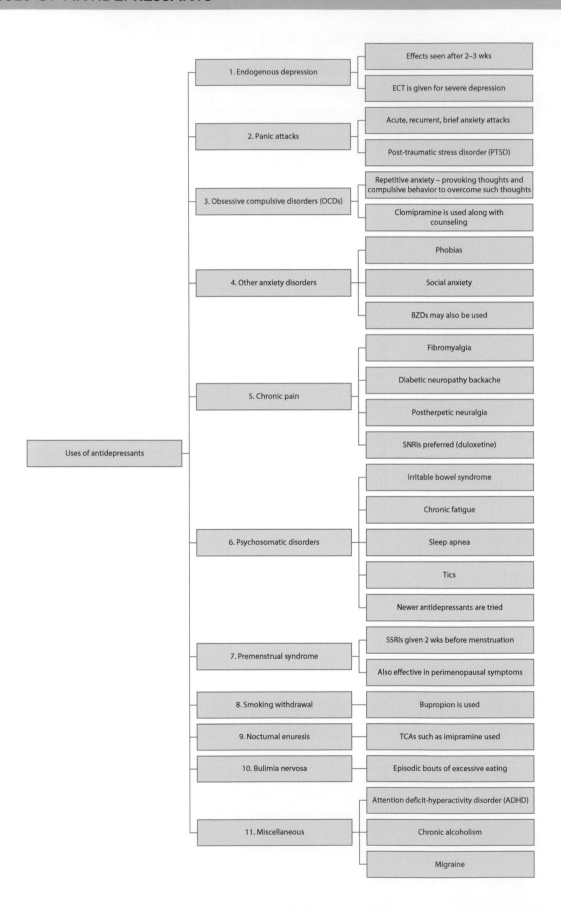

Uses of antidepressants

1. Endogenous depression
- Effects seen after 2–3 wks
- ECT is given for severe depression

2. Panic attacks
- Acute, recurrent, brief anxiety attacks
- Post-traumatic stress disorder (PTSD)

3. Obsessive compulsive disorders (OCDs)
- Repetitive anxiety – provoking thoughts and compulsive behavior to overcome such thoughts
- Clomipramine is used along with counseling

4. Other anxiety disorders
- Phobias
- Social anxiety
- BZDs may also be used

5. Chronic pain
- Fibromyalgia
- Diabetic neuropathy backache
- Postherpetic neuralgia
- SNRIs preferred (duloxetine)

6. Psychosomatic disorders
- Irritable bowel syndrome
- Chronic fatigue
- Sleep apnea
- Tics
- Newer antidepressants are tried

7. Premenstrual syndrome
- SSRIs given 2 wks before menstruation
- Also effective in perimenopausal symptoms

8. Smoking withdrawal
- Bupropion is used

9. Nocturnal enuresis
- TCAs such as imipramine used

10. Bulimia nervosa
- Episodic bouts of excessive eating

11. Miscellaneous
- Attention deficit-hyperactivity disorder (ADHD)
- Chronic alcoholism
- Migraine

24

Mood stabilizers and lithium

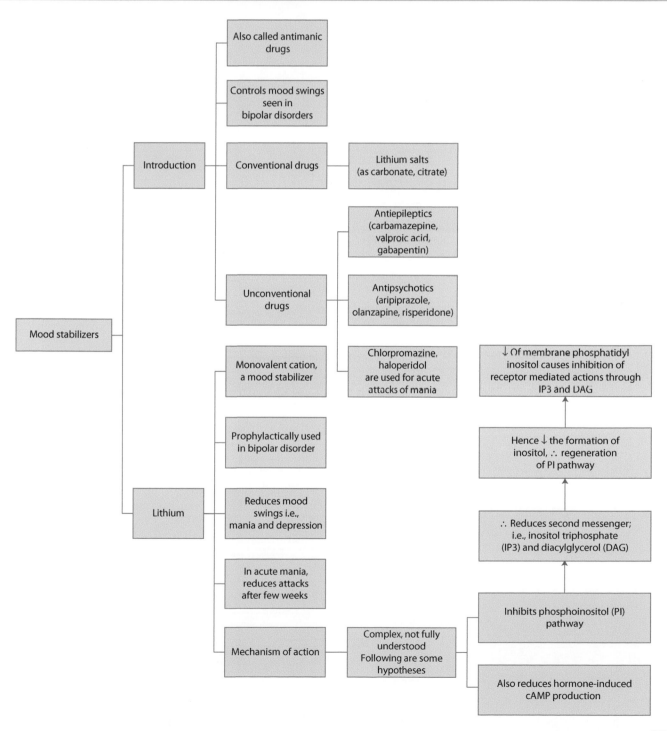

24.2 PHARMACOKINETICS, ADRs, AND USES

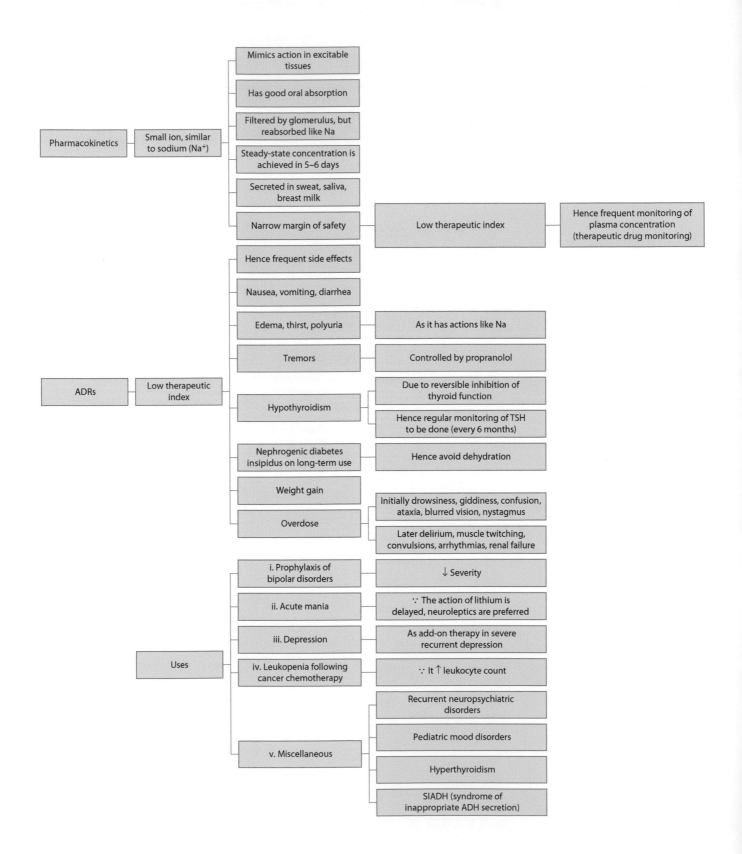

Pharmacokinetics — Small ion, similar to sodium (Na⁺)
- Mimics action in excitable tissues
- Has good oral absorption
- Filtered by glomerulus, but reabsorbed like Na
- Steady-state concentration is achieved in 5–6 days
- Secreted in sweat, saliva, breast milk
- Narrow margin of safety — Low therapeutic index — Hence frequent monitoring of plasma concentration (therapeutic drug monitoring)

ADRs — Low therapeutic index
- Hence frequent side effects
- Nausea, vomiting, diarrhea
- Edema, thirst, polyuria — As it has actions like Na
- Tremors — Controlled by propranolol
- Hypothyroidism
  - Due to reversible inhibition of thyroid function
  - Hence regular monitoring of TSH to be done (every 6 months)
- Nephrogenic diabetes insipidus on long-term use — Hence avoid dehydration
- Weight gain
- Overdose
  - Initially drowsiness, giddiness, confusion, ataxia, blurred vision, nystagmus
  - Later delirium, muscle twitching, convulsions, arrhythmias, renal failure

Uses
- i. Prophylaxis of bipolar disorders — ↓ Severity
- ii. Acute mania — ∵ The action of lithium is delayed, neuroleptics are preferred
- iii. Depression — As add-on therapy in severe recurrent depression
- iv. Leukopenia following cancer chemotherapy — ∵ It ↑ leukocyte count
- v. Miscellaneous
  - Recurrent neuropsychiatric disorders
  - Pediatric mood disorders
  - Hyperthyroidism
  - SIADH (syndrome of inappropriate ADH secretion)

24.3 RILUZOLE AND NONCONVENTIONAL MOOD STABILIZERS

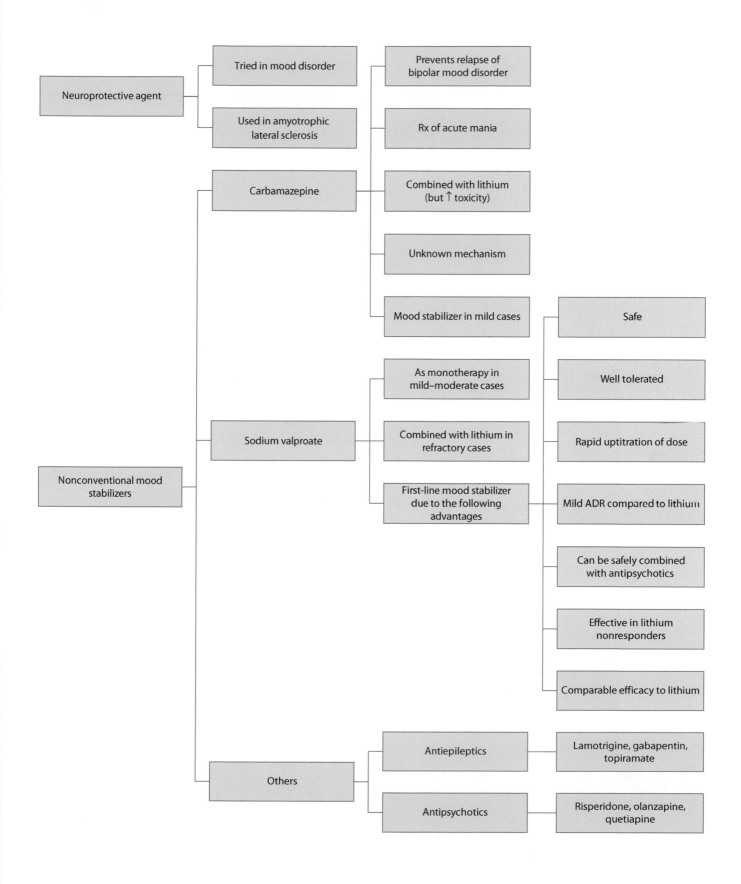

25

Antipsychotics

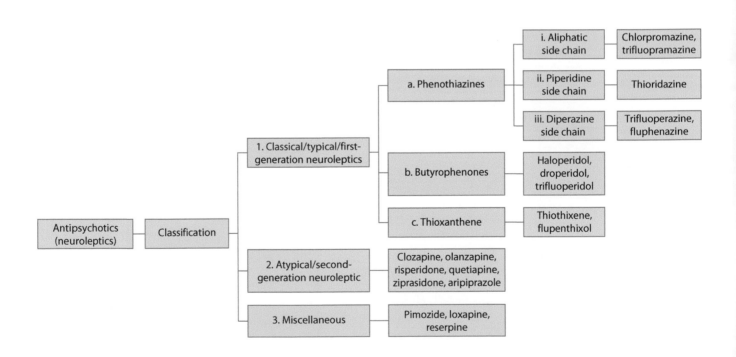

25.2 CHLORPROMAZINE (CPZ) – MECHANISM OF ACTION

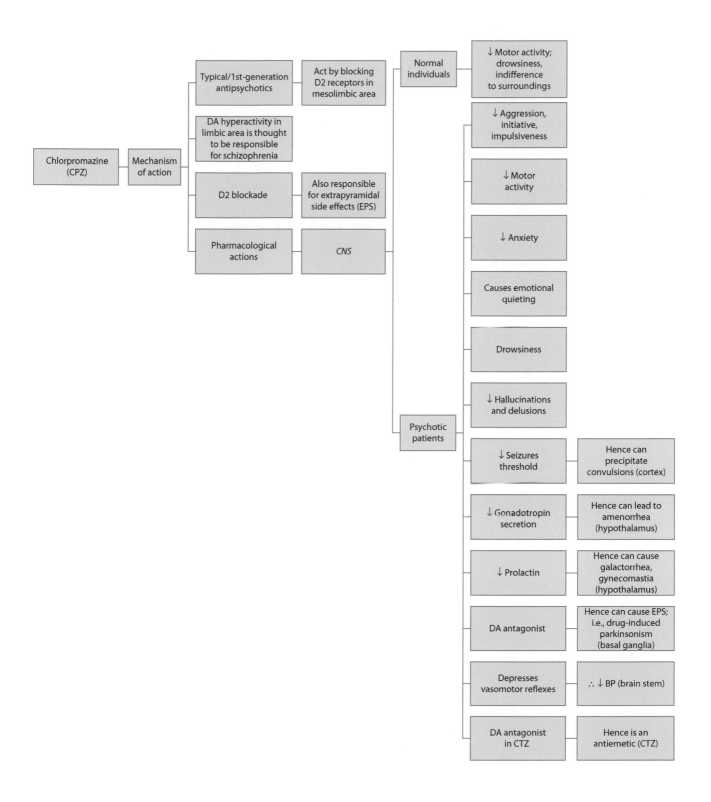

(Continued)

25.2 CHLORPROMAZINE (CPZ) – PHARMACOLOGICAL ACTIONS (Continued)

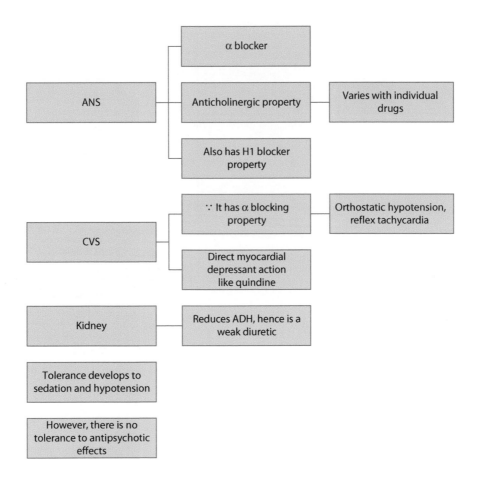

25.3 ADVERSE EFFECTS

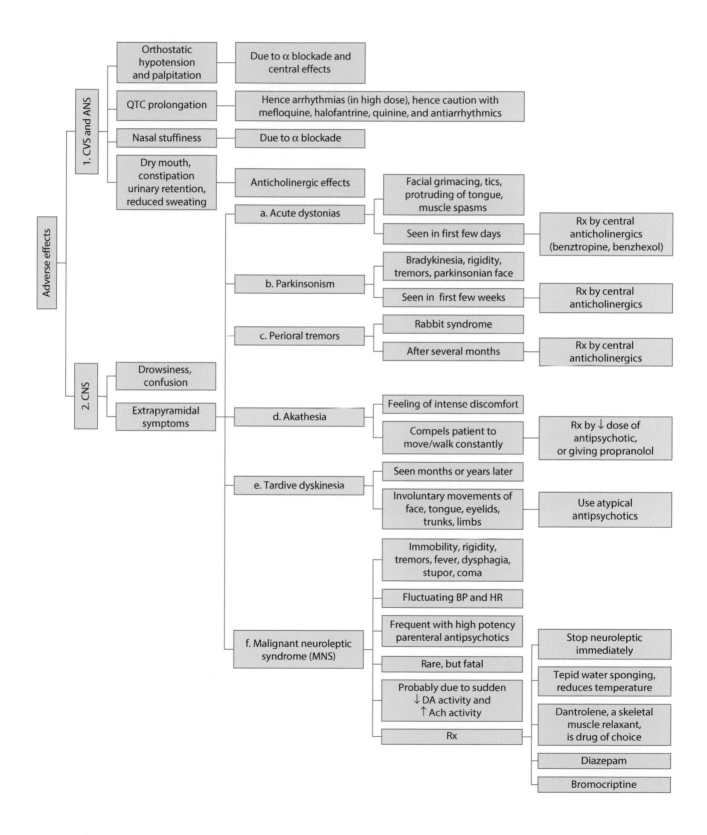

(Continued)

25.3 ADVERSE EFFECTS (Continued)

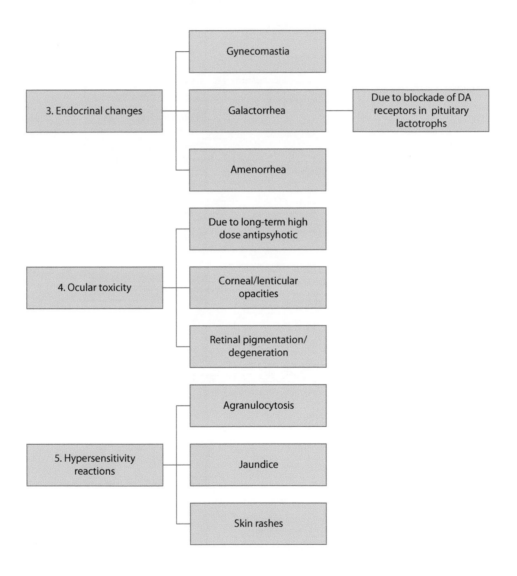

25.4 DRUG INTERACTIONS AND USES

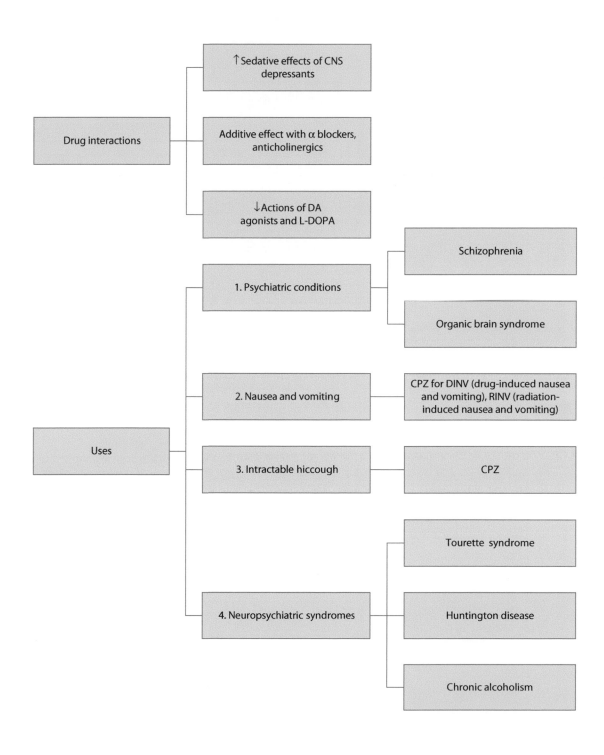

25.5 INDIVIDUAL ANTIPSYCHOTICS

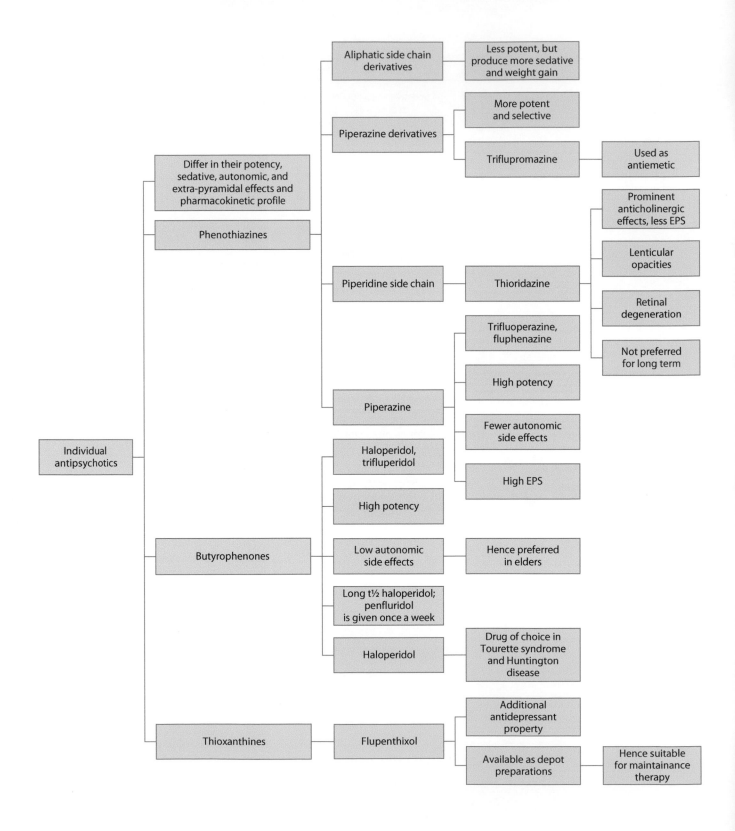

25.6 ATYPICAL ANTIPSYCHOTICS

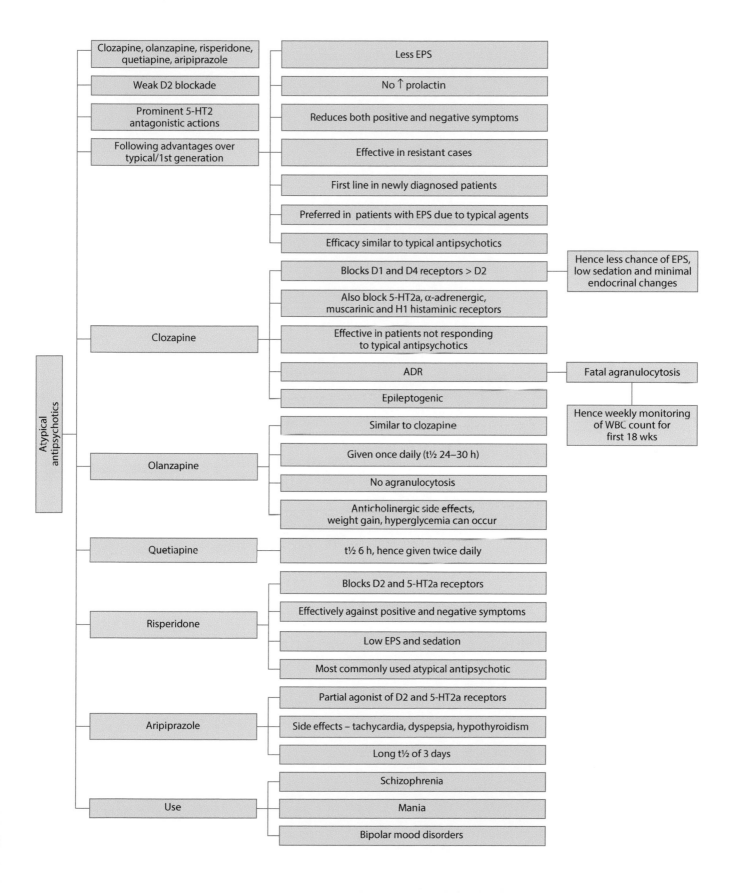

Atypical antipsychotics

- Clozapine, olanzapine, risperidone, quetiapine, aripiprazole
- Weak D2 blockade
- Prominent 5-HT2 antagonistic actions
- Following advantages over typical/1st generation
  - Less EPS
  - No ↑ prolactin
  - Reduces both positive and negative symptoms
  - Effective in resistant cases
  - First line in newly diagnosed patients
  - Preferred in patients with EPS due to typical agents
  - Efficacy similar to typical antipsychotics

- Clozapine
  - Blocks D1 and D4 receptors > D2 → Hence less chance of EPS, low sedation and minimal endocrinal changes
  - Also block 5-HT2a, α-adrenergic, muscarinic and H1 histaminic receptors
  - Effective in patients not responding to typical antipsychotics
  - ADR → Fatal agranulocytosis → Hence weekly monitoring of WBC count for first 18 wks
  - Epileptogenic

- Olanzapine
  - Similar to clozapine
  - Given once daily (t½ 24–30 h)
  - No agranulocytosis
  - Anticholinergic side effects, weight gain, hyperglycemia can occur

- Quetiapine
  - t½ 6 h, hence given twice daily

- Risperidone
  - Blocks D2 and 5-HT2a receptors
  - Effectively against positive and negative symptoms
  - Low EPS and sedation
  - Most commonly used atypical antipsychotic

- Aripiprazole
  - Partial agonist of D2 and 5-HT2a receptors
  - Side effects – tachycardia, dyspepsia, hypothyroidism
  - Long t½ of 3 days

- Use
  - Schizophrenia
  - Mania
  - Bipolar mood disorders

25.7 OTHER ANTIPSYCHOTICS

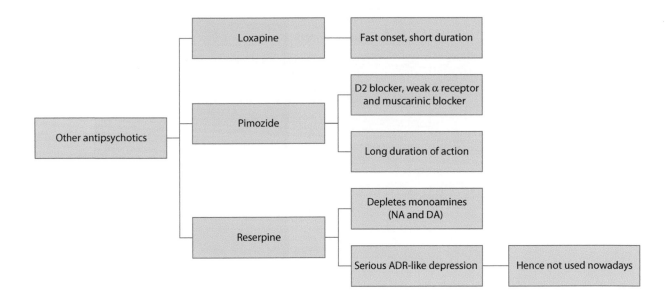

25.8 ANXIOLYTICS (NONBENZODIAZEPINES)

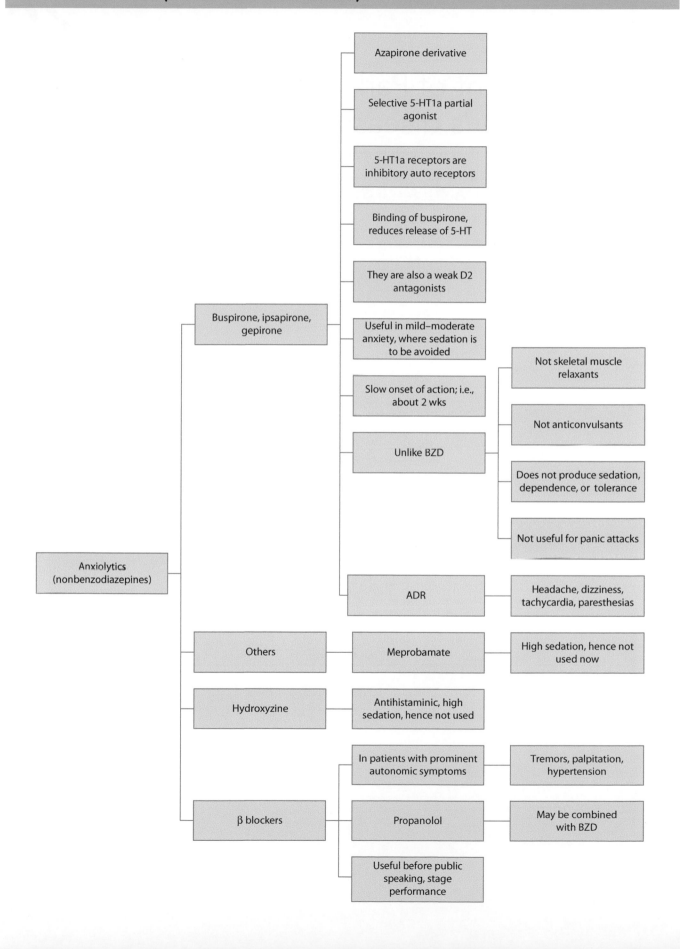

Anxiolytics (nonbenzodiazepines)

- Buspirone, ipsapirone, gepirone
  - Azapirone derivative
  - Selective 5-HT1a partial agonist
  - 5-HT1a receptors are inhibitory auto receptors
  - Binding of buspirone, reduces release of 5-HT
  - They are also a weak D2 antagonists
  - Useful in mild–moderate anxiety, where sedation is to be avoided
  - Slow onset of action; i.e., about 2 wks
  - Unlike BZD
    - Not skeletal muscle relaxants
    - Not anticonvulsants
    - Does not produce sedation, dependence, or tolerance
    - Not useful for panic attacks
  - ADR
    - Headache, dizziness, tachycardia, paresthesias
- Others
  - Meprobamate
    - High sedation, hence not used now
- Hydroxyzine
  - Antihistaminic, high sedation, hence not used
- β blockers
  - In patients with prominent autonomic symptoms
    - Tremors, palpitation, hypertension
  - Propanolol
    - May be combined with BZD
  - Useful before public speaking, stage performance

Drug treatment of Parkinsonism and Alzheimer's disease

26.1 CLASSIFICATION OF ANTIPARKINSONIAN DRUGS

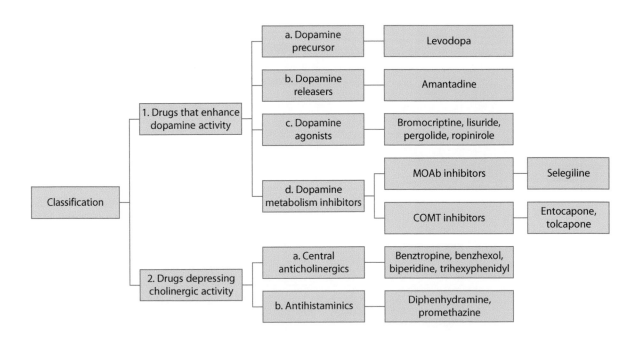

26.2 DOPAMINE PRECURSOR – LEVODOPA

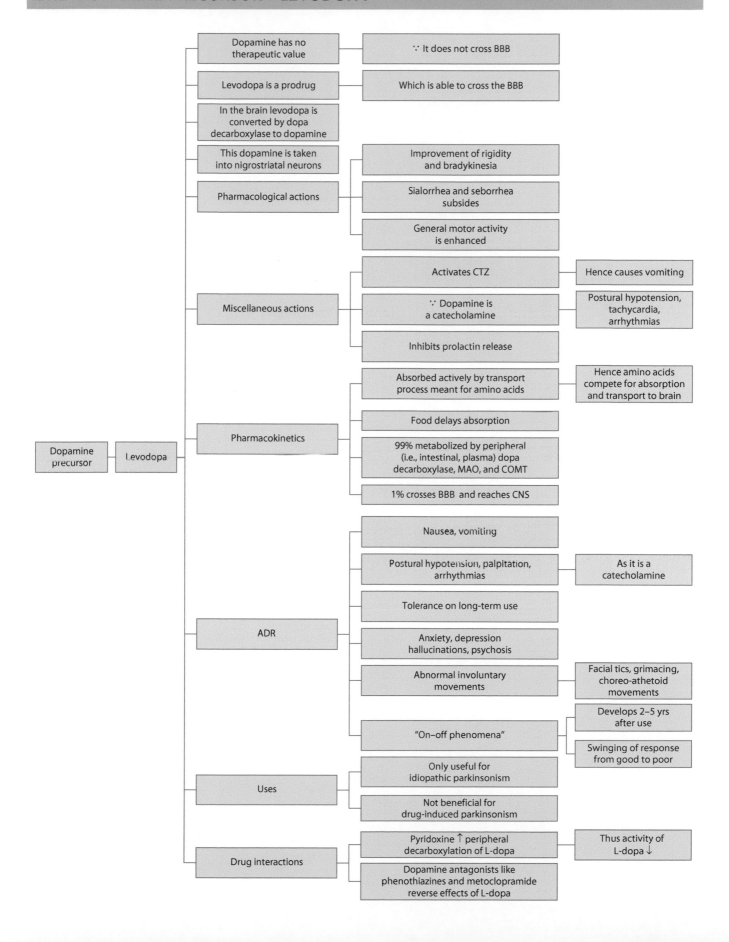

26.3 CARBIDOPA AND BENSERAZIDE, DOPAMINE RELEASERS

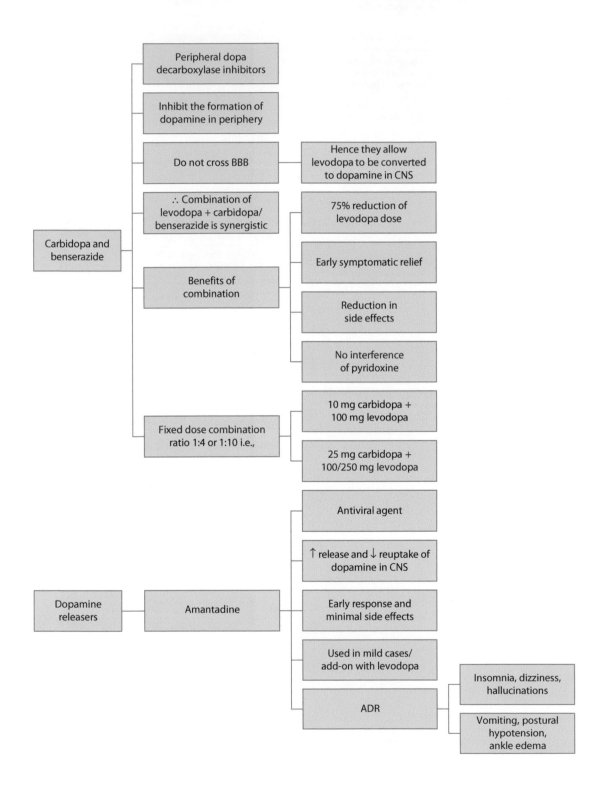

26.4 DOPAMINE RECEPTOR AGONISTS AND DOPAMINE METABOLISM INHIBITORS

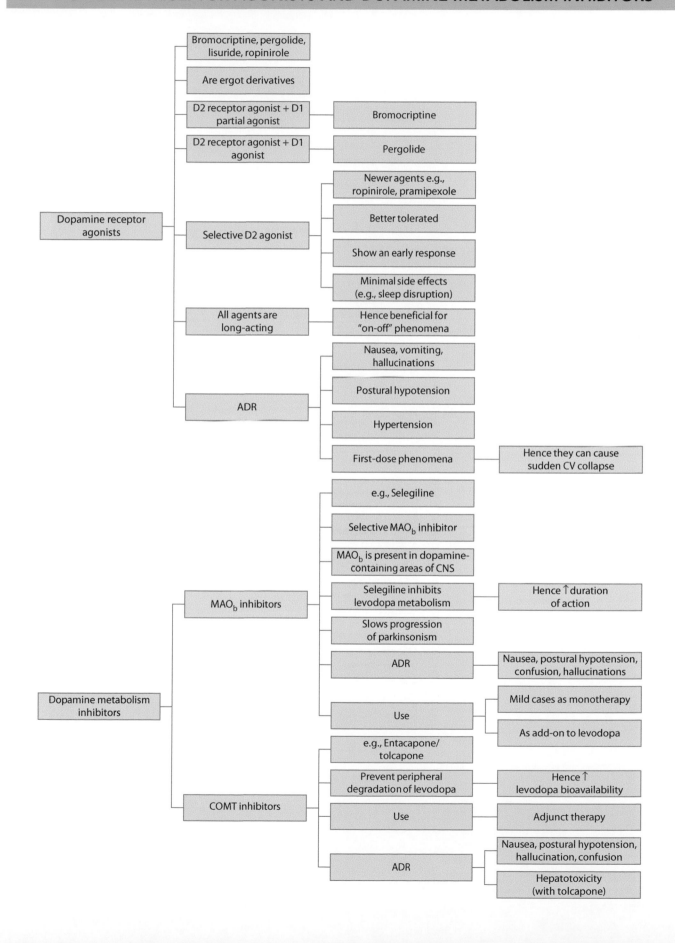

26.5 CENTRAL ANTICHOLINERGICS AND DRUG-INDUCED PARKINSONISM

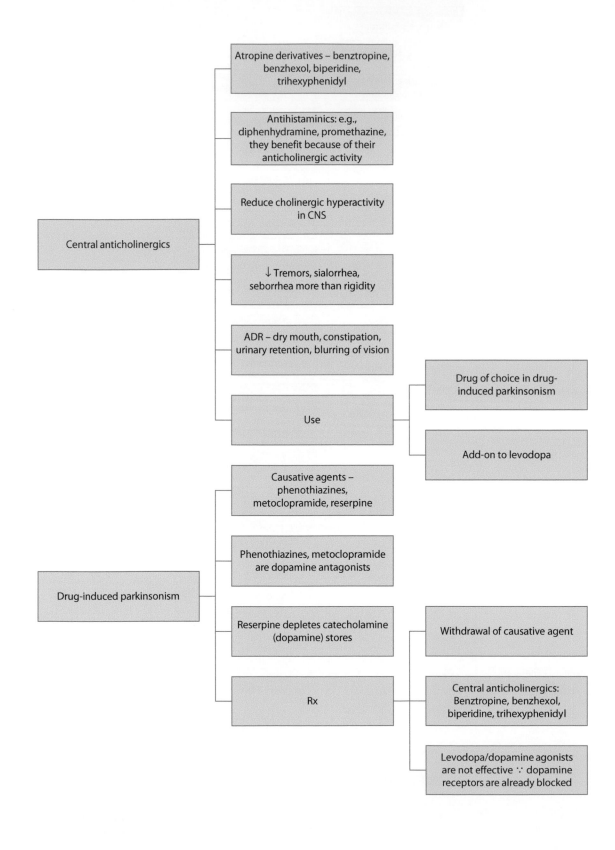

26.6 DRUGS FOR ALZHEIMER'S DISEASE (AD)

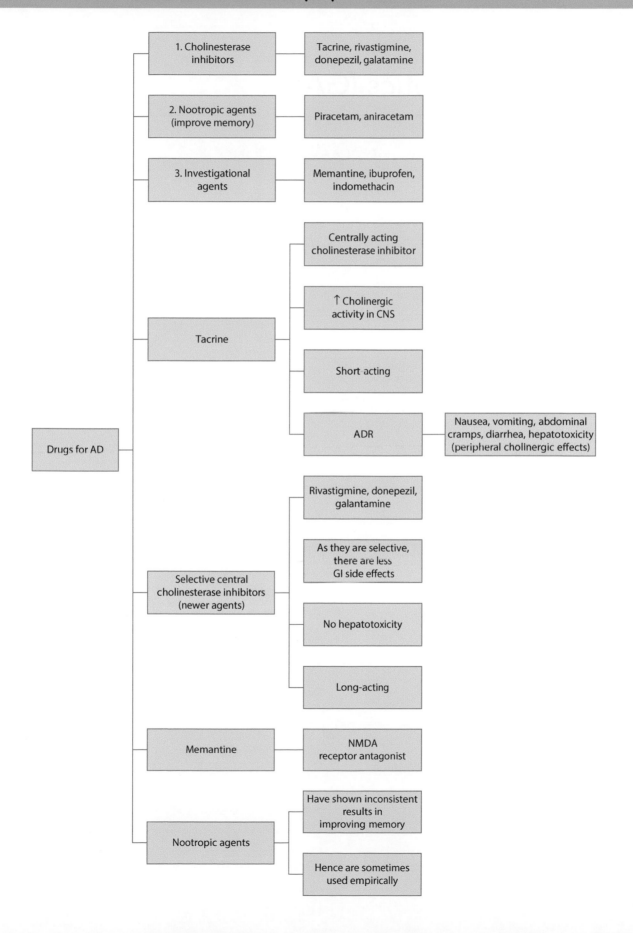

General anesthetics (GA)

27.1 MECHANISM OF ACTION AND CLASSIFICATION

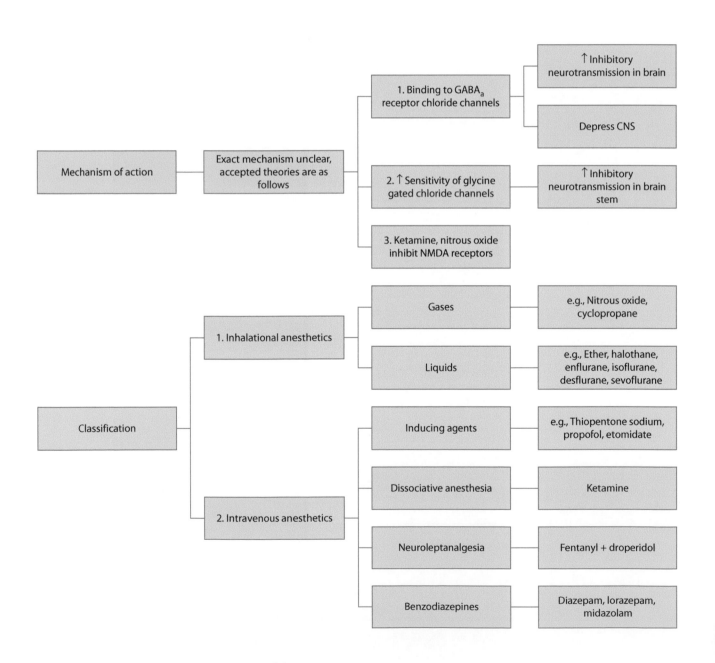

27.2 INHALATIONAL ANESTHETICS AND FACTORS DETERMINING ANESTHETIC PP IN BRAIN

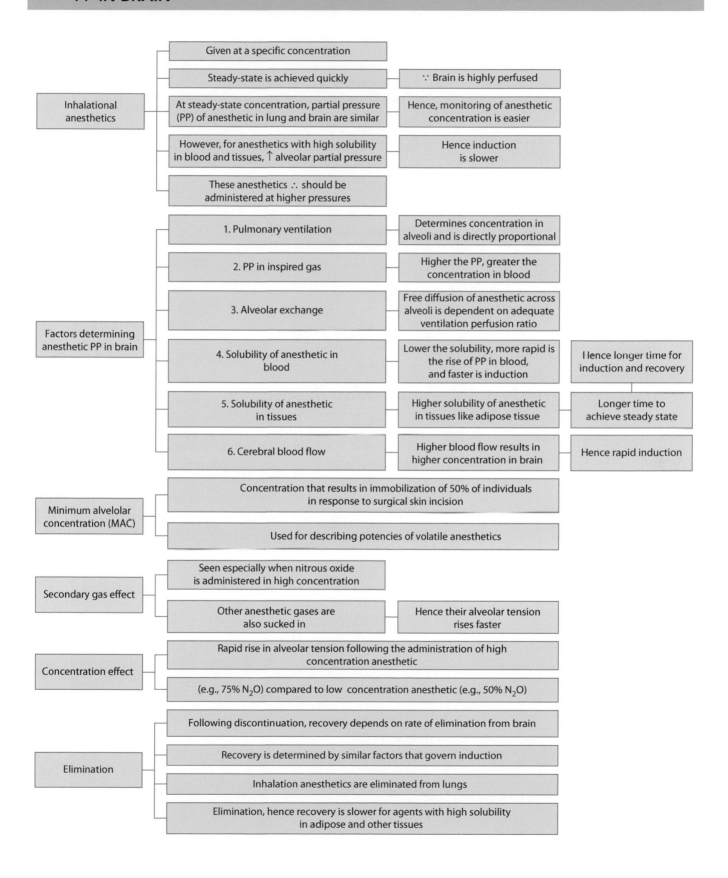

27.3 NITROUS OXIDE

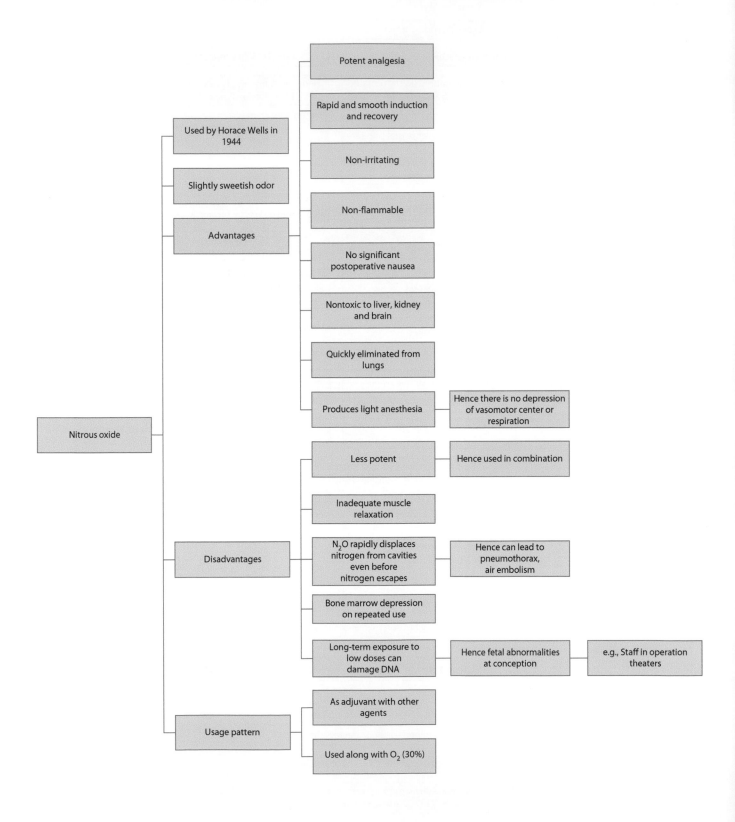

Nitrous oxide

- Used by Horace Wells in 1944
- Slightly sweetish odor
- Advantages
  - Potent analgesia
  - Rapid and smooth induction and recovery
  - Non-irritating
  - Non-flammable
  - No significant postoperative nausea
  - Nontoxic to liver, kidney and brain
  - Quickly eliminated from lungs
  - Produces light anesthesia → Hence there is no depression of vasomotor center or respiration
- Disadvantages
  - Less potent → Hence used in combination
  - Inadequate muscle relaxation
  - N_2O rapidly displaces nitrogen from cavities even before nitrogen escapes → Hence can lead to pneumothorax, air embolism
  - Bone marrow depression on repeated use
  - Long-term exposure to low doses can damage DNA → Hence fetal abnormalities at conception → e.g., Staff in operation theaters
- Usage pattern
  - As adjuvant with other agents
  - Used along with O_2 (30%)

27.4 HALOTHANE AND CONGENERS

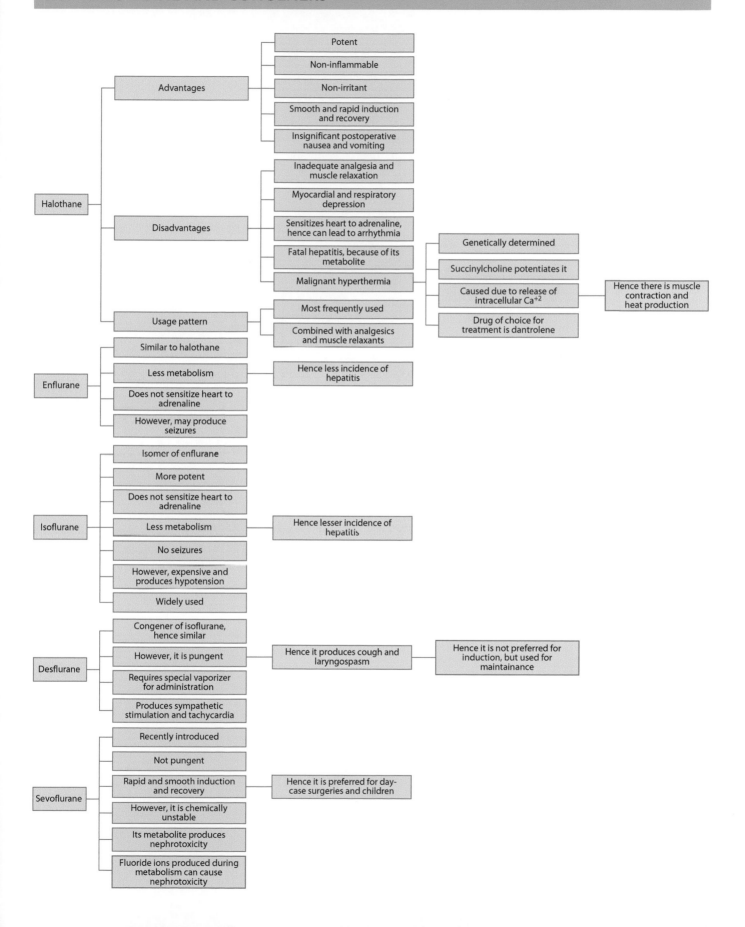

Halothane

Advantages
- Potent
- Non-inflammable
- Non-irritant
- Smooth and rapid induction and recovery
- Insignificant postoperative nausea and vomiting

Disadvantages
- Inadequate analgesia and muscle relaxation
- Myocardial and respiratory depression
- Sensitizes heart to adrenaline, hence can lead to arrhythmia
- Fatal hepatitis, because of its metabolite
- Malignant hyperthermia
  - Genetically determined
  - Succinylcholine potentiates it
  - Caused due to release of intracellular Ca^{+2} — Hence there is muscle contraction and heat production
  - Drug of choice for treatment is dantrolene

Usage pattern
- Most frequently used
- Combined with analgesics and muscle relaxants

Enflurane
- Similar to halothane
- Less metabolism — Hence less incidence of hepatitis
- Does not sensitize heart to adrenaline
- However, may produce seizures

Isoflurane
- Isomer of enflurane
- More potent
- Does not sensitize heart to adrenaline
- Less metabolism — Hence lesser incidence of hepatitis
- No seizures
- However, expensive and produces hypotension
- Widely used

Desflurane
- Congener of isoflurane, hence similar
- However, it is pungent — Hence it produces cough and laryngospasm — Hence it is not preferred for induction, but used for maintainance
- Requires special vaporizer for administration
- Produces sympathetic stimulation and tachycardia

Sevoflurane
- Recently introduced
- Not pungent
- Rapid and smooth induction and recovery — Hence it is preferred for day-case surgeries and children
- However, it is chemically unstable
- Its metabolite produces nephrotoxicity
- Fluoride ions produced during metabolism can cause nephrotoxicity

27.5 INTRAVENOUS ANESTHETICS AND INDUCING AGENTS

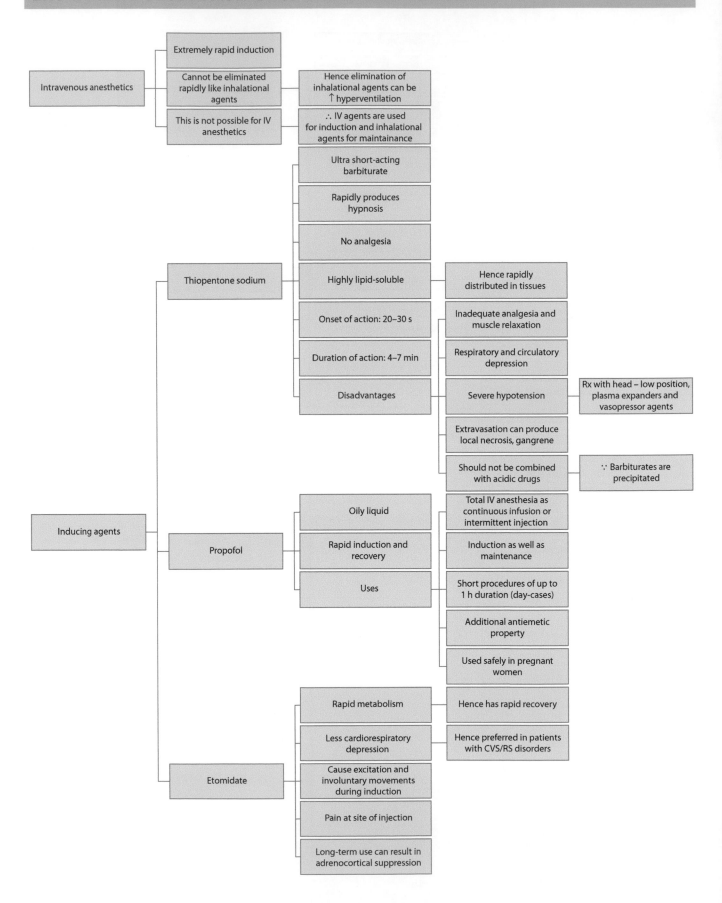

27.6 DISSOCIATIVE ANESTHESIA (KETAMINE)

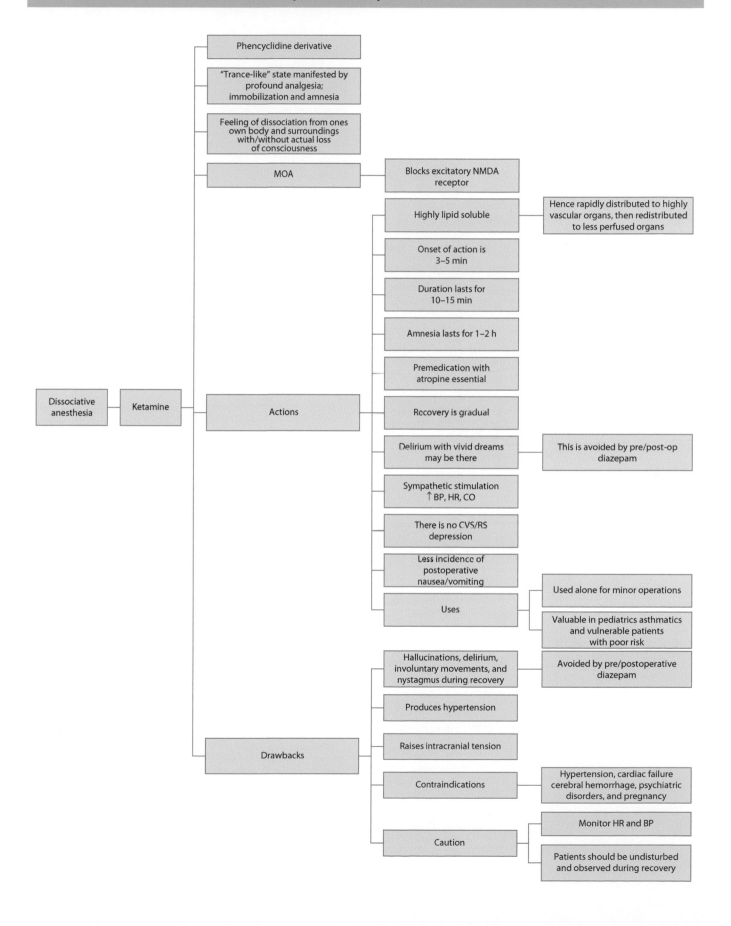

Dissociative anesthesia — Ketamine

- Phencyclidine derivative
- "Trance-like" state manifested by profound analgesia; immobilization and amnesia
- Feeling of dissociation from ones own body and surroundings with/without actual loss of consciousness
- MOA
  - Blocks excitatory NMDA receptor
- Actions
  - Highly lipid soluble — Hence rapidly distributed to highly vascular organs, then redistributed to less perfused organs
  - Onset of action is 3–5 min
  - Duration lasts for 10–15 min
  - Amnesia lasts for 1–2 h
  - Premedication with atropine essential
  - Recovery is gradual
  - Delirium with vivid dreams may be there — This is avoided by pre/post-op diazepam
  - Sympathetic stimulation ↑ BP, HR, CO
  - There is no CVS/RS depression
  - Less incidence of postoperative nausea/vomiting
  - Uses
    - Used alone for minor operations
    - Valuable in pediatrics asthmatics and vulnerable patients with poor risk
- Drawbacks
  - Hallucinations, delirium, involuntary movements, and nystagmus during recovery — Avoided by pre/postoperative diazepam
  - Produces hypertension
  - Raises intracranial tension
  - Contraindications — Hypertension, cardiac failure cerebral hemorrhage, psychiatric disorders, and pregnancy
  - Caution
    - Monitor HR and BP
    - Patients should be undisturbed and observed during recovery

27.7 NEUROLEPTANALGESIA AND BENZODIAZEPINES

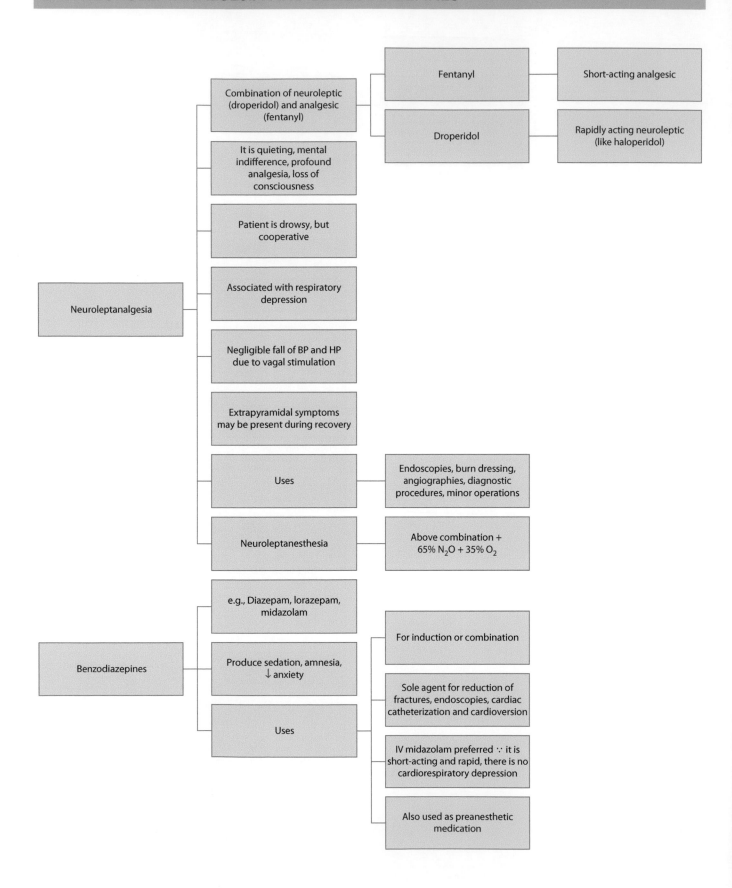

27.8 PREANESTHETIC MEDICATION AND BALANCED ANESTHESIA

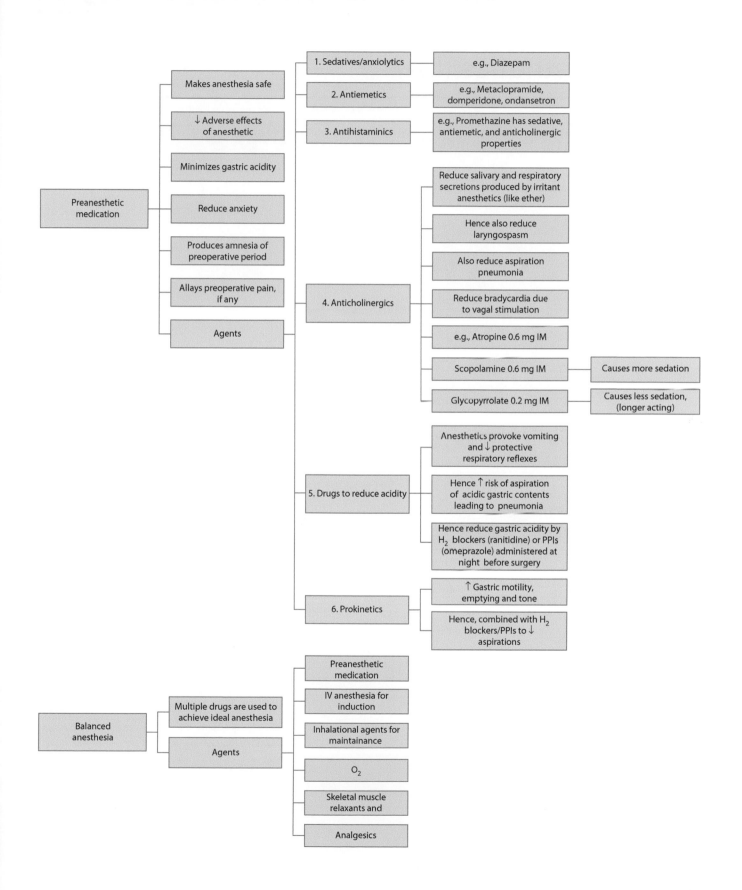

Local anesthetics (LA)

28.1 LOCAL ANESTHETICS (LA) – INTRODUCTION, HISTORY, AND CLASSIFICATION

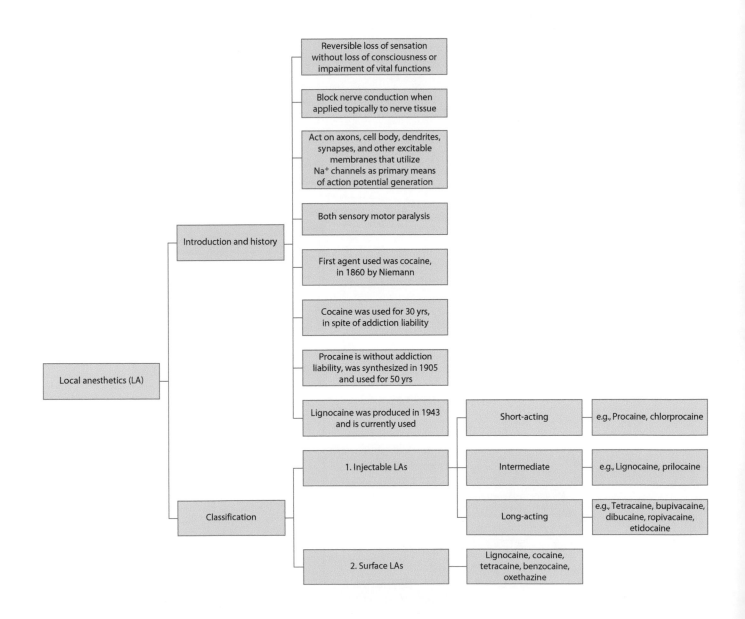

Local anesthetics (LA)

Introduction and history
- Reversible loss of sensation without loss of consciousness or impairment of vital functions
- Block nerve conduction when applied topically to nerve tissue
- Act on axons, cell body, dendrites, synapses, and other excitable membranes that utilize Na⁺ channels as primary means of action potential generation
- Both sensory motor paralysis
- First agent used was cocaine, in 1860 by Niemann
- Cocaine was used for 30 yrs, in spite of addiction liability
- Procaine is without addiction liability, was synthesized in 1905 and used for 50 yrs
- Lignocaine was produced in 1943 and is currently used

Classification
- 1. Injectable LAs
  - Short-acting — e.g., Procaine, chlorprocaine
  - Intermediate — e.g., Lignocaine, prilocaine
  - Long-acting — e.g., Tetracaine, bupivacaine, dibucaine, ropivacaine, etidocaine
- 2. Surface LAs
  - Lignocaine, cocaine, tetracaine, benzocaine, oxethazine

28.2 CHEMISTRY AND MECHANISM OF ACTION

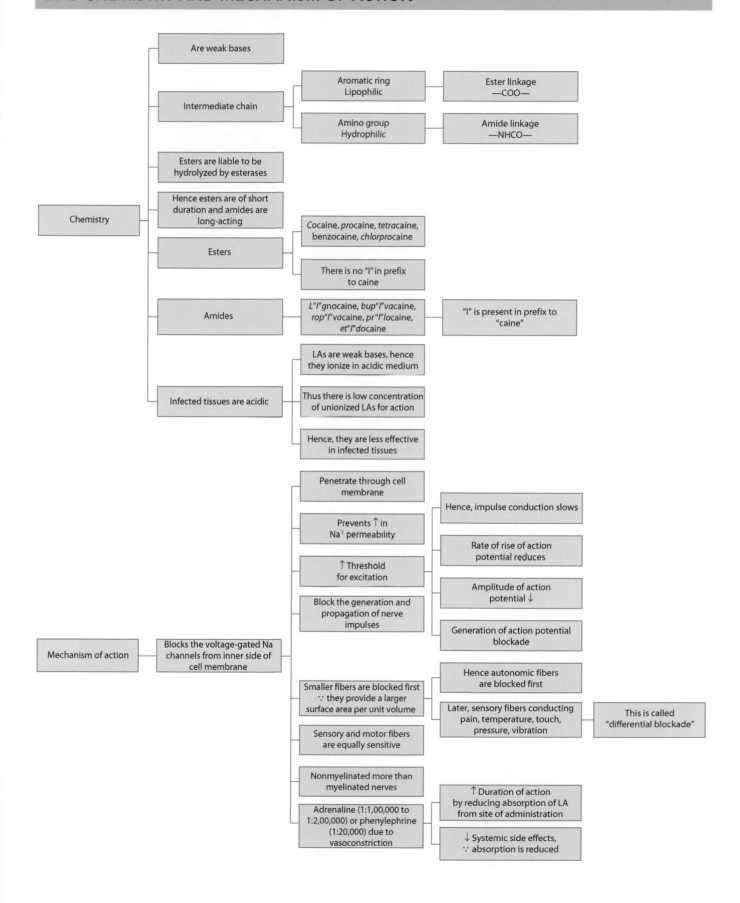

28.3 ACTIONS, PHARMACOKINETICS, AND ADRs

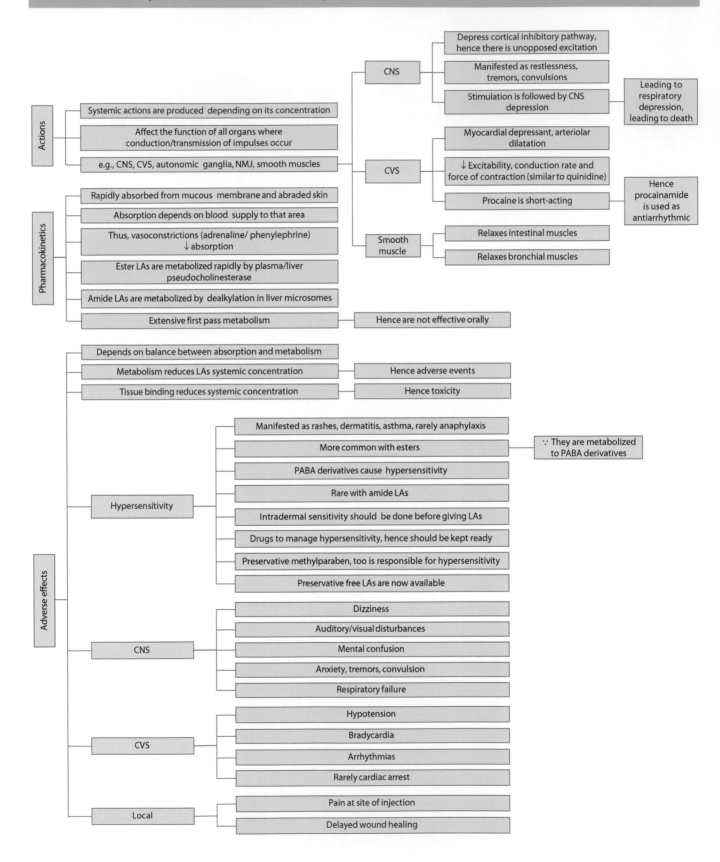

Actions

- Systemic actions are produced depending on its concentration
- Affect the function of all organs where conduction/transmission of impulses occur
- e.g., CNS, CVS, autonomic ganglia, NMJ, smooth muscles

CNS
- Depress cortical inhibitory pathway, hence there is unopposed excitation
- Manifested as restlessness, tremors, convulsions
- Stimulation is followed by CNS depression — Leading to respiratory depression, leading to death

CVS
- Myocardial depressant, arteriolar dilatation
- ↓ Excitability, conduction rate and force of contraction (similar to quinidine)
- Procaine is short-acting — Hence procainamide is used as antiarrhythmic

Smooth muscle
- Relaxes intestinal muscles
- Relaxes bronchial muscles

Pharmacokinetics

- Rapidly absorbed from mucous membrane and abraded skin
- Absorption depends on blood supply to that area
- Thus, vasoconstrictions (adrenaline/ phenylephrine) ↓ absorption
- Ester LAs are metabolized rapidly by plasma/liver pseudocholinesterase
- Amide LAs are metabolized by dealkylation in liver microsomes
- Extensive first pass metabolism — Hence are not effective orally
- Depends on balance between absorption and metabolism
- Metabolism reduces LAs systemic concentration — Hence adverse events
- Tissue binding reduces systemic concentration — Hence toxicity

Adverse effects

Hypersensitivity
- Manifested as rashes, dermatitis, asthma, rarely anaphylaxis
- More common with esters — ∵ They are metabolized to PABA derivatives
- PABA derivatives cause hypersensitivity
- Rare with amide LAs
- Intradermal sensitivity should be done before giving LAs
- Drugs to manage hypersensitivity, hence should be kept ready
- Preservative methylparaben, too is responsible for hypersensitivity
- Preservative free LAs are now available

CNS
- Dizziness
- Auditory/visual disturbances
- Mental confusion
- Anxiety, tremors, convulsion
- Respiratory failure

CVS
- Hypotension
- Bradycardia
- Arrhythmias
- Rarely cardiac arrest

Local
- Pain at site of injection
- Delayed wound healing

28.4 INDIVIDUAL AGENTS

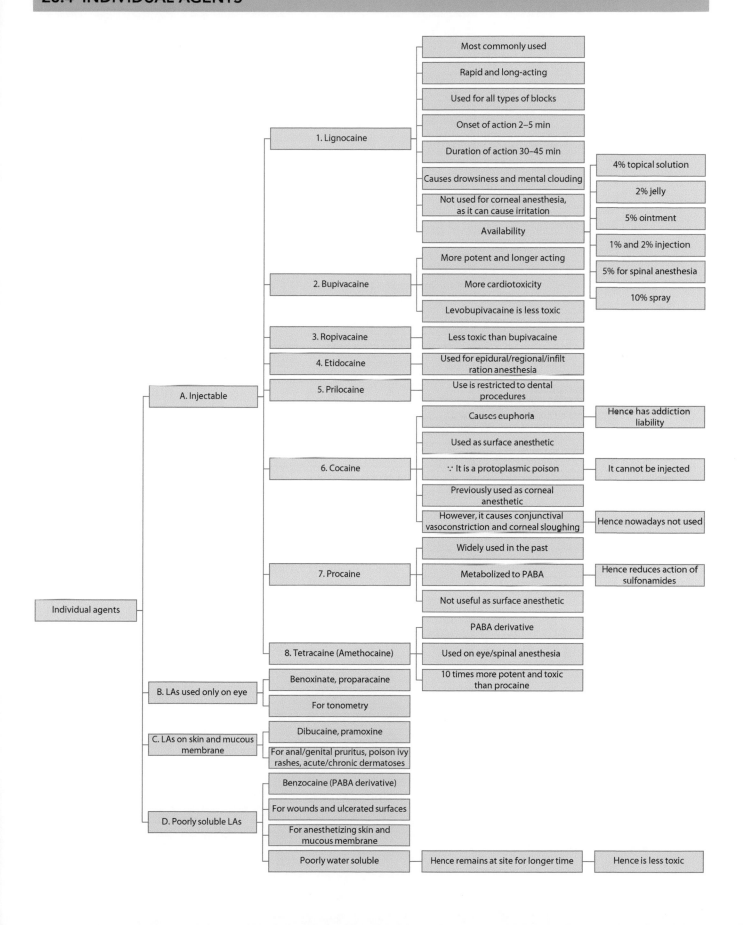

28.5 USES OF LAs

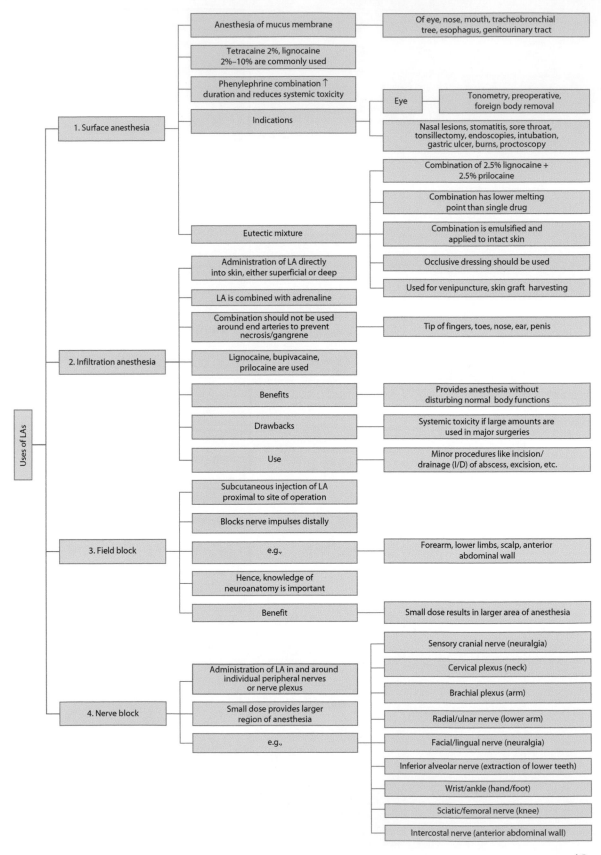

(Continued)

28.5 USES OF LAs (Continued)

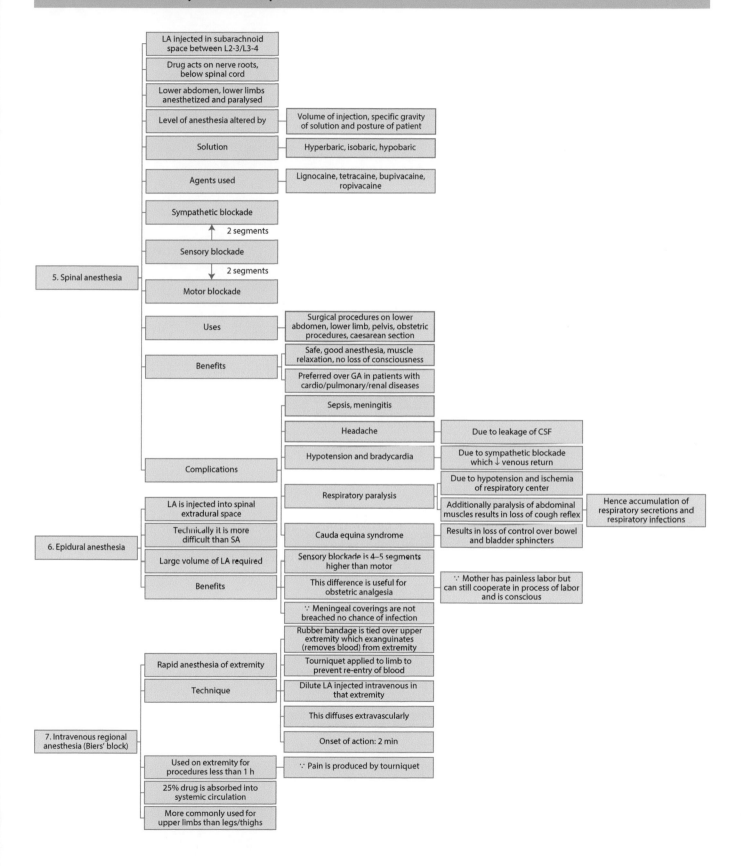

5. Spinal anesthesia

- LA injected in subarachnoid space between L2-3/L3-4
- Drug acts on nerve roots, below spinal cord
- Lower abdomen, lower limbs anesthetized and paralysed
- Level of anesthesia altered by — Volume of injection, specific gravity of solution and posture of patient
- Solution — Hyperbaric, isobaric, hypobaric
- Agents used — Lignocaine, tetracaine, bupivacaine, ropivacaine
- Sympathetic blockade
  - ↑ 2 segments
- Sensory blockade
  - ↓ 2 segments
- Motor blockade
- Uses — Surgical procedures on lower abdomen, lower limb, pelvis, obstetric procedures, caesarean section
- Benefits
  - Safe, good anesthesia, muscle relaxation, no loss of consciousness
  - Preferred over GA in patients with cardio/pulmonary/renal diseases
- Complications
  - Sepsis, meningitis
  - Headache — Due to leakage of CSF
  - Hypotension and bradycardia — Due to sympathetic blockade which ↓ venous return
  - Respiratory paralysis
    - Due to hypotension and ischemia of respiratory center
    - Additionally paralysis of abdominal muscles results in loss of cough reflex — Hence accumulation of respiratory secretions and respiratory infections
  - Cauda equina syndrome — Results in loss of control over bowel and bladder sphincters

6. Epidural anesthesia

- LA is injected into spinal extradural space
- Technically it is more difficult than SA
- Large volume of LA required
- Benefits
  - Sensory blockade is 4–5 segments higher than motor
  - This difference is useful for obstetric analgesia — ∵ Mother has painless labor but can still cooperate in process of labor and is conscious
  - ∵ Meningeal coverings are not breached no chance of infection

7. Intravenous regional anesthesia (Biers' block)

- Rapid anesthesia of extremity
- Technique
  - Rubber bandage is tied over upper extremity which exanguinates (removes blood) from extremity
  - Tourniquet applied to limb to prevent re-entry of blood
  - Dilute LA injected intravenous in that extremity
  - This diffuses extravascularly
  - Onset of action: 2 min
- Used on extremity for procedures less than 1 h — ∵ Pain is produced by tourniquet
- 25% drug is absorbed into systemic circulation
- More commonly used for upper limbs than legs/thighs

Opioid analgesics

29

29.1 OPIOID ANALGESICS CLASSIFICATION

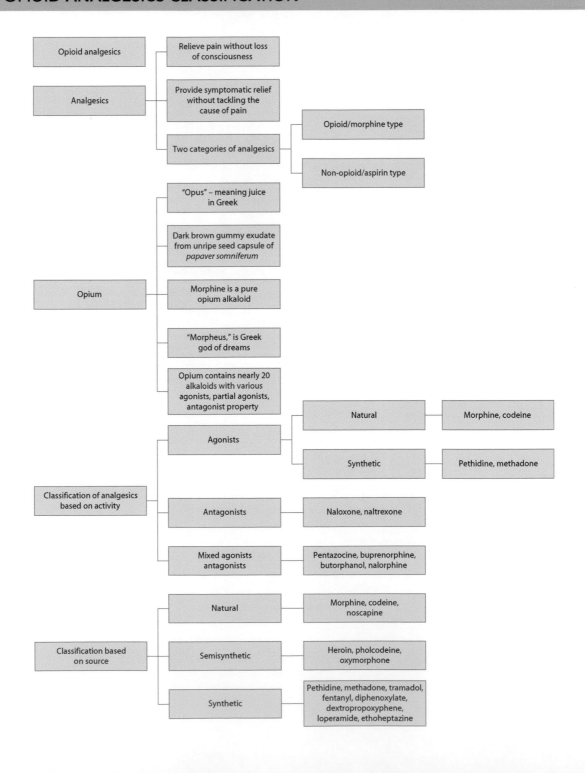

Opioid analgesics → Relieve pain without loss of consciousness

Analgesics → Provide symptomatic relief without tackling the cause of pain

Two categories of analgesics → Opioid/morphine type; Non-opioid/aspirin type

Opium:
- "Opus" – meaning juice in Greek
- Dark brown gummy exudate from unripe seed capsule of *papaver somniferum*
- Morphine is a pure opium alkaloid
- "Morpheus," is Greek god of dreams
- Opium contains nearly 20 alkaloids with various agonists, partial agonists, antagonist property

Classification of analgesics based on activity:
- Agonists → Natural → Morphine, codeine; Synthetic → Pethidine, methadone
- Antagonists → Naloxone, naltrexone
- Mixed agonists antagonists → Pentazocine, buprenorphine, butorphanol, nalorphine

Classification based on source:
- Natural → Morphine, codeine, noscapine
- Semisynthetic → Heroin, pholcodeine, oxymorphone
- Synthetic → Pethidine, methadone, tramadol, fentanyl, diphenoxylate, dextropropoxyphene, loperamide, ethoheptazine

29.2 MORPHINE AND MECHANISM OF ACTION

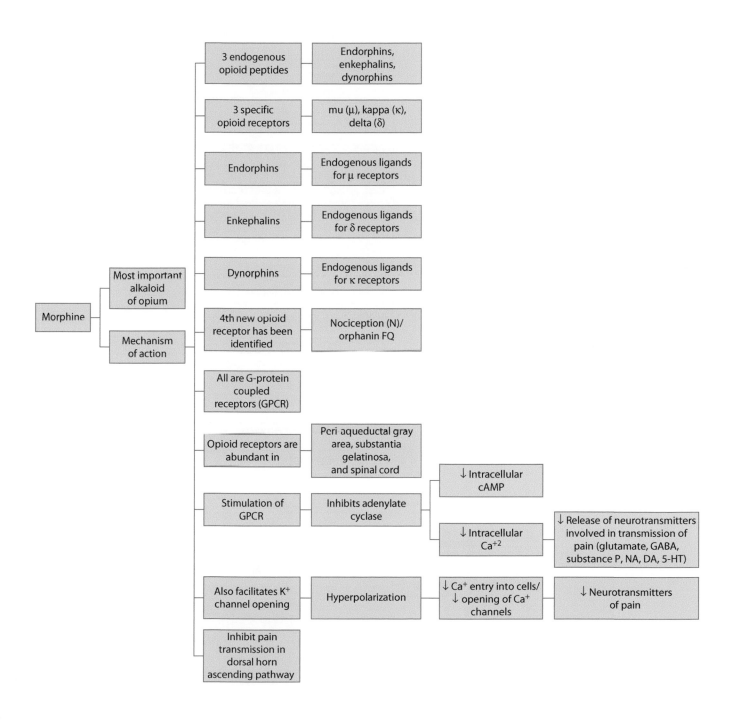

29.3 PHARMACOLOGICAL ACTIONS

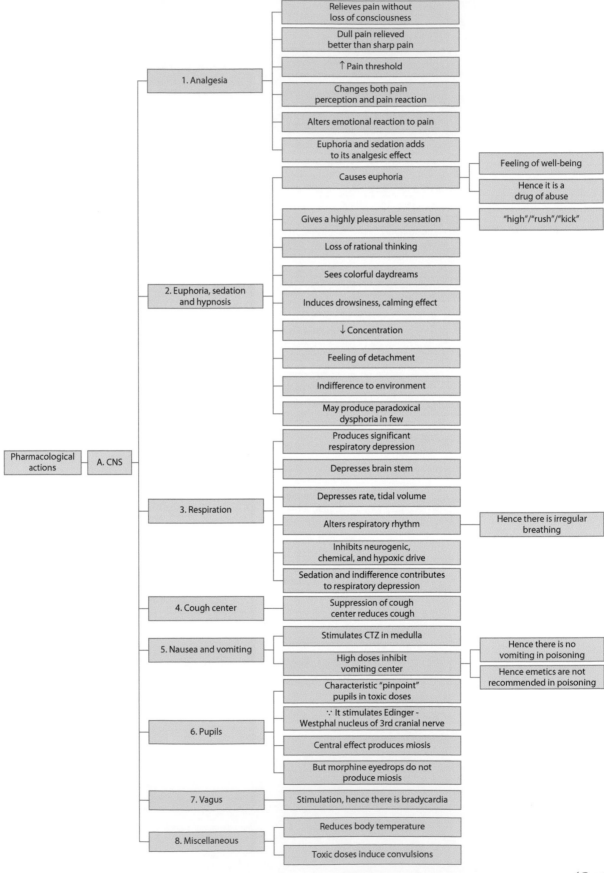

(Continued)

29.3 PHARMACOLOGICAL ACTIONS (Continued)

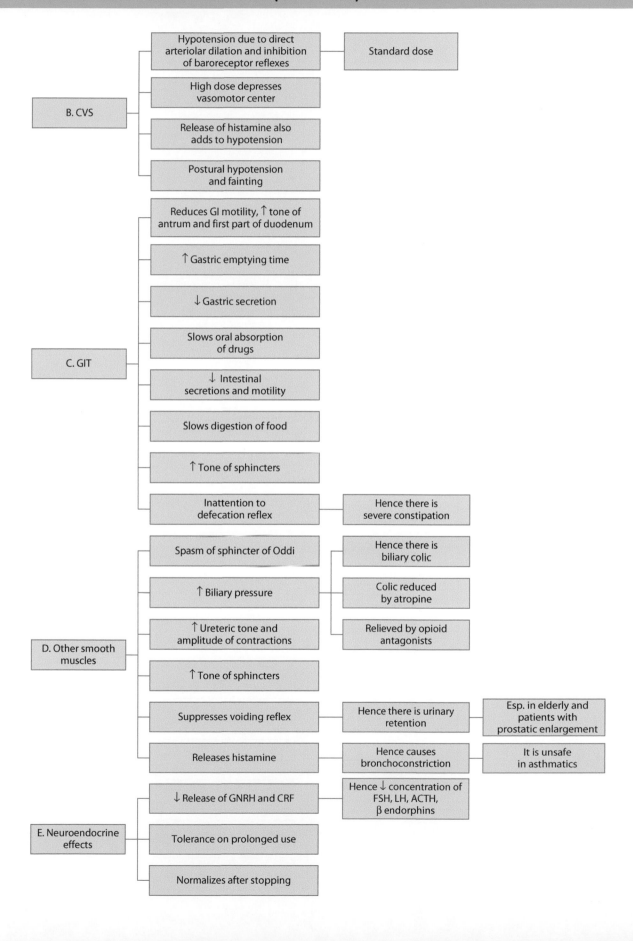

B. CVS
- Hypotension due to direct arteriolar dilation and inhibition of baroreceptor reflexes — Standard dose
- High dose depresses vasomotor center
- Release of histamine also adds to hypotension
- Postural hypotension and fainting

C. GIT
- Reduces GI motility, ↑ tone of antrum and first part of duodenum
- ↑ Gastric emptying time
- ↓ Gastric secretion
- Slows oral absorption of drugs
- ↓ Intestinal secretions and motility
- Slows digestion of food
- ↑ Tone of sphincters
- Inattention to defecation reflex — Hence there is severe constipation

D. Other smooth muscles
- Spasm of sphincter of Oddi
- ↑ Biliary pressure — Hence there is biliary colic / Colic reduced by atropine / Relieved by opioid antagonists
- ↑ Ureteric tone and amplitude of contractions
- ↑ Tone of sphincters
- Suppresses voiding reflex — Hence there is urinary retention — Esp. in elderly and patients with prostatic enlargement
- Releases histamine — Hence causes bronchoconstriction — It is unsafe in asthmatics

E. Neuroendocrine effects
- ↓ Release of GNRH and CRF — Hence ↓ concentration of FSH, LH, ACTH, β endorphins
- Tolerance on prolonged use
- Normalizes after stopping

29.4 PHARMACOKINETICS AND ADVERSE EFFECTS

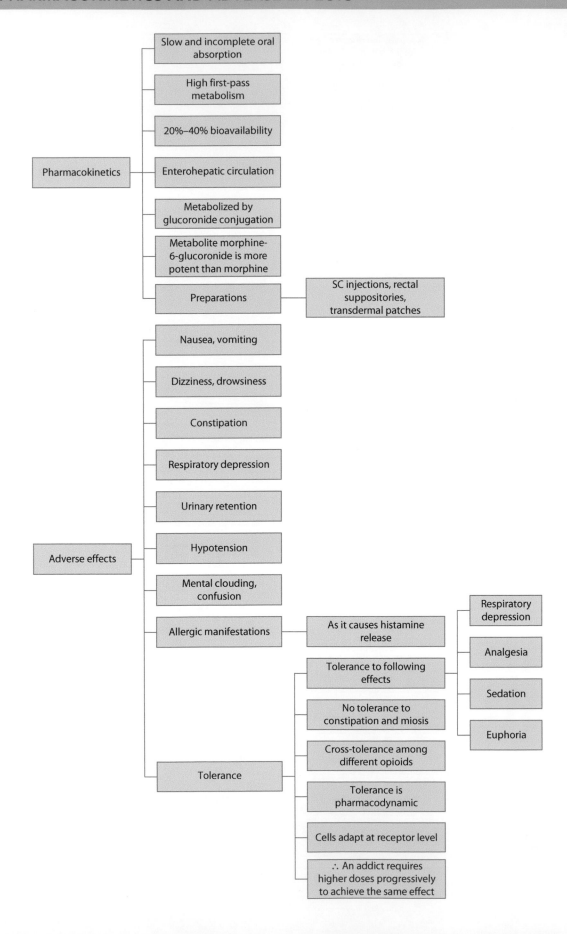

29.5 DEPENDENCE

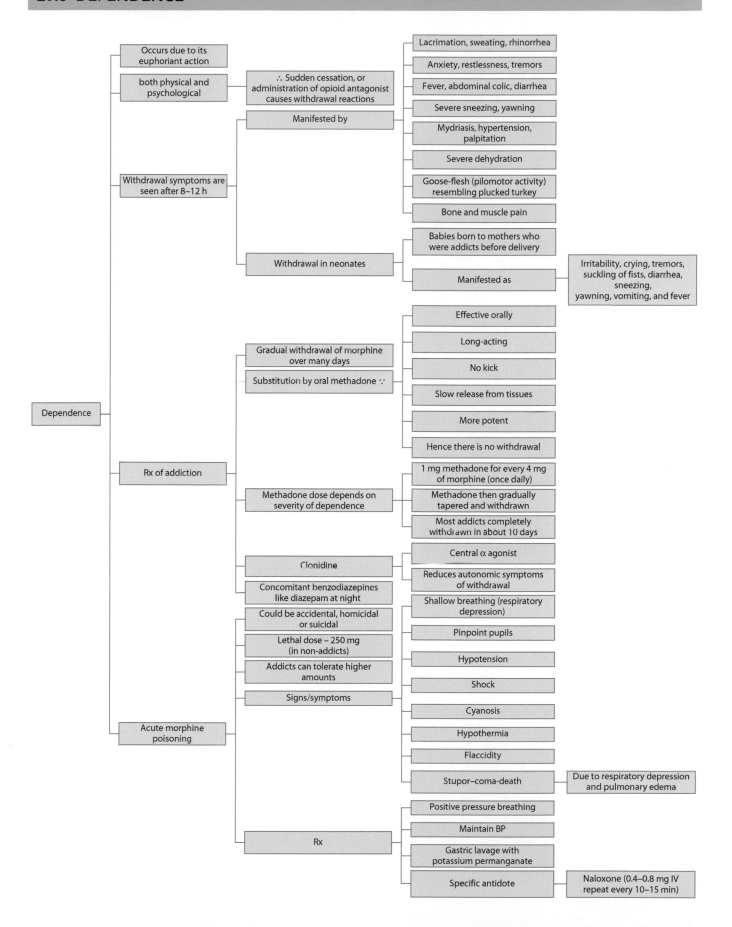

Dependence

- Occurs due to its euphoriant action
- both physical and psychological
- Withdrawal symptoms are seen after 8–12 h
  - ∴ Sudden cessation, or administration of opioid antagonist causes withdrawal reactions
  - Manifested by
    - Lacrimation, sweating, rhinorrhea
    - Anxiety, restlessness, tremors
    - Fever, abdominal colic, diarrhea
    - Severe sneezing, yawning
    - Mydriasis, hypertension, palpitation
    - Severe dehydration
    - Goose-flesh (pilomotor activity) resembling plucked turkey
    - Bone and muscle pain
  - Withdrawal in neonates
    - Babies born to mothers who were addicts before delivery
    - Manifested as
      - Irritability, crying, tremors, suckling of fists, diarrhea, sneezing, yawning, vomiting, and fever
- Rx of addiction
  - Gradual withdrawal of morphine over many days
  - Substitution by oral methadone ∵
    - Effective orally
    - Long-acting
    - No kick
    - Slow release from tissues
    - More potent
    - Hence there is no withdrawal
  - Methadone dose depends on severity of dependence
    - 1 mg methadone for every 4 mg of morphine (once daily)
    - Methadone then gradually tapered and withdrawn
    - Most addicts completely withdrawn in about 10 days
  - Clonidine
    - Central α agonist
    - Reduces autonomic symptoms of withdrawal
  - Concomitant benzodiazepines like diazepam at night
- Acute morphine poisoning
  - Could be accidental, homicidal or suicidal
  - Lethal dose – 250 mg (in non-addicts)
  - Addicts can tolerate higher amounts
  - Signs/symptoms
    - Shallow breathing (respiratory depression)
    - Pinpoint pupils
    - Hypotension
    - Shock
    - Cyanosis
    - Hypothermia
    - Flaccidity
    - Stupor–coma-death
      - Due to respiratory depression and pulmonary edema
  - Rx
    - Positive pressure breathing
    - Maintain BP
    - Gastric lavage with potassium permanganate
    - Specific antidote
      - Naloxone (0.4–0.8 mg IV repeat every 10–15 min)

29.6 PRECAUTIONS AND CONTRAINDICATIONS

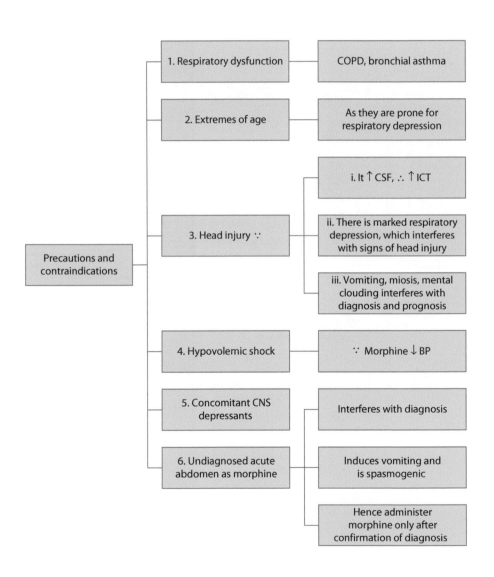

Precautions and contraindications

1. Respiratory dysfunction — COPD, bronchial asthma

2. Extremes of age — As they are prone for respiratory depression

3. Head injury ∵
- i. It ↑ CSF, ∴ ↑ ICT
- ii. There is marked respiratory depression, which interferes with signs of head injury
- iii. Vomiting, miosis, mental clouding interferes with diagnosis and prognosis

4. Hypovolemic shock — ∵ Morphine ↓ BP

5. Concomitant CNS depressants — Interferes with diagnosis

6. Undiagnosed acute abdomen as morphine
- Induces vomiting and is spasmogenic
- Hence administer morphine only after confirmation of diagnosis

29.7 OTHER OPIOIDS

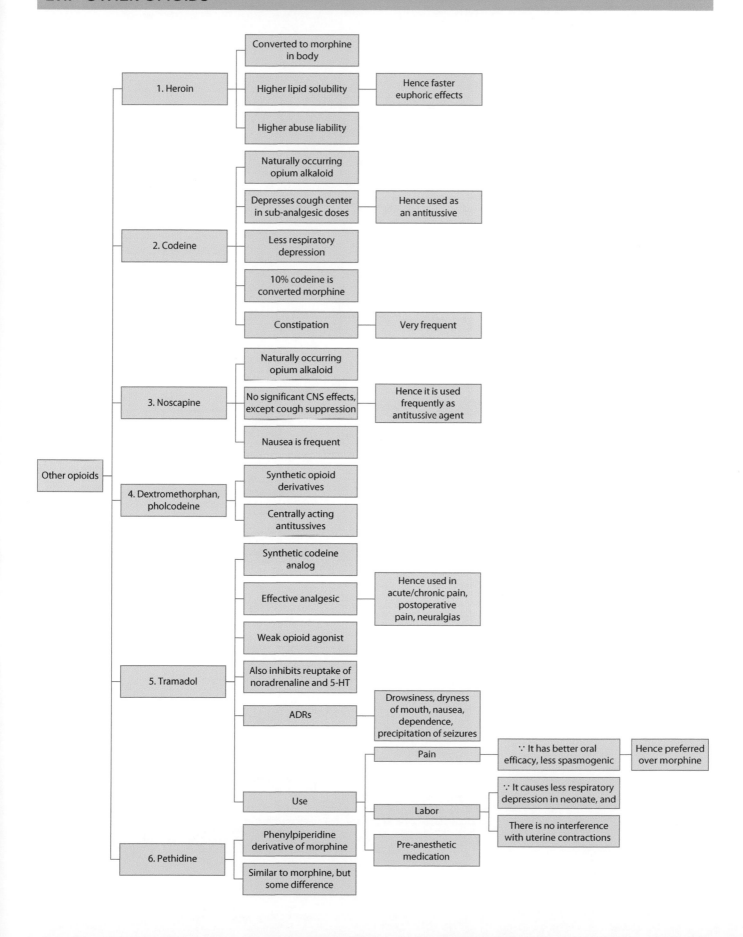

29.8 PETHIDINE DERIVATIVES – FENTANYL

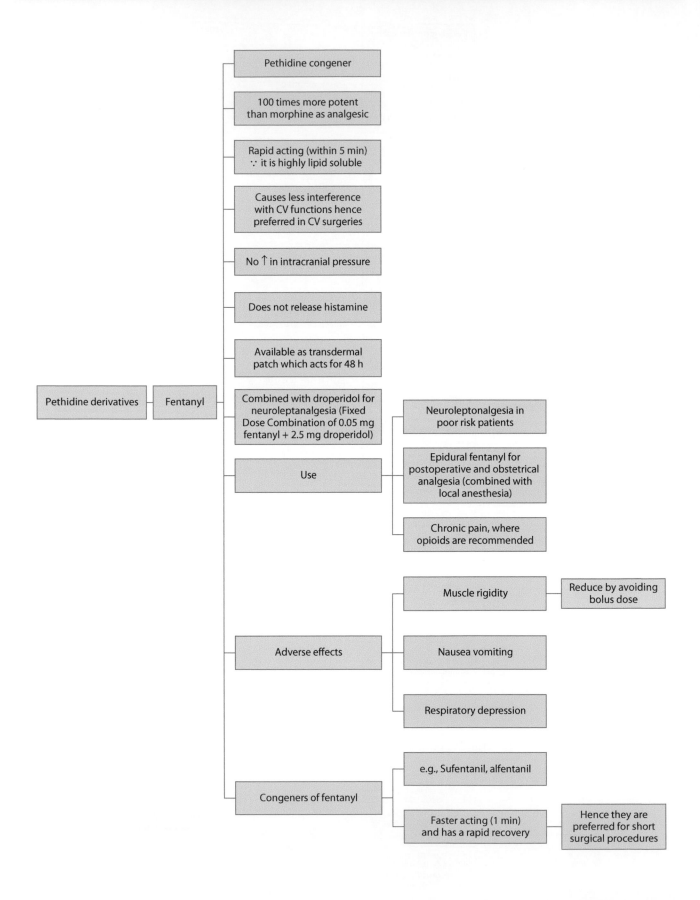

29.9 METHADONE, DEXTROPROPOXYPHENE, AND ETHOHEPTAZINE

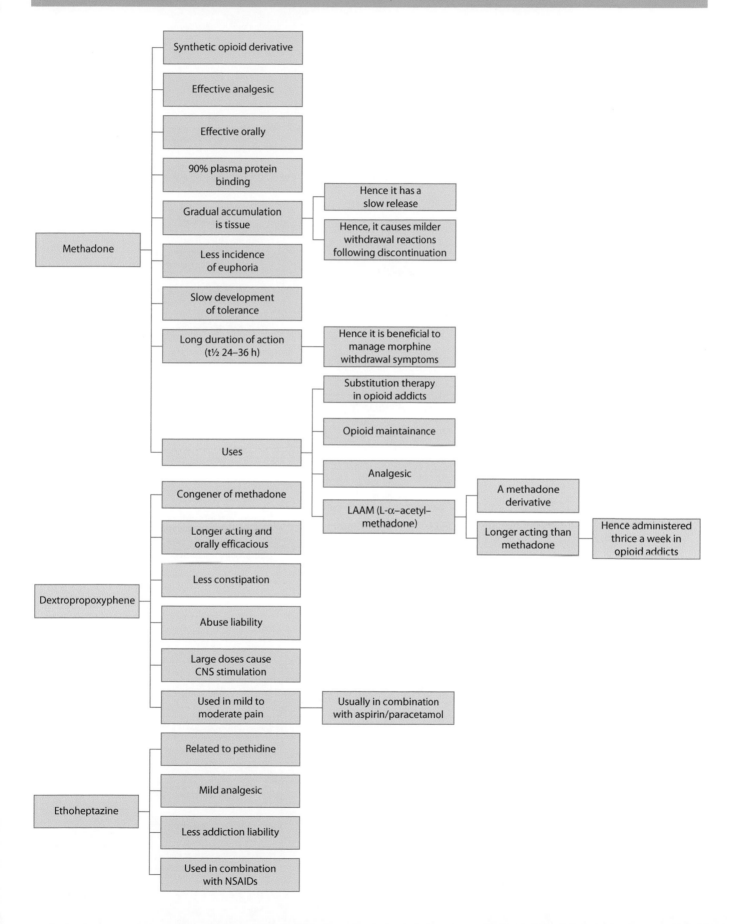

Methadone
- Synthetic opioid derivative
- Effective analgesic
- Effective orally
- 90% plasma protein binding
- Gradual accumulation is tissue
  - Hence it has a slow release
  - Hence, it causes milder withdrawal reactions following discontinuation
- Less incidence of euphoria
- Slow development of tolerance
- Long duration of action (t½ 24–36 h)
  - Hence it is beneficial to manage morphine withdrawal symptoms
- Uses
  - Substitution therapy in opioid addicts
  - Opioid maintainance
  - Analgesic
  - LAAM (L-α–acetyl–methadone)
    - A methadone derivative
    - Longer acting than methadone
      - Hence administered thrice a week in opioid addicts

Dextropropoxyphene
- Congener of methadone
- Longer acting and orally efficacious
- Less constipation
- Abuse liability
- Large doses cause CNS stimulation
- Used in mild to moderate pain
  - Usually in combination with aspirin/paracetamol

Ethoheptazine
- Related to pethidine
- Mild analgesic
- Less addiction liability
- Used in combination with NSAIDs

29.10 USES OF MORPHINE AND CONGENERS

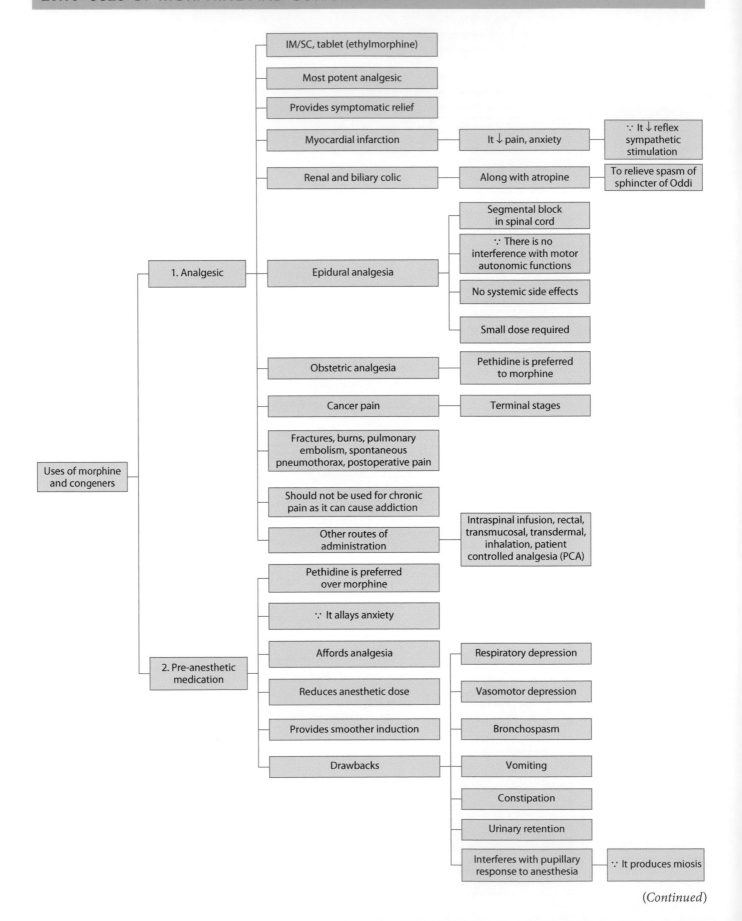

Uses of morphine and congeners

1. Analgesic
- IM/SC, tablet (ethylmorphine)
- Most potent analgesic
- Provides symptomatic relief
- Myocardial infarction → It ↓ pain, anxiety → ∵ It ↓ reflex sympathetic stimulation
- Renal and biliary colic → Along with atropine → To relieve spasm of sphincter of Oddi
- Epidural analgesia
  - Segmental block in spinal cord
  - ∵ There is no interference with motor autonomic functions
  - No systemic side effects
  - Small dose required
- Obstetric analgesia → Pethidine is preferred to morphine
- Cancer pain → Terminal stages
- Fractures, burns, pulmonary embolism, spontaneous pneumothorax, postoperative pain
- Should not be used for chronic pain as it can cause addiction
- Other routes of administration → Intraspinal infusion, rectal, transmucosal, transdermal, inhalation, patient controlled analgesia (PCA)

2. Pre-anesthetic medication
- Pethidine is preferred over morphine
- ∵ It allays anxiety
- Affords analgesia
- Reduces anesthetic dose
- Provides smoother induction
- Drawbacks
  - Respiratory depression
  - Vasomotor depression
  - Bronchospasm
  - Vomiting
  - Constipation
  - Urinary retention
  - Interferes with pupillary response to anesthesia → ∵ It produces miosis

(Continued)

29.10 USES OF MORPHINE AND CONGENERS (Continued)

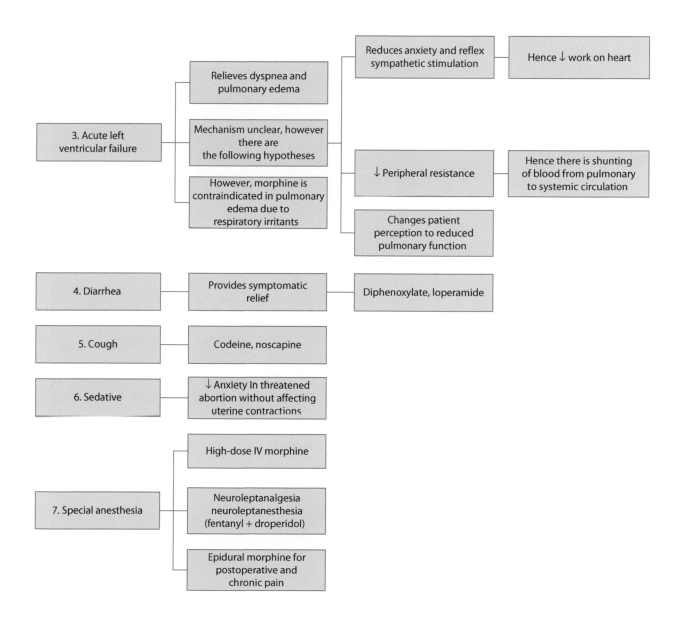

3. Acute left ventricular failure
- Relieves dyspnea and pulmonary edema
- Mechanism unclear, however there are the following hypotheses
  - Reduces anxiety and reflex sympathetic stimulation → Hence ↓ work on heart
  - ↓ Peripheral resistance → Hence there is shunting of blood from pulmonary to systemic circulation
  - Changes patient perception to reduced pulmonary function
- However, morphine is contraindicated in pulmonary edema due to respiratory irritants

4. Diarrhea
- Provides symptomatic relief → Diphenoxylate, loperamide

5. Cough
- Codeine, noscapine

6. Sedative
- ↓ Anxiety In threatened abortion without affecting uterine contractions

7. Special anesthesia
- High-dose IV morphine
- Neuroleptanalgesia neuroleptanesthesia (fentanyl + droperidol)
- Epidural morphine for postoperative and chronic pain

29.11 MIXED AGONISTS AND ANTAGONISTS

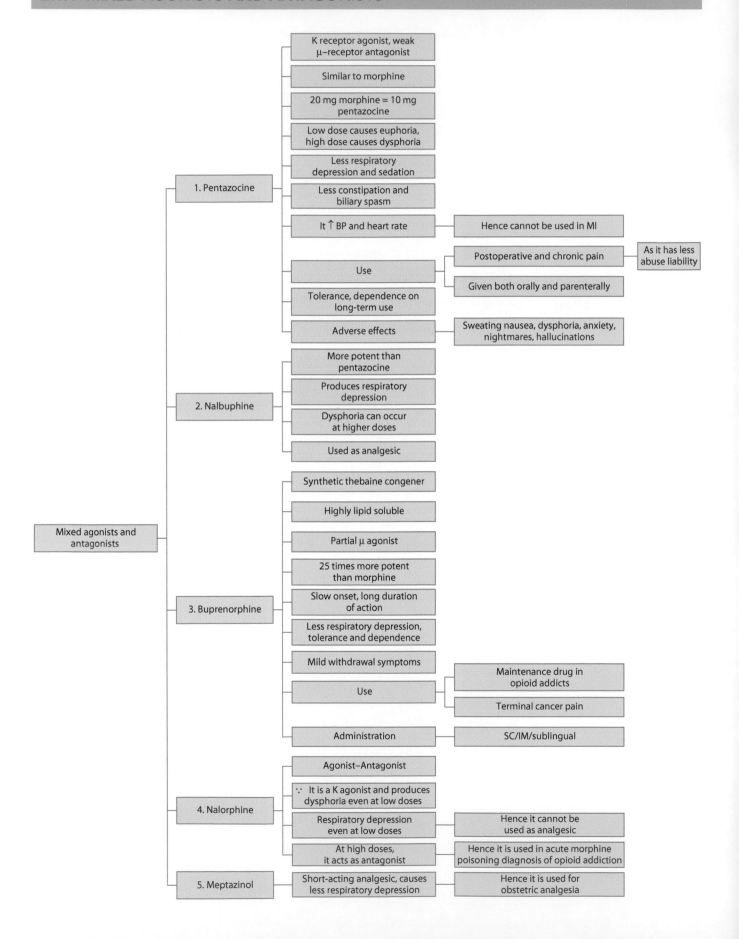

Mixed agonists and antagonists

1. Pentazocine
- K receptor agonist, weak μ–receptor antagonist
- Similar to morphine
- 20 mg morphine = 10 mg pentazocine
- Low dose causes euphoria, high dose causes dysphoria
- Less respiratory depression and sedation
- Less constipation and biliary spasm
- It ↑ BP and heart rate — Hence cannot be used in MI
- Use
  - Postoperative and chronic pain — As it has less abuse liability
  - Given both orally and parenterally
- Tolerance, dependence on long-term use
- Adverse effects — Sweating nausea, dysphoria, anxiety, nightmares, hallucinations

2. Nalbuphine
- More potent than pentazocine
- Produces respiratory depression
- Dysphoria can occur at higher doses
- Used as analgesic

3. Buprenorphine
- Synthetic thebaine congener
- Highly lipid soluble
- Partial μ agonist
- 25 times more potent than morphine
- Slow onset, long duration of action
- Less respiratory depression, tolerance and dependence
- Mild withdrawal symptoms
- Use
  - Maintenance drug in opioid addicts
  - Terminal cancer pain
- Administration — SC/IM/sublingual

4. Nalorphine
- Agonist–Antagonist
- ∵ It is a K agonist and produces dysphoria even at low doses
- Respiratory depression even at low doses — Hence it cannot be used as analgesic
- At high doses, it acts as antagonist — Hence it is used in acute morphine poisoning diagnosis of opioid addiction

5. Meptazinol
- Short-acting analgesic, causes less respiratory depression — Hence it is used for obstetric analgesia

29.12 OPIOID ANTAGONISTS

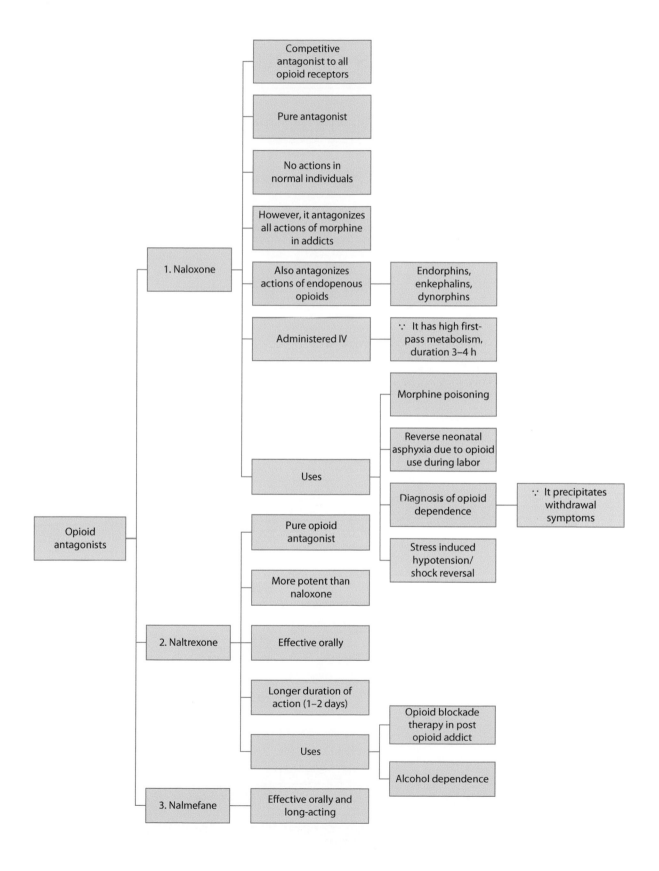

CNS stimulants/drugs of abuse

30.1 CNS STIMULANTS – CLASSIFICATION AND RESPIRATORY STIMULANTS

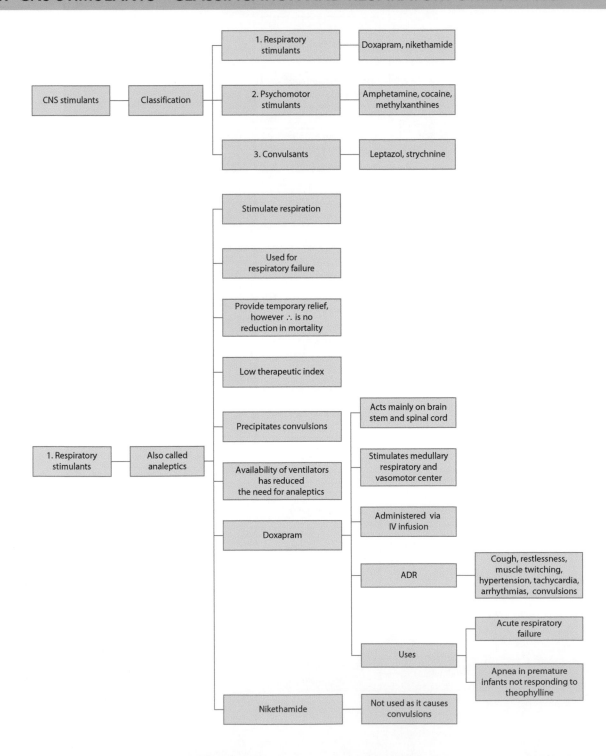

30.2 PSYCHOMOTOR STIMULANTS/METHYLXANTHINES – ACTIONS

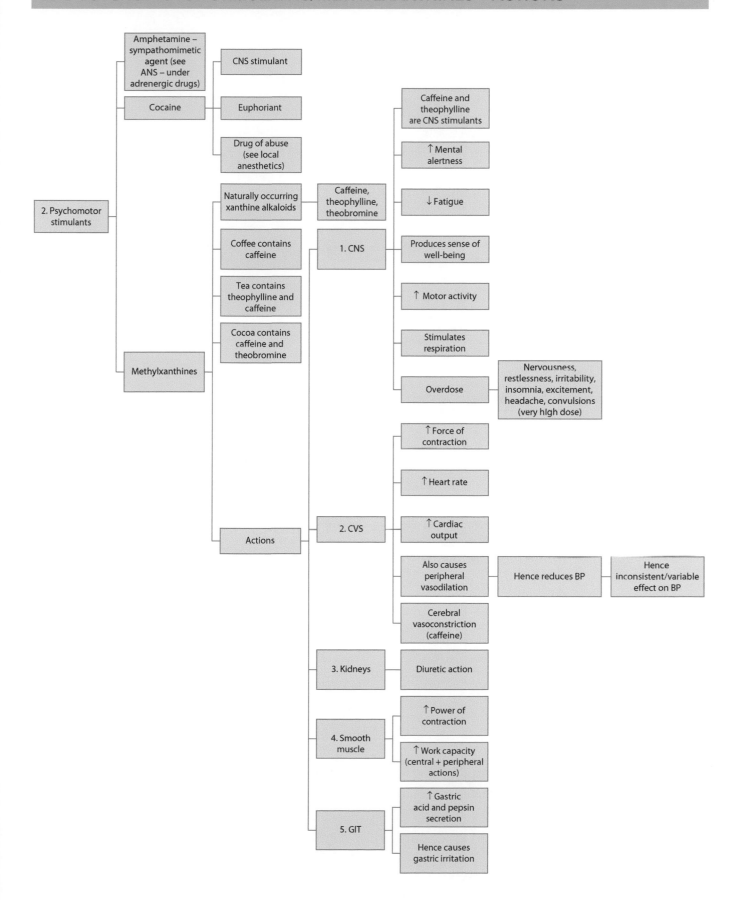

30.3 METHYLXANTHINES – PHARMACOKINETICS, ADVERSE EFFECTS, AND USES

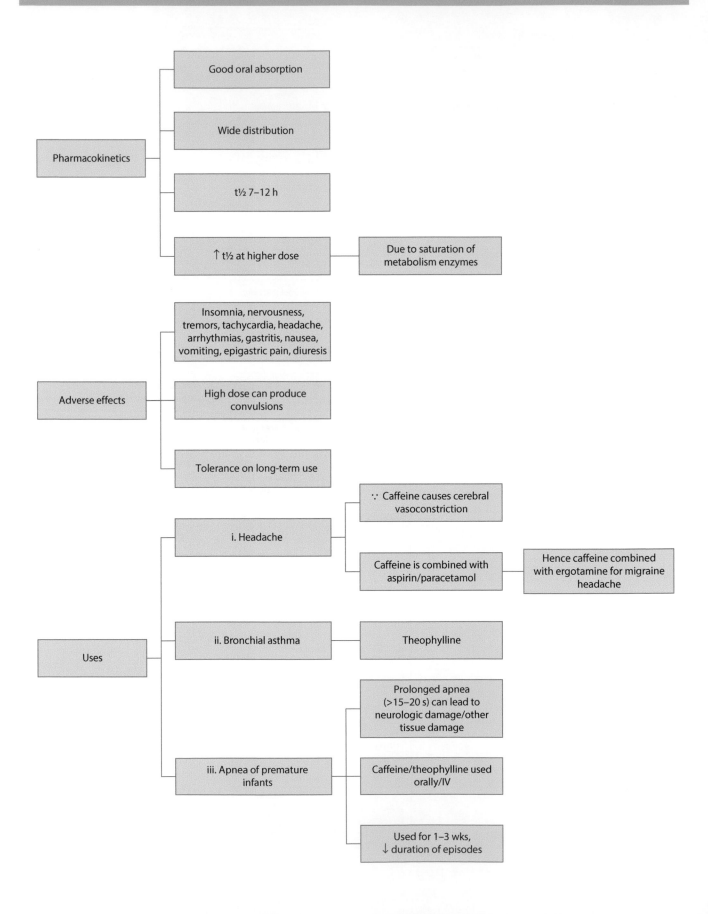

Pharmacokinetics
- Good oral absorption
- Wide distribution
- t½ 7–12 h
- ↑ t½ at higher dose — Due to saturation of metabolism enzymes

Adverse effects
- Insomnia, nervousness, tremors, tachycardia, headache, arrhythmias, gastritis, nausea, vomiting, epigastric pain, diuresis
- High dose can produce convulsions
- Tolerance on long-term use

Uses
- i. Headache
  - ∵ Caffeine causes cerebral vasoconstriction
  - Caffeine is combined with aspirin/paracetamol — Hence caffeine combined with ergotamine for migraine headache
- ii. Bronchial asthma — Theophylline
- iii. Apnea of premature infants
  - Prolonged apnea (>15–20 s) can lead to neurologic damage/other tissue damage
  - Caffeine/theophylline used orally/IV
  - Used for 1–3 wks, ↓ duration of episodes

30.4 NOOTROPICS

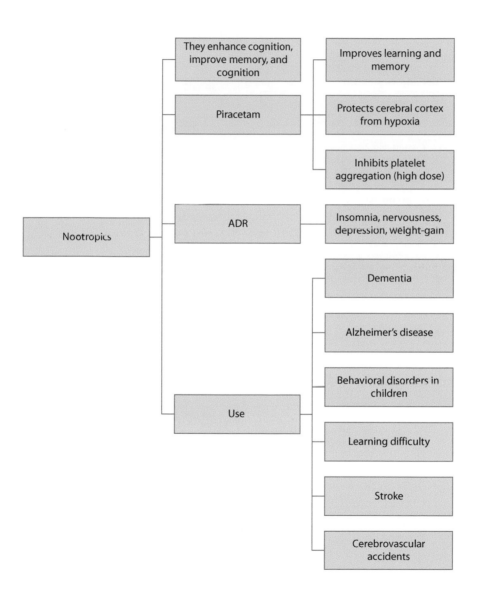

Nootropics

- They enhance cognition, improve memory, and cognition
- Piracetam
  - Improves learning and memory
  - Protects cerebral cortex from hypoxia
  - Inhibits platelet aggregation (high dose)
- ADR
  - Insomnia, nervousness, depression, weight-gain
- Use
  - Dementia
  - Alzheimer's disease
  - Behavioral disorders in children
  - Learning difficulty
  - Stroke
  - Cerebrovascular accidents

30.5 DRUGS OF ABUSE – OPIOIDS, CNS STIMULANTS, AND CNS DEPRESSANTS

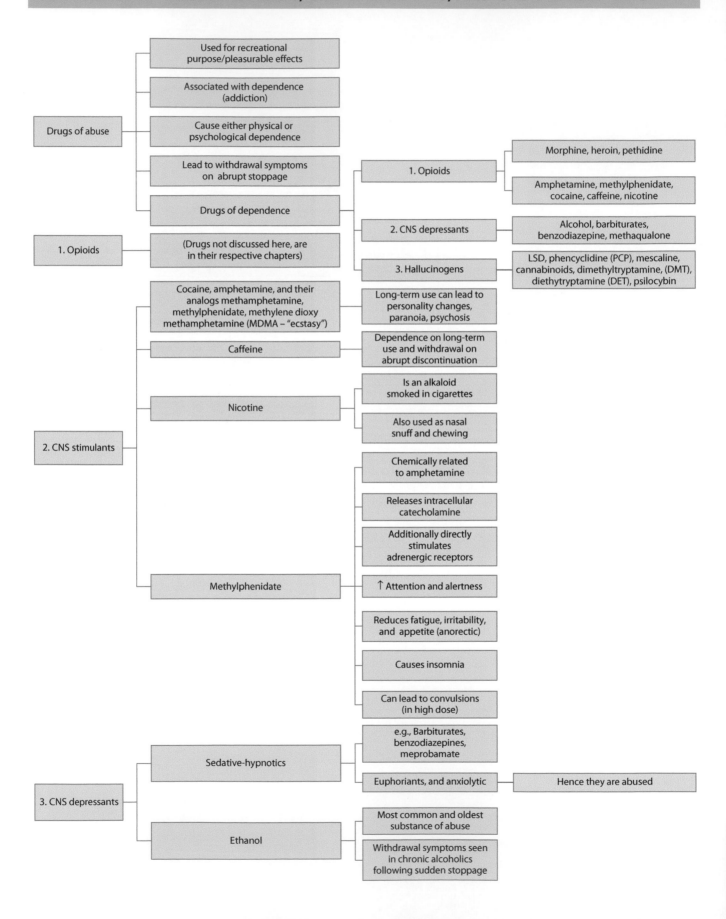

Drugs of abuse
- Used for recreational purpose/pleasurable effects
- Associated with dependence (addiction)
- Cause either physical or psychological dependence
- Lead to withdrawal symptoms on abrupt stoppage
- Drugs of dependence
  - 1. Opioids
    - Morphine, heroin, pethidine
    - Amphetamine, methylphenidate, cocaine, caffeine, nicotine
  - 2. CNS depressants
    - Alcohol, barbiturates, benzodiazepine, methaqualone
  - 3. Hallucinogens
    - LSD, phencyclidine (PCP), mescaline, cannabinoids, dimethyltryptamine, (DMT), diethytryptamine (DET), psilocybin

1. Opioids
- (Drugs not discussed here, are in their respective chapters)

2. CNS stimulants
- Cocaine, amphetamine, and their analogs methamphetamine, methylphenidate, methylene dioxy methamphetamine (MDMA – "ecstasy")
  - Long-term use can lead to personality changes, paranoia, psychosis
- Caffeine
  - Dependence on long-term use and withdrawal on abrupt discontinuation
- Nicotine
  - Is an alkaloid smoked in cigarettes
  - Also used as nasal snuff and chewing
- Methylphenidate
  - Chemically related to amphetamine
  - Releases intracellular catecholamine
  - Additionally directly stimulates adrenergic receptors
  - ↑ Attention and alertness
  - Reduces fatigue, irritability, and appetite (anorectic)
  - Causes insomnia
  - Can lead to convulsions (in high dose)

3. CNS depressants
- Sedative-hypnotics
  - e.g., Barbiturates, benzodiazepines, meprobamate
  - Euphoriants, and anxiolytic → Hence they are abused
- Ethanol
  - Most common and oldest substance of abuse
  - Withdrawal symptoms seen in chronic alcoholics following sudden stoppage

30.6 HALLUCINOGENS

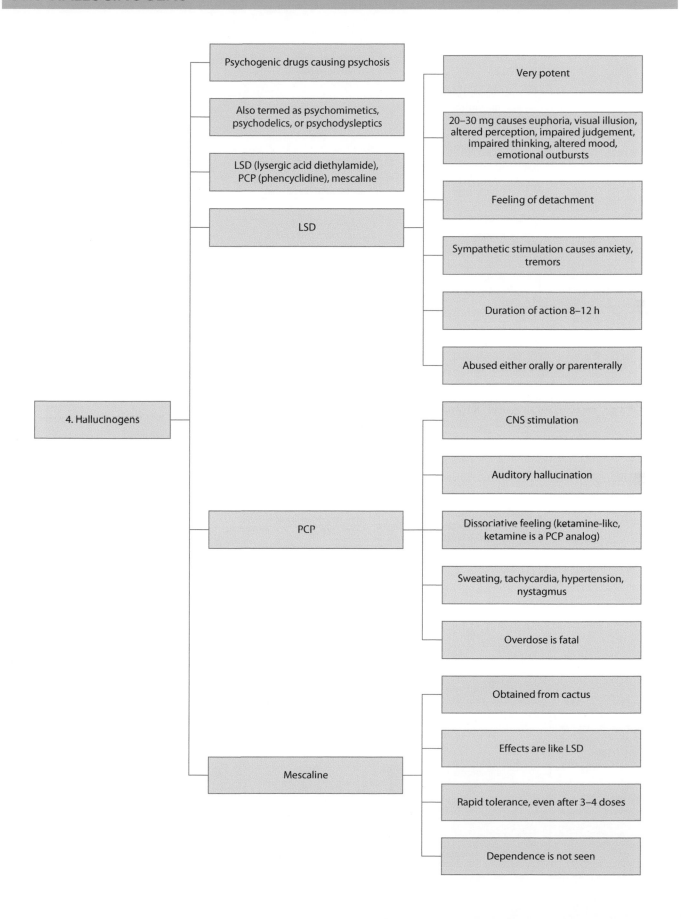

4. Hallucinogens

- Psychogenic drugs causing psychosis
- Also termed as psychomimetics, psychodelics, or psychodysleptics
- LSD (lysergic acid diethylamide), PCP (phencyclidine), mescaline
- LSD
  - Very potent
  - 20–30 mg causes euphoria, visual illusion, altered perception, impaired judgement, impaired thinking, altered mood, emotional outbursts
  - Feeling of detachment
  - Sympathetic stimulation causes anxiety, tremors
  - Duration of action 8–12 h
  - Abused either orally or parenterally
- PCP
  - CNS stimulation
  - Auditory hallucination
  - Dissociative feeling (ketamine-like, ketamine is a PCP analog)
  - Sweating, tachycardia, hypertension, nystagmus
  - Overdose is fatal
- Mescaline
  - Obtained from cactus
  - Effects are like LSD
  - Rapid tolerance, even after 3–4 doses
  - Dependence is not seen

30.7 CANNABINOIDS AND DRUGS FOR TOBACCO WITHDRAWAL

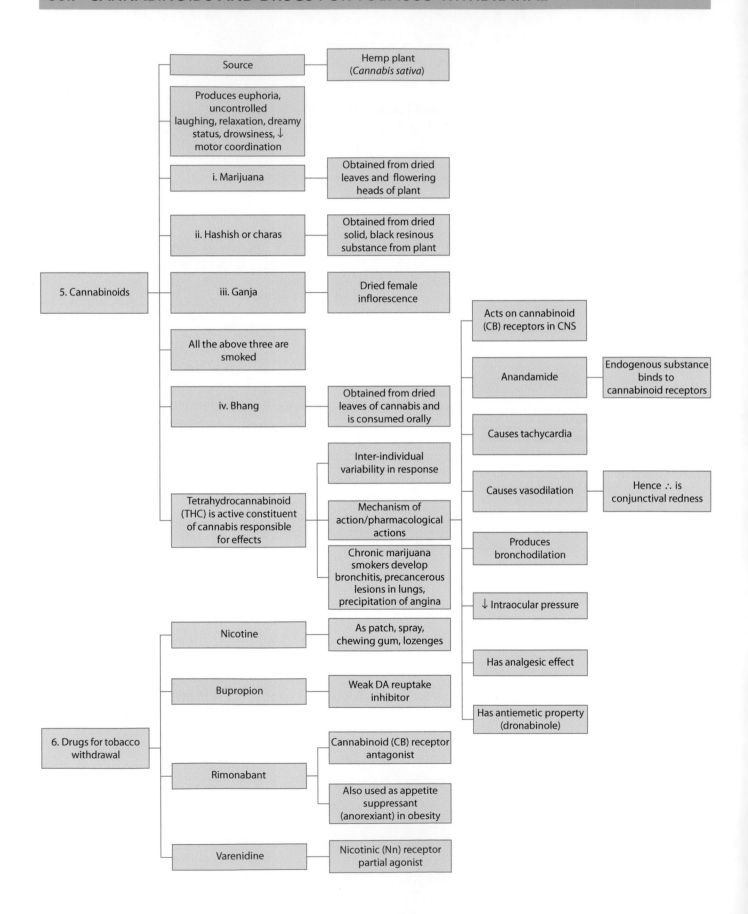

5. Cannabinoids

- Source — Hemp plant (*Cannabis sativa*)
- Produces euphoria, uncontrolled laughing, relaxation, dreamy status, drowsiness, ↓ motor coordination
- i. Marijuana — Obtained from dried leaves and flowering heads of plant
- ii. Hashish or charas — Obtained from dried solid, black resinous substance from plant
- iii. Ganja — Dried female inflorescence
- All the above three are smoked
- iv. Bhang — Obtained from dried leaves of cannabis and is consumed orally
- Tetrahydrocannabinoid (THC) is active constituent of cannabis responsible for effects
  - Inter-individual variability in response
  - Mechanism of action/pharmacological actions
    - Acts on cannabinoid (CB) receptors in CNS
    - Anandamide — Endogenous substance binds to cannabinoid receptors
    - Causes tachycardia
    - Causes vasodilation — Hence ∴ is conjunctival redness
    - Produces bronchodilation
    - ↓ Intraocular pressure
    - Has analgesic effect
    - Has antiemetic property (dronabinole)
  - Chronic marijuana smokers develop bronchitis, precancerous lesions in lungs, precipitation of angina

6. Drugs for tobacco withdrawal

- Nicotine — As patch, spray, chewing gum, lozenges
- Bupropion — Weak DA reuptake inhibitor
- Rimonabant
  - Cannabinoid (CB) receptor antagonist
  - Also used as appetite suppressant (anorexiant) in obesity
- Varenidine — Nicotinic (Nn) receptor partial agonist

PART V

Autacoid pharmacology

31

Autacoids, histamine and antihistaminics

31.1 AUTACOIDS – INTRODUCTION, CLASSIFICATION OF AUTACOIDS AND HISTAMINE

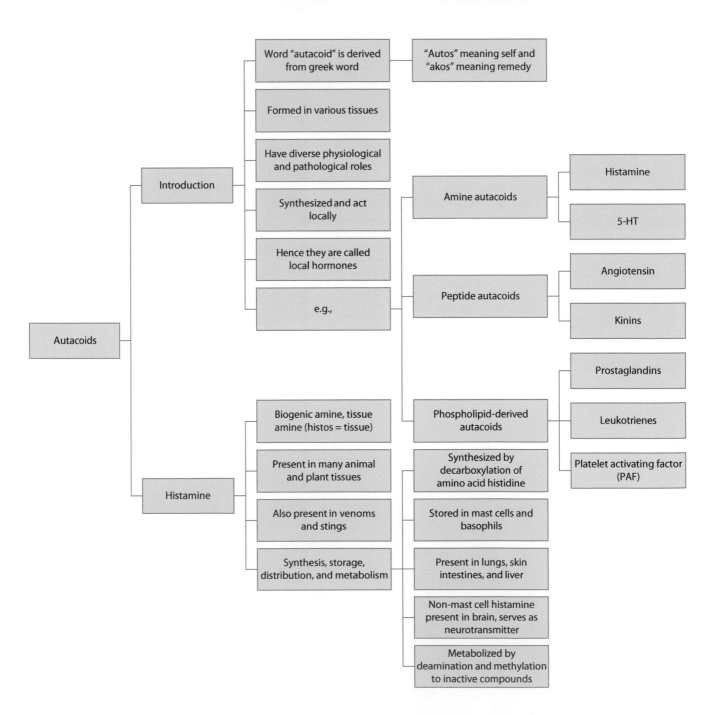

31.2 MECHANISM OF ACTION AND HISTAMINE RELEASERS

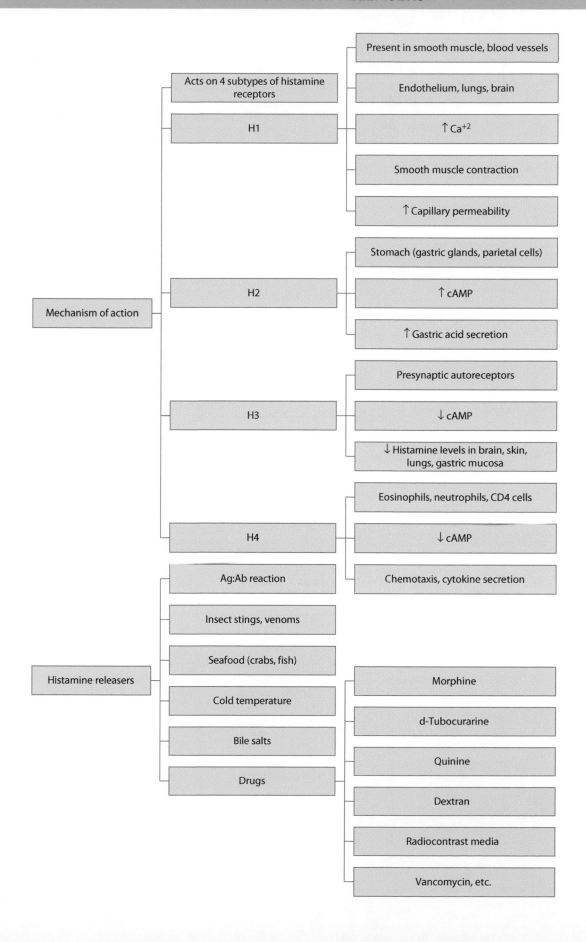

31.3 ACTIONS, USES, AND ADRs

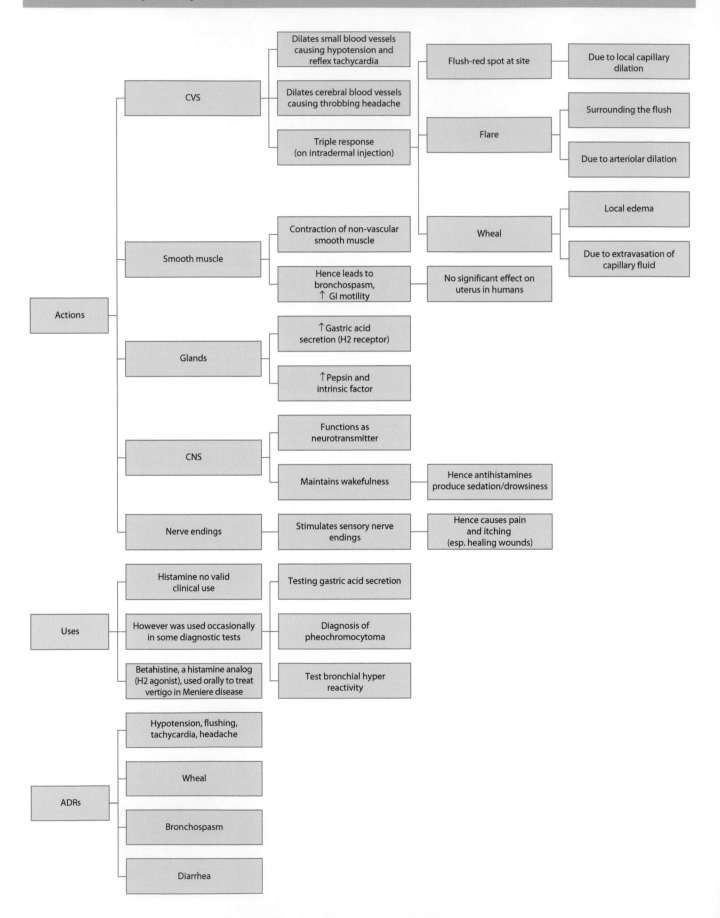

31.4 ANTIHISTAMINES – CLASSIFICATION AND PHARMACOLOGICAL ACTIONS

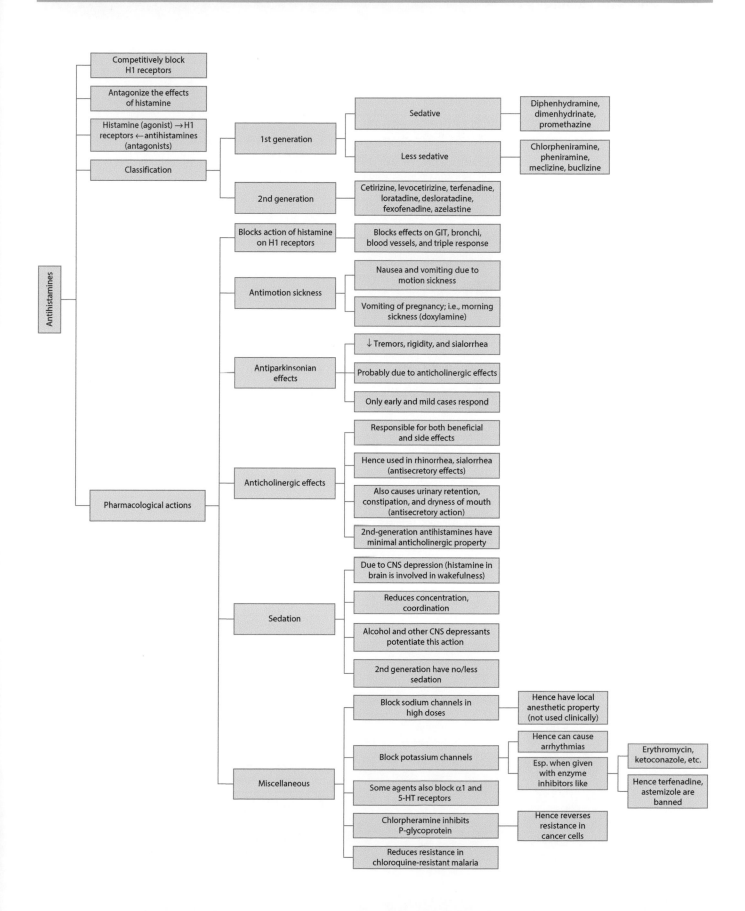

31.5 ADVERSE EFFECTS, DRUG INTERACTIONS, AND SECOND-GENERATION ANTIHISTAMINICS

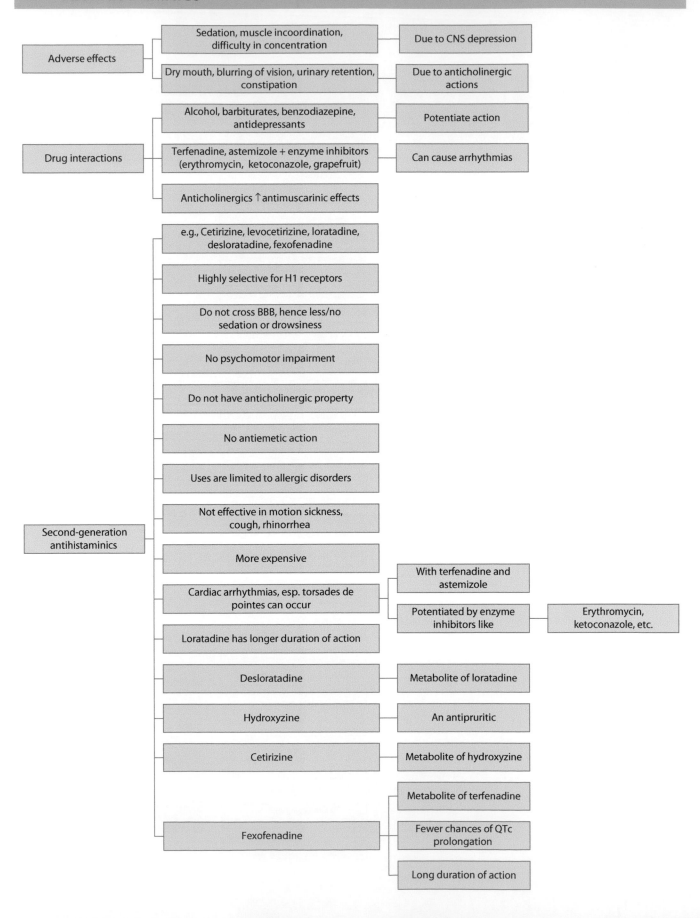

31.6 USES OF ANTIHISTAMINICS

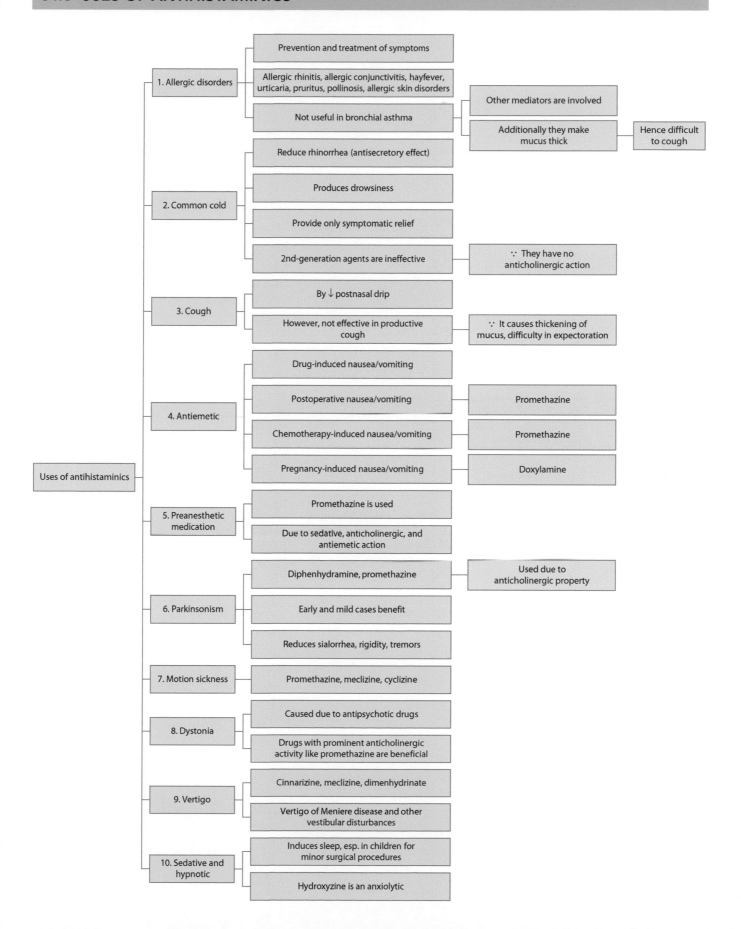

31.7 DRUGS FOR VERTIGO

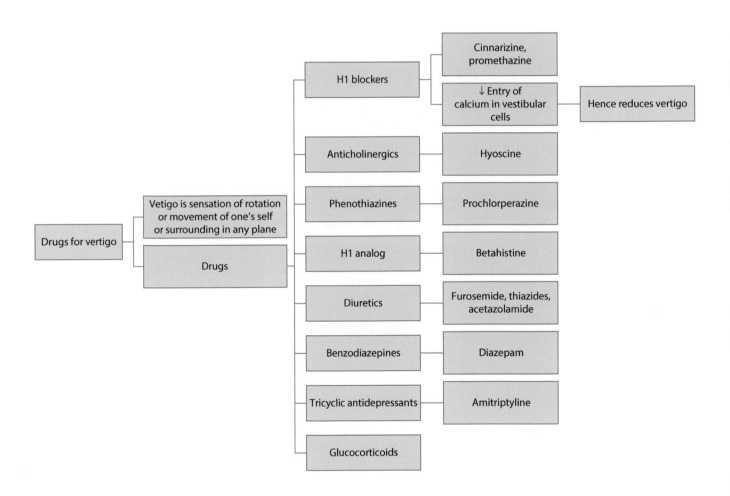

32

5-Hydroxytryptamine agonists and antagonists and drug treatment of migraine

32.1 5-HYDROXYTRYPTAMINE – INTRODUCTION

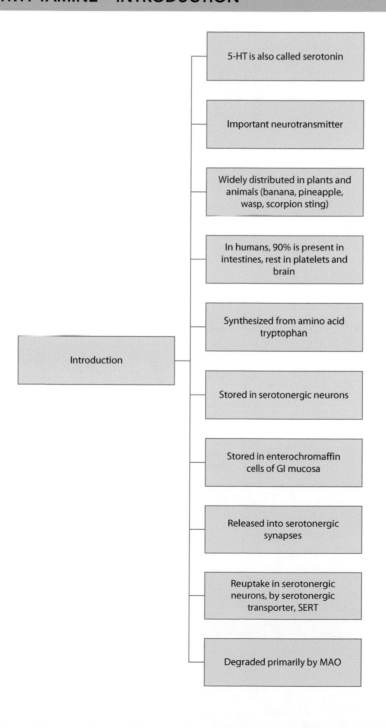

Introduction

- 5-HT is also called serotonin
- Important neurotransmitter
- Widely distributed in plants and animals (banana, pineapple, wasp, scorpion sting)
- In humans, 90% is present in intestines, rest in platelets and brain
- Synthesized from amino acid tryptophan
- Stored in serotonergic neurons
- Stored in enterochromaffin cells of GI mucosa
- Released into serotonergic synapses
- Reuptake in serotonergic neurons, by serotonergic transporter, SERT
- Degraded primarily by MAO

32.2 5-HT RECEPTORS

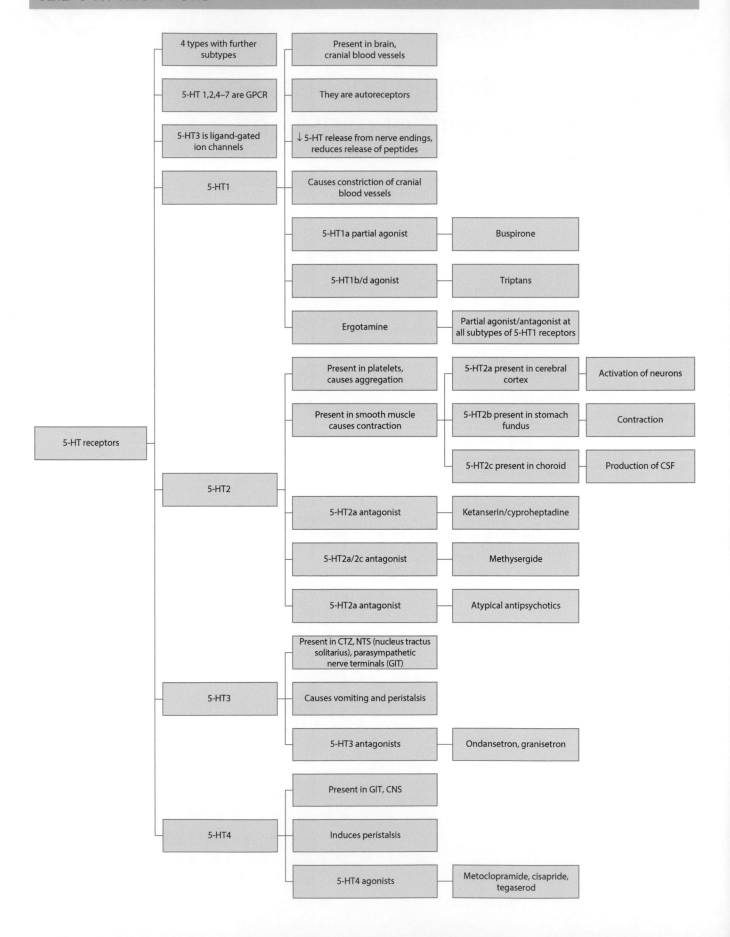

32.3 5-HT AGONISTS

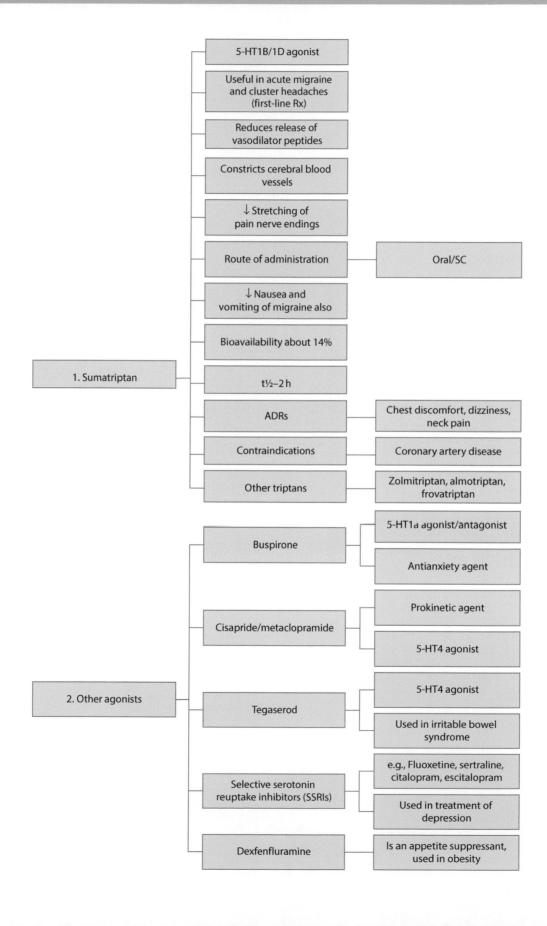

32.4 5-HT ANTAGONISTS

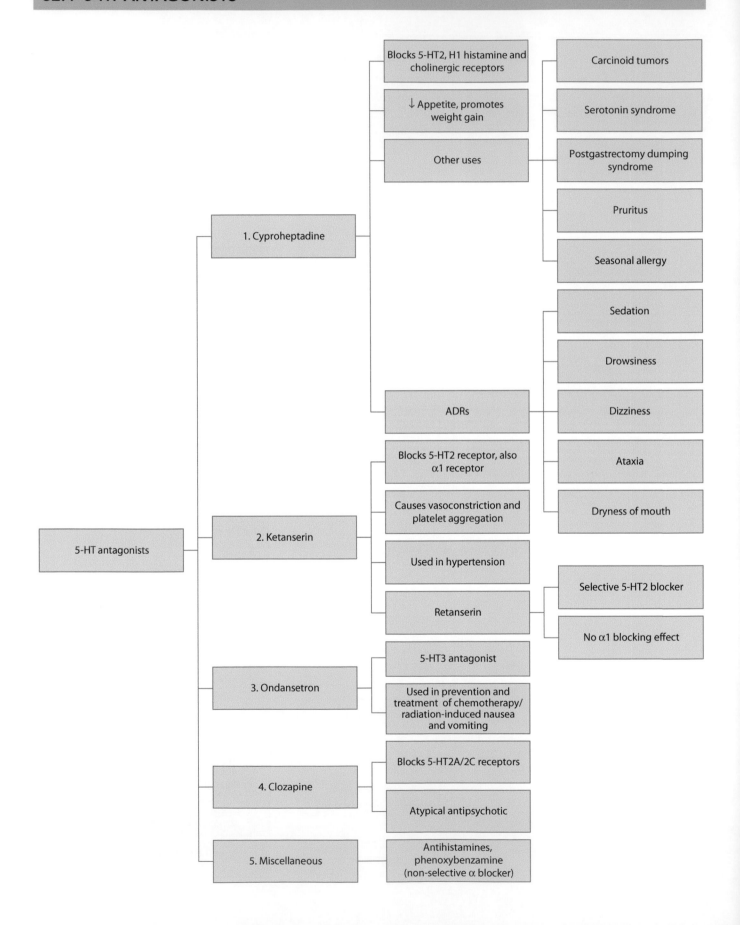

32.5 ERGOT ALKALOIDS

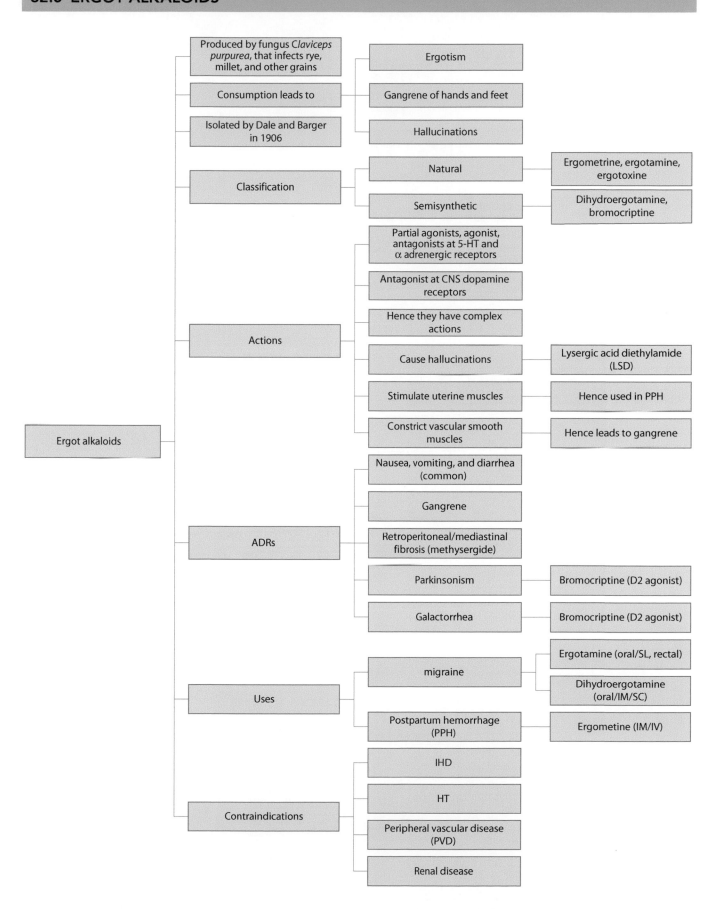

32.6 DRUG TREATMENT OF MIGRAINE

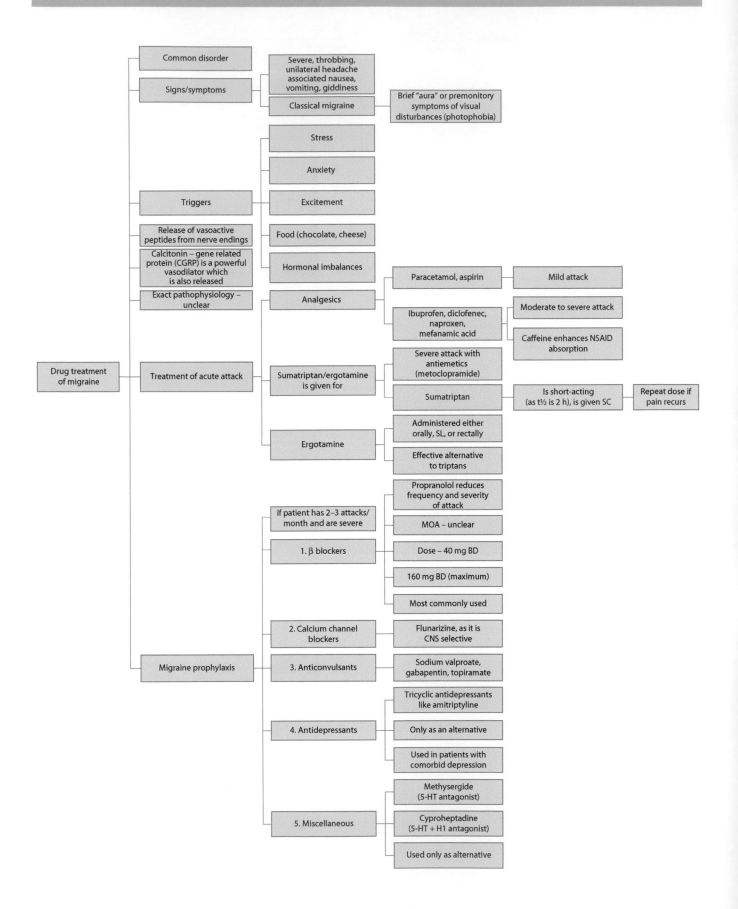

Eicosanoids and leukotrienes

33.1 EICOSANOIDS – INTRODUCTION AND SYNTHESIS

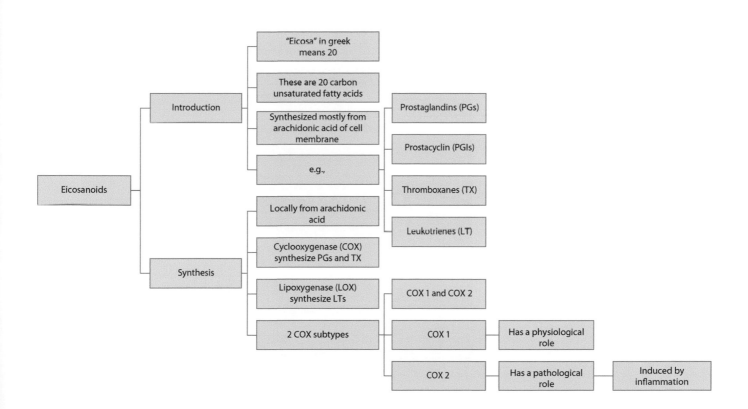

33.2 PROSTAGLANDINS AND THROMBOXANES – MECHANISM OF ACTION AND ACTIONS

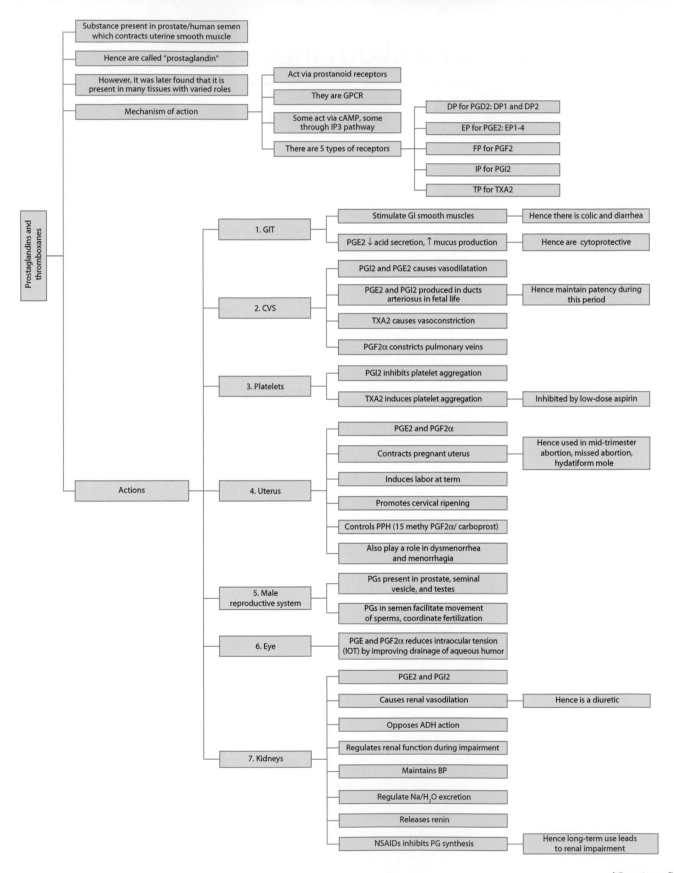

(Continued)

33.2 PROSTAGLANDINS AND THROMBOXANES – MECHANISM OF ACTION AND ACTIONS (Continued)

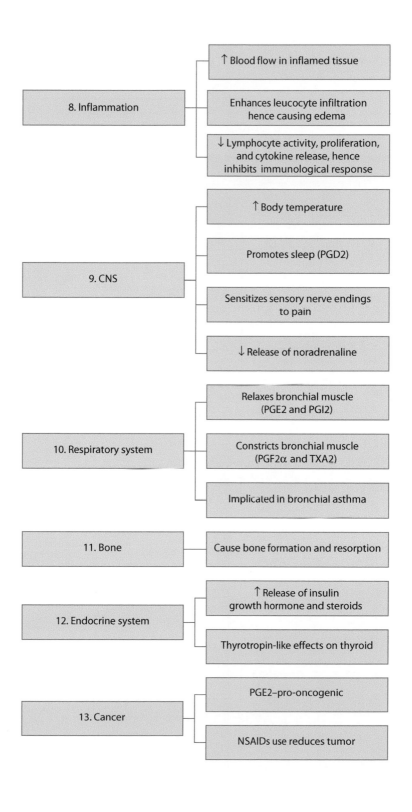

8. Inflammation
- ↑ Blood flow in inflamed tissue
- Enhances leucocyte infiltration hence causing edema
- ↓ Lymphocyte activity, proliferation, and cytokine release, hence inhibits immunological response

9. CNS
- ↑ Body temperature
- Promotes sleep (PGD2)
- Sensitizes sensory nerve endings to pain
- ↓ Release of noradrenaline

10. Respiratory system
- Relaxes bronchial muscle (PGE2 and PGI2)
- Constricts bronchial muscle (PGF2α and TXA2)
- Implicated in bronchial asthma

11. Bone
- Cause bone formation and resorption

12. Endocrine system
- ↑ Release of insulin growth hormone and steroids
- Thyrotropin-like effects on thyroid

13. Cancer
- PGE2–pro-oncogenic
- NSAIDs use reduces tumor

33.3 ADR

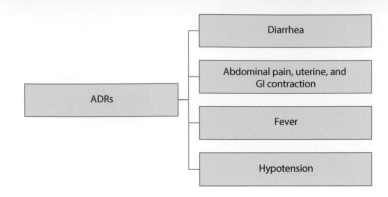

33.4 USES

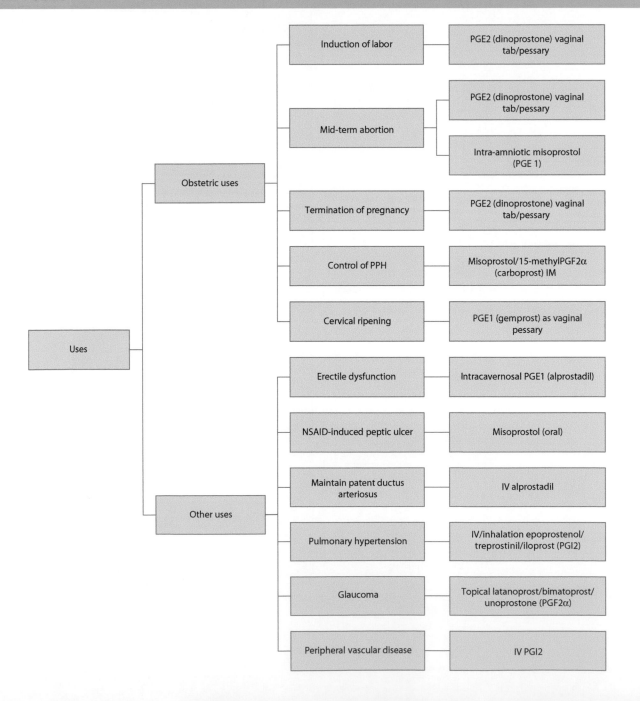

33.5 LEUKOTRIENES – INTRODUCTION, ACTIONS, LEUKOTRIENE ANTAGONISTS AND PLATELET-ACTIVATING FACTOR

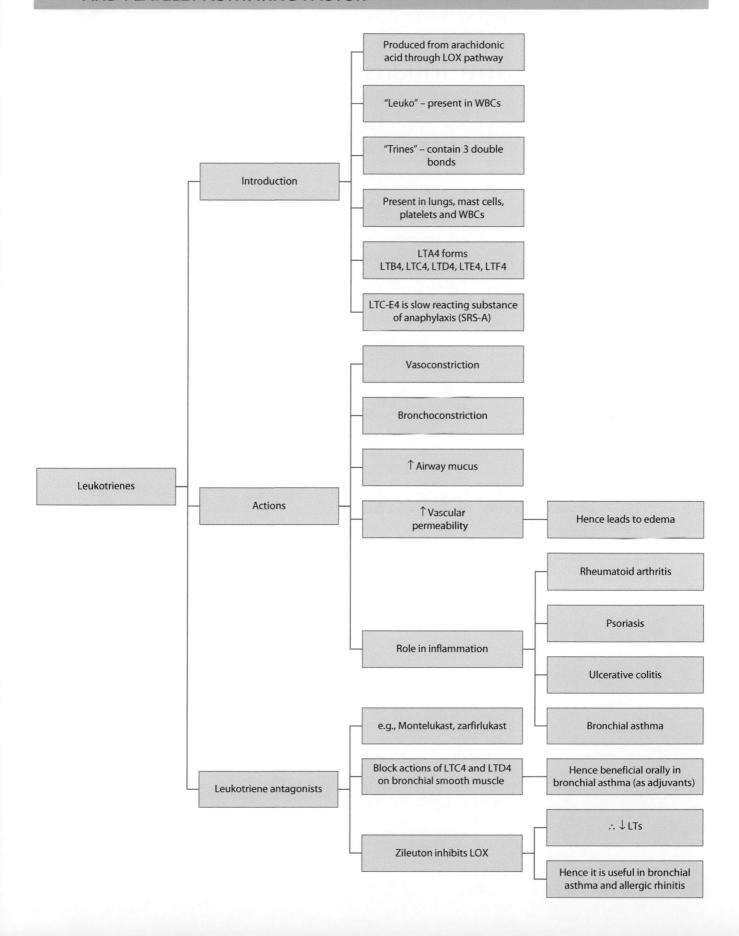

34

Nonsteroidal anti-inflammatory drugs (NSAIDs)

34.1 ANALGESICS

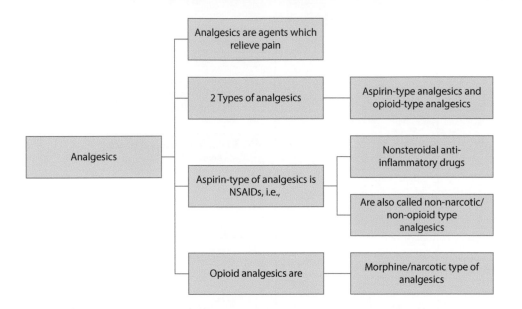

34.2 ASPIRIN-TYPE OF ANALGESICS vs. OPIOID-TYPE OF ANALGESICS

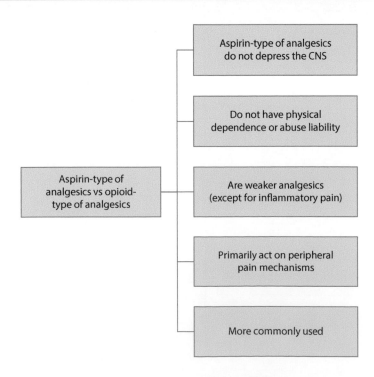

34.3 NSAIDs CLASSIFICATION

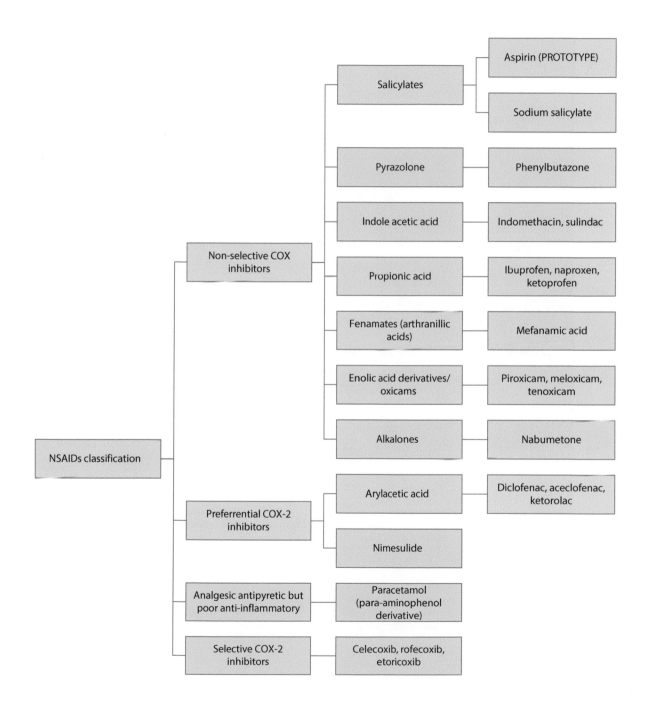

34.4 MECHANISM OF ACTION

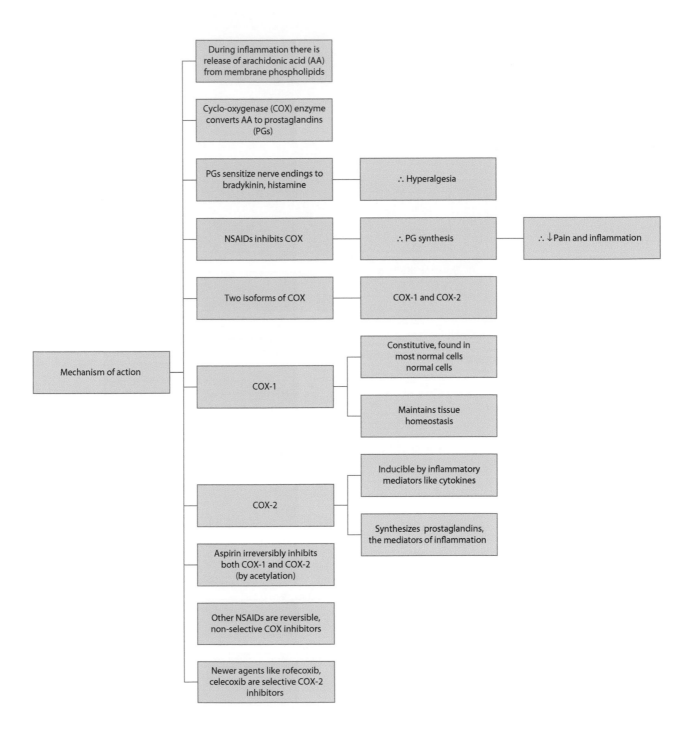

34.5 SALICYLATES

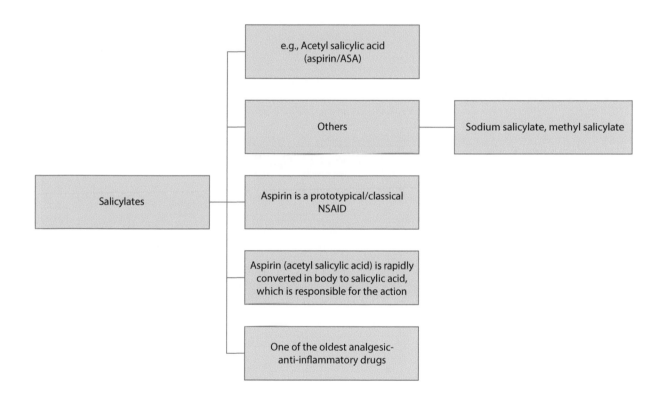

34.6 PHARMACOLOGICAL ACTIONS

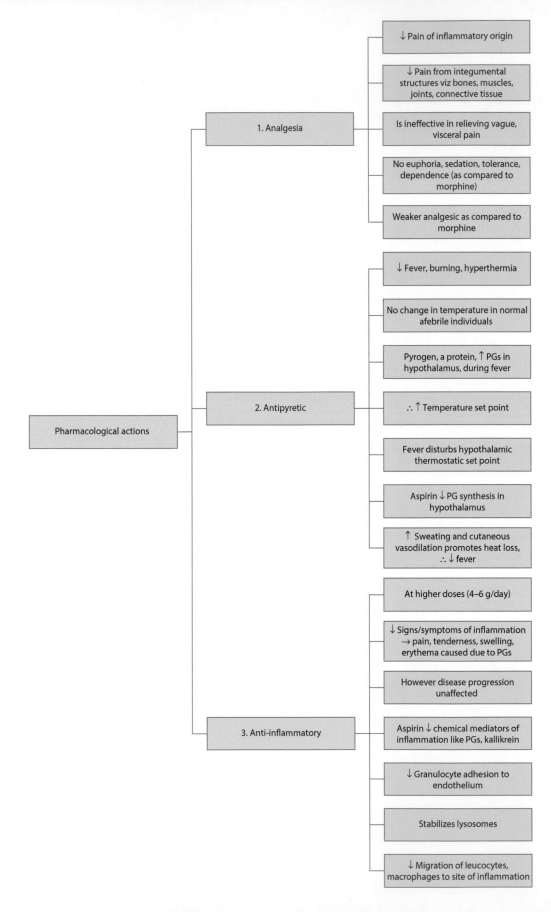

Pharmacological actions

1. Analgesia
- ↓ Pain of inflammatory origin
- ↓ Pain from integumental structures viz bones, muscles, joints, connective tissue
- Is ineffective in relieving vague, visceral pain
- No euphoria, sedation, tolerance, dependence (as compared to morphine)
- Weaker analgesic as compared to morphine

2. Antipyretic
- ↓ Fever, burning, hyperthermia
- No change in temperature in normal afebrile individuals
- Pyrogen, a protein, ↑ PGs in hypothalamus, during fever
- ∴ ↑ Temperature set point
- Fever disturbs hypothalamic thermostatic set point
- Aspirin ↓ PG synthesis in hypothalamus
- ↑ Sweating and cutaneous vasodilation promotes heat loss, ∴ ↓ fever

3. Anti-inflammatory
- At higher doses (4–6 g/day)
- ↓ Signs/symptoms of inflammation → pain, tenderness, swelling, erythema caused due to PGs
- However disease progression unaffected
- Aspirin ↓ chemical mediators of inflammation like PGs, kallikrein
- ↓ Granulocyte adhesion to endothelium
- Stabilizes lysosomes
- ↓ Migration of leucocytes, macrophages to site of inflammation

(Continued)

34.6 PHARMACOLOGICAL ACTIONS (Continued)

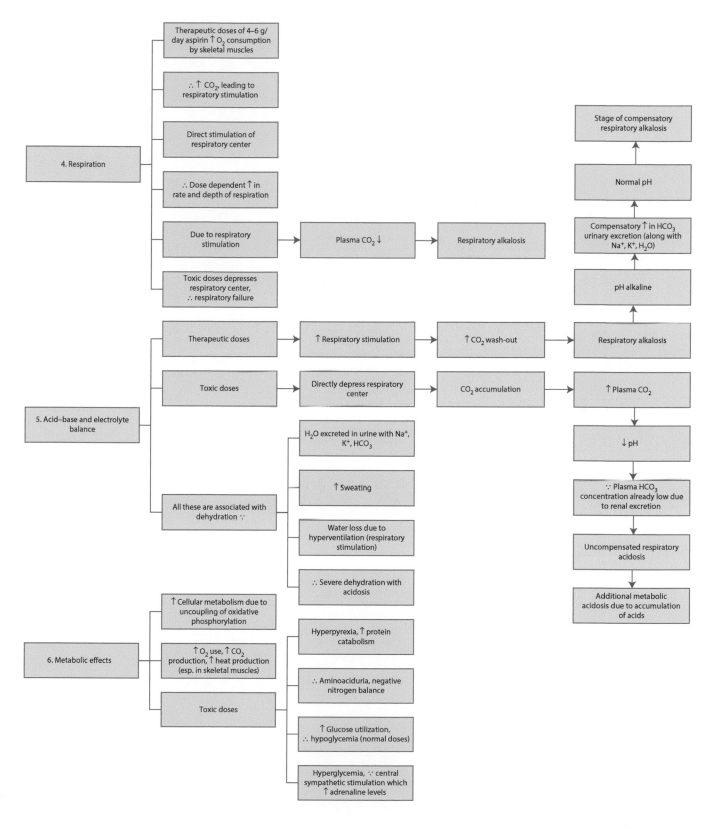

(Continued)

34.6 PHARMACOLOGICAL ACTIONS (Continued)

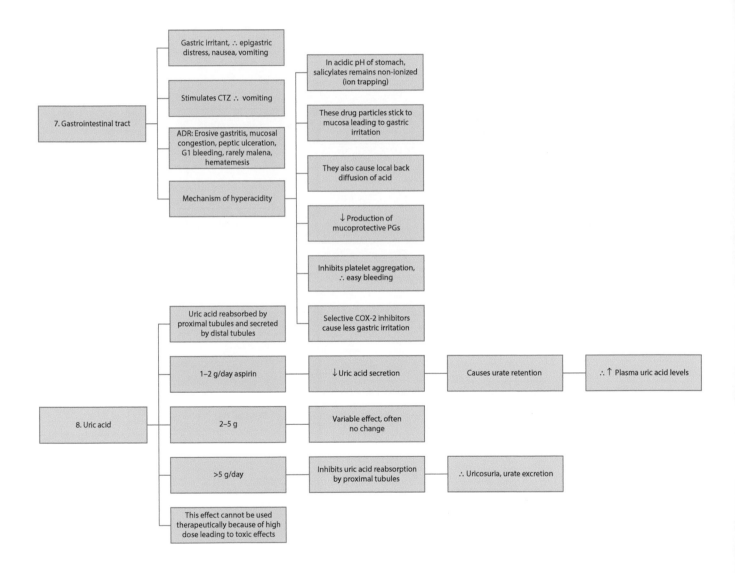

(Continued)

34.6 PHARMACOLOGICAL ACTIONS (Continued)

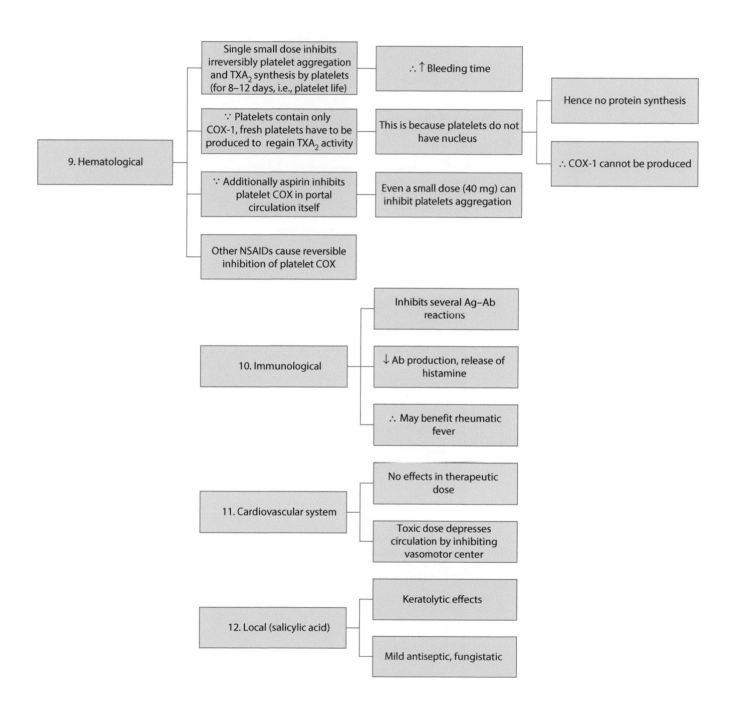

34.7 IMPORTANT PHARMACOKINETIC ASPECTS AND DOSES

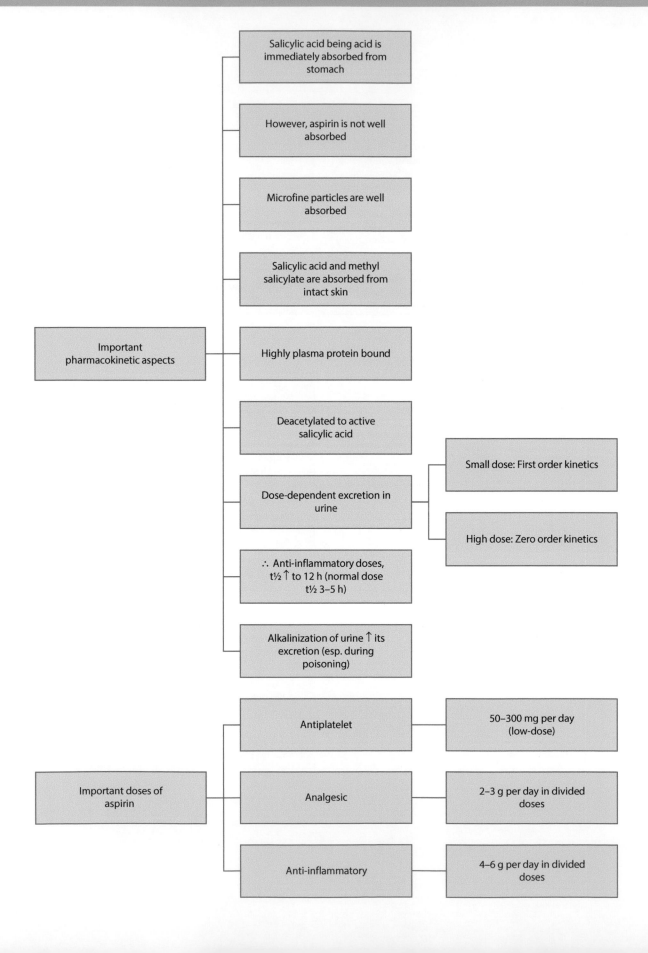

Important pharmacokinetic aspects
- Salicylic acid being acid is immediately absorbed from stomach
- However, aspirin is not well absorbed
- Microfine particles are well absorbed
- Salicylic acid and methyl salicylate are absorbed from intact skin
- Highly plasma protein bound
- Deacetylated to active salicylic acid
- Dose-dependent excretion in urine
  - Small dose: First order kinetics
  - High dose: Zero order kinetics
- ∴ Anti-inflammatory doses, t½ ↑ to 12 h (normal dose t½ 3–5 h)
- Alkalinization of urine ↑ its excretion (esp. during poisoning)

Important doses of aspirin
- Antiplatelet — 50–300 mg per day (low-dose)
- Analgesic — 2–3 g per day in divided doses
- Anti-inflammatory — 4–6 g per day in divided doses

34.8 MAJOR ADVERSE EFFECTS

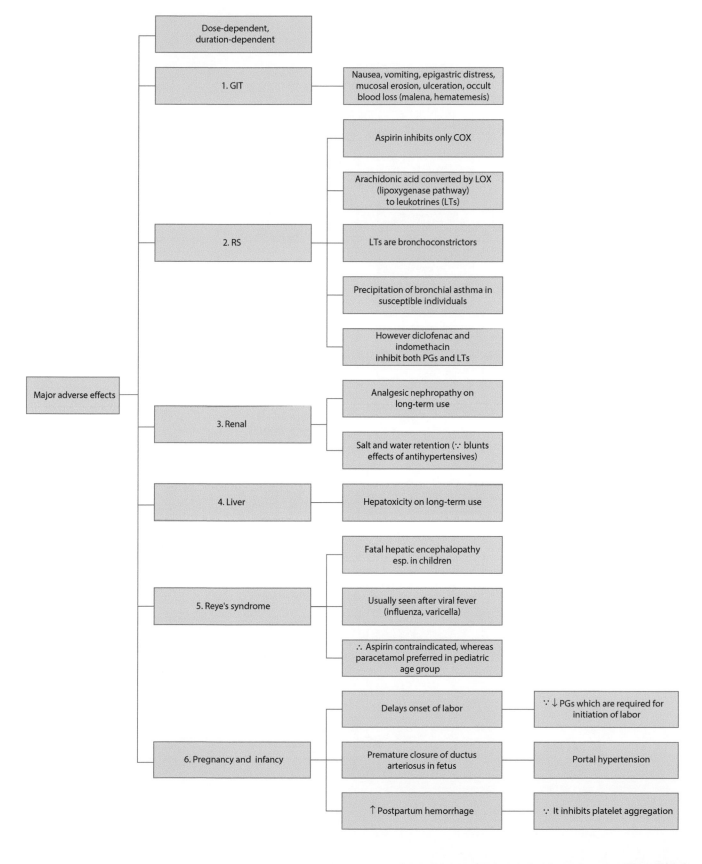

34.8 MAJOR ADVERSE EFFECTS (Continued)

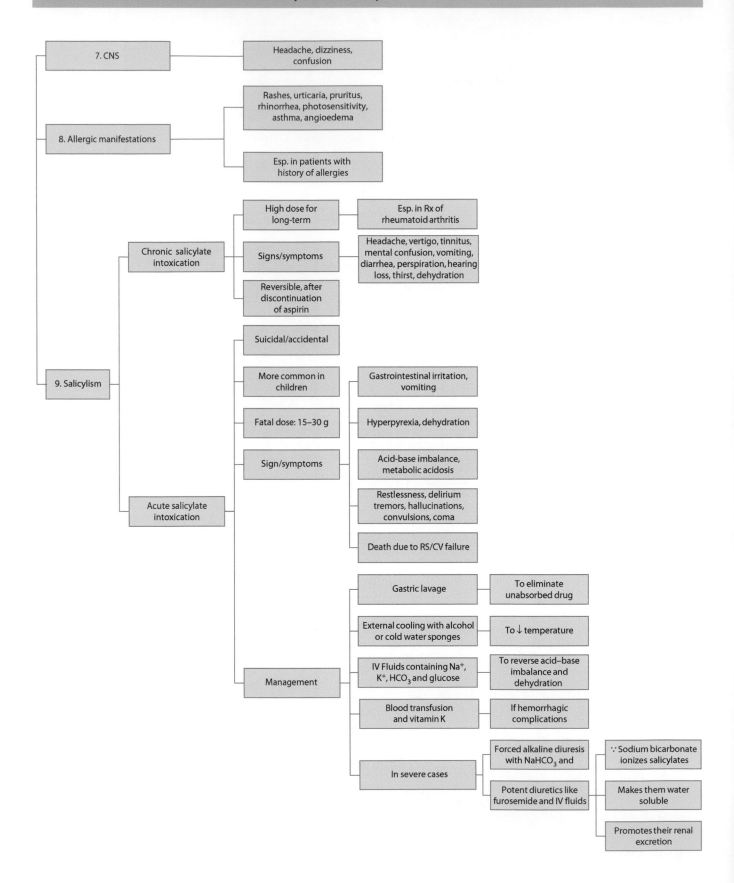

7. CNS — Headache, dizziness, confusion

8. Allergic manifestations
- Rashes, urticaria, pruritus, rhinorrhea, photosensitivity, asthma, angioedema
- Esp. in patients with history of allergies

9. Salicylism

Chronic salicylate intoxication
- High dose for long-term — Esp. in Rx of rheumatoid arthritis
- Signs/symptoms — Headache, vertigo, tinnitus, mental confusion, vomiting, diarrhea, perspiration, hearing loss, thirst, dehydration
- Reversible, after discontinuation of aspirin

Acute salicylate intoxication
- Suicidal/accidental
- More common in children
- Fatal dose: 15–30 g
- Sign/symptoms
  - Gastrointestinal irritation, vomiting
  - Hyperpyrexia, dehydration
  - Acid-base imbalance, metabolic acidosis
  - Restlessness, delirium tremors, hallucinations, convulsions, coma
  - Death due to RS/CV failure
- Management
  - Gastric lavage — To eliminate unabsorbed drug
  - External cooling with alcohol or cold water sponges — To ↓ temperature
  - IV Fluids containing Na$^+$, K$^+$, HCO$_3$ and glucose — To reverse acid–base imbalance and dehydration
  - Blood transfusion and vitamin K — If hemorrhagic complications
  - In severe cases
    - Forced alkaline diuresis with NaHCO$_3$ and
    - Potent diuretics like furosemide and IV fluids
    - ∴ Sodium bicarbonate ionizes salicylates
    - Makes them water soluble
    - Promotes their renal excretion

34.9 PRECAUTIONS AND CONTRAINDICATIONS

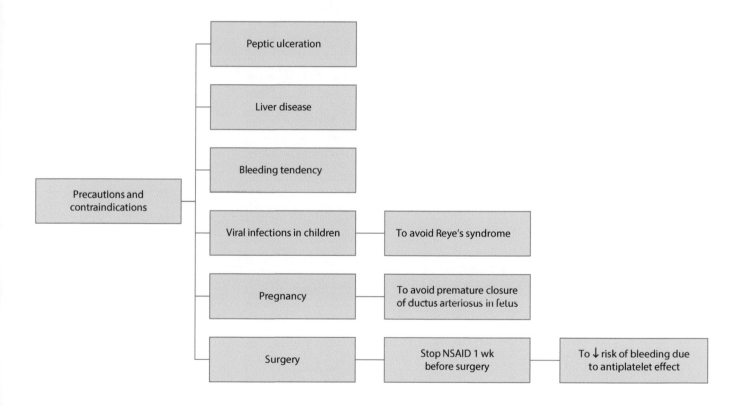

34.10 INDICATIONS

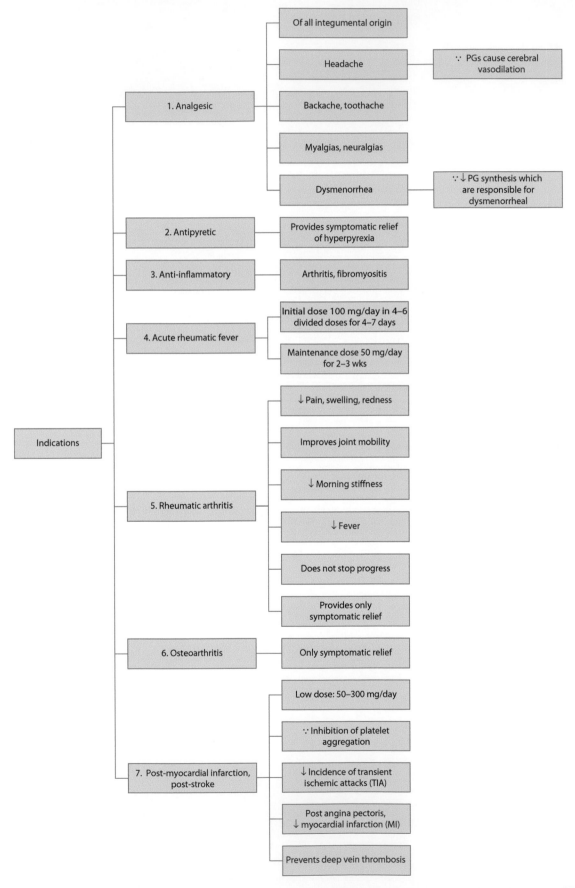

(Continued)

34.10 INDICATIONS (Continued)

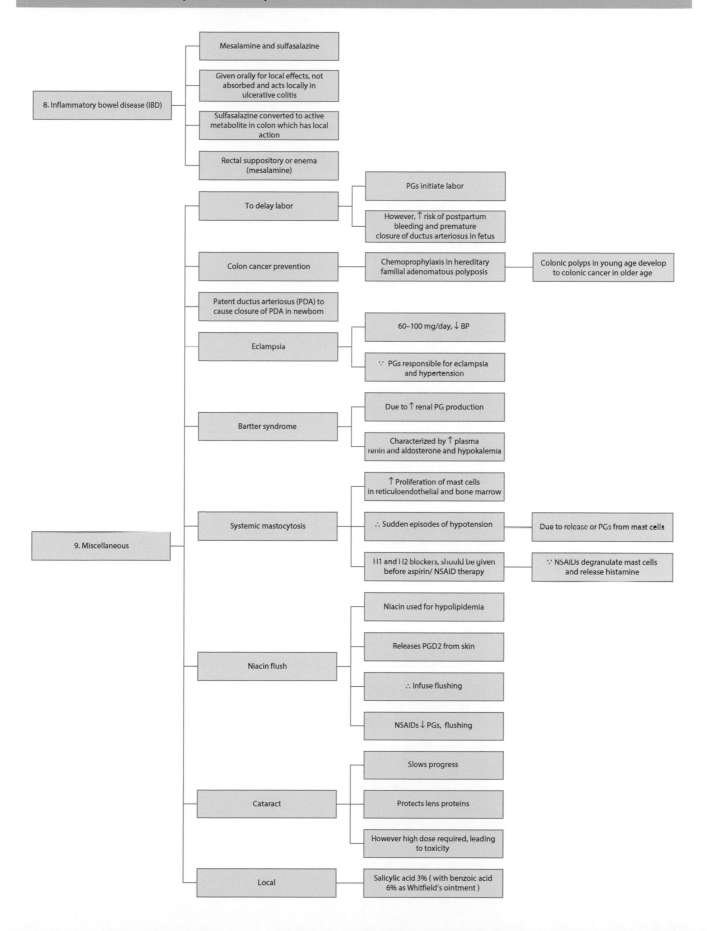

34.11 WHY USE OF ASPIRIN IS CURRENTLY RESTRICTED AND DRUG INTERACTIONS

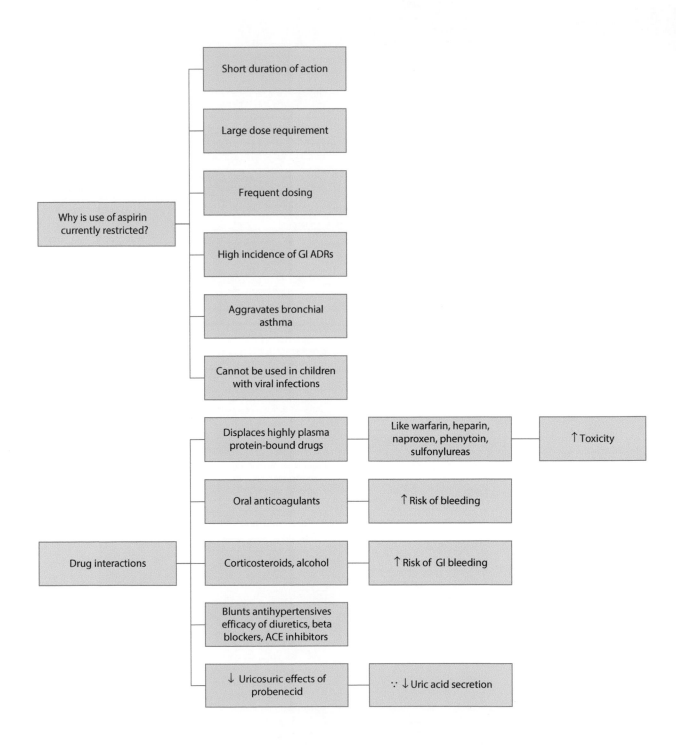

34.12 PYRAZOLONE DERIVATIVES

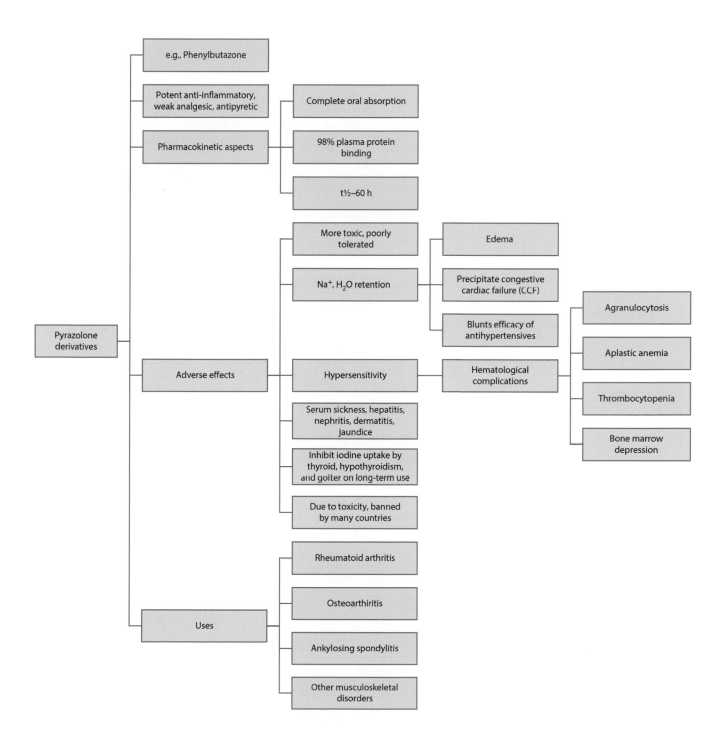

34.13 INDOLE ACETIC ACID DERIVATIVES

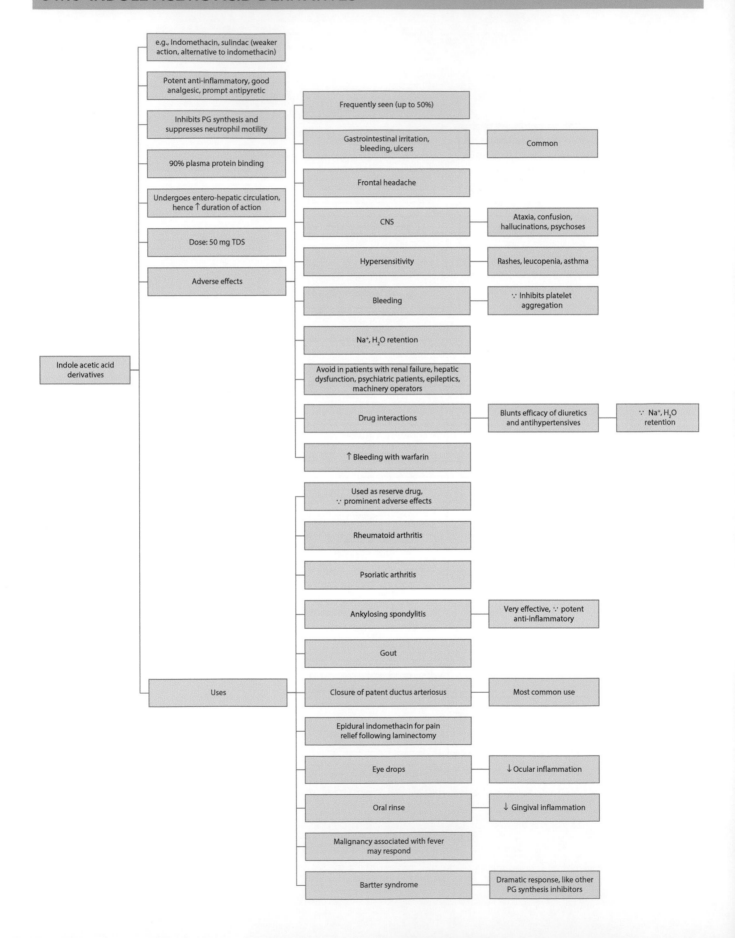

34.14 PROPIONIC ACID DERIVATIVES

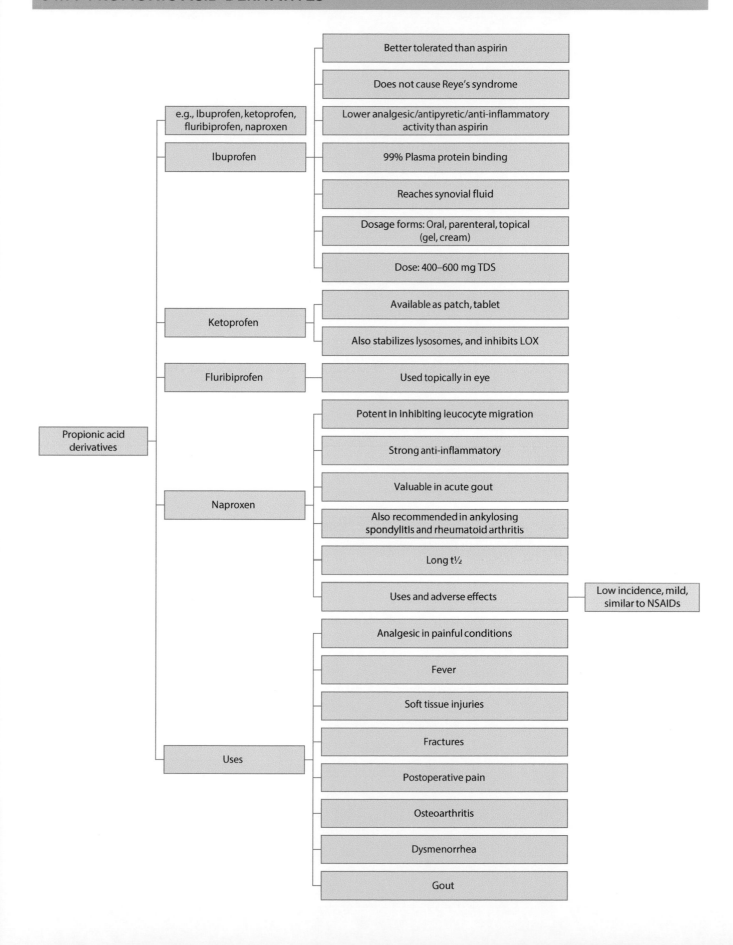

34.15 ANTHRANILIC ACID DERIVATIVES

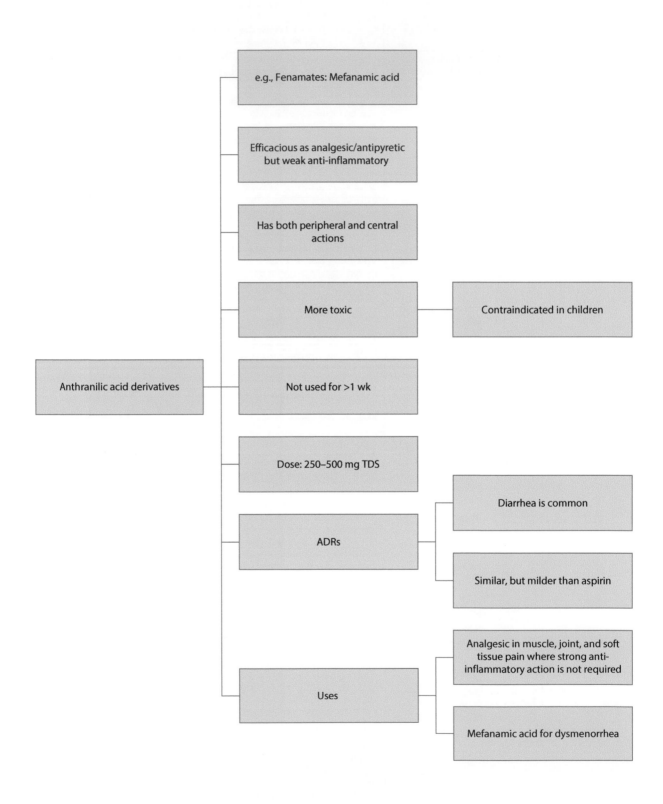

34.16 ENOLIC ACID DERIVATIVES

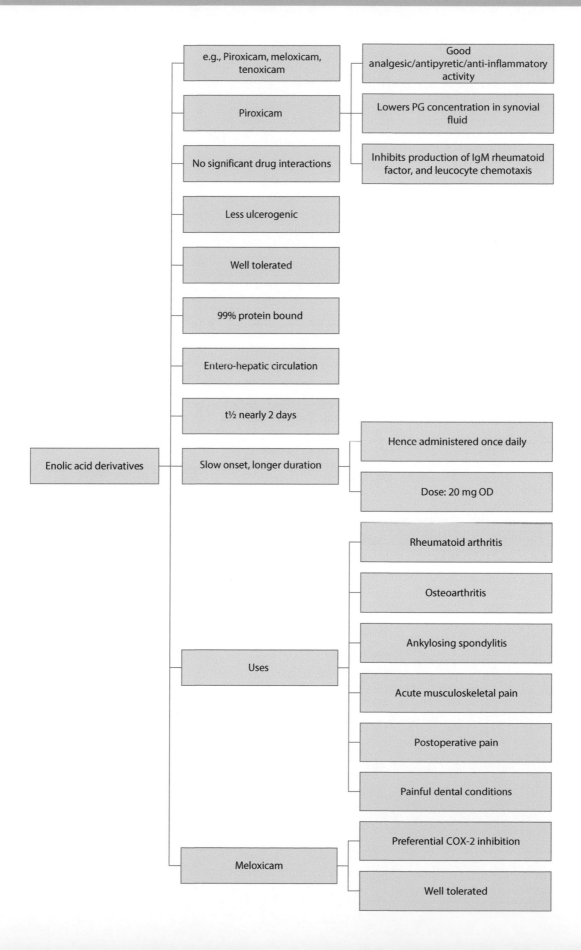

34.17 ALKALONES

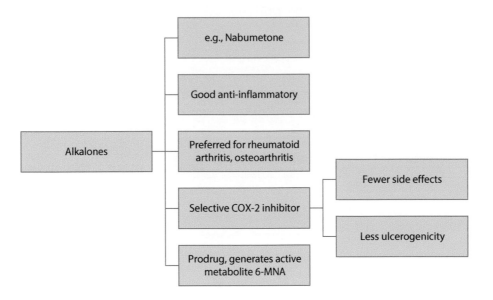

34.18 ARYL-ACTETIC ACID DERIVATIVES

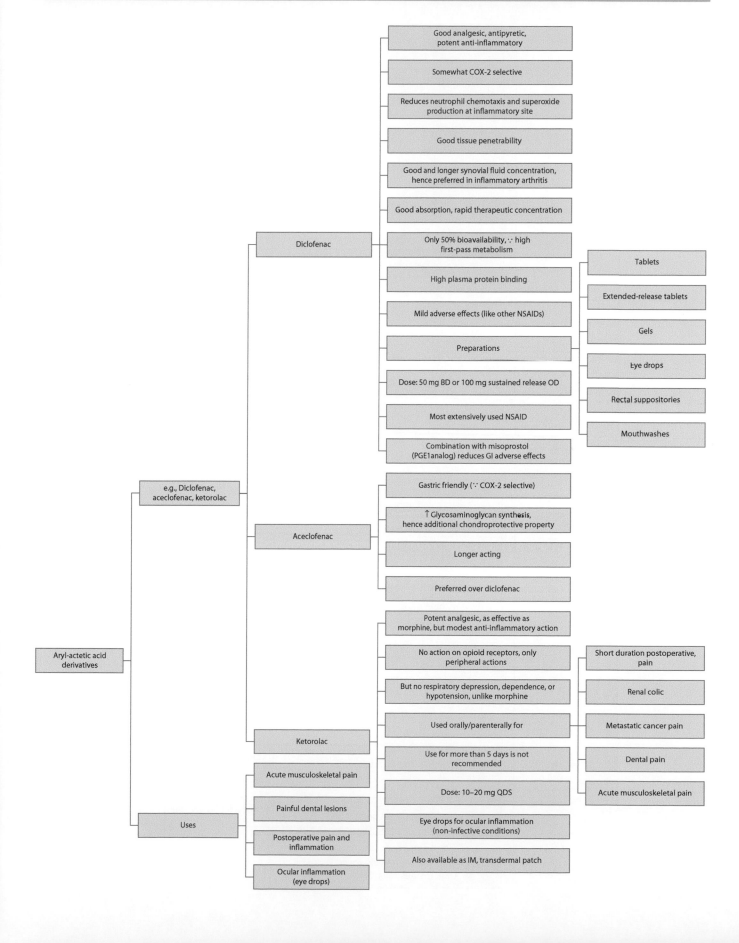

34.19 PREFERRENTIAL COX-2 INHIBITORS

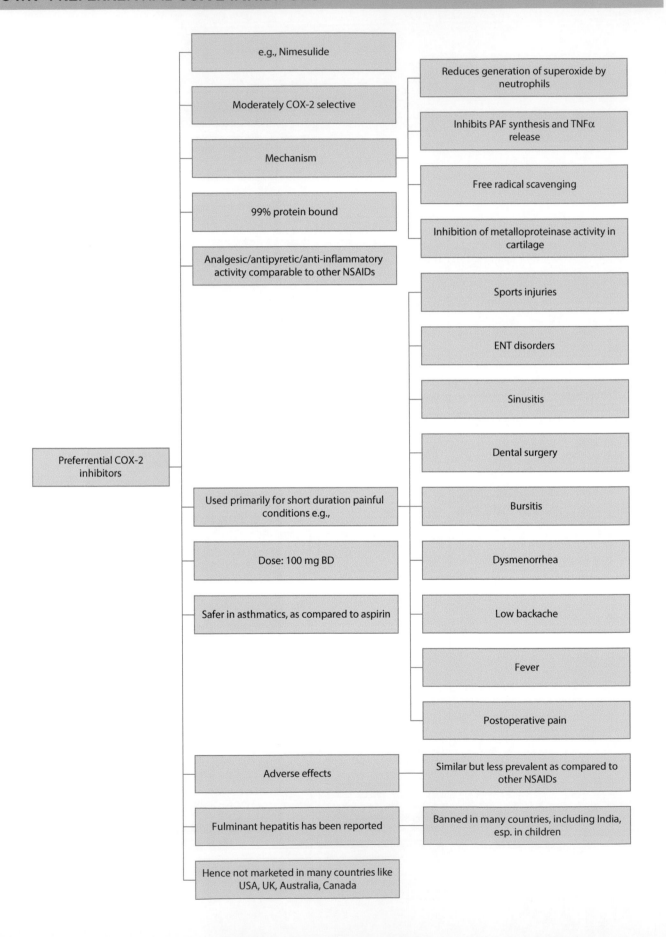

34.20 PARA–AMINOPHENOL DERIVATIVES, PARACETAMOL AND PHARMACOKINETIC ASPECTS

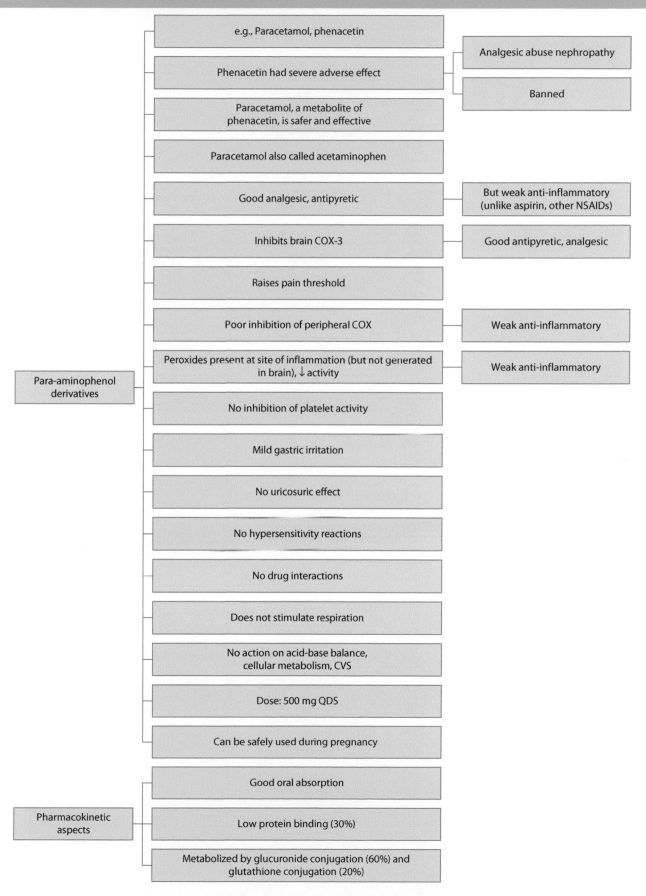

34.21 ADVERSE EFFECTS

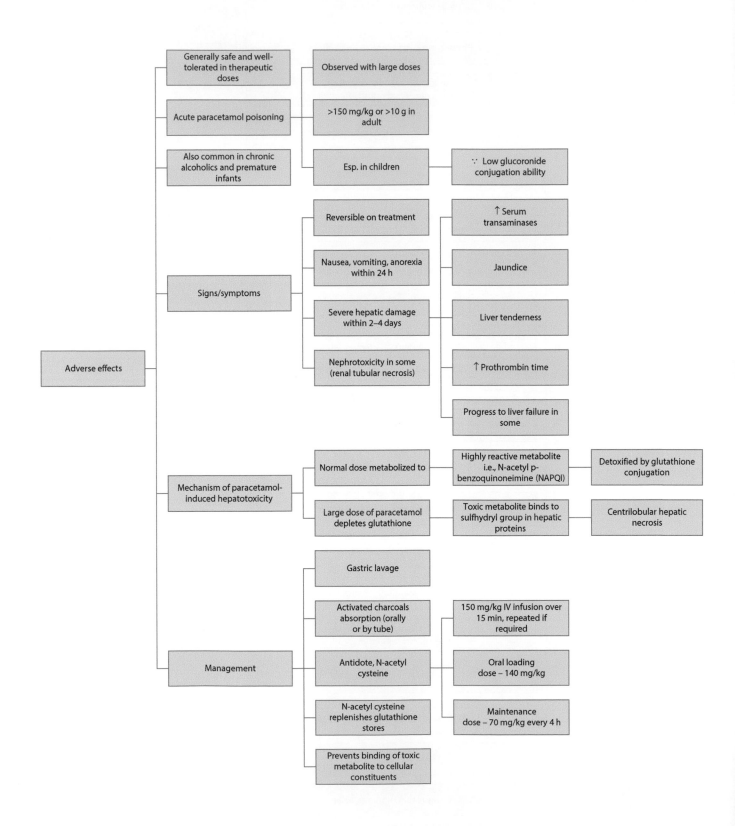

34.22 USES

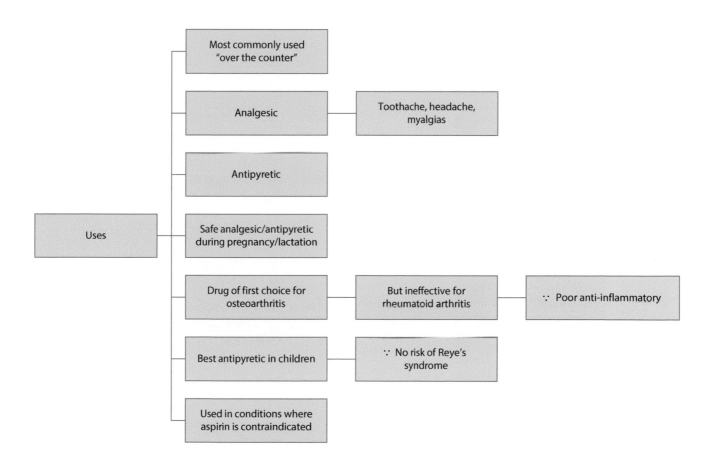

34.23 SELECTIVE COX-2 INHIBITORS

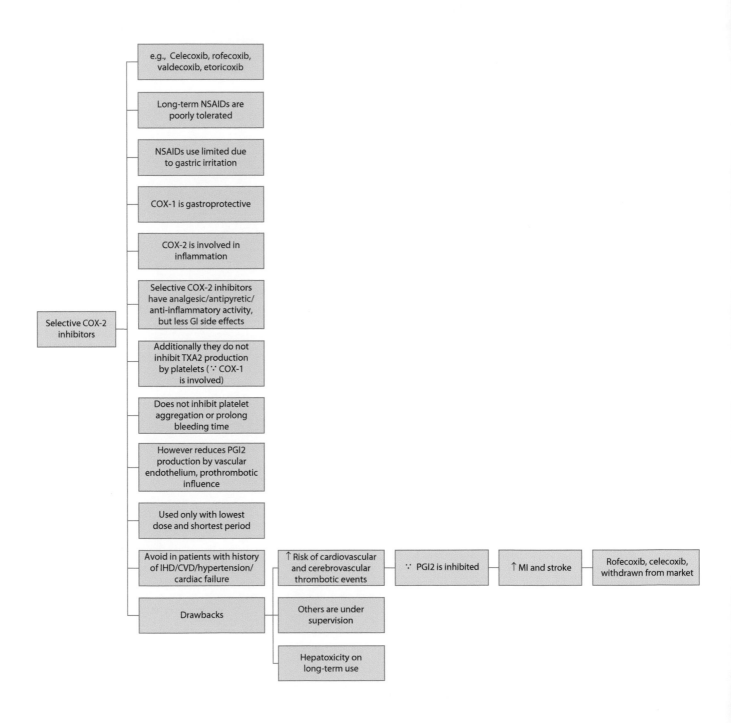

34.24 CHOICE OF NSAIDs

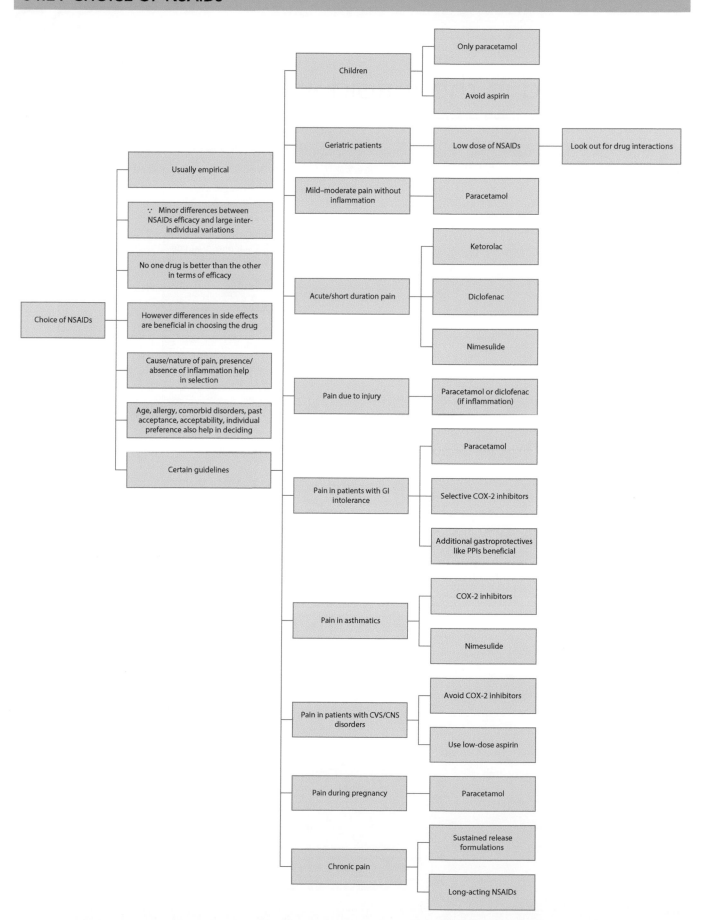

Drugs used in rheumtoid arthritis and gout

35.1 DRUGS USED IN RHEUMATOID ARTHRITIS – CLASSIFICATION

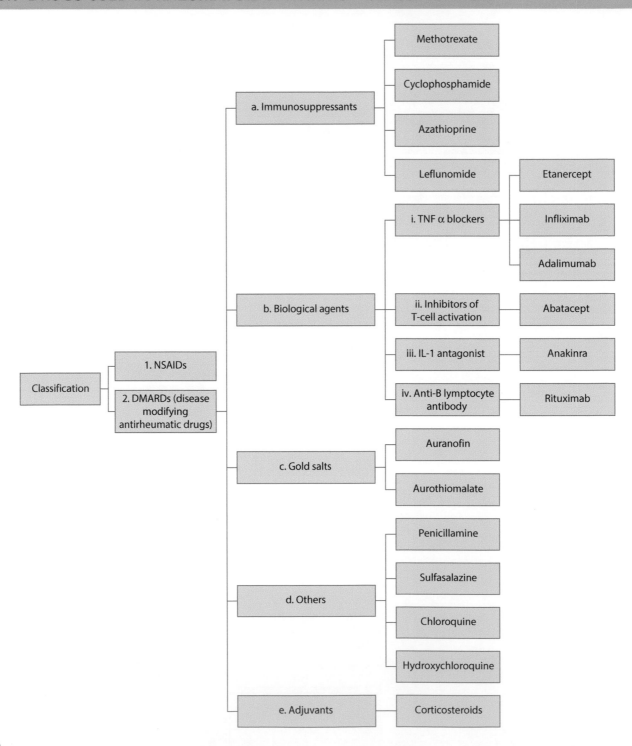

35.2 NSAIDs AND IMMUNOSUPPRESSANTS

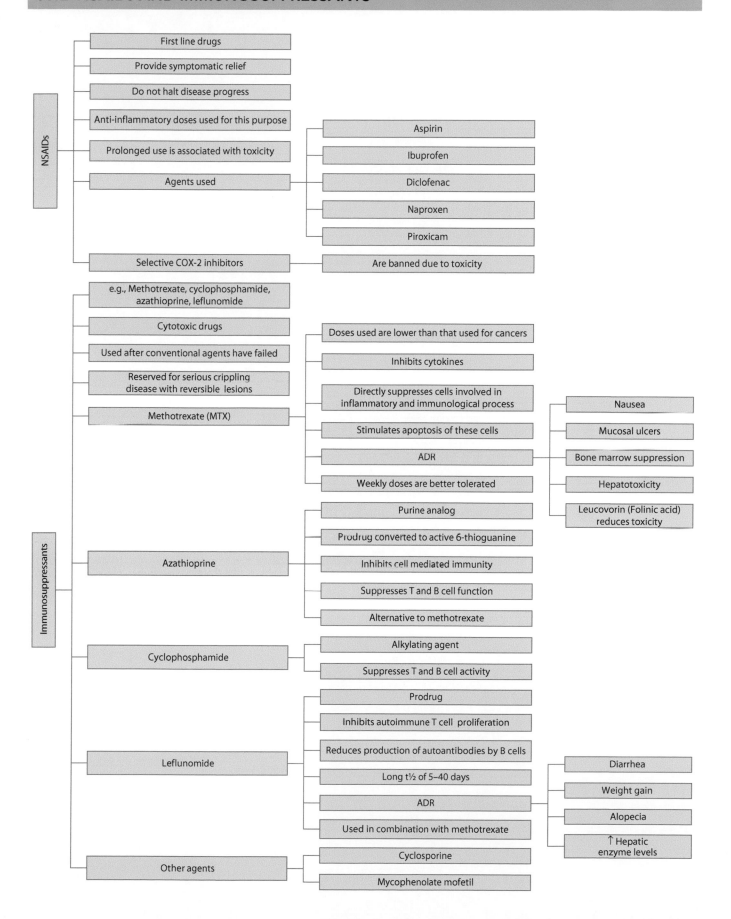

NSAIDs
- First line drugs
- Provide symptomatic relief
- Do not halt disease progress
- Anti-inflammatory doses used for this purpose
- Prolonged use is associated with toxicity
- Agents used
  - Aspirin
  - Ibuprofen
  - Diclofenac
  - Naproxen
  - Piroxicam
- Selective COX-2 inhibitors
  - Are banned due to toxicity

Immunosuppressants
- e.g., Methotrexate, cyclophosphamide, azathioprine, leflunomide
- Cytotoxic drugs
- Used after conventional agents have failed
- Reserved for serious crippling disease with reversible lesions
- Methotrexate (MTX)
  - Doses used are lower than that used for cancers
  - Inhibits cytokines
  - Directly suppresses cells involved in inflammatory and immunological process
  - Stimulates apoptosis of these cells
  - ADR
    - Nausea
    - Mucosal ulcers
    - Bone marrow suppression
    - Hepatotoxicity
    - Leucovorin (Folinic acid) reduces toxicity
  - Weekly doses are better tolerated
- Azathioprine
  - Purine analog
  - Prodrug converted to active 6-thioguanine
  - Inhibits cell mediated immunity
  - Suppresses T and B cell function
  - Alternative to methotrexate
- Cyclophosphamide
  - Alkylating agent
  - Suppresses T and B cell activity
- Leflunomide
  - Prodrug
  - Inhibits autoimmune T cell proliferation
  - Reduces production of autoantibodies by B cells
  - Long t½ of 5–40 days
  - ADR
    - Diarrhea
    - Weight gain
    - Alopecia
    - ↑ Hepatic enzyme levels
  - Used in combination with methotrexate
- Other agents
  - Cyclosporine
  - Mycophenolate mofetil

35.3 BIOLOGICAL AGENTS

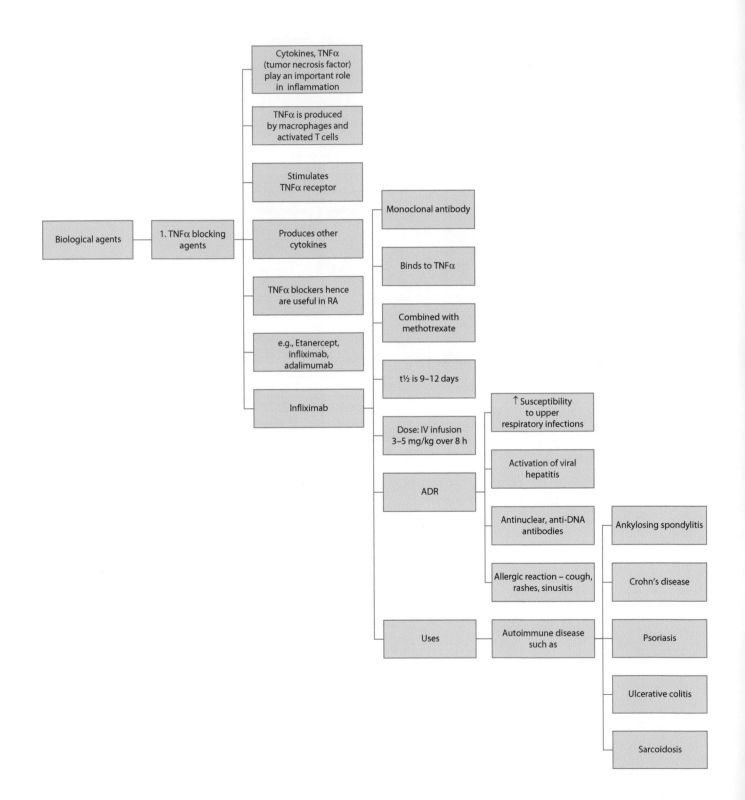

(Continued)

35.3 BIOLOGICAL AGENTS (Continued)

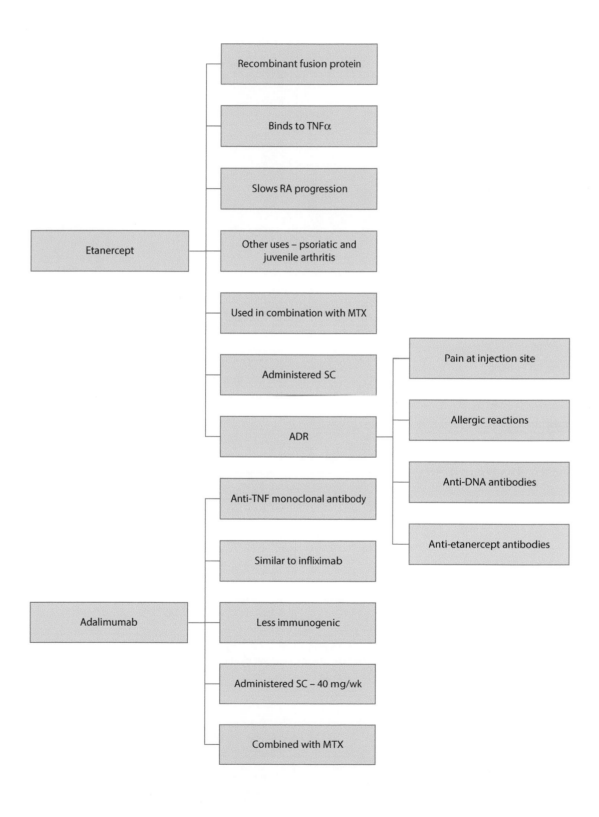

Etanercept
- Recombinant fusion protein
- Binds to TNFα
- Slows RA progression
- Other uses – psoriatic and juvenile arthritis
- Used in combination with MTX
- Administered SC
- ADR
  - Pain at injection site
  - Allergic reactions
  - Anti-DNA antibodies
  - Anti-etanercept antibodies

Adalimumab
- Anti-TNF monoclonal antibody
- Similar to infliximab
- Less immunogenic
- Administered SC – 40 mg/wk
- Combined with MTX

35.4 INHIBITORS OF T-CELL ACTIVATION, IL-1 ANTAGONIST, AND ANTI-B LYMPHOCYTE ANTIBODY

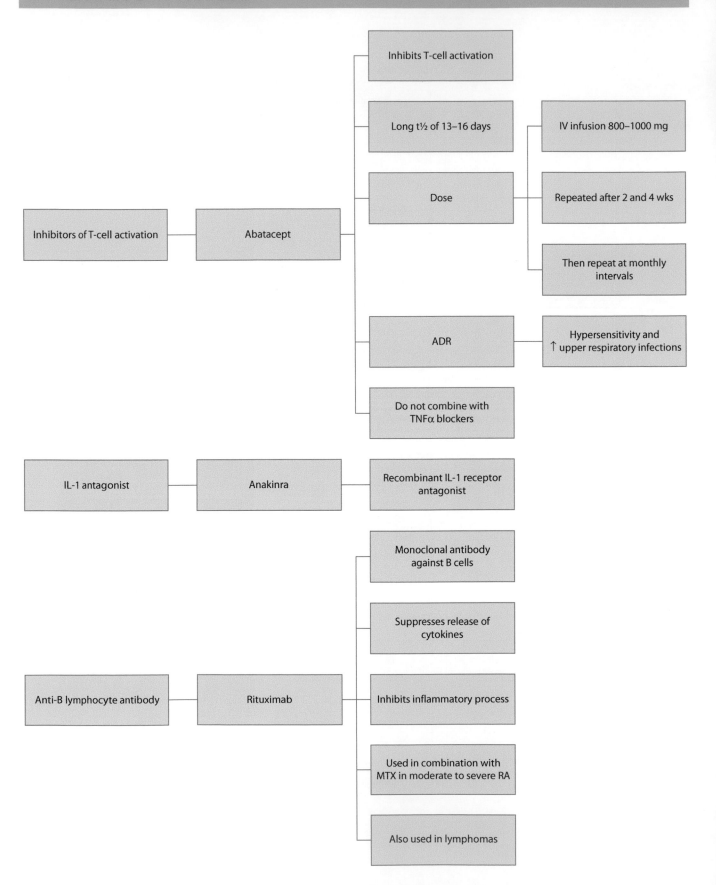

Inhibitors of T-cell activation — Abatacept
- Inhibits T-cell activation
- Long t½ of 13–16 days
- Dose
  - IV infusion 800–1000 mg
  - Repeated after 2 and 4 wks
  - Then repeat at monthly intervals
- ADR
  - Hypersensitivity and ↑ upper respiratory infections
- Do not combine with TNFα blockers

IL-1 antagonist — Anakinra — Recombinant IL-1 receptor antagonist

Anti-B lymphocyte antibody — Rituximab
- Monoclonal antibody against B cells
- Suppresses release of cytokines
- Inhibits inflammatory process
- Used in combination with MTX in moderate to severe RA
- Also used in lymphomas

35.5 GOLD SALTS

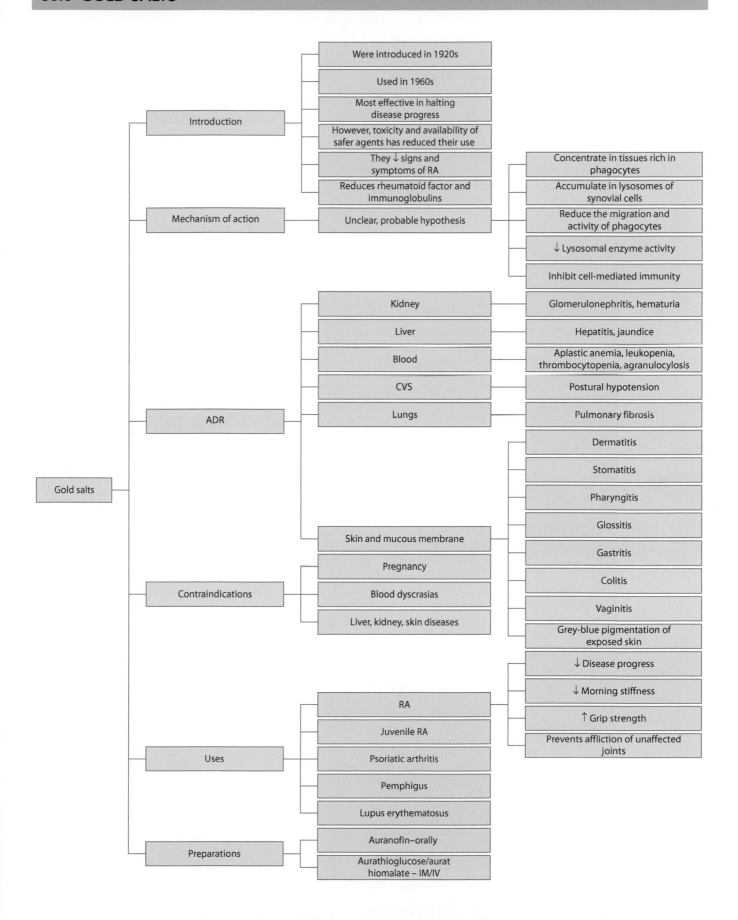

35.6 OTHER ANTIRHEUMATIC DRUGS

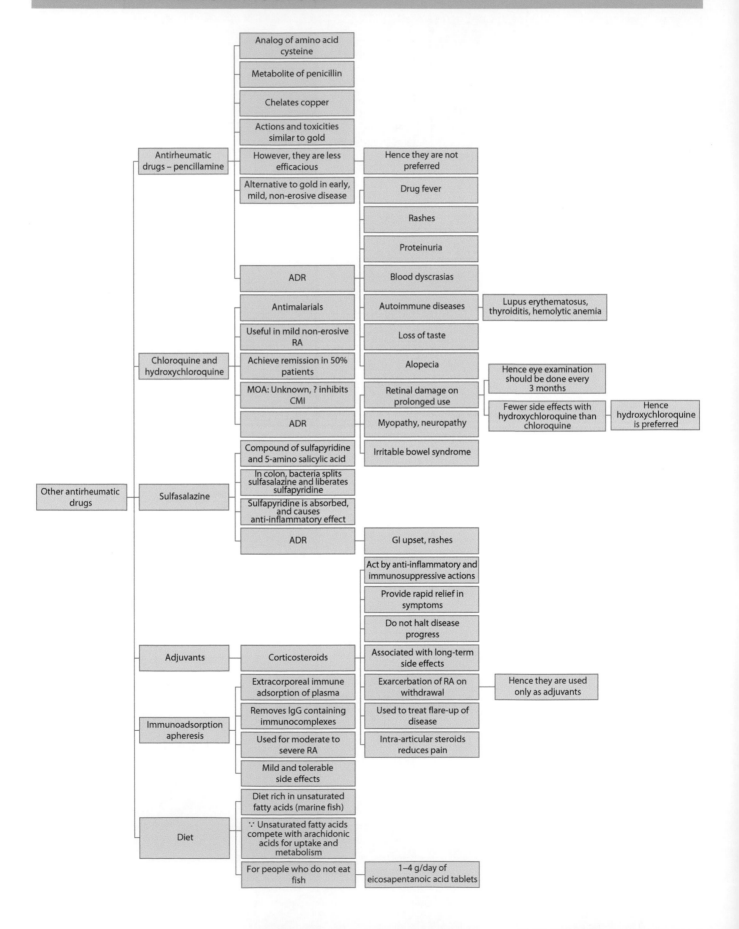

35.7 CLASSIFICATION OF DRUGS FOR GOUT AND COLCHICINE

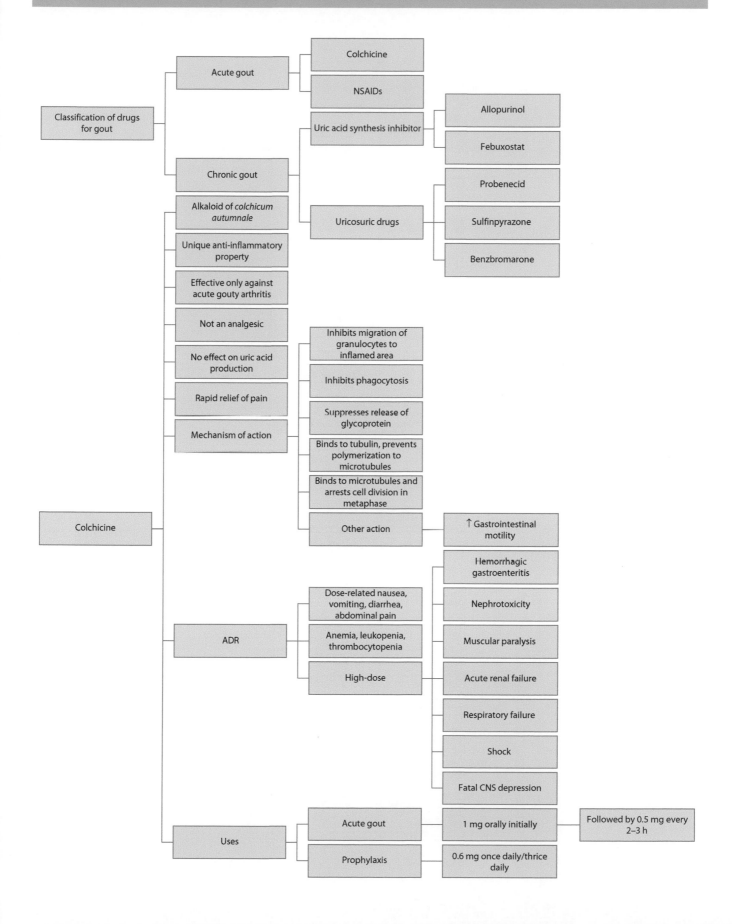

35.8 NSAIDs, ALLOPURINOL, AND FEBUXOSTAT

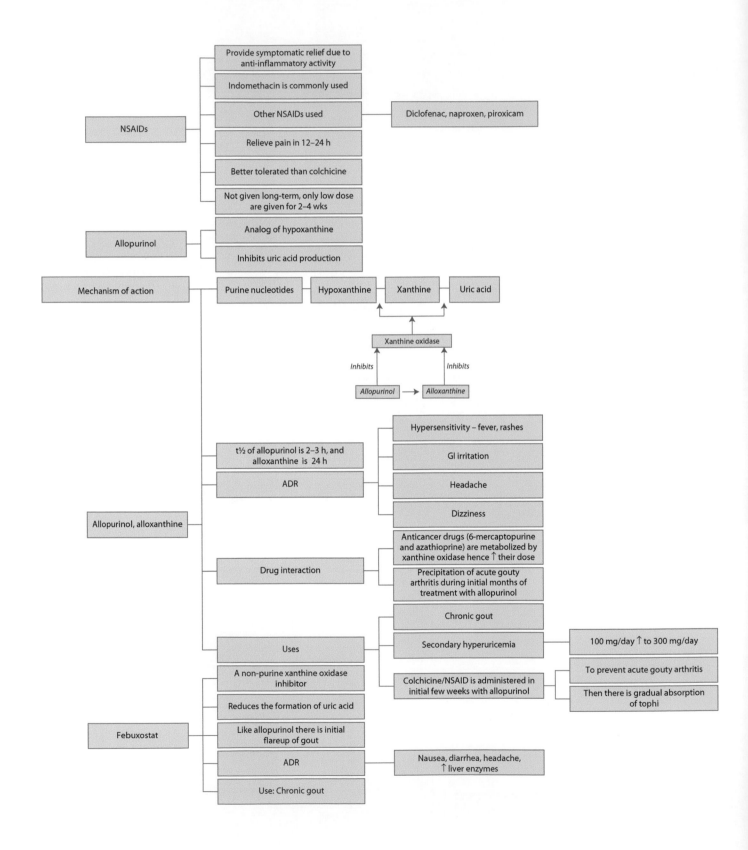

35.9 URICOSURIC DRUGS

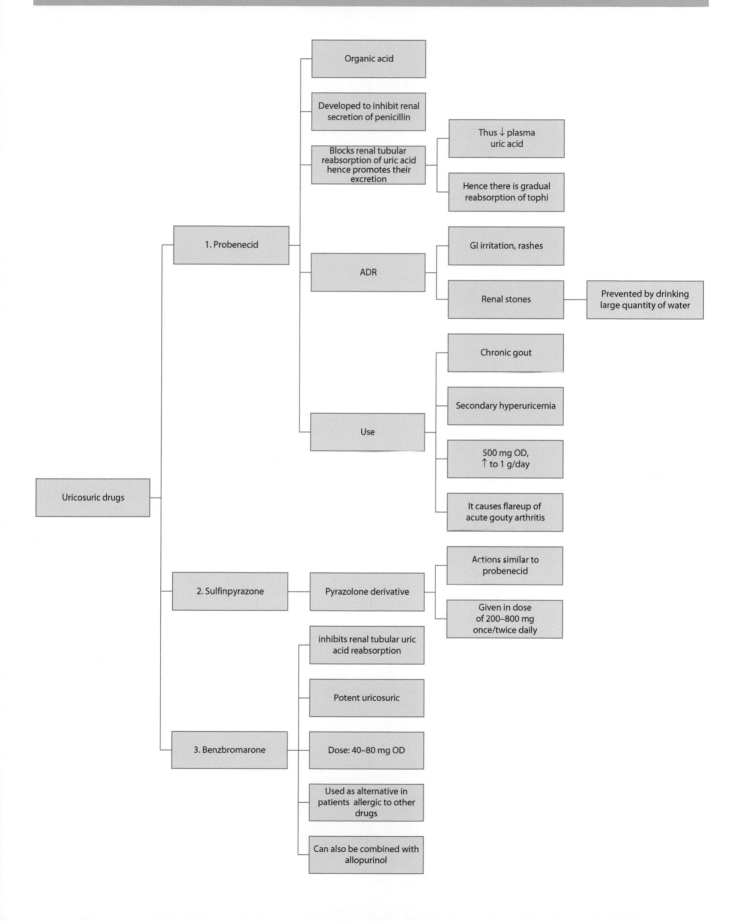

Uricosuric drugs

1. Probenecid
- Organic acid
- Developed to inhibit renal secretion of penicillin
- Blocks renal tubular reabsorption of uric acid hence promotes their excretion
  - Thus ↓ plasma uric acid
  - Hence there is gradual reabsorption of tophi
- ADR
  - GI irritation, rashes
  - Renal stones → Prevented by drinking large quantity of water
- Use
  - Chronic gout
  - Secondary hyperuricemia
  - 500 mg OD, ↑ to 1 g/day
  - It causes flareup of acute gouty arthritis

2. Sulfinpyrazone
- Pyrazolone derivative
  - Actions similar to probenecid
  - Given in dose of 200–800 mg once/twice daily

3. Benzbromarone
- inhibits renal tubular uric acid reabsorption
- Potent uricosuric
- Dose: 40–80 mg OD
- Used as alternative in patients allergic to other drugs
- Can also be combined with allopurinol

PART VI

Respiratory pharmacology

Drugs used in the treatment of bronchial asthma and chronic obstuctive pulmonary disorders (COPD)

36.1 CLASSIFICATION OF DRUGS FOR BRONCHIAL ASTHMA

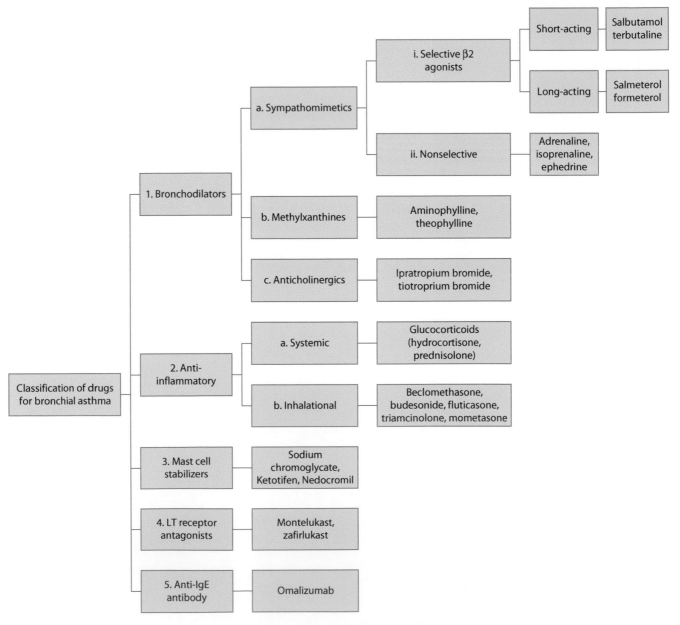

36.2 SYMPATHOMIMETICS

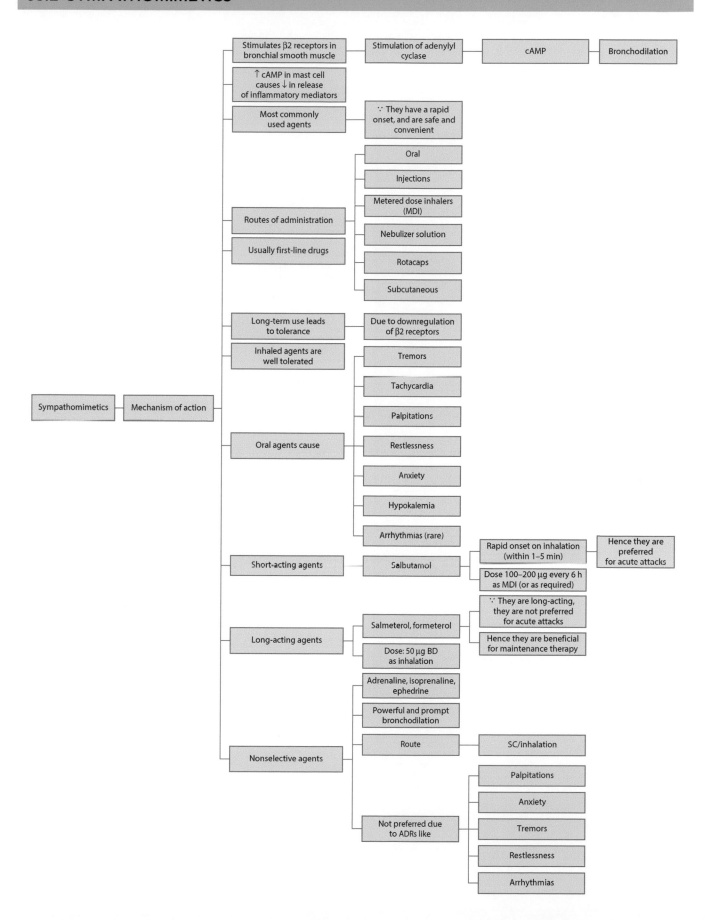

36.3 METHYLXANTHINES

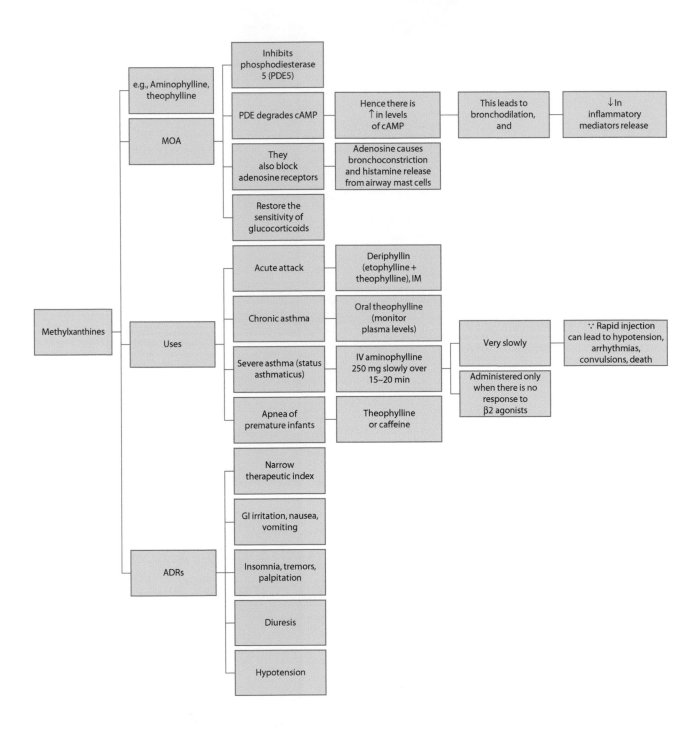

36.4 ANTICHOLINERGICS

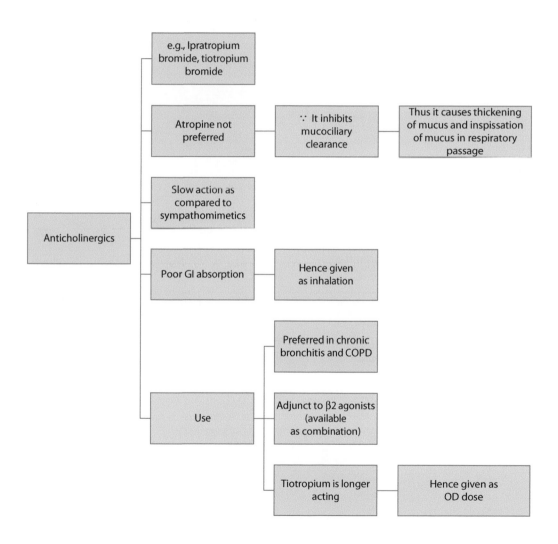

36.5 ANTI-INFLAMMATORY DRUGS

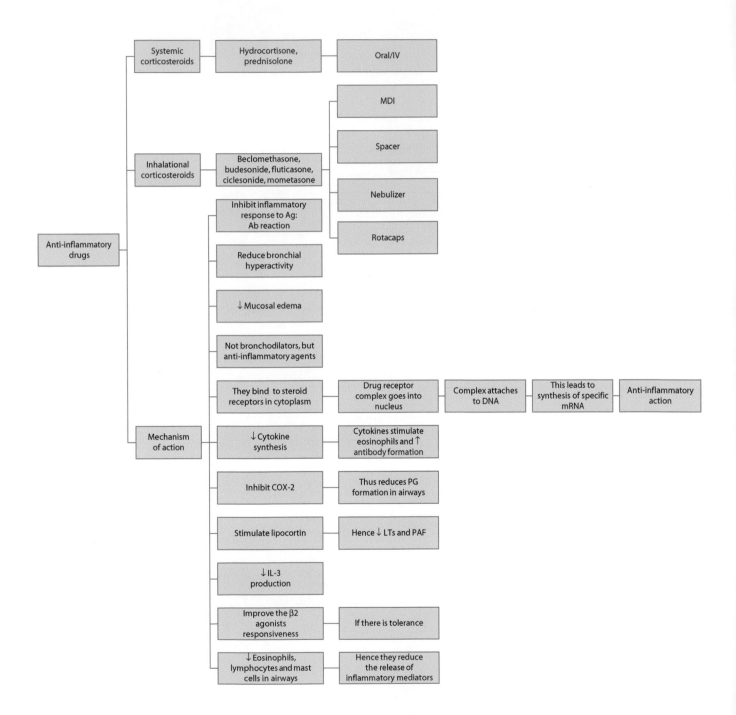

36.6 ANTI-INFLAMMATORY DRUGS – USES, INHALATION STEROIDS

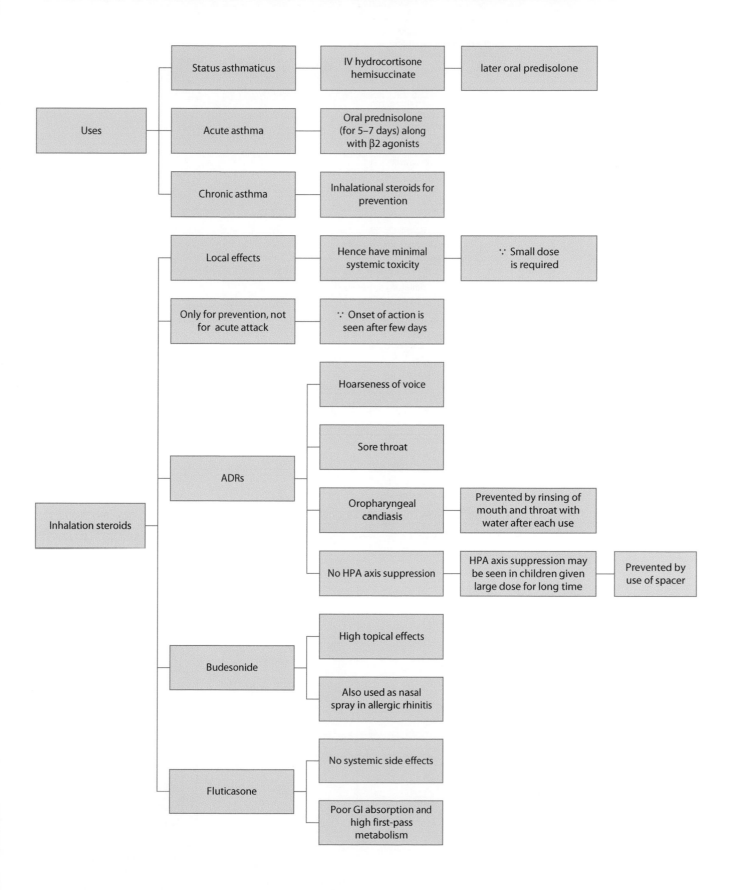

36.7 MAST CELL STABILIZERS

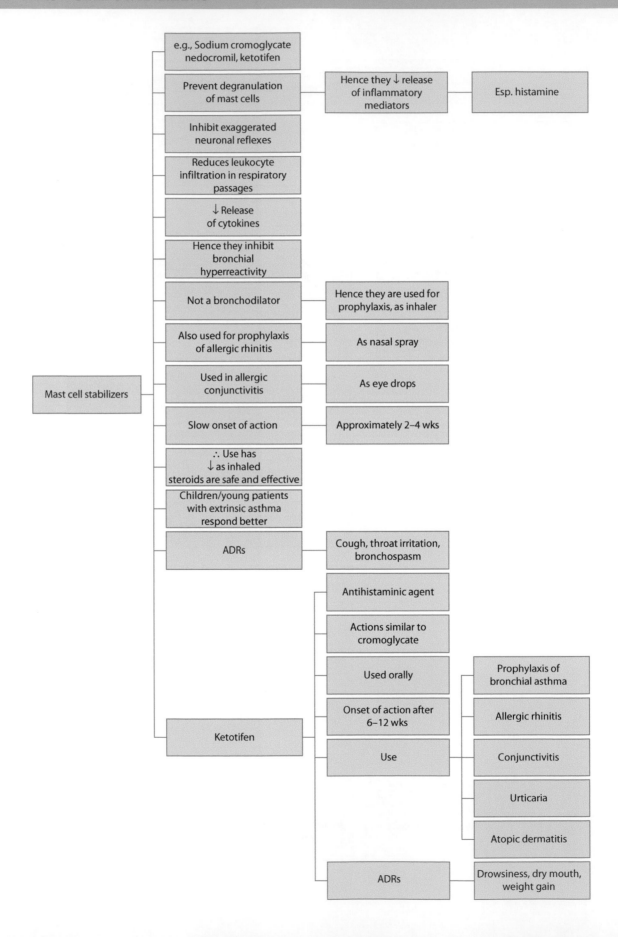

36.8 LEUKOTRIENE RECEPTOR ANTAGONISTS (LRA) AND ANTI-IgE ANTIBODY

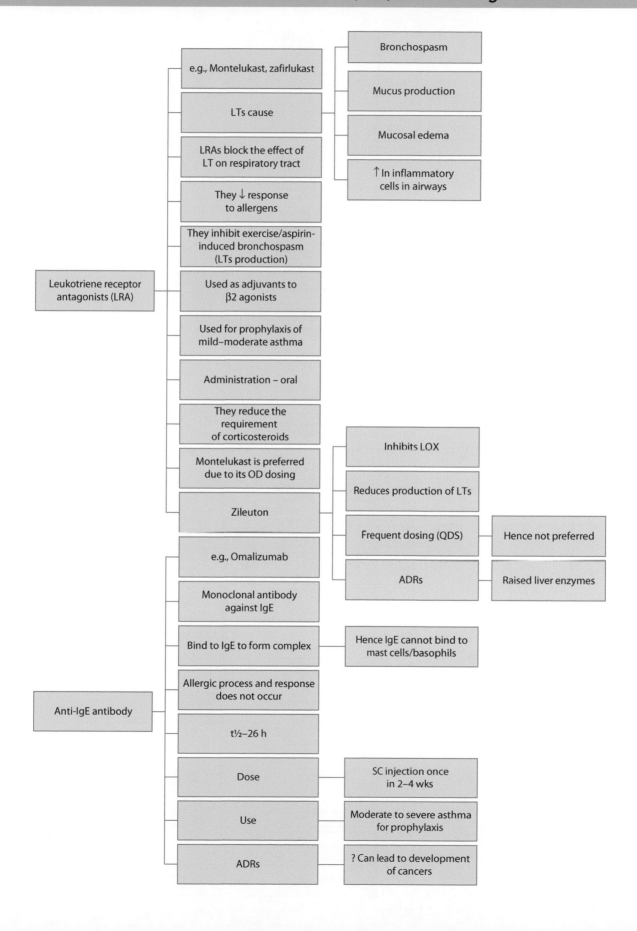

Leukotriene receptor antagonists (LRA)
- e.g., Montelukast, zafirlukast
- LTs cause
  - Bronchospasm
  - Mucus production
  - Mucosal edema
  - ↑ In inflammatory cells in airways
- LRAs block the effect of LT on respiratory tract
- They ↓ response to allergens
- They inhibit exercise/aspirin-induced bronchospasm (LTs production)
- Used as adjuvants to β2 agonists
- Used for prophylaxis of mild–moderate asthma
- Administration – oral
- They reduce the requirement of corticosteroids
- Montelukast is preferred due to its OD dosing
- Zileuton
  - Inhibits LOX
  - Reduces production of LTs
  - Frequent dosing (QDS) — Hence not preferred
  - ADRs — Raised liver enzymes

Anti-IgE antibody
- e.g., Omalizumab
- Monoclonal antibody against IgE
- Bind to IgE to form complex — Hence IgE cannot bind to mast cells/basophils
- Allergic process and response does not occur
- t½–26 h
- Dose — SC injection once in 2–4 wks
- Use — Moderate to severe asthma for prophylaxis
- ADRs — ? Can lead to development of cancers

36.9 TREATMENT OF BRONCHIAL ASTHMA

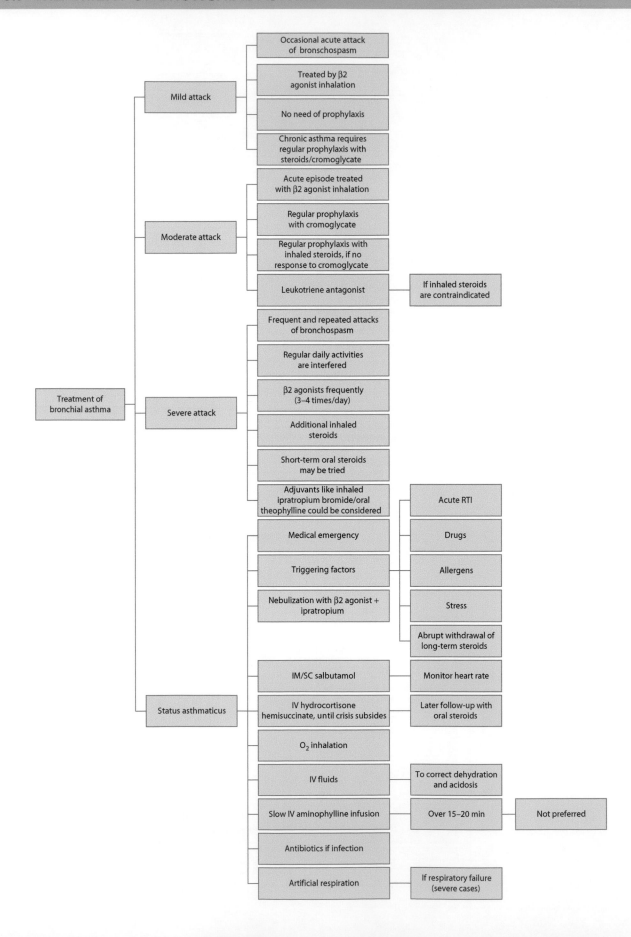

36.10 MANAGEMENT OF CHRONIC OBSTRUCTIVE PULMONARY DISEASE (COPD)/CHRONIC OBSTRUCTIVE LUNG DISEASE (COLD)

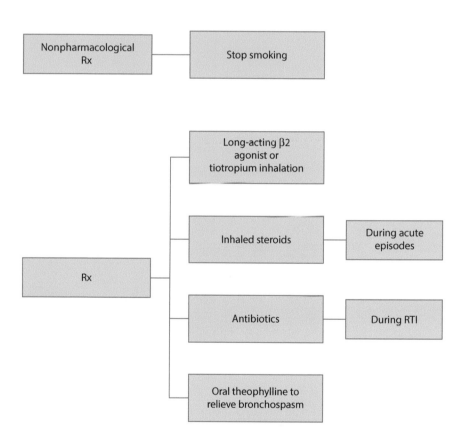

36.11 AEROSOLS IN ASTHMA

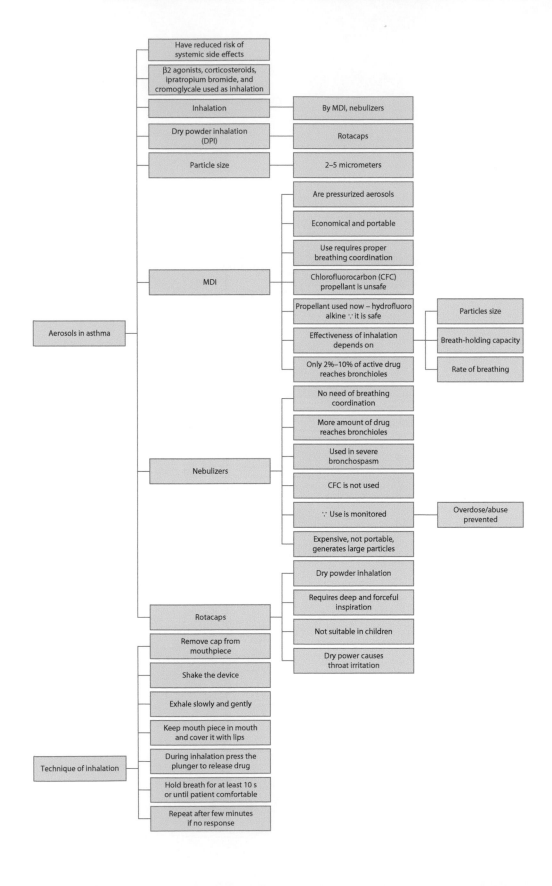

Drugs used in the treatment of cough

37.1 ANTITUSSIVES AND CENTRAL COUGH SUPPRESSANTS

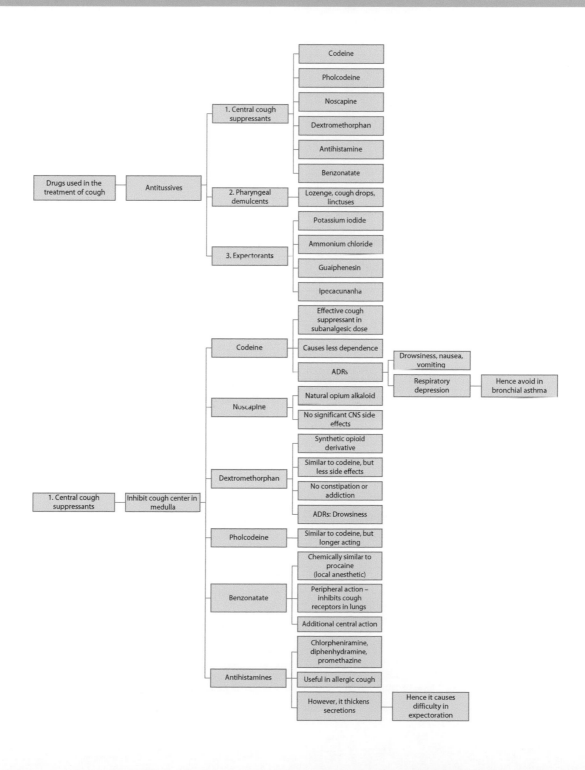

37.2 PHARYNGEAL DEMULCENTS AND EXPECTORANTS

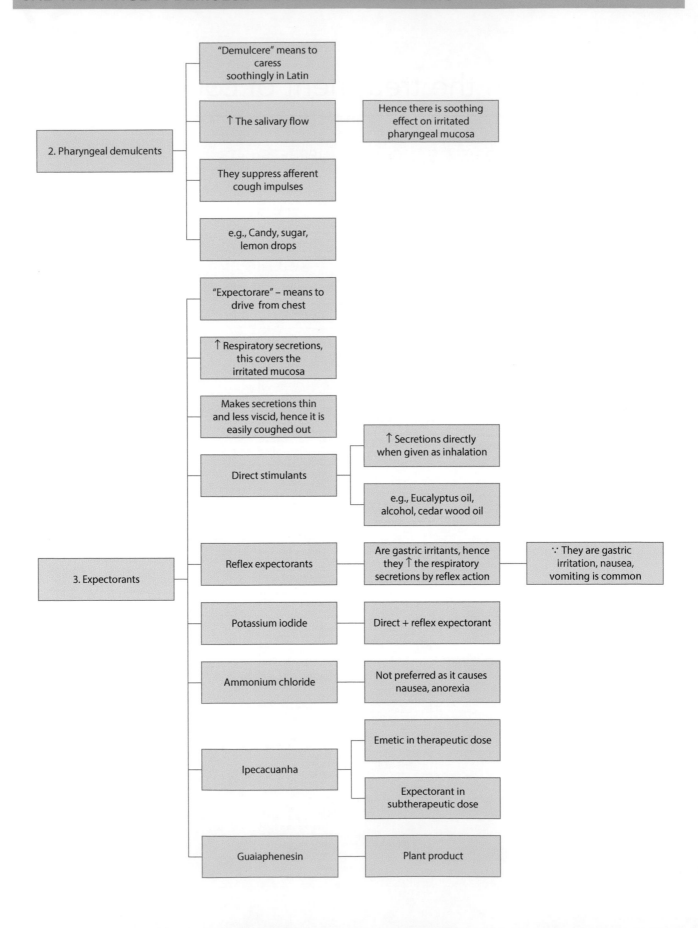

2. Pharyngeal demulcents

- "Demulcere" means to caress soothingly in Latin
- ↑ The salivary flow → Hence there is soothing effect on irritated pharyngeal mucosa
- They suppress afferent cough impulses
- e.g., Candy, sugar, lemon drops

3. Expectorants

- "Expectorare" – means to drive from chest
- ↑ Respiratory secretions, this covers the irritated mucosa
- Makes secretions thin and less viscid, hence it is easily coughed out
- Direct stimulants
  - ↑ Secretions directly when given as inhalation
  - e.g., Eucalyptus oil, alcohol, cedar wood oil
- Reflex expectorants → Are gastric irritants, hence they ↑ the respiratory secretions by reflex action → ∵ They are gastric irritation, nausea, vomiting is common
- Potassium iodide → Direct + reflex expectorant
- Ammonium chloride → Not preferred as it causes nausea, anorexia
- Ipecacuanha
  - Emetic in therapeutic dose
  - Expectorant in subtherapeutic dose
- Guaiaphenesin → Plant product

37.3 MUCOLYTICS AND DRUGS CAUSING COUGH

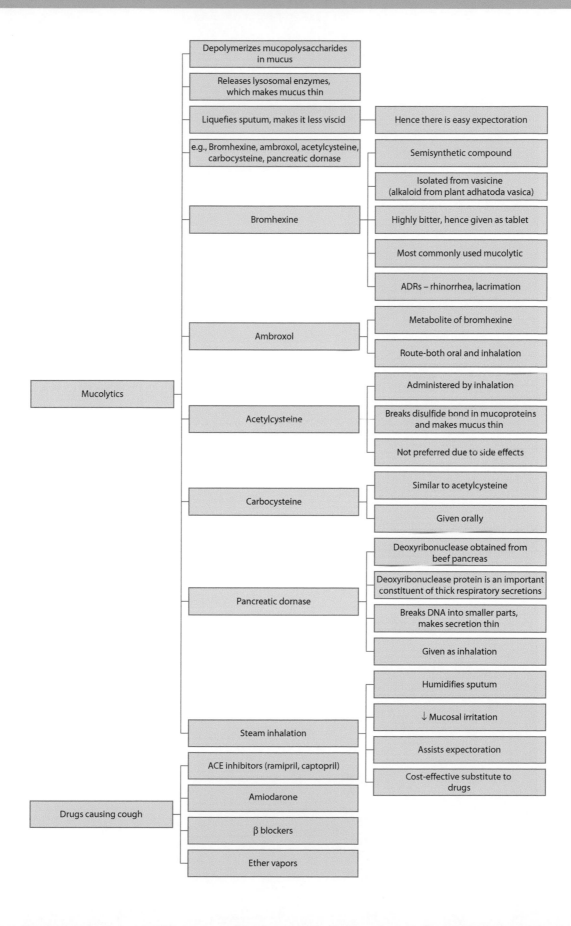

- Mucolytics
  - Depolymerizes mucopolysaccharides in mucus
  - Releases lysosomal enzymes, which makes mucus thin
  - Liquefies sputum, makes it less viscid
    - Hence there is easy expectoration
  - e.g., Bromhexine, ambroxol, acetylcysteine, carbocysteine, pancreatic dornase
  - Bromhexine
    - Semisynthetic compound
    - Isolated from vasicine (alkaloid from plant adhatoda vasica)
    - Highly bitter, hence given as tablet
    - Most commonly used mucolytic
    - ADRs – rhinorrhea, lacrimation
  - Ambroxol
    - Metabolite of bromhexine
    - Route-both oral and inhalation
  - Acetylcysteine
    - Administered by inhalation
    - Breaks disulfide bond in mucoproteins and makes mucus thin
    - Not preferred due to side effects
  - Carbocysteine
    - Similar to acetylcysteine
    - Given orally
  - Pancreatic dornase
    - Deoxyribonuclease obtained from beef pancreas
    - Deoxyribonuclease protein is an important constituent of thick respiratory secretions
    - Breaks DNA into smaller parts, makes secretion thin
    - Given as inhalation
  - Steam inhalation
    - Humidifies sputum
    - ↓ Mucosal irritation
    - Assists expectoration
    - Cost-effective substitute to drugs
- Drugs causing cough
  - ACE inhibitors (ramipril, captopril)
  - Amiodarone
  - β blockers
  - Ether vapors

PART VII

Hematological pharmacology

Hematinics

38.1 INTRODUCTION AND IRON ABSORPTION

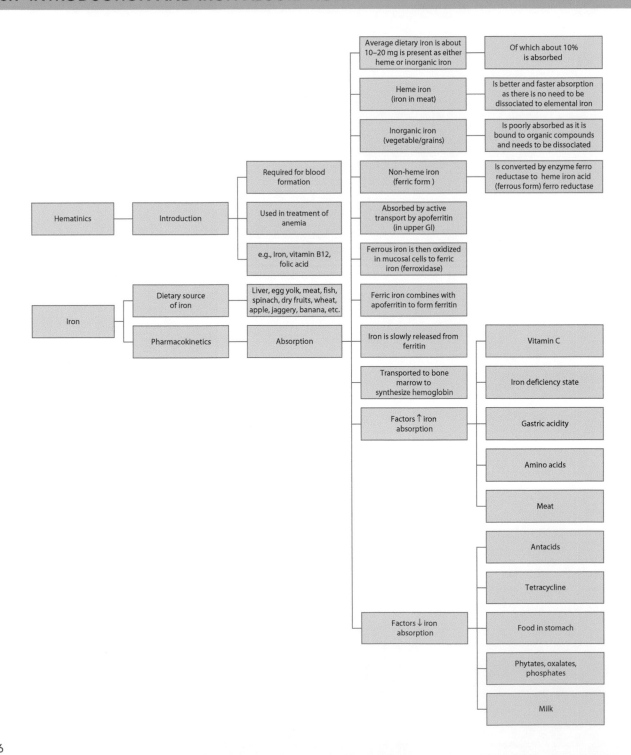

38.2 IRON METABOLISM AND REQUIREMENTS

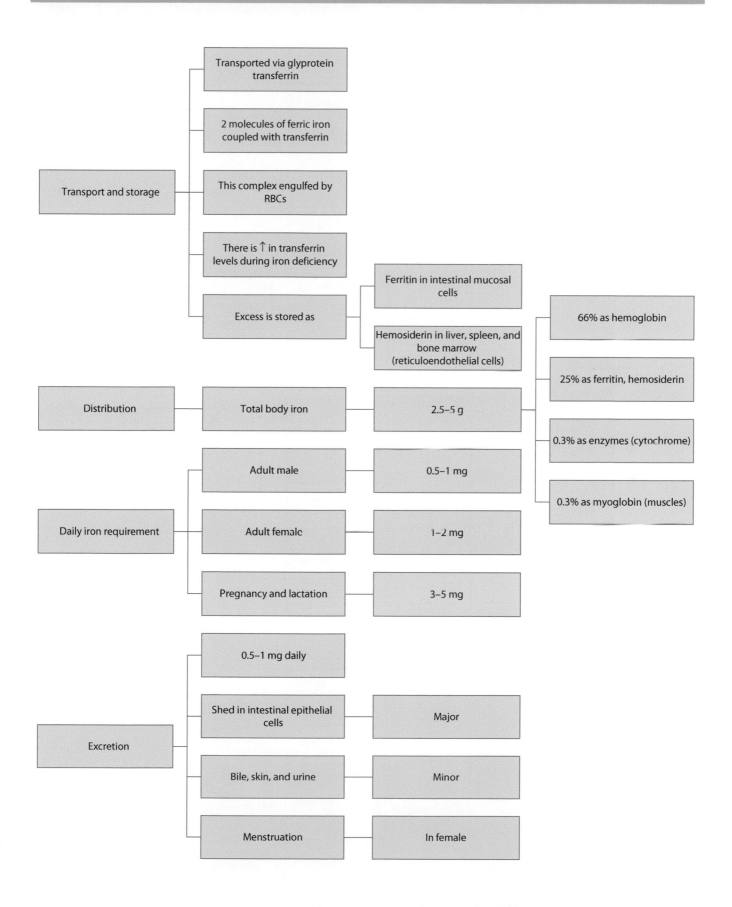

38.3 IRON PREPARATIONS – ORAL AND PARENTERAL

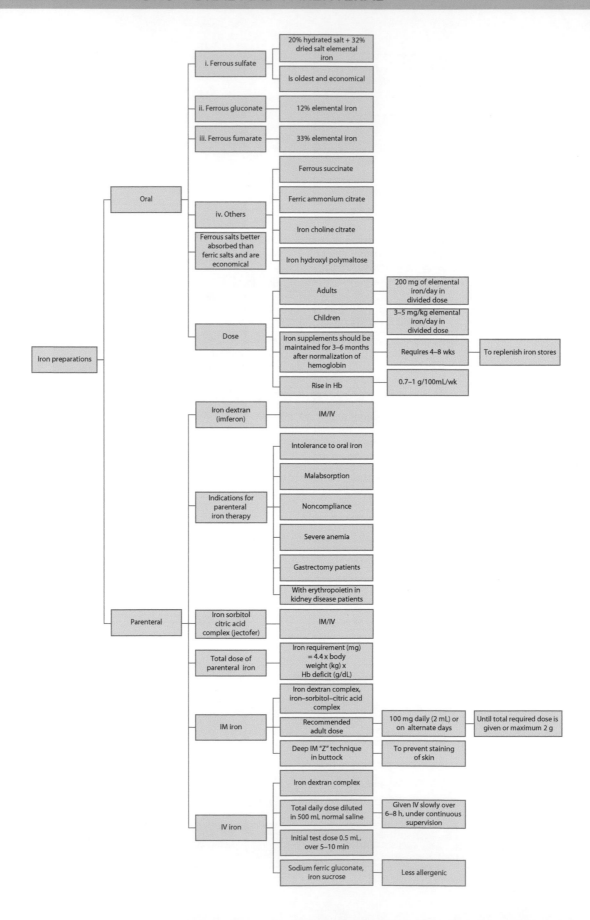

38.4 USES OF IRON AND ADRs

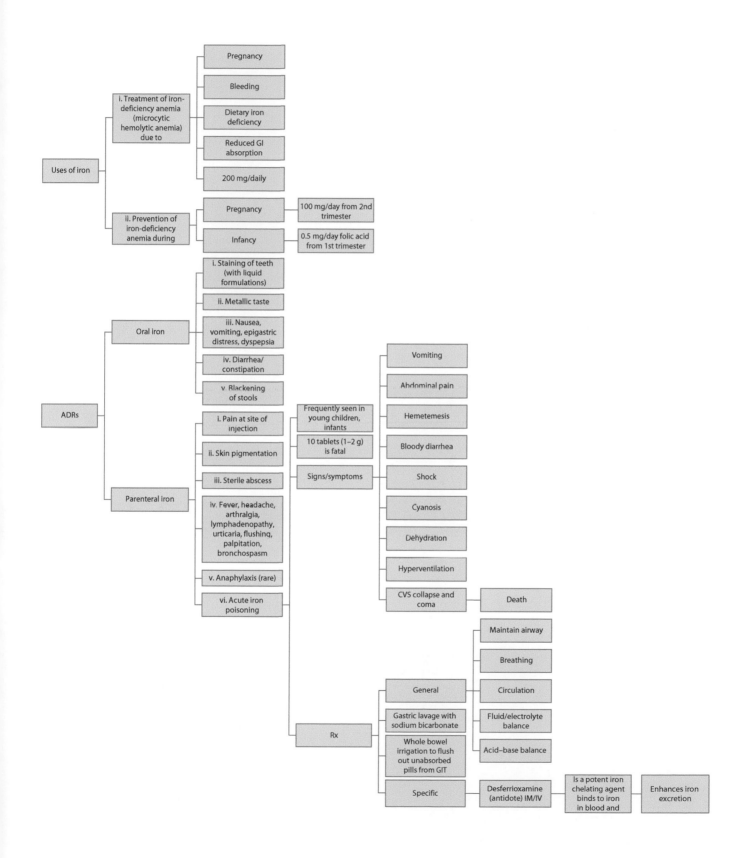

38.5 MATURATION FACTORS AND VITAMIN B12

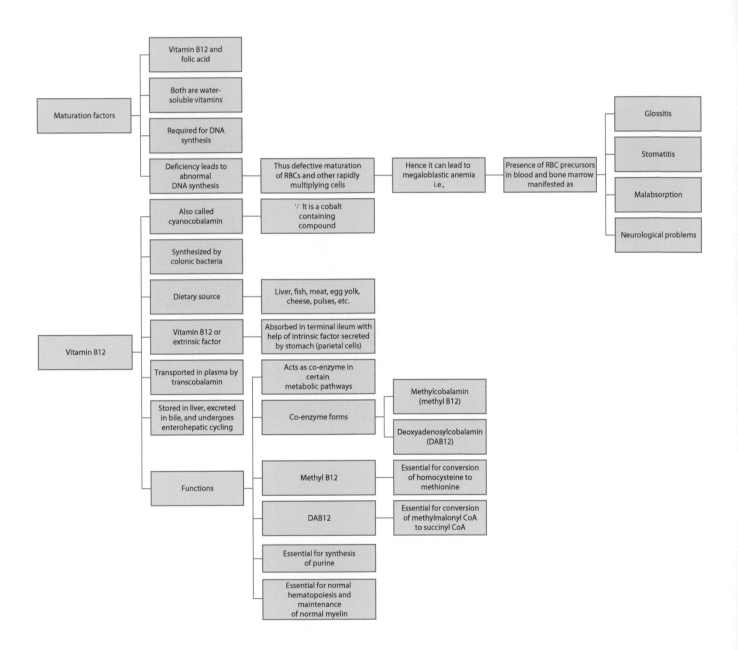

Maturation factors
- Vitamin B12 and folic acid
- Both are water-soluble vitamins
- Required for DNA synthesis
- Deficiency leads to abnormal DNA synthesis → Thus defective maturation of RBCs and other rapidly multiplying cells → Hence it can lead to megaloblastic anemia i.e., → Presence of RBC precursors in blood and bone marrow manifested as
  - Glossitis
  - Stomatitis
  - Malabsorption
  - Neurological problems

Vitamin B12
- Also called cyanocobalamin → ∵ It is a cobalt containing compound
- Synthesized by colonic bacteria
- Dietary source → Liver, fish, meat, egg yolk, cheese, pulses, etc.
- Vitamin B12 or extrinsic factor → Absorbed in terminal ileum with help of intrinsic factor secreted by stomach (parietal cells)
- Transported in plasma by transcobalamin
- Stored in liver, excreted in bile, and undergoes enterohepatic cycling
- Functions
  - Acts as co-enzyme in certain metabolic pathways
  - Co-enzyme forms
    - Methylcobalamin (methyl B12)
    - Deoxyadenosylcobalamin (DAB12)
  - Methyl B12 → Essential for conversion of homocysteine to methionine
  - DAB12 → Essential for conversion of methylmalonyl CoA to succinyl CoA
  - Essential for synthesis of purine
  - Essential for normal hematopoiesis and maintenance of normal myelin

38.6 DEFICIENCY, PREPARATIONS, AND USES

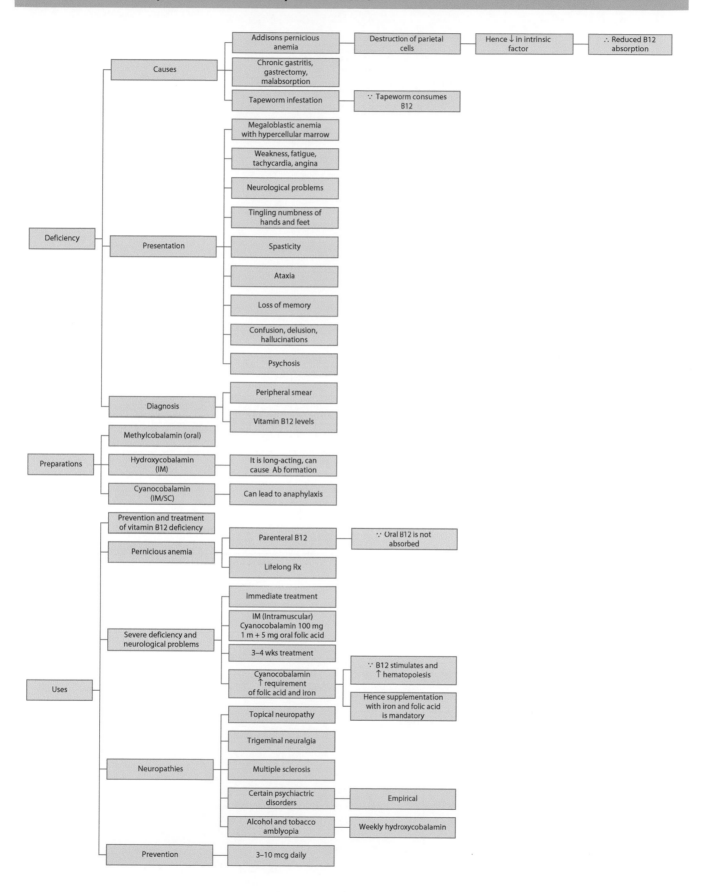

38.7 FOLIC ACID (FA)

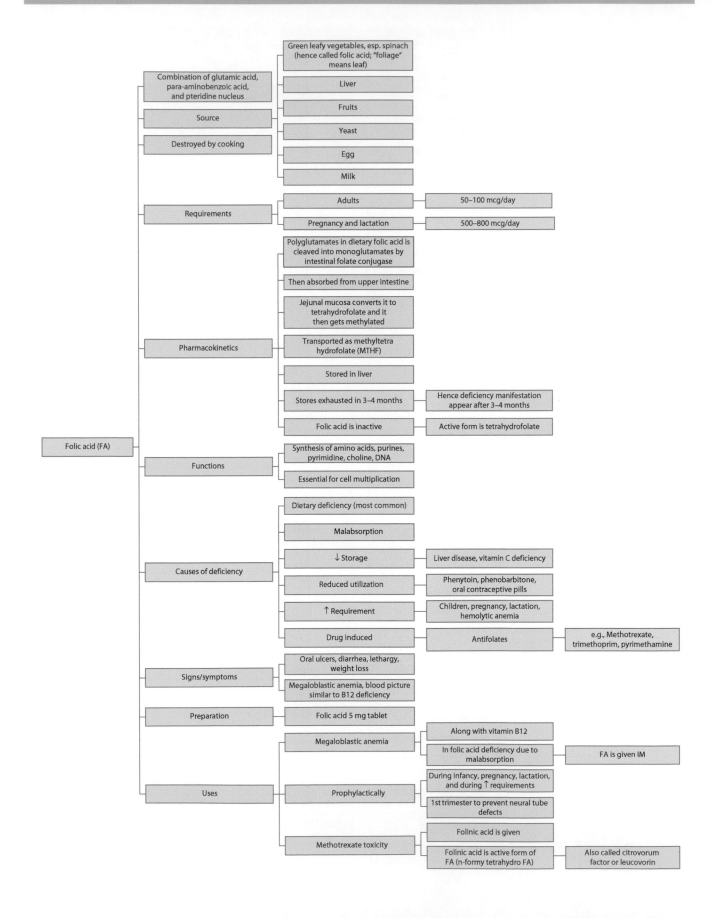

Folic acid (FA)

- Combination of glutamic acid, para-aminobenzoic acid, and pteridine nucleus
- Source
  - Green leafy vegetables, esp. spinach (hence called folic acid; "foliage" means leaf)
  - Liver
  - Fruits
  - Yeast
  - Egg
  - Milk
- Destroyed by cooking
- Requirements
  - Adults → 50–100 mcg/day
  - Pregnancy and lactation → 500–800 mcg/day
- Pharmacokinetics
  - Polyglutamates in dietary folic acid is cleaved into monoglutamates by intestinal folate conjugase
  - Then absorbed from upper intestine
  - Jejunal mucosa converts it to tetrahydrofolate and it then gets methylated
  - Transported as methyltetra hydrofolate (MTHF)
  - Stored in liver
  - Stores exhausted in 3–4 months → Hence deficiency manifestation appear after 3–4 months
  - Folic acid is inactive → Active form is tetrahydrofolate
- Functions
  - Synthesis of amino acids, purines, pyrimidine, choline, DNA
  - Essential for cell multiplication
- Causes of deficiency
  - Dietary deficiency (most common)
  - Malabsorption
  - ↓ Storage → Liver disease, vitamin C deficiency
  - Reduced utilization → Phenytoin, phenobarbitone, oral contraceptive pills
  - ↑ Requirement → Children, pregnancy, lactation, hemolytic anemia
  - Drug induced → Antifolates → e.g., Methotrexate, trimethoprim, pyrimethamine
- Signs/symptoms
  - Oral ulcers, diarrhea, lethargy, weight loss
  - Megaloblastic anemia, blood picture similar to B12 deficiency
- Preparation → Folic acid 5 mg tablet
- Uses
  - Megaloblastic anemia
    - Along with vitamin B12
    - In folic acid deficiency due to malabsorption → FA is given IM
  - Prophylactically
    - During infancy, pregnancy, lactation, and during ↑ requirements
    - 1st trimester to prevent neural tube defects
  - Methotrexate toxicity
    - Folinic acid is given
    - Folinic acid is active form of FA (n-formy tetrahydro FA) → Also called citrovorum factor or leucovorin

38.8 HEMATOPOIETIC GROWTH FACTOR AND ERYTHROPOIETIN

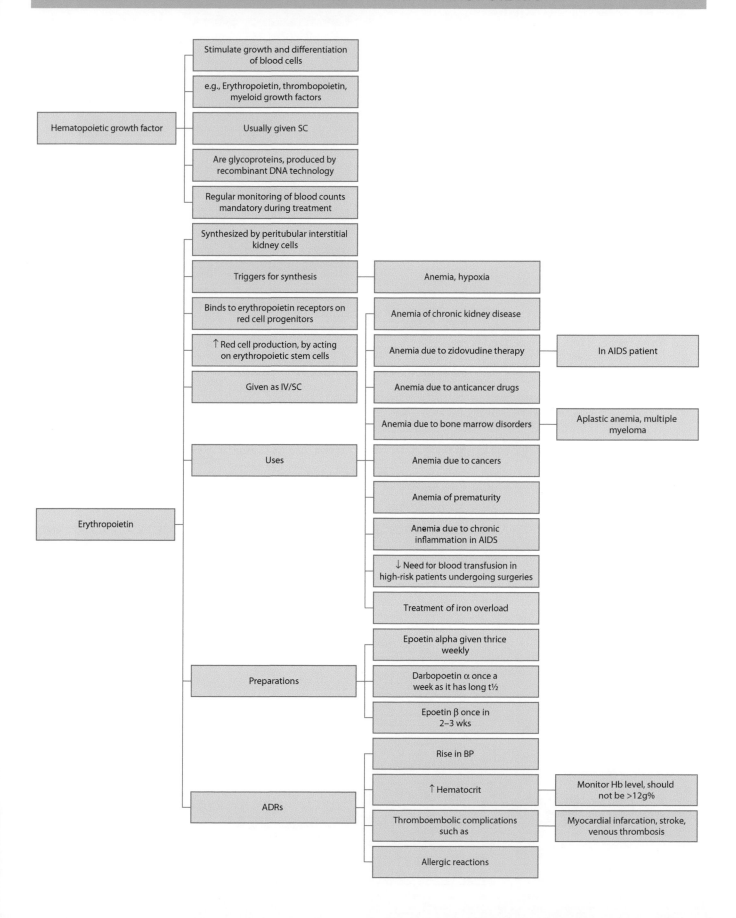

38.9 MYELOID GROWTH FACTORS, MEGAKARYOCYTE GROWTH FACTORS, AND INTERLEUKINS

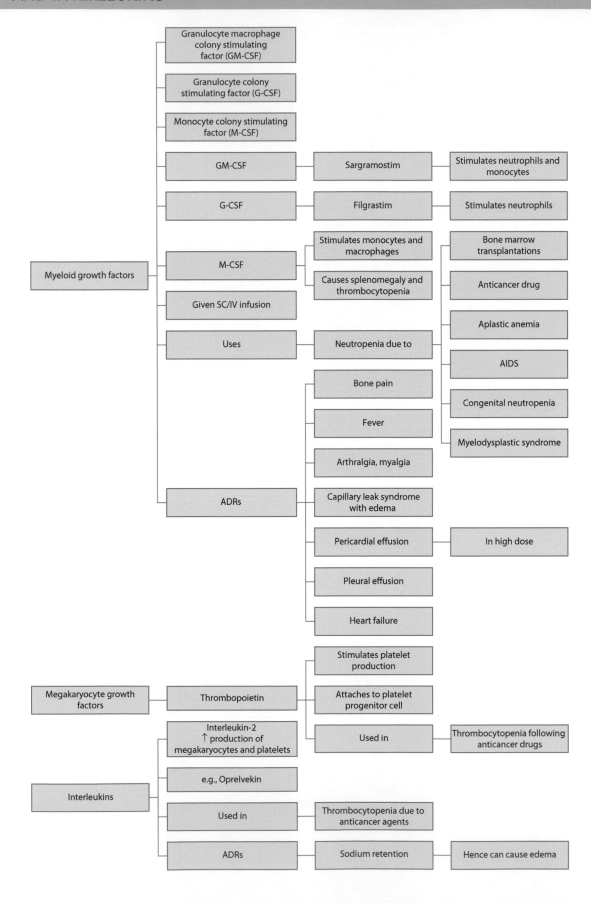

39

Hemostatic agents

39.1 LOCAL AGENTS/STYPTICS

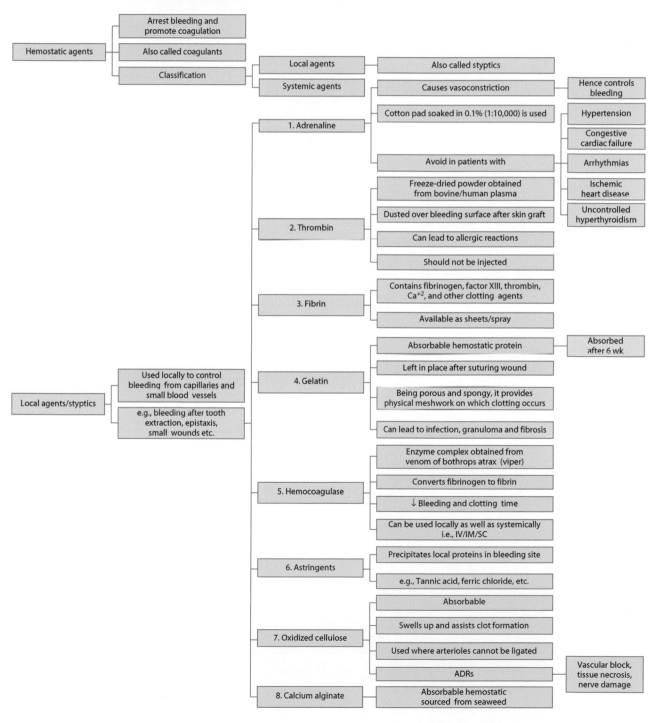

39.2 SYSTEMIC AGENTS

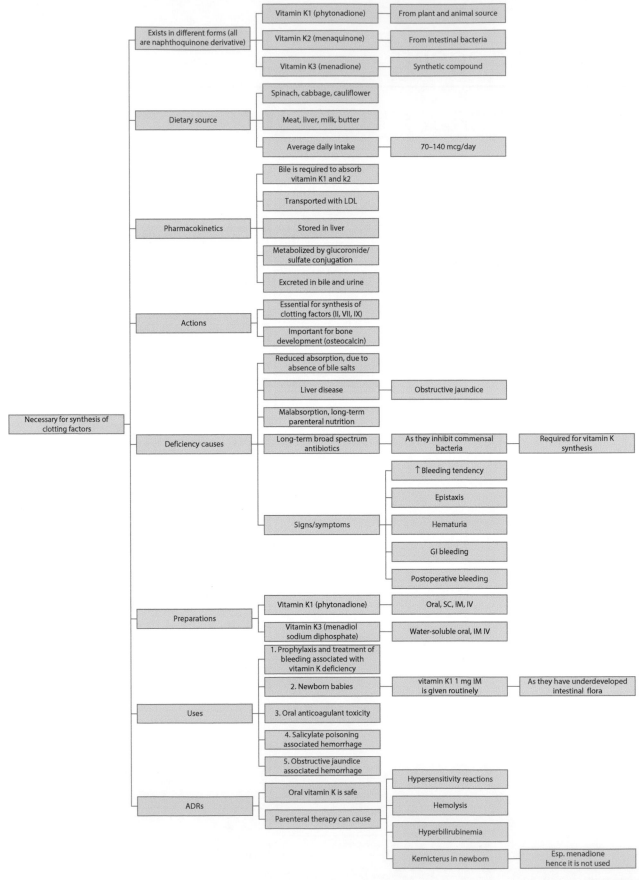

Necessary for synthesis of clotting factors

- **Exists in different forms (all are naphthoquinone derivative)**
  - Vitamin K1 (phytonadione) — From plant and animal source
  - Vitamin K2 (menaquinone) — From intestinal bacteria
  - Vitamin K3 (menadione) — Synthetic compound

- **Dietary source**
  - Spinach, cabbage, cauliflower
  - Meat, liver, milk, butter
  - Average daily intake — 70–140 mcg/day

- **Pharmacokinetics**
  - Bile is required to absorb vitamin K1 and k2
  - Transported with LDL
  - Stored in liver
  - Metabolized by glucoronide/sulfate conjugation
  - Excreted in bile and urine

- **Actions**
  - Essential for synthesis of clotting factors (II, VII, IX)
  - Important for bone development (osteocalcin)

- **Deficiency causes**
  - Reduced absorption, due to absence of bile salts
  - Liver disease — Obstructive jaundice
  - Malabsorption, long-term parenteral nutrition
  - Long-term broad spectrum antibiotics — As they inhibit commensal bacteria — Required for vitamin K synthesis
  - Signs/symptoms
    - ↑ Bleeding tendency
    - Epistaxis
    - Hematuria
    - GI bleeding
    - Postoperative bleeding

- **Preparations**
  - Vitamin K1 (phytonadione) — Oral, SC, IM, IV
  - Vitamin K3 (menadiol sodium diphosphate) — Water-soluble oral, IM IV

- **Uses**
  - 1. Prophylaxis and treatment of bleeding associated with vitamin K deficiency
  - 2. Newborn babies — vitamin K1 1 mg IM is given routinely — As they have underdeveloped intestinal flora
  - 3. Oral anticoagulant toxicity
  - 4. Salicylate poisoning associated hemorrhage
  - 5. Obstructive jaundice associated hemorrhage

- **ADRs**
  - Oral vitamin K is safe
  - Parenteral therapy can cause
    - Hypersensitivity reactions
    - Hemolysis
    - Hyperbilirubinemia
    - Kernicterus in newborn — Esp. menadione hence it is not used

(Continued)

39.2 SYSTEMIC AGENTS (Continued)

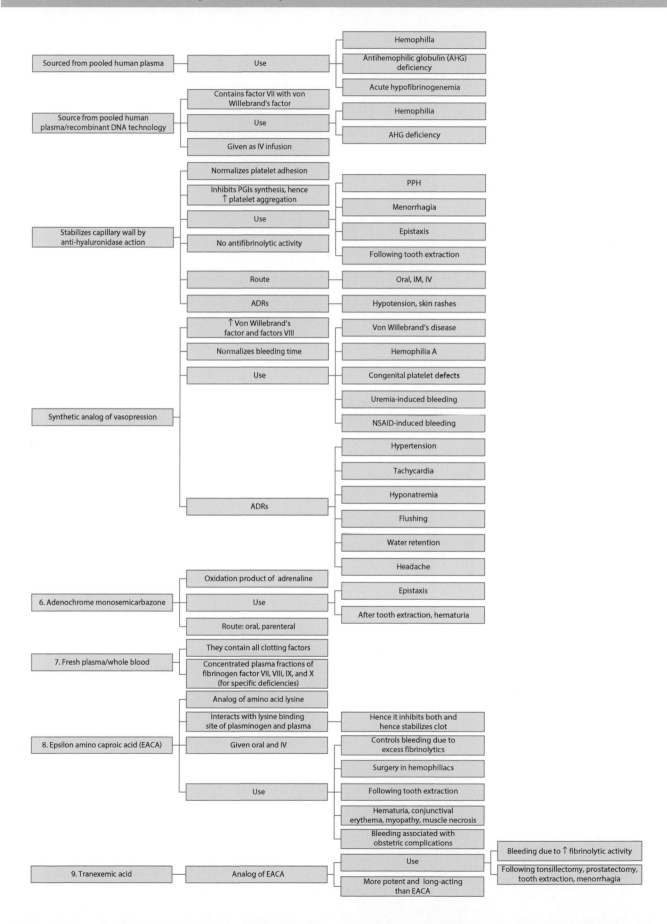

Sourced from pooled human plasma — Use — Hemophilla
— Antihemophilic globulin (AHG) deficiency
— Acute hypofibrinogenemia

Source from pooled human plasma/recombinant DNA technology
— Contains factor VII with von Willebrand's factor
— Use — Hemophilia
— AHG deficiency
— Given as IV infusion

Stabilizes capillary wall by anti-hyaluronidase action
— Normalizes platelet adhesion
— Inhibits PGIs synthesis, hence ↑ platelet aggregation
— Use — PPH
— Menorrhagia
— Epistaxis
— Following tooth extraction
— No antifibrinolytic activity
— Route — Oral, IM, IV
— ADRs — Hypotension, skin rashes

Synthetic analog of vasopression
— ↑ Von Willebrand's factor and factors VIII
— Normalizes bleeding time
— Use — Von Willebrand's disease
— Hemophilia A
— Congenital platelet defects
— Uremia-induced bleeding
— NSAID-induced bleeding
— ADRs — Hypertension
— Tachycardia
— Hyponatremia
— Flushing
— Water retention
— Headache

6. Adenochrome monosemicarbazone
— Oxidation product of adrenaline
— Use — Epistaxis
— After tooth extraction, hematuria
— Route: oral, parenteral

7. Fresh plasma/whole blood
— They contain all clotting factors
— Concentrated plasma fractions of fibrinogen factor VII, VIII, IX, and X (for specific deficiencies)

8. Epsilon amino caproic acid (EACA)
— Analog of amino acid lysine
— Interacts with lysine binding site of plasminogen and plasma — Hence it inhibits both and hence stabilizes clot
— Given oral and IV
— Use — Controls bleeding due to excess fibrinolytics
— Surgery in hemophiliacs
— Following tooth extraction
— Hematuria, conjunctival erythema, myopathy, muscle necrosis
— Bleeding associated with obstetric complications

9. Tranexemic acid
— Analog of EACA — Use — Bleeding due to ↑ fibrinolytic activity
— Following tonsillectomy, prostatectomy, tooth extraction, menorrhagia
— More potent and long-acting than EACA

39.3 SCLEROSING AGENTS

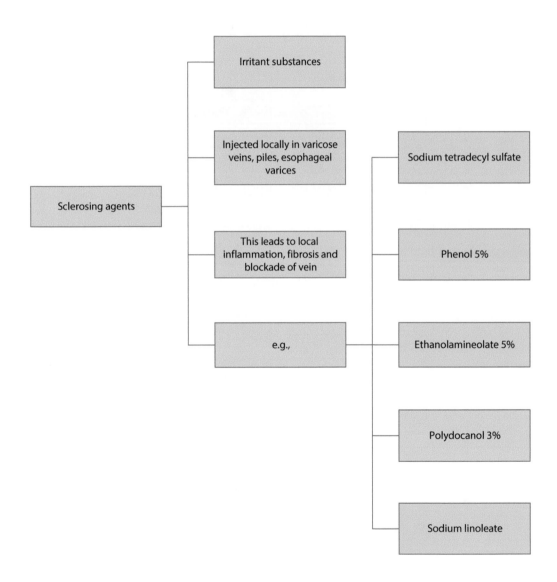

40

Anticoagulants

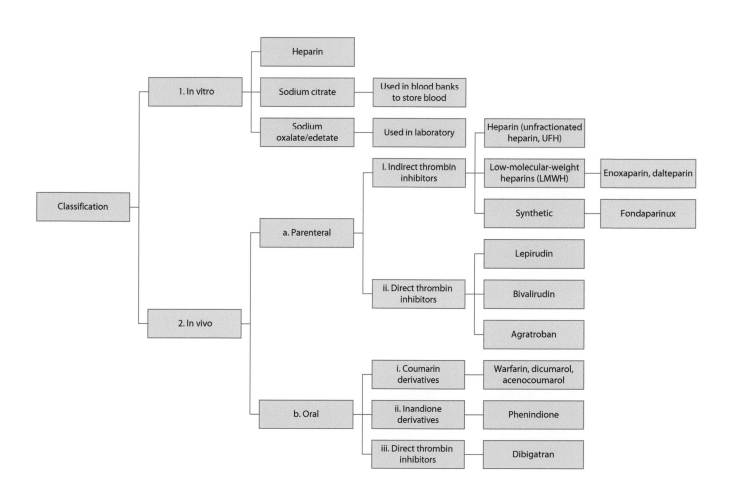

40.2 PARENTERAL ANTICOAGULANTS – HEPARIN

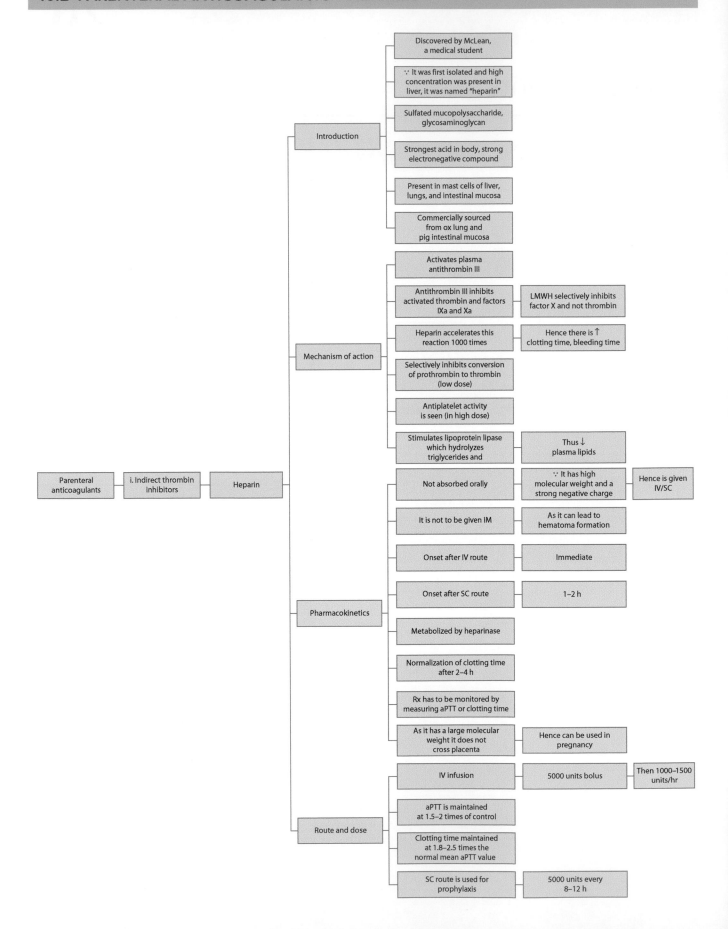

Parenteral anticoagulants → **i. Indirect thrombin inhibitors** → **Heparin**

Introduction
- Discovered by McLean, a medical student
- ∵ It was first isolated and high concentration was present in liver, it was named "heparin"
- Sulfated mucopolysaccharide, glycosaminoglycan
- Strongest acid in body, strong electronegative compound
- Present in mast cells of liver, lungs, and intestinal mucosa
- Commercially sourced from ox lung and pig intestinal mucosa

Mechanism of action
- Activates plasma antithrombin III
- Antithrombin III inhibits activated thrombin and factors IXa and Xa → LMWH selectively inhibits factor X and not thrombin
- Heparin accelerates this reaction 1000 times → Hence there is ↑ clotting time, bleeding time
- Selectively inhibits conversion of prothrombin to thrombin (low dose)
- Antiplatelet activity is seen (in high dose)
- Stimulates lipoprotein lipase which hydrolyzes triglycerides and → Thus ↓ plasma lipids

Pharmacokinetics
- Not absorbed orally → ∵ It has high molecular weight and a strong negative charge → Hence is given IV/SC
- It is not to be given IM → As it can lead to hematoma formation
- Onset after IV route → Immediate
- Onset after SC route → 1–2 h
- Metabolized by heparinase
- Normalization of clotting time after 2–4 h
- Rx has to be monitored by measuring aPTT or clotting time
- As it has a large molecular weight it does not cross placenta → Hence can be used in pregnancy

Route and dose
- IV infusion → 5000 units bolus → Then 1000–1500 units/hr
- aPTT is maintained at 1.5–2 times of control
- Clotting time maintained at 1.8–2.5 times the normal mean aPTT value
- SC route is used for prophylaxis → 5000 units every 8–12 h

40.3 ADRs AND CONTRAINDICATIONS OF HEPARIN

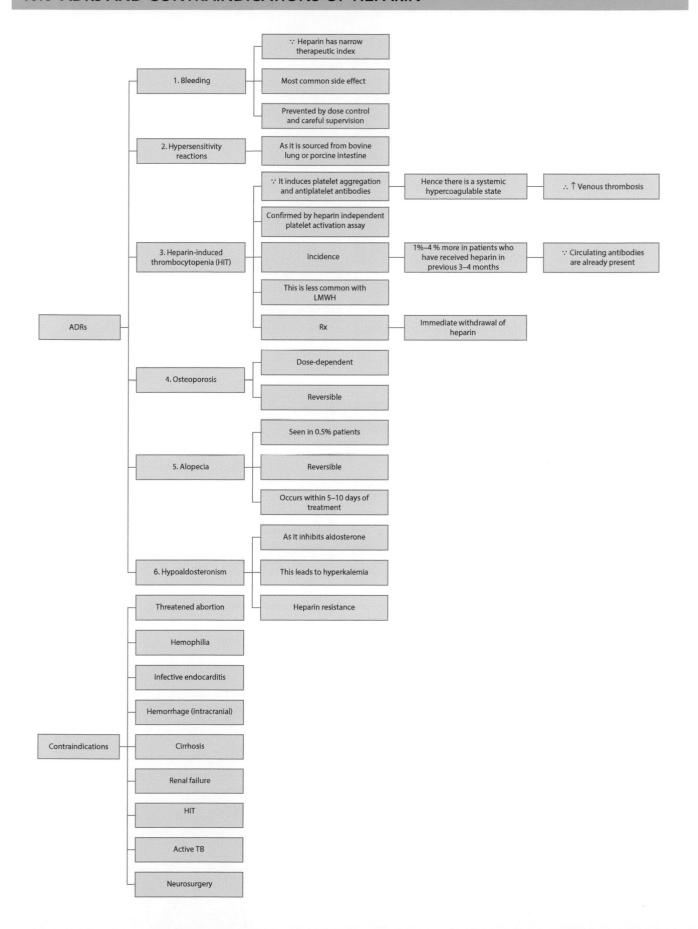

40.4 LOW-MOLECULAR-WEIGHT HEPARINS (LMWHs) AND HEPARIN ANTAGONIST

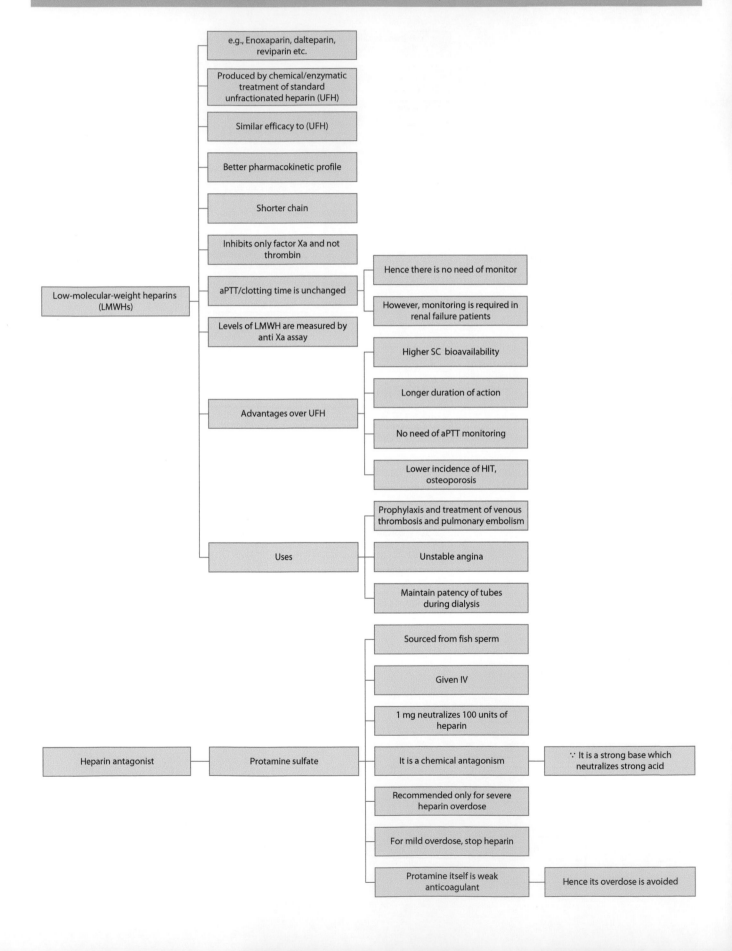

Low-molecular-weight heparins (LMWHs)

- e.g., Enoxaparin, dalteparin, reviparin etc.
- Produced by chemical/enzymatic treatment of standard unfractionated heparin (UFH)
- Similar efficacy to (UFH)
- Better pharmacokinetic profile
- Shorter chain
- Inhibits only factor Xa and not thrombin
- aPTT/clotting time is unchanged
  - Hence there is no need of monitor
  - However, monitoring is required in renal failure patients
- Levels of LMWH are measured by anti Xa assay
- Advantages over UFH
  - Higher SC bioavailability
  - Longer duration of action
  - No need of aPTT monitoring
  - Lower incidence of HIT, osteoporosis
- Uses
  - Prophylaxis and treatment of venous thrombosis and pulmonary embolism
  - Unstable angina
  - Maintain patency of tubes during dialysis

Heparin antagonist — **Protamine sulfate**

- Sourced from fish sperm
- Given IV
- 1 mg neutralizes 100 units of heparin
- It is a chemical antagonism
  - ∴ It is a strong base which neutralizes strong acid
- Recommended only for severe heparin overdose
- For mild overdose, stop heparin
- Protamine itself is weak anticoagulant
  - Hence its overdose is avoided

40.5 SYNTHETIC HEPARIN DERIVATIVES, HEPARINOIDS, AND PARENTERAL DIRECT THROMBIN INHIBITORS

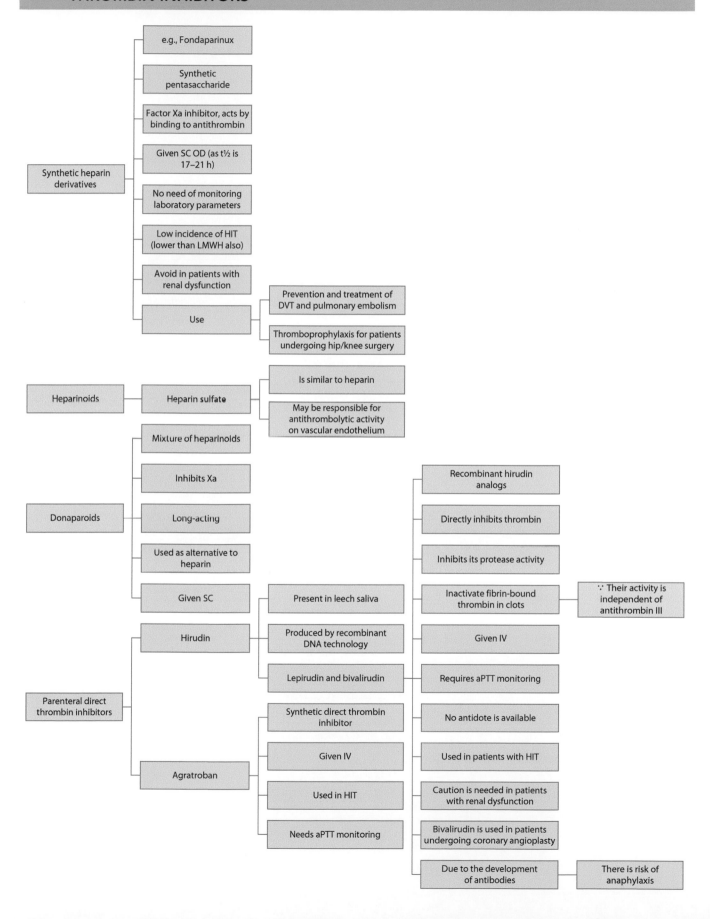

40.6 ORAL ANTICOAGULANTS – MECHANISM OF ACTION AND PHARMACOKINETICS (WARFARIN)

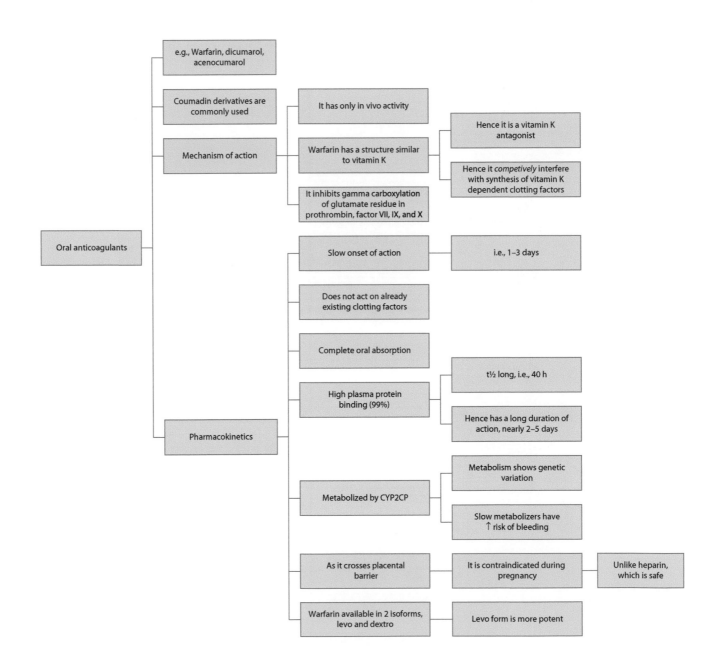

Oral anticoagulants

- e.g., Warfarin, dicumarol, acenocumarol
- Coumadin derivatives are commonly used
- Mechanism of action
  - It has only in vivo activity
  - Warfarin has a structure similar to vitamin K
    - Hence it is a vitamin K antagonist
    - Hence it *competively* interfere with synthesis of vitamin K dependent clotting factors
  - It inhibits gamma carboxylation of glutamate residue in prothrombin, factor VII, IX, and X
- Pharmacokinetics
  - Slow onset of action
    - i.e., 1–3 days
  - Does not act on already existing clotting factors
  - Complete oral absorption
  - High plasma protein binding (99%)
    - t½ long, i.e., 40 h
    - Hence has a long duration of action, nearly 2–5 days
  - Metabolized by CYP2CP
    - Metabolism shows genetic variation
    - Slow metabolizers have ↑ risk of bleeding
  - As it crosses placental barrier
    - It is contraindicated during pregnancy
      - Unlike heparin, which is safe
  - Warfarin available in 2 isoforms, levo and dextro
    - Levo form is more potent

40.7 USES AND ADRs OF WARFARIN

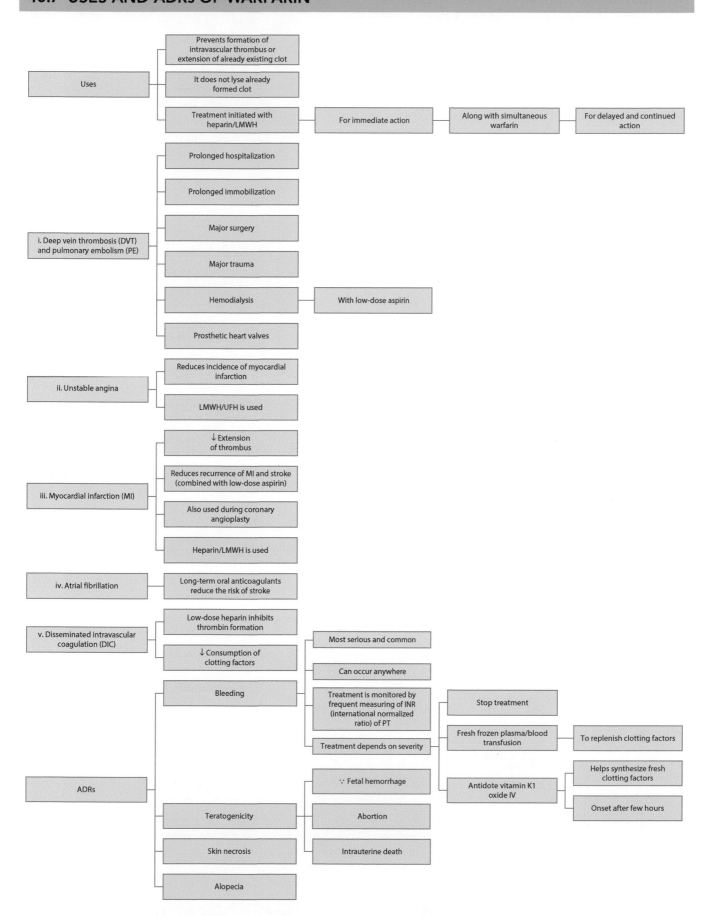

Uses
- Prevents formation of intravascular thrombus or extension of already existing clot
- It does not lyse already formed clot
- Treatment initiated with heparin/LMWH
  - For immediate action
  - Along with simultaneous warfarin
  - For delayed and continued action

i. Deep vein thrombosis (DVT) and pulmonary embolism (PE)
- Prolonged hospitalization
- Prolonged immobilization
- Major surgery
- Major trauma
- Hemodialysis
  - With low-dose aspirin
- Prosthetic heart valves

ii. Unstable angina
- Reduces incidence of myocardial infarction
- LMWH/UFH is used

iii. Myocardial infarction (MI)
- ↓ Extension of thrombus
- Reduces recurrence of MI and stroke (combined with low-dose aspirin)
- Also used during coronary angioplasty
- Heparin/LMWH is used

iv. Atrial fibrillation
- Long-term oral anticoagulants reduce the risk of stroke

v. Disseminated intravascular coagulation (DIC)
- Low-dose heparin inhibits thrombin formation
- ↓ Consumption of clotting factors

ADRs
- Bleeding
  - Most serious and common
  - Can occur anywhere
  - Treatment is monitored by frequent measuring of INR (international normalized ratio) of PT
  - Treatment depends on severity
    - Stop treatment
    - Fresh frozen plasma/blood transfusion
      - To replenish clotting factors
    - Antidote vitamin K1 oxide IV
      - Helps synthesize fresh clotting factors
      - Onset after few hours
- Teratogenicity
  - ∵ Fetal hemorrhage
  - Abortion
  - Intrauterine death
- Skin necrosis
- Alopecia

40.8 DRUG INTERACTIONS OF WARFARIN

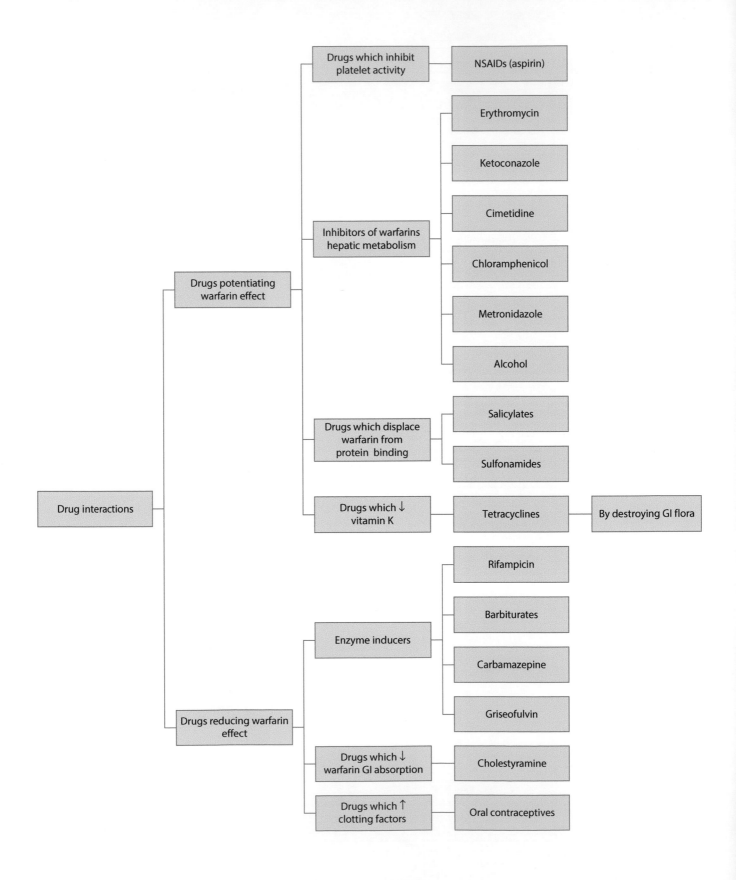

40.9 ORAL DIRECT THROMBIN INHIBITORS

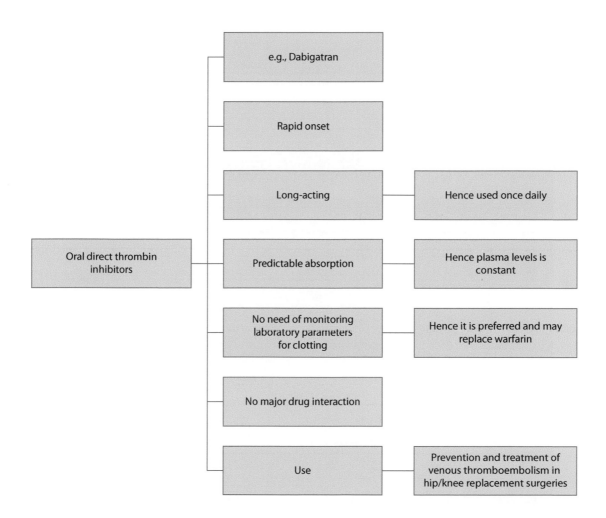

40.10 DIFFERENCES BETWEEN HEPARIN vs. LMW HEPARIN

	Heparin	Low-molecular-weight heparin
1. Mol wt	High	Low
2. Source	Natural	Semi-synthetic
3. Thrombin inhibition	Present	Absent
4. Clotting parameters	Effected	Not effected
5. Laboratory monitoring	Needed	Not needed
6. SC bioavailability	Low	High
7. Duration of action	2–4 h (Short)	18–24 h (long)
8. Dose	4–6/day	Once daily
9. Bleeding complications	High	Minimal
10. Thrombocytopenia	High	Low

40.11 DIFFERENCES BETWEEN HEPARIN AND DICUMAROL/WARFARIN

	Heparin	Dicaumarol/warfarin
1. Source	Natural	Synthetic
2. Chemistry	Mucopolysaccharide	Coumarin
3. Action	In vitro and in vivo	Only in vivo
4. Administration	Parenteral (IV/SC)	Oral
5. Onset	Rapid (3–6 h)	Slow (1–3 days)
6. Duration	Short (2–4 h)	Long (4–7 days)
7. Mechanism	Stimulates antithrombin III	Inhibits clotting factors
8. Antidote	Protamine sulfate	Vitamin K1 oxide
9. Usage	For initiation	For maintenance
10. Usage in pregnancy	Used	Not used as it is teratogenic
11. Cost	Expensive	Economical
12. Monitoring	Measuring aPTT/clotting time	Synthetic

Antiplatelet agents

41.1 CLASSIFICATION AND ASPIRIN

Antiplatelet agents → Classification

- i. Thromboxane synthesis (TXA2) inhibitors → Low-dose aspirin
- ii. Purnergic (P2Y12) receptor antagonists/ADP antagonists → Ticlopidine, clopidogrel
- iii. Phosphodiesterase inhibitor → Dipyridamole
- iv. Glycoprotein IIb/IIIa receptor antagonists → Abciximab, eptifibatide, tirofiban
- v. Miscellaneous → PGI2, cilostazol

Aspirin

- Thromboxane A2 (TXA2) causes platelet aggregation
- Low-dose aspirin (50–325 mg)
  - Irreversibly acetylates cyclooxygenase-1
  - Hence inhibits the formation of TXA2
- This effect lasts for 7–10 days → Until fresh platelets are produced
- PGI2 is responsible for platelet inhibition
- High dose aspirin inhibits both TXA2 and PGI2 → Hence efficacy ↓
- When thrombosis occurs in spite of aspirin → Termed aspirin resistance (30% incidence)
- Use → Prophylaxis of MI and stroke
- ADRs → GI irritation and bleeding (dose related)

41.2 PURINERGIC RECEPTOR (P2Y12) ANTAGONISTS/ADP ANTIGONISTS AND PHOSPHODIESTERASE (PDE) INHIBITORS

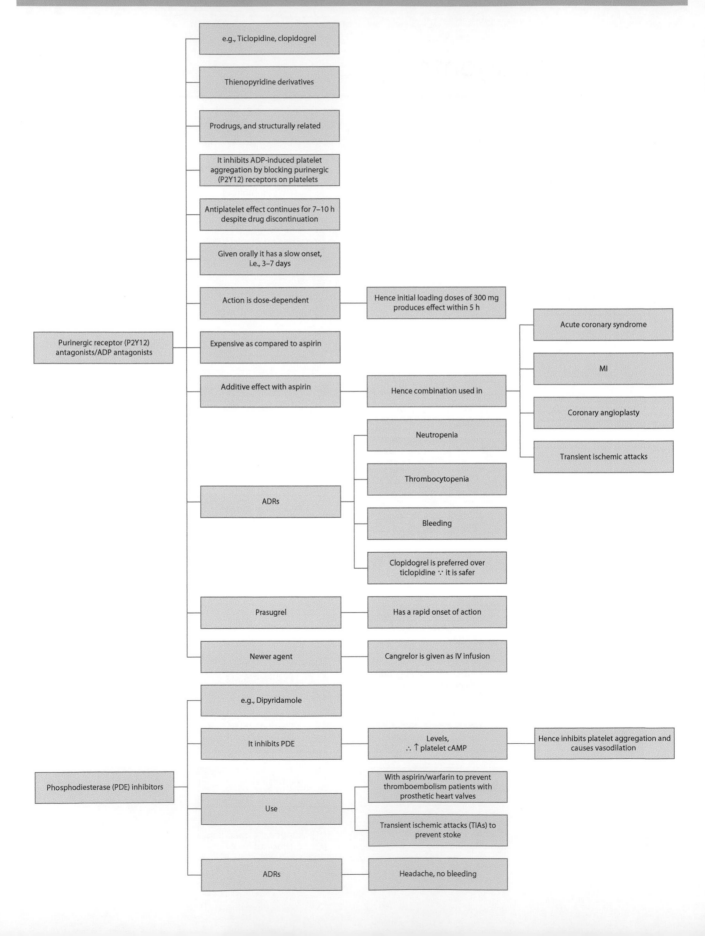

41.3 GLYCOPROTEIN IIB/IIIA RECEPTOR ANTAGONISTS AND MISCELLANEOUS

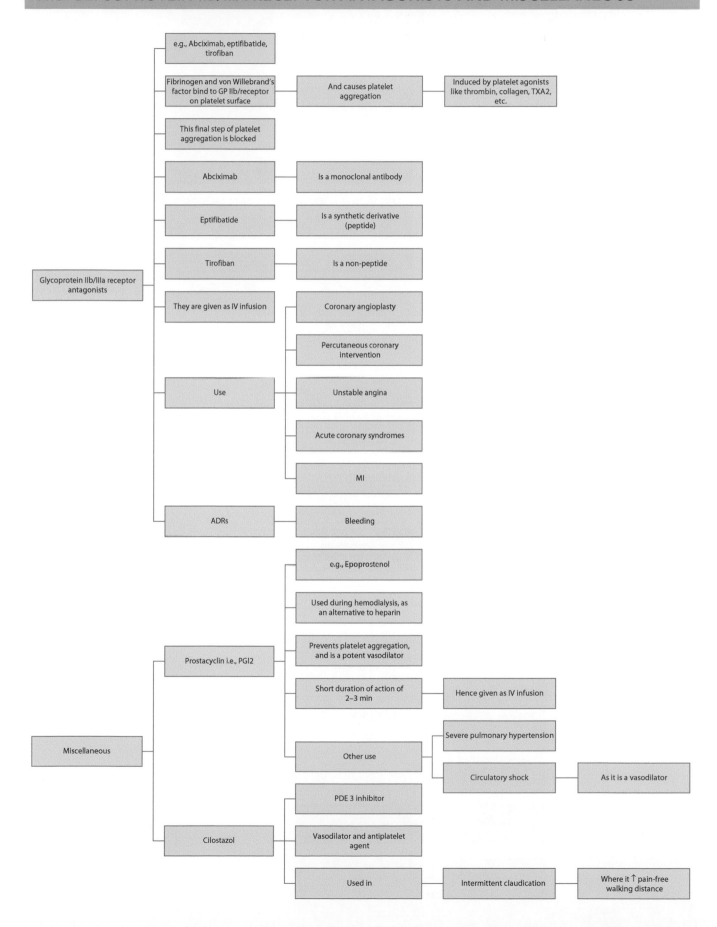

41.4 USES OF ANTIPLATELET AGENTS

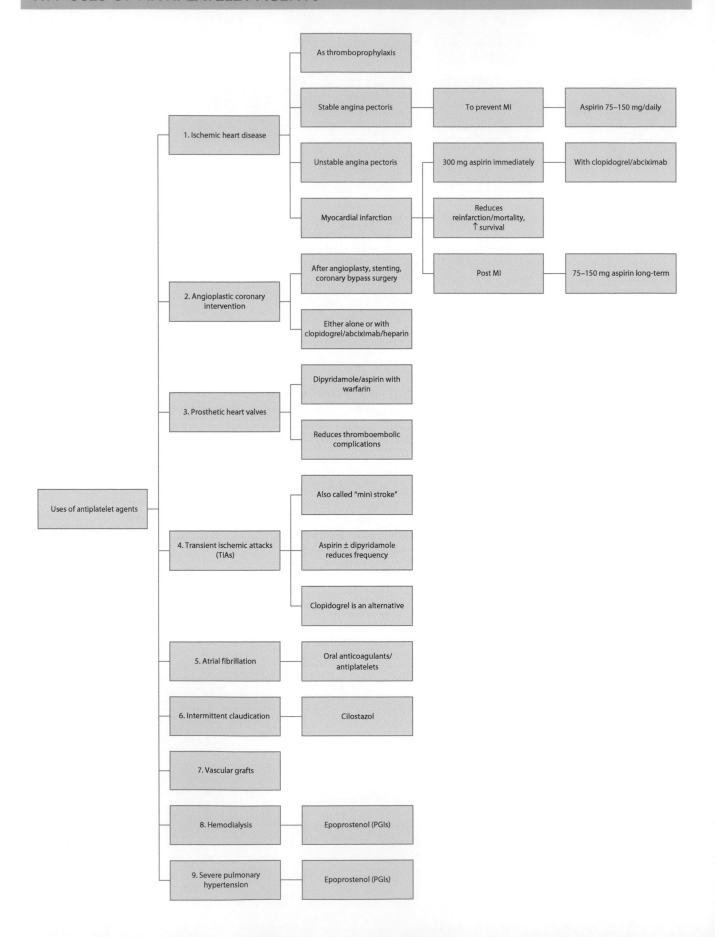

Uses of antiplatelet agents

1. Ischemic heart disease
- As thromboprophylaxis
- Stable angina pectoris → To prevent MI → Aspirin 75–150 mg/daily
- Unstable angina pectoris
- Myocardial infarction
  - 300 mg aspirin immediately → With clopidogrel/abciximab
  - Reduces reinfarction/mortality, ↑ survival
  - Post MI → 75–150 mg aspirin long-term

2. Angioplastic coronary intervention
- After angioplasty, stenting, coronary bypass surgery
- Either alone or with clopidogrel/abciximab/heparin

3. Prosthetic heart valves
- Dipyridamole/aspirin with warfarin
- Reduces thromboembolic complications

4. Transient ischemic attacks (TIAs)
- Also called "mini stroke"
- Aspirin ± dipyridamole reduces frequency
- Clopidogrel is an alternative

5. Atrial fibrillation
- Oral anticoagulants/antiplatelets

6. Intermittent claudication
- Cilostazol

7. Vascular grafts

8. Hemodialysis
- Epoprostenol (PGIs)

9. Severe pulmonary hypertension
- Epoprostenol (PGIs)

42

Thrombolytics (fibrinolytics) and antifibrinolytics

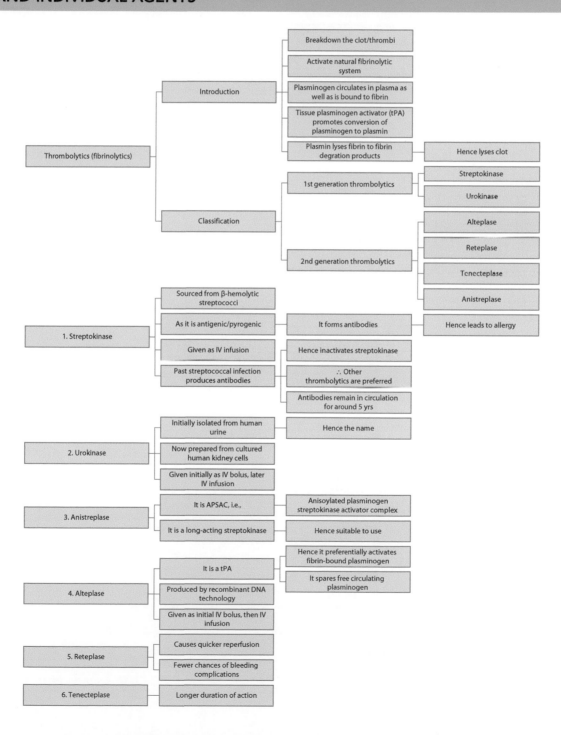

42.2 USES, ADRs, AND CONTRAINDICATIONS

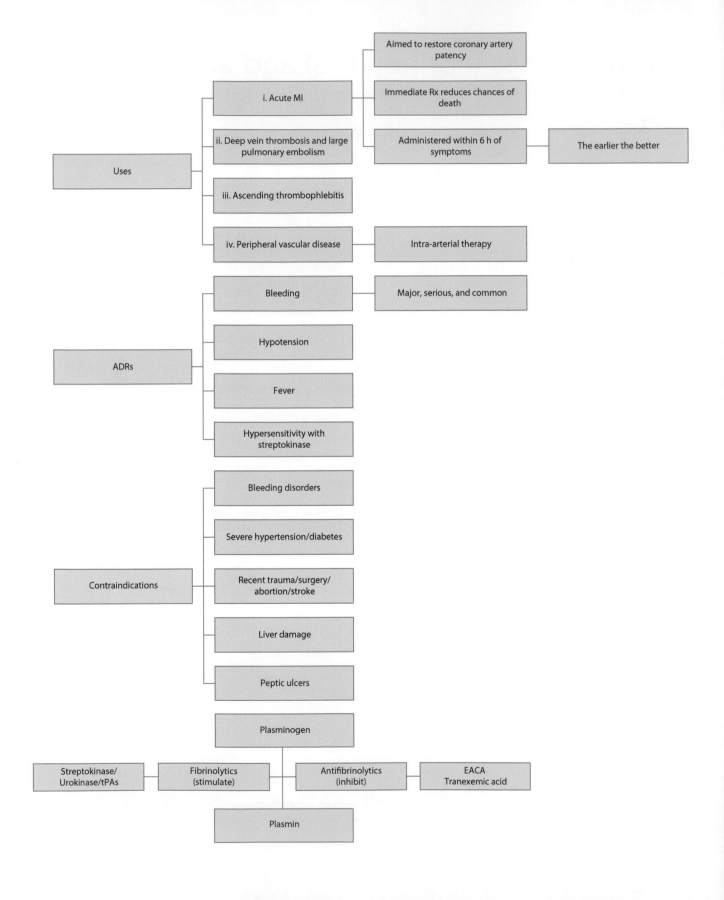

42.3 ANTIFIBRINOLYTICS – USES AND CONTRAINDICATIONS

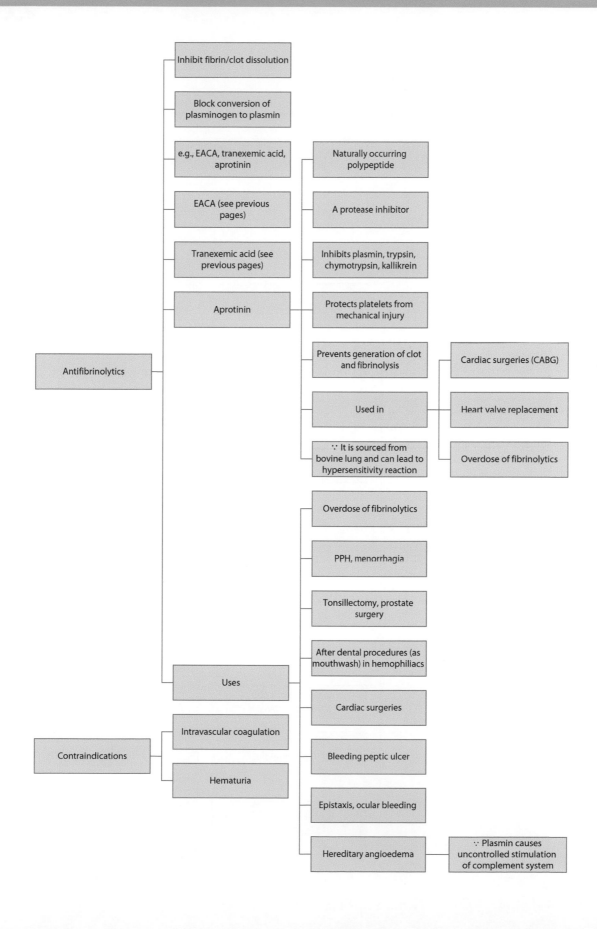

Hypolipidemic drugs

43.1 CLASSIFICATION OF HYPOLIPIDEMICS

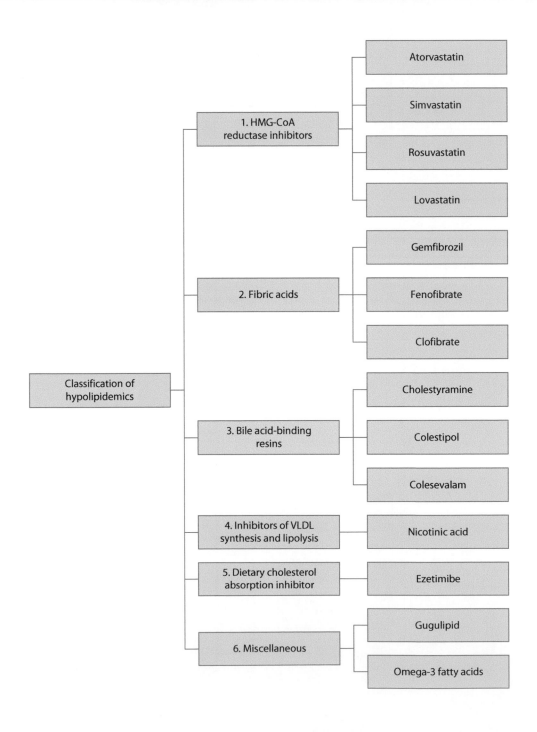

43.2 HMG-CoA REDUCTASE INHIBITORS (STATINS)

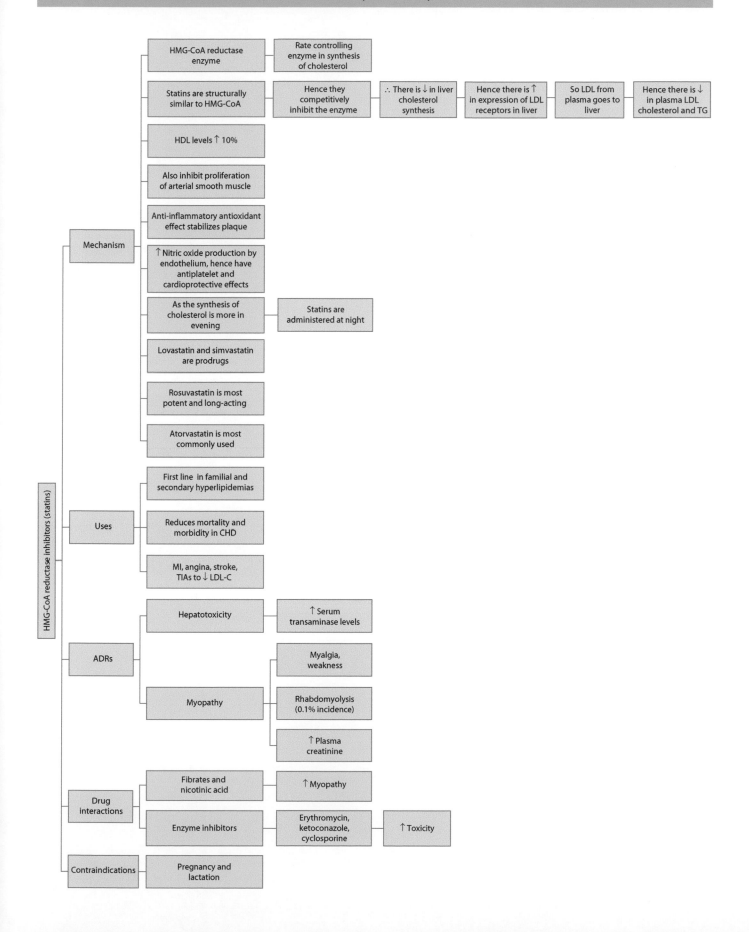

43.3 FIBRIC ACIDS (FIBRATES)

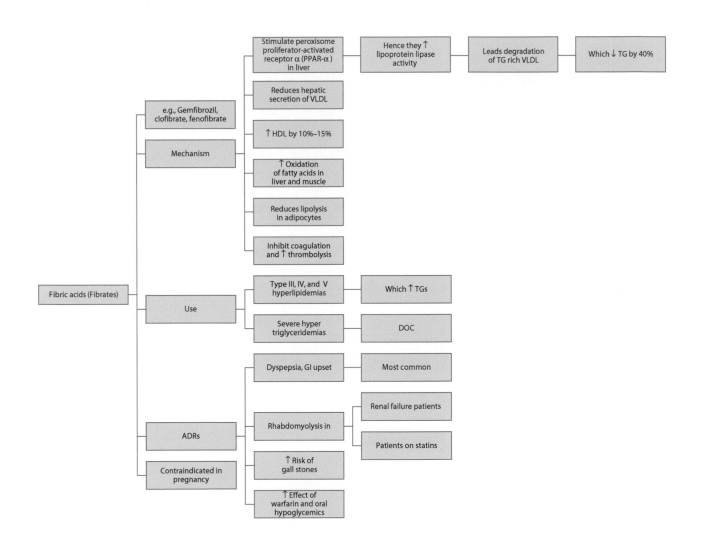

Fibric acids (Fibrates)

- e.g., Gemfibrozil, clofibrate, fenofibrate
- Mechanism
  - Stimulate peroxisome proliferator-activated receptor α (PPAR-α) in liver → Hence they ↑ lipoprotein lipase activity → Leads degradation of TG rich VLDL → Which ↓ TG by 40%
  - Reduces hepatic secretion of VLDL
  - ↑ HDL by 10%–15%
  - ↑ Oxidation of fatty acids in liver and muscle
  - Reduces lipolysis in adipocytes
  - Inhibit coagulation and ↑ thrombolysis
- Use
  - Type III, IV, and V hyperlipidemias → Which ↑ TGs
  - Severe hyper triglyceridemias → DOC
- ADRs
  - Dyspepsia, GI upset → Most common
  - Rhabdomyolysis in → Renal failure patients / Patients on statins
  - ↑ Risk of gall stones
  - ↑ Effect of warfarin and oral hypoglycemics
- Contraindicated in pregnancy

43.4 BILE ACID-BINDING RESINS (BAB – RESINS)

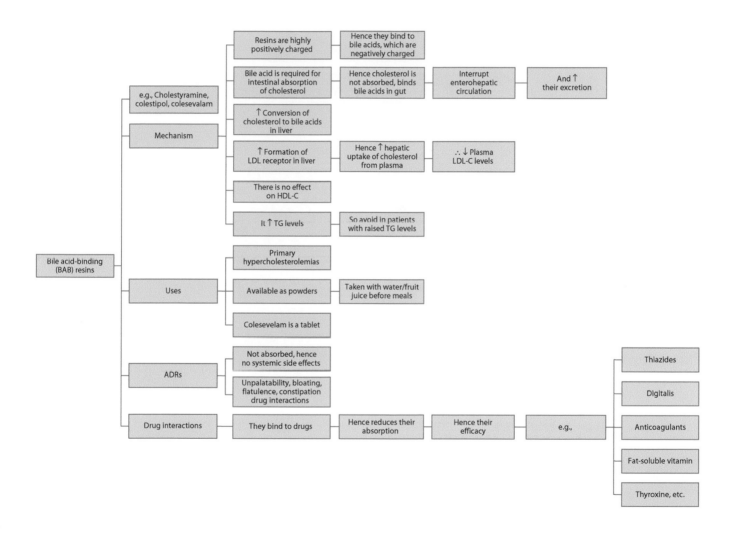

43.5 NICOTINIC ACID OR NIACIN

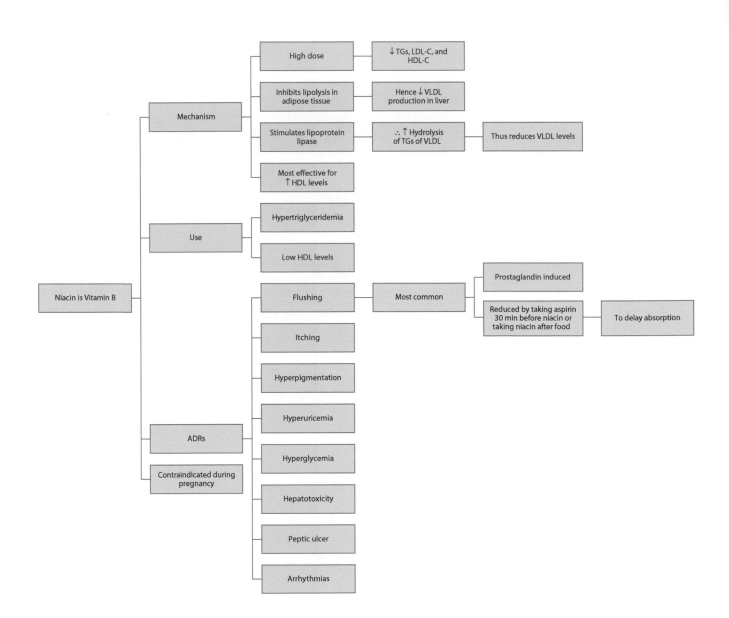

43.6 DIETARY CHOLESTEROL ABSORPTION INHIBITOR, GUGULIPID, AND OMEGA-3 FATTY ACIDS

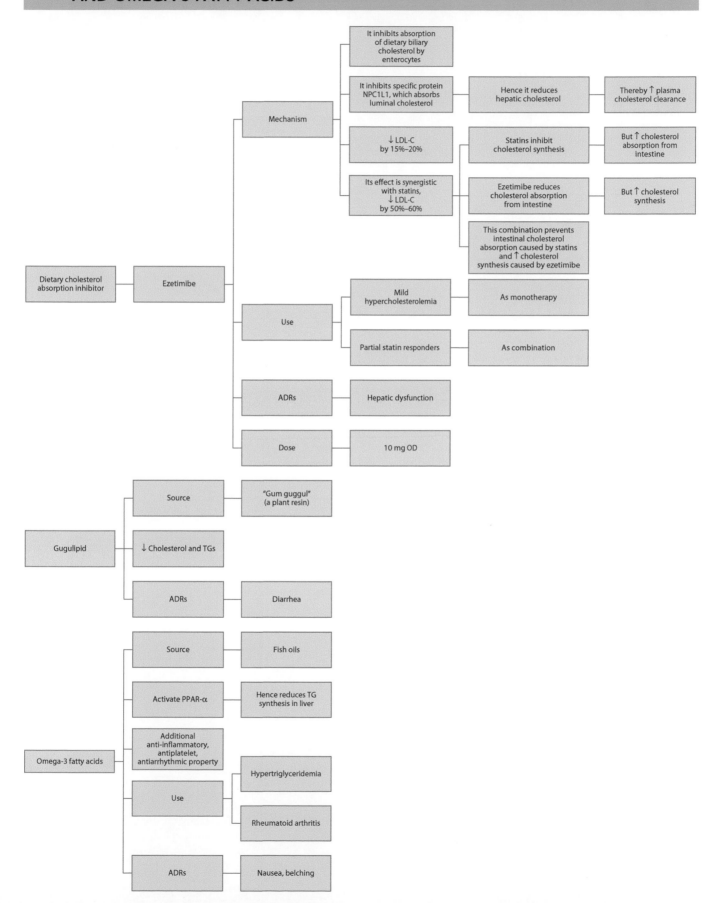

PART VIII

Gastrointestinal pharmacology

Drug therapy of peptic ulcer and GERD

44.1 CLASSIFICATION OF DRUGS USED FOR PEPTIC ULCER

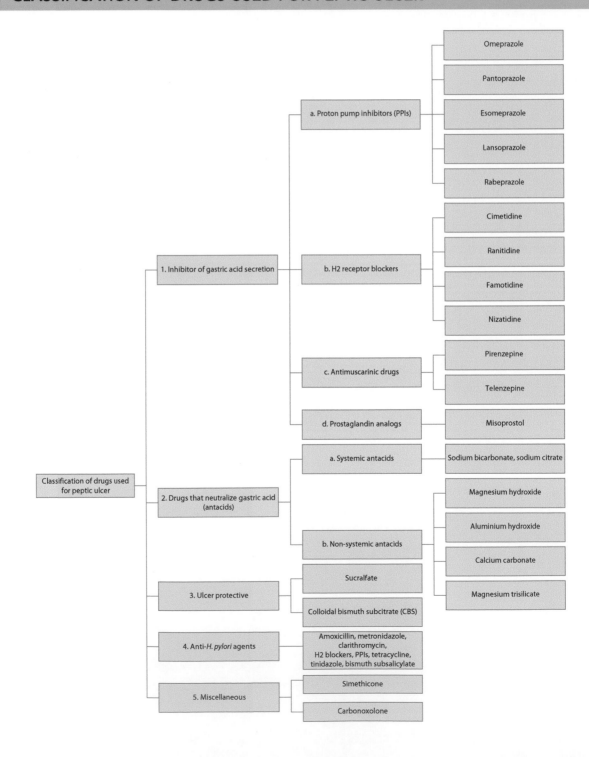

44.2 ANTACIDS – INTRODUCTION, TYPES, AND SYSTEMIC ANTACIDS

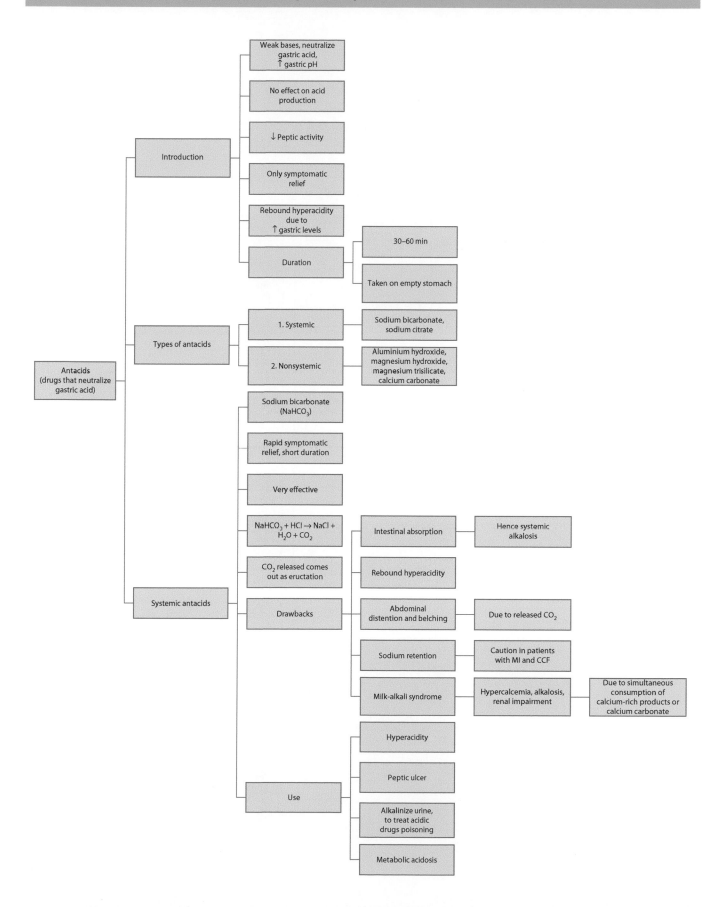

44.3 NONSYSTEMIC ANTACIDS

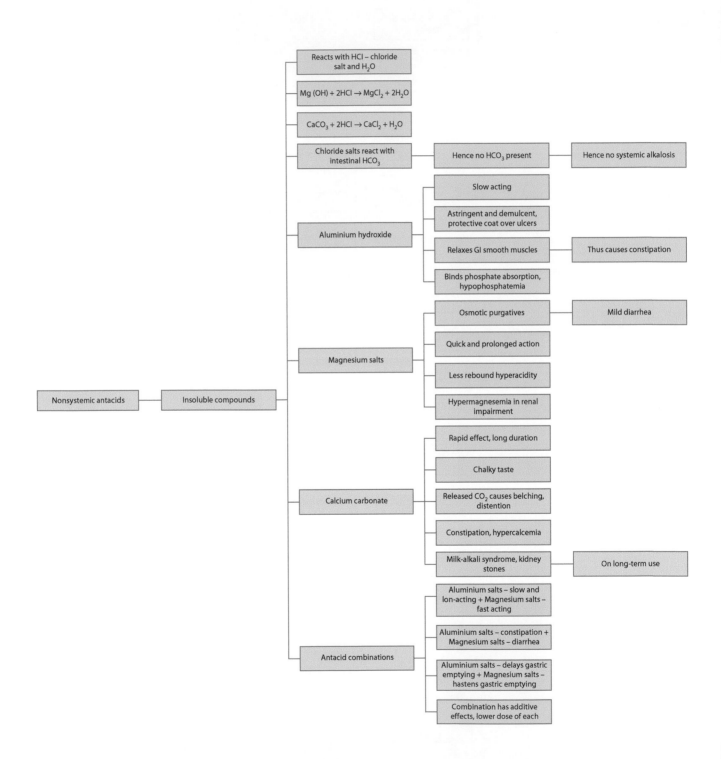

Nonsystemic antacids → Insoluble compounds

- Reacts with HCl – chloride salt and H_2O
- $Mg(OH) + 2HCl \rightarrow MgCl_2 + 2H_2O$
- $CaCO_3 + 2HCl \rightarrow CaCl_2 + H_2O$
- Chloride salts react with intestinal HCO_3 → Hence no HCO_3 present → Hence no systemic alkalosis

Aluminium hydroxide
- Slow acting
- Astringent and demulcent, protective coat over ulcers
- Relaxes GI smooth muscles → Thus causes constipation
- Binds phosphate absorption, hypophosphatemia

Magnesium salts
- Osmotic purgatives → Mild diarrhea
- Quick and prolonged action
- Less rebound hyperacidity
- Hypermagnesemia in renal impairment

Calcium carbonate
- Rapid effect, long duration
- Chalky taste
- Released CO_2 causes belching, distention
- Constipation, hypercalcemia
- Milk-alkali syndrome, kidney stones → On long-term use

Antacid combinations
- Aluminium salts – slow and lon-acting + Magnesium salts – fast acting
- Aluminium salts – constipation + Magnesium salts – diarrhea
- Aluminium salts – delays gastric emptying + Magnesium salts – hastens gastric emptying
- Combination has additive effects, lower dose of each

44.4 USE, ADRs, AND DRUG INTERACTIONS

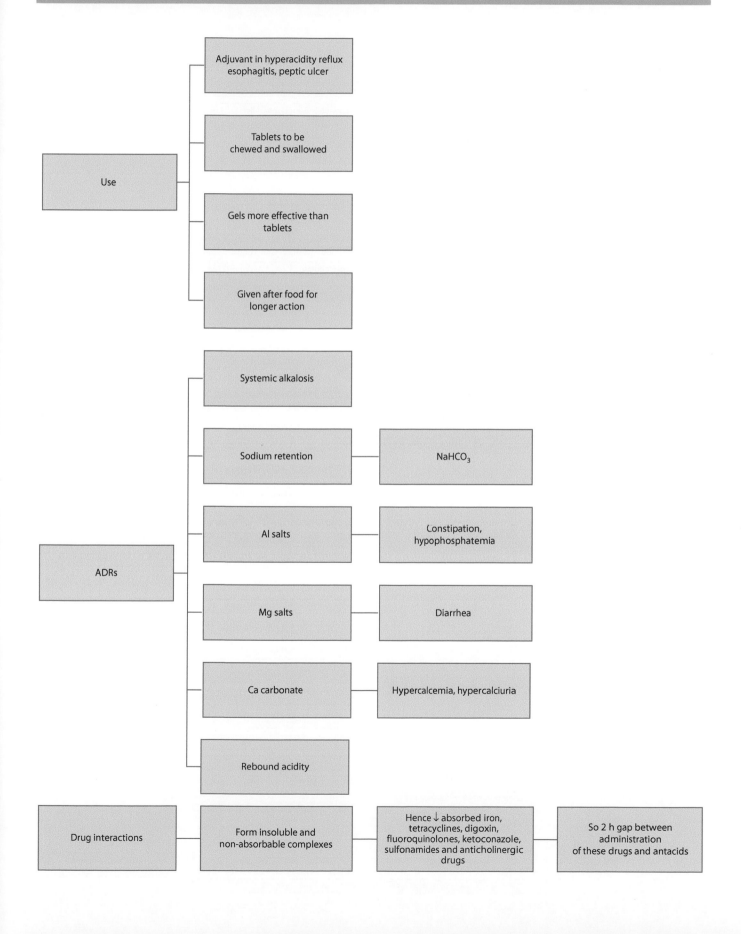

Use
- Adjuvant in hyperacidity reflux esophagitis, peptic ulcer
- Tablets to be chewed and swallowed
- Gels more effective than tablets
- Given after food for longer action

ADRs
- Systemic alkalosis
- Sodium retention — NaHCO₃
- Al salts — Constipation, hypophosphatemia
- Mg salts — Diarrhea
- Ca carbonate — Hypercalcemia, hypercalciuria
- Rebound acidity

Drug interactions — Form insoluble and non-absorbable complexes — Hence ↓ absorbed iron, tetracyclines, digoxin, fluoroquinolones, ketoconazole, sulfonamides and anticholinergic drugs — So 2 h gap between administration of these drugs and antacids

44.5 PROTON PUMP INHIBITORS (PPIs)

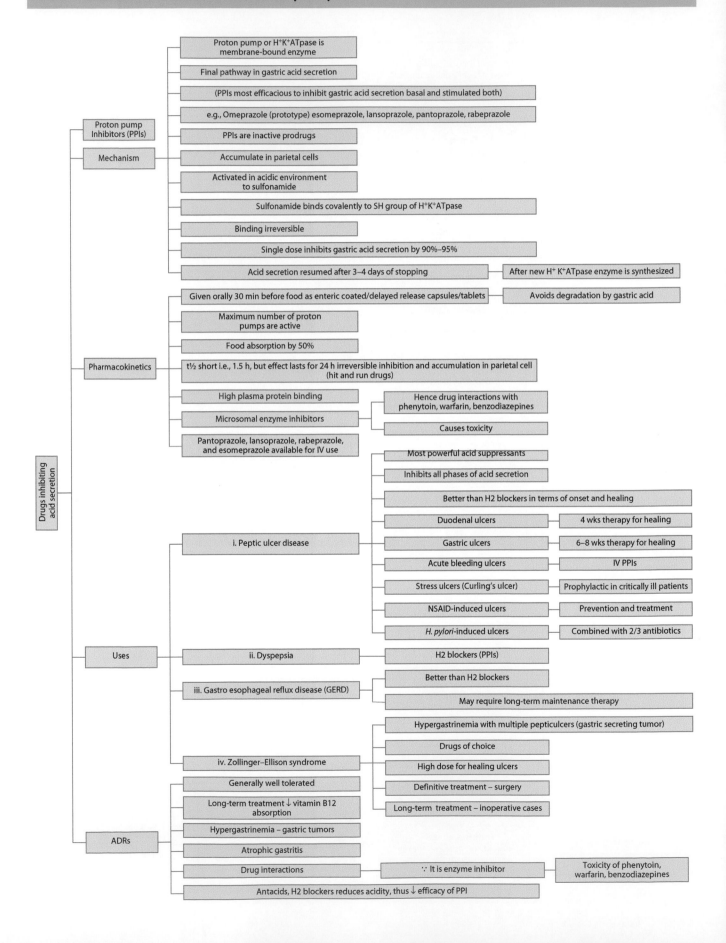

Drugs inhibiting acid secretion

Proton pump Inhibitors (PPIs)

Mechanism
- Proton pump or H⁺K⁺ATpase is membrane-bound enzyme
- Final pathway in gastric acid secretion
- (PPIs most efficacious to inhibit gastric acid secretion basal and stimulated both)
- e.g., Omeprazole (prototype) esomeprazole, lansoprazole, pantoprazole, rabeprazole
- PPIs are inactive prodrugs
- Accumulate in parietal cells
- Activated in acidic environment to sulfonamide
- Sulfonamide binds covalently to SH group of H⁺K⁺ATpase
- Binding irreversible
- Single dose inhibits gastric acid secretion by 90%–95%
- Acid secretion resumed after 3–4 days of stopping — After new H⁺ K⁺ATpase enzyme is synthesized

Pharmacokinetics
- Given orally 30 min before food as enteric coated/delayed release capsules/tablets — Avoids degradation by gastric acid
- Maximum number of proton pumps are active
- Food absorption by 50%
- t½ short i.e., 1.5 h, but effect lasts for 24 h irreversible inhibition and accumulation in parietal cell (hit and run drugs)
- High plasma protein binding
- Microsomal enzyme inhibitors — Hence drug interactions with phenytoin, warfarin, benzodiazepines / Causes toxicity
- Pantoprazole, lansoprazole, rabeprazole, and esomeprazole available for IV use

Uses
- i. Peptic ulcer disease
  - Most powerful acid suppressants
  - Inhibits all phases of acid secretion
  - Better than H2 blockers in terms of onset and healing
  - Duodenal ulcers — 4 wks therapy for healing
  - Gastric ulcers — 6–8 wks therapy for healing
  - Acute bleeding ulcers — IV PPIs
  - Stress ulcers (Curling's ulcer) — Prophylactic in critically ill patients
  - NSAID-induced ulcers — Prevention and treatment
  - *H. pylori*-induced ulcers — Combined with 2/3 antibiotics
- ii. Dyspepsia — H2 blockers (PPIs)
- iii. Gastro esophageal reflux disease (GERD)
  - Better than H2 blockers
  - May require long-term maintenance therapy
- iv. Zollinger–Ellison syndrome
  - Hypergastrinemia with multiple pepticulcers (gastric secreting tumor)
  - Drugs of choice
  - High dose for healing ulcers
  - Definitive treatment – surgery
  - Long-term treatment – inoperative cases

ADRs
- Generally well tolerated
- Long-term treatment ↓ vitamin B12 absorption
- Hypergastrinemia – gastric tumors
- Atrophic gastritis
- Drug interactions — ∵ It is enzyme inhibitor — Toxicity of phenytoin, warfarin, benzodiazepines
- Antacids, H2 blockers reduces acidity, thus ↓ efficacy of PPI

44.6 H2-RECEPTOR BLOCKERS

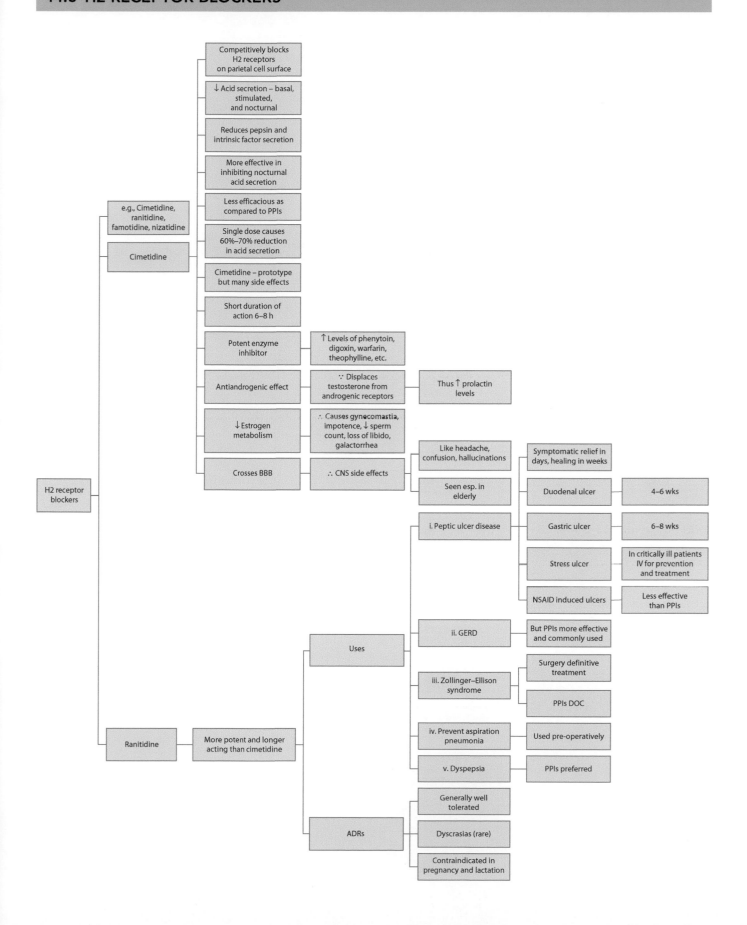

H2 receptor blockers

- e.g., Cimetidine, ranitidine, famotidine, nizatidine
- Cimetidine
  - Competitively blocks H2 receptors on parietal cell surface
  - ↓ Acid secretion – basal, stimulated, and nocturnal
  - Reduces pepsin and intrinsic factor secretion
  - More effective in inhibiting nocturnal acid secretion
  - Less efficacious as compared to PPIs
  - Single dose causes 60%–70% reduction in acid secretion
  - Cimetidine – prototype but many side effects
  - Short duration of action 6–8 h
  - Potent enzyme inhibitor → ↑ Levels of phenytoin, digoxin, warfarin, theophylline, etc.
  - Antiandrogenic effect → ∵ Displaces testosterone from androgenic receptors → Thus ↑ prolactin levels
  - ↓ Estrogen metabolism → ∴ Causes gynecomastia, impotence, ↓ sperm count, loss of libido, galactorrhea
  - Crosses BBB → ∴ CNS side effects → Like headache, confusion, hallucinations / Seen esp. in elderly

- Ranitidine
  - More potent and longer acting than cimetidine
  - Uses
    - i. Peptic ulcer disease
      - Symptomatic relief in days, healing in weeks
      - Duodenal ulcer → 4–6 wks
      - Gastric ulcer → 6–8 wks
      - Stress ulcer → In critically ill patients IV for prevention and treatment
      - NSAID induced ulcers → Less effective than PPIs
    - ii. GERD → But PPIs more effective and commonly used
    - iii. Zollinger–Ellison syndrome
      - Surgery definitive treatment
      - PPIs DOC
    - iv. Prevent aspiration pneumonia → Used pre-operatively
    - v. Dyspepsia → PPIs preferred
  - ADRs
    - Generally well tolerated
    - Dyscrasias (rare)
    - Contraindicated in pregnancy and lactation

44.7 ANTIMUSCARINIC AGENTS AND PROSTAGLANDIN ANALOGS

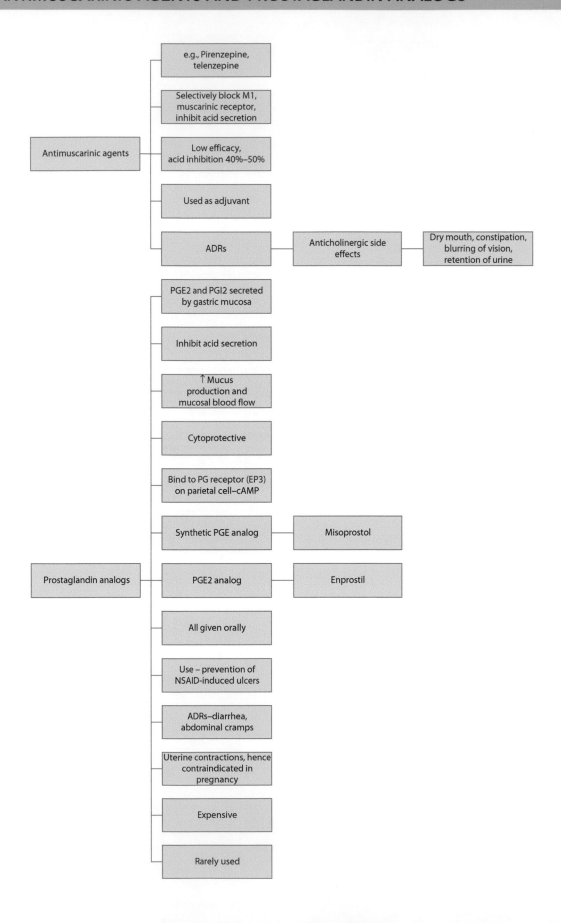

Antimuscarinic agents
- e.g., Pirenzepine, telenzepine
- Selectively block M1, muscarinic receptor, inhibit acid secretion
- Low efficacy, acid inhibition 40%–50%
- Used as adjuvant
- ADRs — Anticholinergic side effects — Dry mouth, constipation, blurring of vision, retention of urine

Prostaglandin analogs
- PGE2 and PGI2 secreted by gastric mucosa
- Inhibit acid secretion
- ↑ Mucus production and mucosal blood flow
- Cytoprotective
- Bind to PG receptor (EP3) on parietal cell–cAMP
- Synthetic PGE analog — Misoprostol
- PGE2 analog — Enprostil
- All given orally
- Use – prevention of NSAID-induced ulcers
- ADRs–diarrhea, abdominal cramps
- Uterine contractions, hence contraindicated in pregnancy
- Expensive
- Rarely used

44.8 ULCER PROTECTIVES

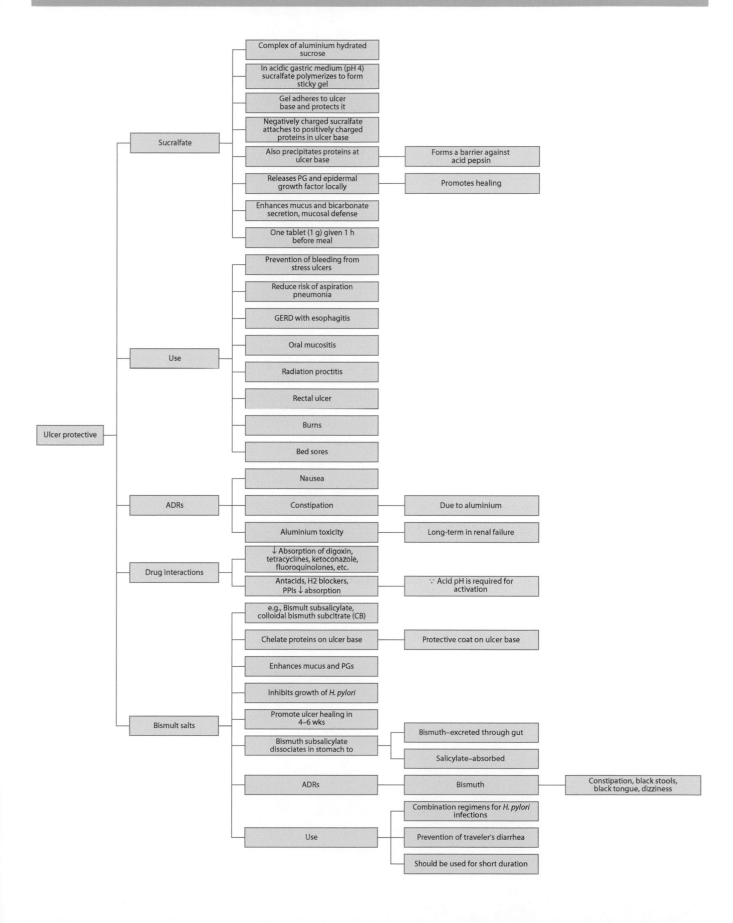

44.9 MISCELLANEOUS AGENTS

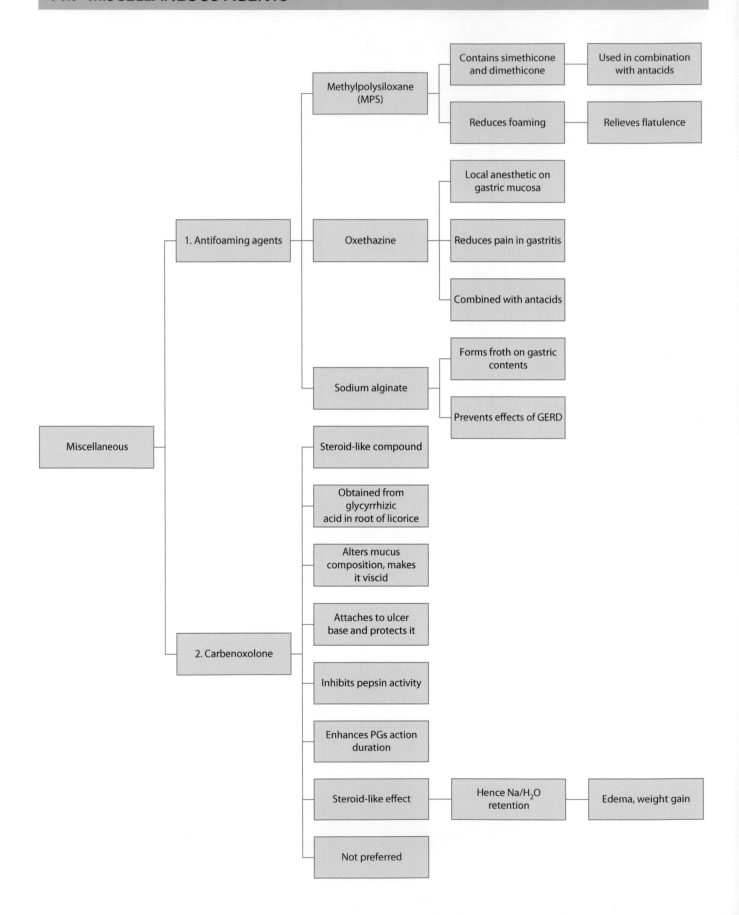

44.10 ANTI-*H. PYLORI* AGENTS

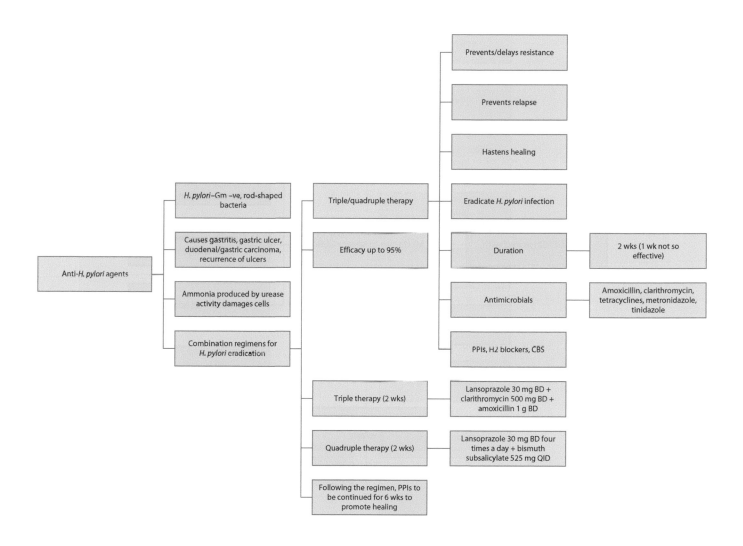

45.2 EMETICS

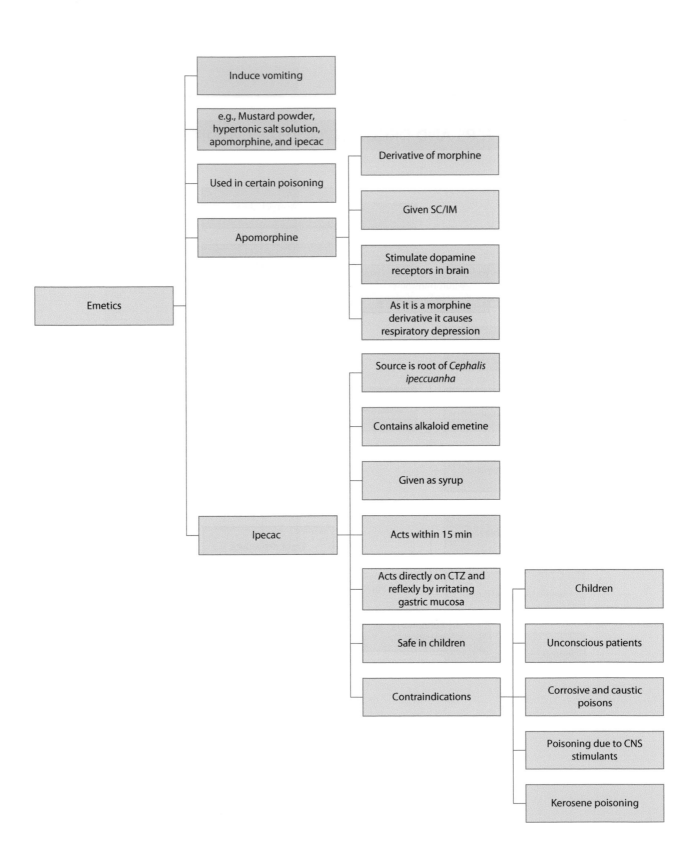

Emetics
- Induce vomiting
- e.g., Mustard powder, hypertonic salt solution, apomorphine, and ipecac
- Used in certain poisoning
- Apomorphine
  - Derivative of morphine
  - Given SC/IM
  - Stimulate dopamine receptors in brain
  - As it is a morphine derivative it causes respiratory depression
- Ipecac
  - Source is root of *Cephalis ipeccuanha*
  - Contains alkaloid emetine
  - Given as syrup
  - Acts within 15 min
  - Acts directly on CTZ and reflexly by irritating gastric mucosa
  - Safe in children
  - Contraindications
    - Children
    - Unconscious patients
    - Corrosive and caustic poisons
    - Poisoning due to CNS stimulants
    - Kerosene poisoning

45.3 CLASSIFICATIONS OF ANTIEMETICS

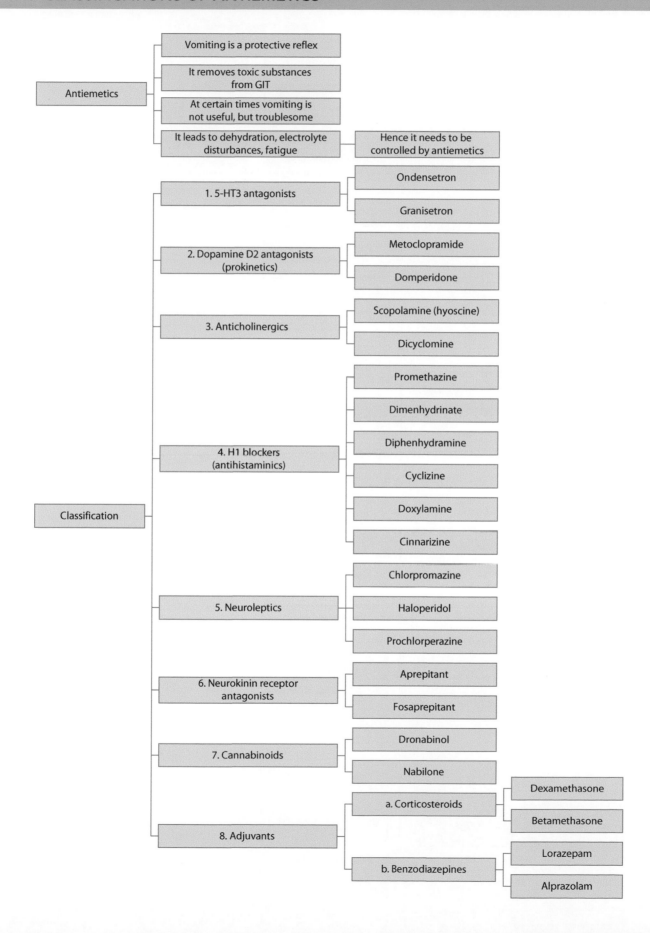

Antiemetics
- Vomiting is a protective reflex
- It removes toxic substances from GIT
- At certain times vomiting is not useful, but troublesome
- It leads to dehydration, electrolyte disturbances, fatigue → Hence it needs to be controlled by antiemetics

Classification
1. 5-HT3 antagonists
   - Ondensetron
   - Granisetron
2. Dopamine D2 antagonists (prokinetics)
   - Metoclopramide
   - Domperidone
3. Anticholinergics
   - Scopolamine (hyoscine)
   - Dicyclomine
4. H1 blockers (antihistaminics)
   - Promethazine
   - Dimenhydrinate
   - Diphenhydramine
   - Cyclizine
   - Doxylamine
   - Cinnarizine
5. Neuroleptics
   - Chlorpromazine
   - Haloperidol
   - Prochlorperazine
6. Neurokinin receptor antagonists
   - Aprepitant
   - Fosaprepitant
7. Cannabinoids
   - Dronabinol
   - Nabilone
8. Adjuvants
   - a. Corticosteroids
     - Dexamethasone
     - Betamethasone
   - b. Benzodiazepines
     - Lorazepam
     - Alprazolam

45.4 5-HT3 RECEPTOR ANTAGONISTS (5-HT3RA)

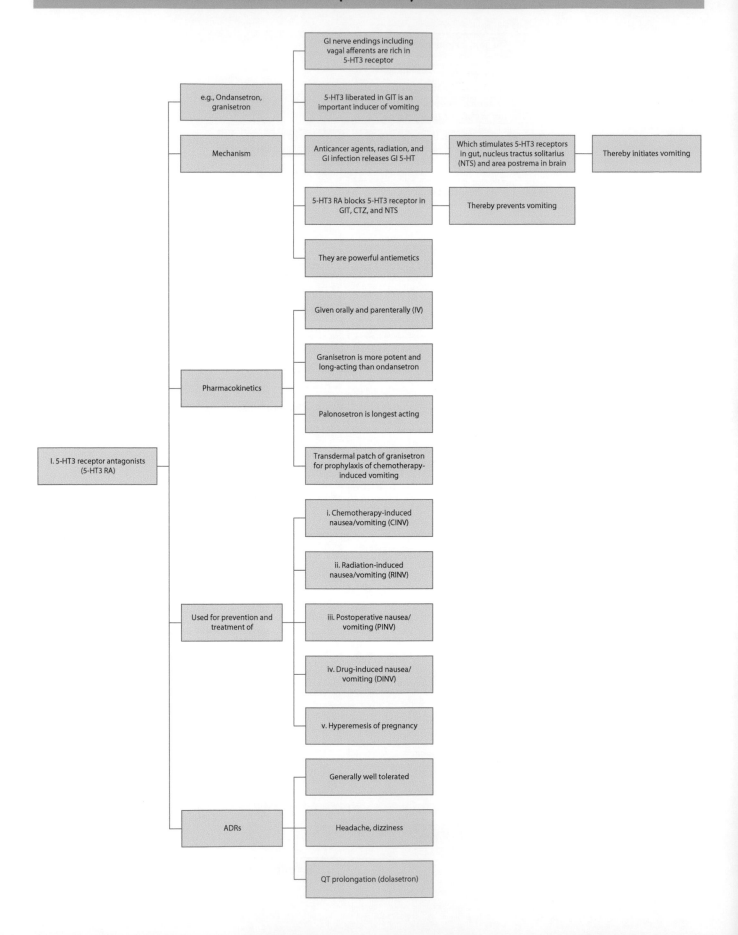

I. 5-HT3 receptor antagonists (5-HT3 RA)

Mechanism
e.g., Ondansetron, granisetron

GI nerve endings including vagal afferents are rich in 5-HT3 receptor

5-HT3 liberated in GIT is an important inducer of vomiting

Anticancer agents, radiation, and GI infection releases GI 5-HT → Which stimulates 5-HT3 receptors in gut, nucleus tractus solitarius (NTS) and area postrema in brain → Thereby initiates vomiting

5-HT3 RA blocks 5-HT3 receptor in GIT, CTZ, and NTS → Thereby prevents vomiting

They are powerful antiemetics

Pharmacokinetics

Given orally and parenterally (IV)

Granisetron is more potent and long-acting than ondansetron

Palonosetron is longest acting

Transdermal patch of granisetron for prophylaxis of chemotherapy-induced vomiting

Used for prevention and treatment of

i. Chemotherapy-induced nausea/vomiting (CINV)

ii. Radiation-induced nausea/vomiting (RINV)

iii. Postoperative nausea/vomiting (PINV)

iv. Drug-induced nausea/vomiting (DINV)

v. Hyperemesis of pregnancy

ADRs

Generally well tolerated

Headache, dizziness

QT prolongation (dolasetron)

45.5 DOPAMINE D2 RECEPTOR ANTAGONISTS (PROKINETICS)

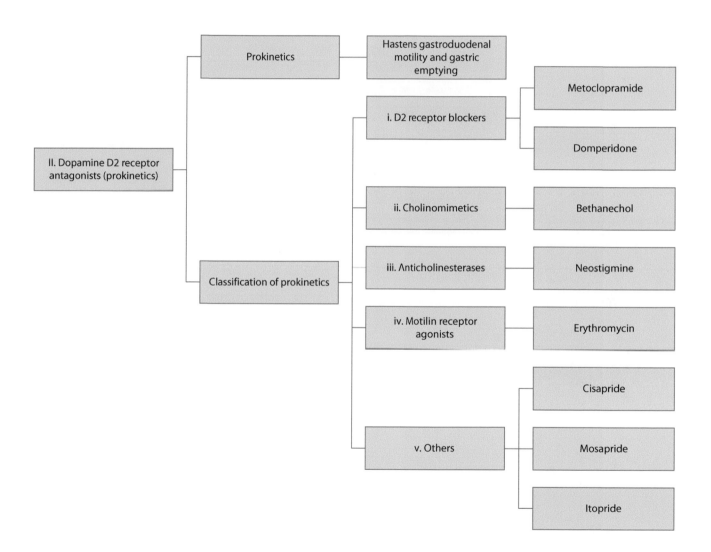

45.6 METOCLOPRAMIDE

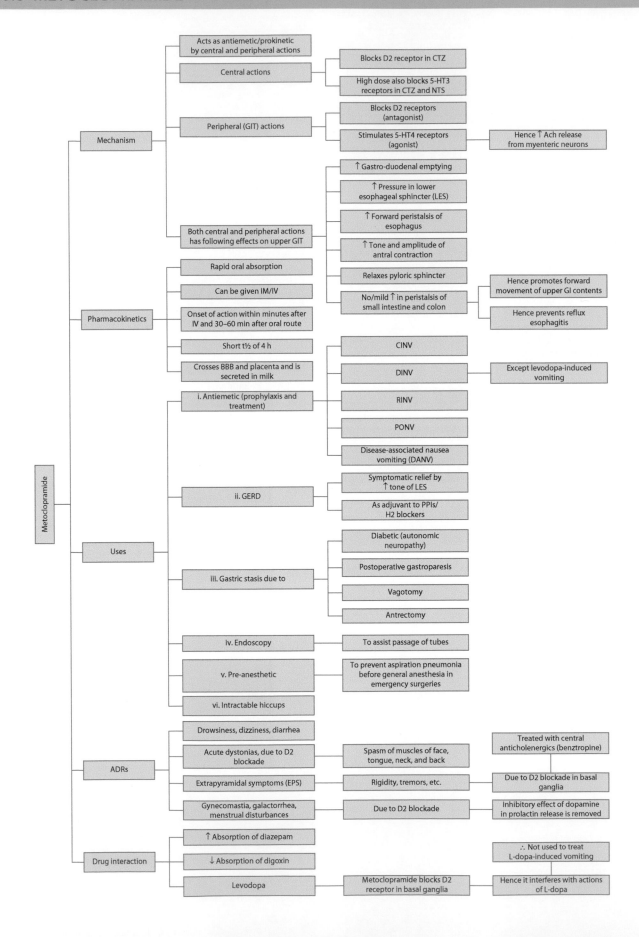

45.7 DOMPERIDONE, CHOLINOMIMETICS, ANTICHOLINESTERASES, AND MOTILIN RECEPTOR AGONISTS

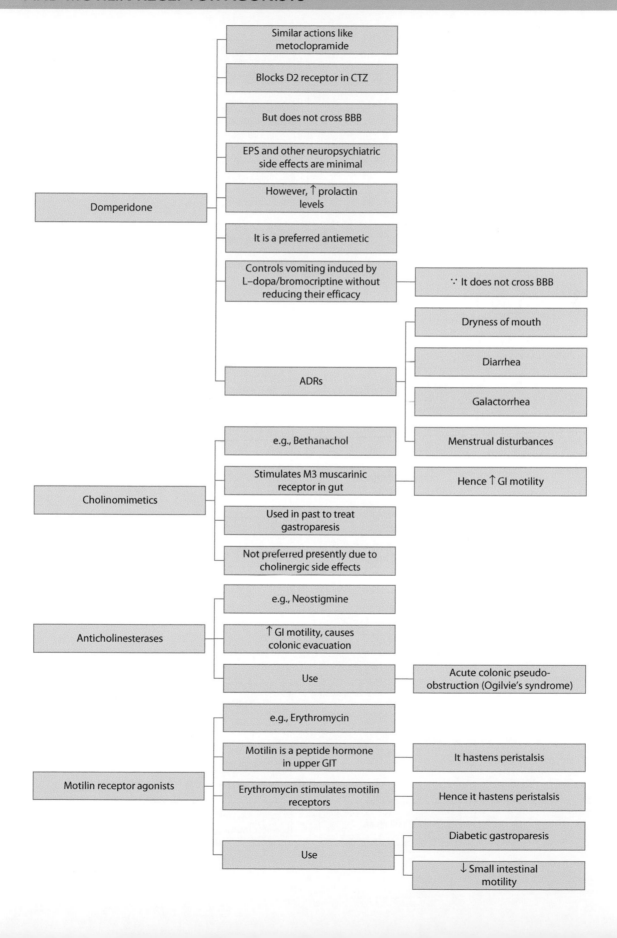

45.8 ANTICHOLINERGICS AND ANTIHISTAMINICS (H1 BLOCKERS)

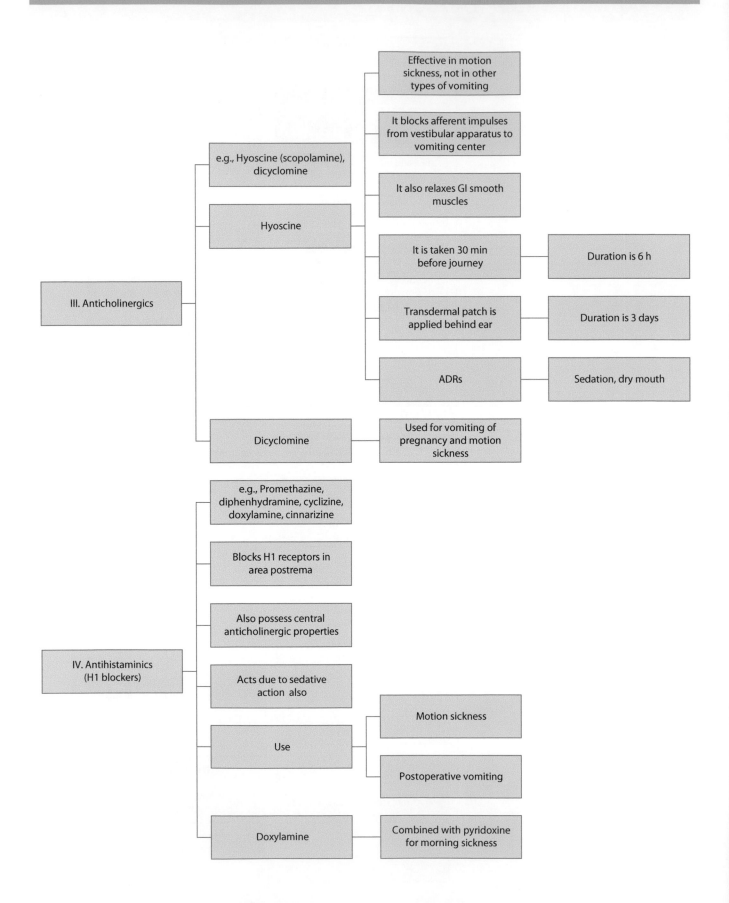

45.9 NEUROLEPTIC, NEUROKININ RECEPTOR ANTAGONISTS, AND CANNABINOIDS

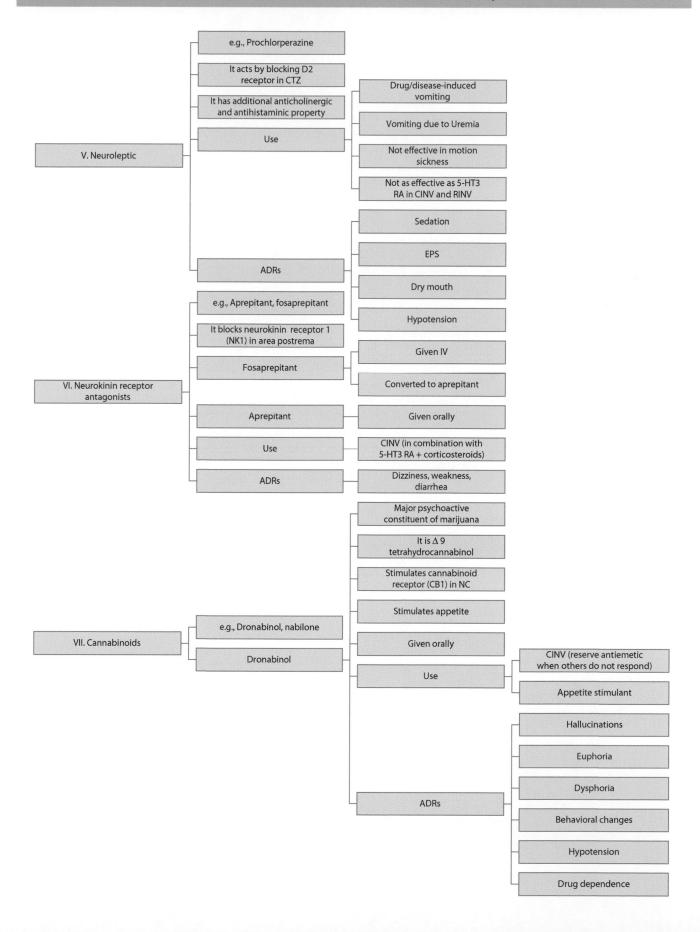

45.10 ADJUVANTS AND PREFERRED ANTIEMETICS

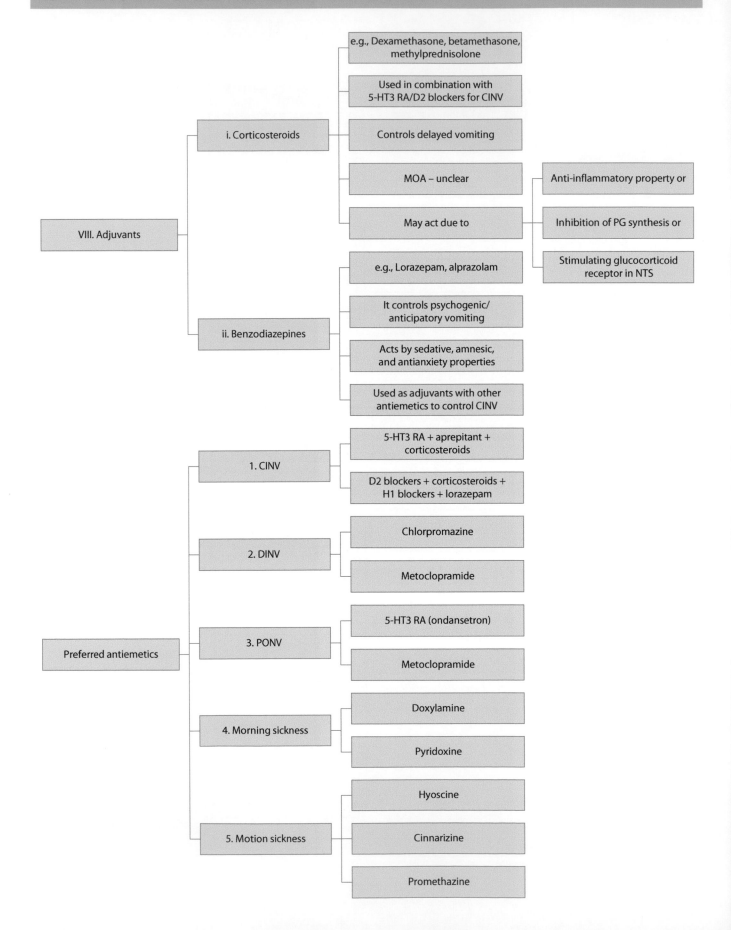

VIII. Adjuvants

i. Corticosteroids
- e.g., Dexamethasone, betamethasone, methylprednisolone
- Used in combination with 5-HT3 RA/D2 blockers for CINV
- Controls delayed vomiting
- MOA – unclear
- May act due to
  - Anti-inflammatory property or
  - Inhibition of PG synthesis or
  - Stimulating glucocorticoid receptor in NTS

ii. Benzodiazepines
- e.g., Lorazepam, alprazolam
- It controls psychogenic/anticipatory vomiting
- Acts by sedative, amnesic, and antianxiety properties
- Used as adjuvants with other antiemetics to control CINV

Preferred antiemetics

1. CINV
- 5-HT3 RA + aprepitant + corticosteroids
- D2 blockers + corticosteroids + H1 blockers + lorazepam

2. DINV
- Chlorpromazine
- Metoclopramide

3. PONV
- 5-HT3 RA (ondansetron)
- Metoclopramide

4. Morning sickness
- Doxylamine
- Pyridoxine

5. Motion sickness
- Hyoscine
- Cinnarizine
- Promethazine

46

Drug treatment of constipation, treatment of IBS, and IBD

46.1 INTRODUCTION AND CLASSIFICATION

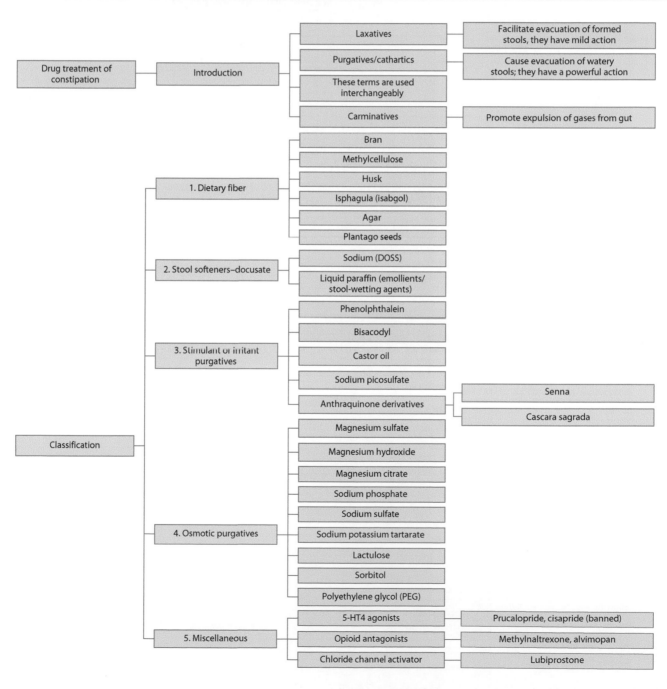

46.2 BULK LAXATIVES

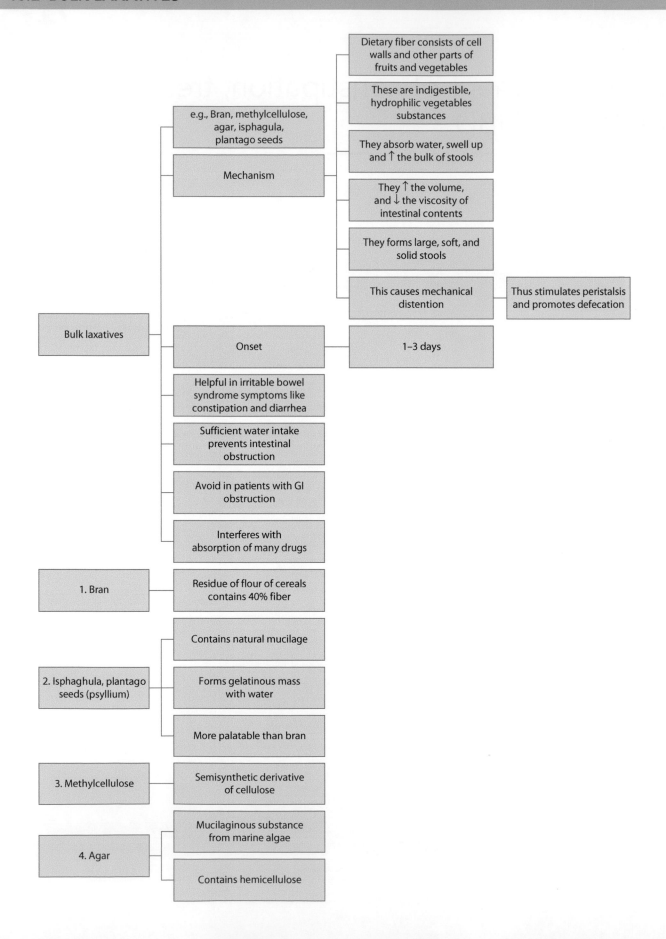

e.g., Bran, methylcellulose, agar, isphagula, plantago seeds

Mechanism
- Dietary fiber consists of cell walls and other parts of fruits and vegetables
- These are indigestible, hydrophilic vegetables substances
- They absorb water, swell up and ↑ the bulk of stools
- They ↑ the volume, and ↓ the viscosity of intestinal contents
- They forms large, soft, and solid stools
- This causes mechanical distention → Thus stimulates peristalsis and promotes defecation

Onset → 1–3 days

Bulk laxatives
- Helpful in irritable bowel syndrome symptoms like constipation and diarrhea
- Sufficient water intake prevents intestinal obstruction
- Avoid in patients with GI obstruction
- Interferes with absorption of many drugs

1. Bran → Residue of flour of cereals contains 40% fiber

2. Isphaghula, plantago seeds (psyllium)
- Contains natural mucilage
- Forms gelatinous mass with water
- More palatable than bran

3. Methylcellulose → Semisynthetic derivative of cellulose

4. Agar
- Mucilaginous substance from marine algae
- Contains hemicellulose

46.3 STOOL SOFTENERS

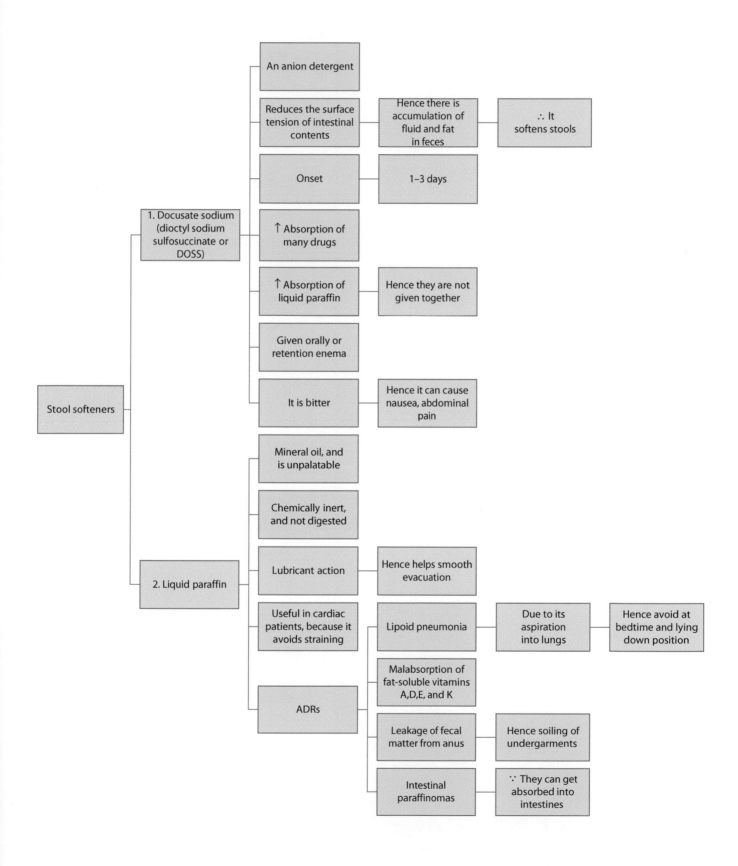

46.4 STIMULANT PURGATIVES

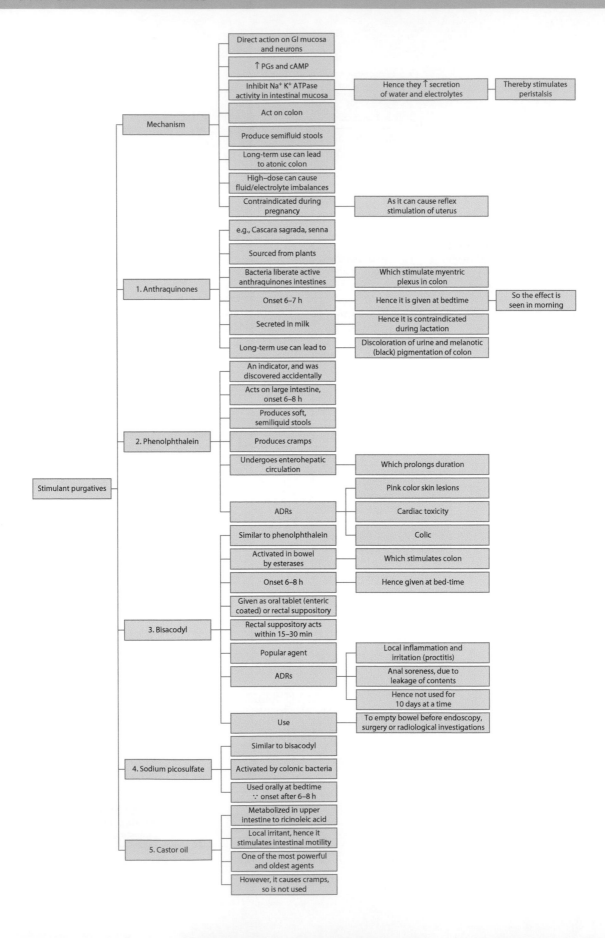

Stimulant purgatives

Mechanism
- Direct action on GI mucosa and neurons
- ↑ PGs and cAMP
- Inhibit Na⁺ K⁺ ATPase activity in intestinal mucosa → Hence they ↑ secretion of water and electrolytes → Thereby stimulates peristalsis
- Act on colon
- Produce semifluid stools
- Long-term use can lead to atonic colon
- High–dose can cause fluid/electrolyte imbalances
- Contraindicated during pregnancy → As it can cause reflex stimulation of uterus

1. Anthraquinones
- e.g., Cascara sagrada, senna
- Sourced from plants
- Bacteria liberate active anthraquinones intestines → Which stimulate myentric plexus in colon
- Onset 6–7 h → Hence it is given at bedtime → So the effect is seen in morning
- Secreted in milk → Hence it is contraindicated during lactation
- Long-term use can lead to → Discoloration of urine and melanotic (black) pigmentation of colon

2. Phenolphthalein
- An indicator, and was discovered accidentally
- Acts on large intestine, onset 6–8 h
- Produces soft, semiliquid stools
- Produces cramps
- Undergoes enterohepatic circulation → Which prolongs duration
- ADRs
  - Pink color skin lesions
  - Cardiac toxicity
  - Colic

3. Bisacodyl
- Similar to phenolphthalein
- Activated in bowel by esterases → Which stimulates colon
- Onset 6–8 h → Hence given at bed-time
- Given as oral tablet (enteric coated) or rectal suppository
- Rectal suppository acts within 15–30 min
- Popular agent
- ADRs
  - Local inflammation and irritation (proctitis)
  - Anal soreness, due to leakage of contents
  - Hence not used for 10 days at a time
- Use → To empty bowel before endoscopy, surgery or radiological investigations

4. Sodium picosulfate
- Similar to bisacodyl
- Activated by colonic bacteria
- Used orally at bedtime ∵ onset after 6–8 h

5. Castor oil
- Metabolized in upper intestine to ricinoleic acid
- Local irritant, hence it stimulates intestinal motility
- One of the most powerful and oldest agents
- However, it causes cramps, so is not used

46.5 OSMOTIC PURGATIVES

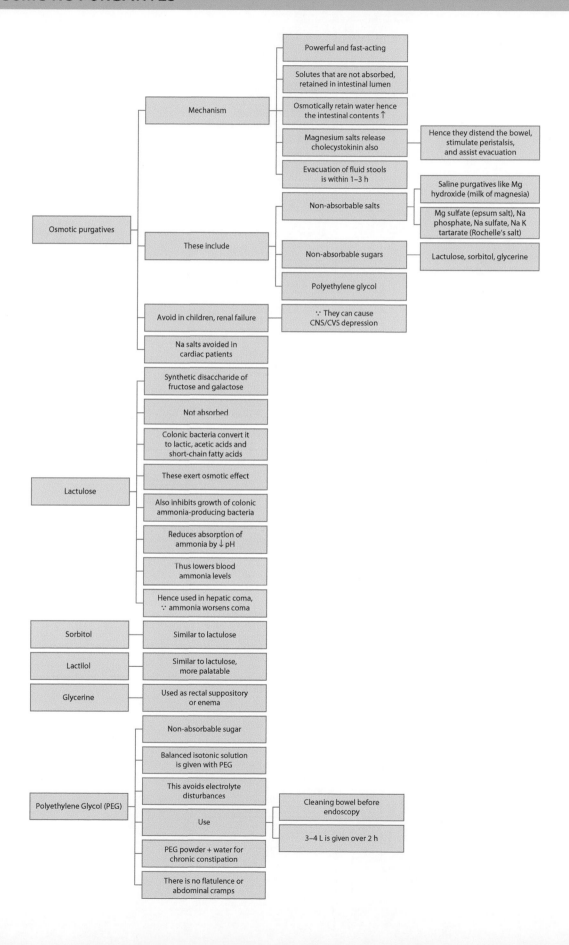

Osmotic purgatives

Mechanism
- Powerful and fast-acting
- Solutes that are not absorbed, retained in intestinal lumen
- Osmotically retain water hence the intestinal contents ↑
- Magnesium salts release cholecystokinin also → Hence they distend the bowel, stimulate peristalsis, and assist evacuation
- Evacuation of fluid stools is within 1–3 h

These include
- Non-absorbable salts
  - Saline purgatives like Mg hydroxide (milk of magnesia)
  - Mg sulfate (epsum salt), Na phosphate, Na sulfate, Na K tartarate (Rochelle's salt)
- Non-absorbable sugars → Lactulose, sorbitol, glycerine
- Polyethylene glycol

Avoid in children, renal failure → ∵ They can cause CNS/CVS depression

Na salts avoided in cardiac patients

Lactulose
- Synthetic disaccharide of fructose and galactose
- Not absorbed
- Colonic bacteria convert it to lactic, acetic acids and short-chain fatty acids
- These exert osmotic effect
- Also inhibits growth of colonic ammonia-producing bacteria
- Reduces absorption of ammonia by ↓ pH
- Thus lowers blood ammonia levels
- Hence used in hepatic coma, ∵ ammonia worsens coma

Sorbitol — Similar to lactulose

Lactilol — Similar to lactulose, more palatable

Glycerine — Used as rectal suppository or enema

Polyethylene Glycol (PEG)
- Non-absorbable sugar
- Balanced isotonic solution is given with PEG
- This avoids electrolyte disturbances
- Use
  - Cleaning bowel before endoscopy
  - 3–4 L is given over 2 h
- PEG powder + water for chronic constipation
- There is no flatulence or abdominal cramps

46.6 MISCELLANEOUS AGENTS AND USE OF LAXATIVES/PURGATIVES

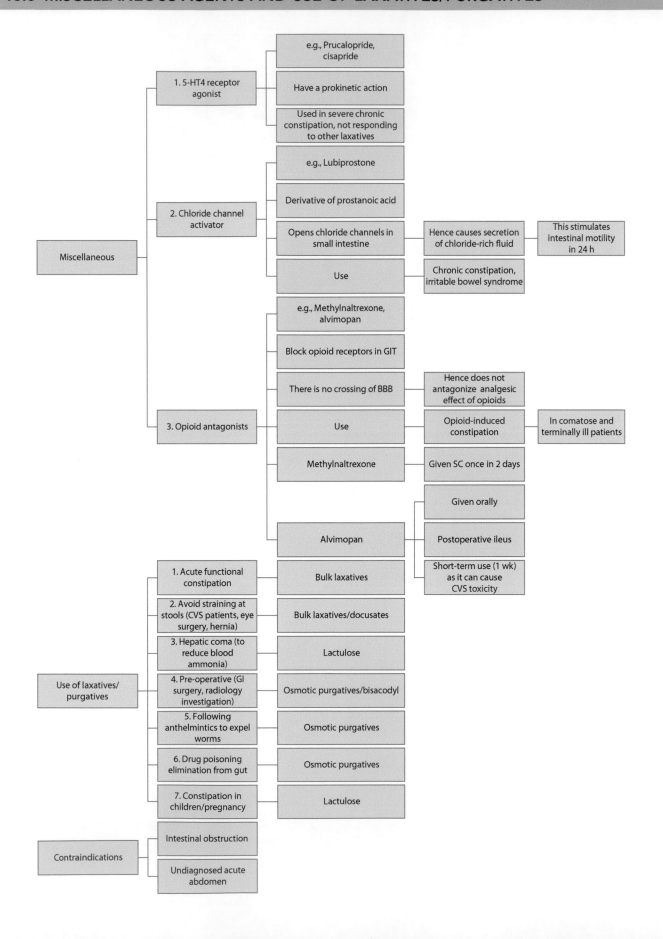

46.7 DRUGS CAUSING CONSTIPATION, LAXATIVE ABUSE, AND NONPHARMACOLOGICAL MEASURES

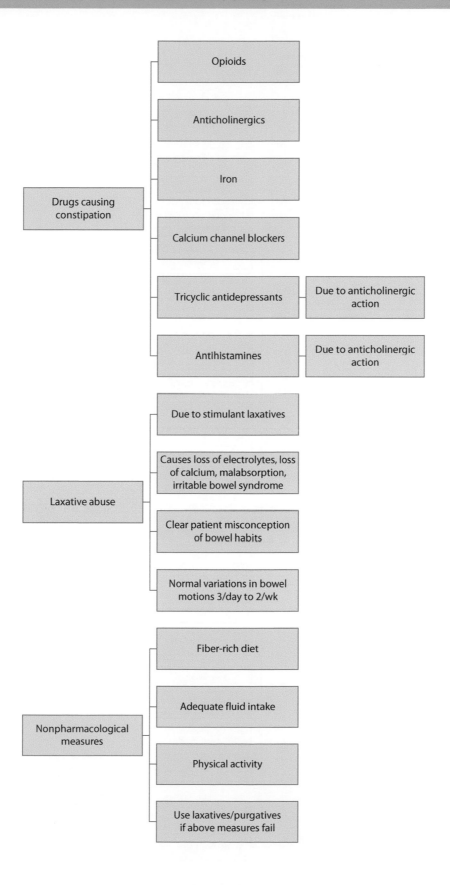

46.8 TREATMENT OF IRRITABLE BOWEL SYNDROME (IBS)

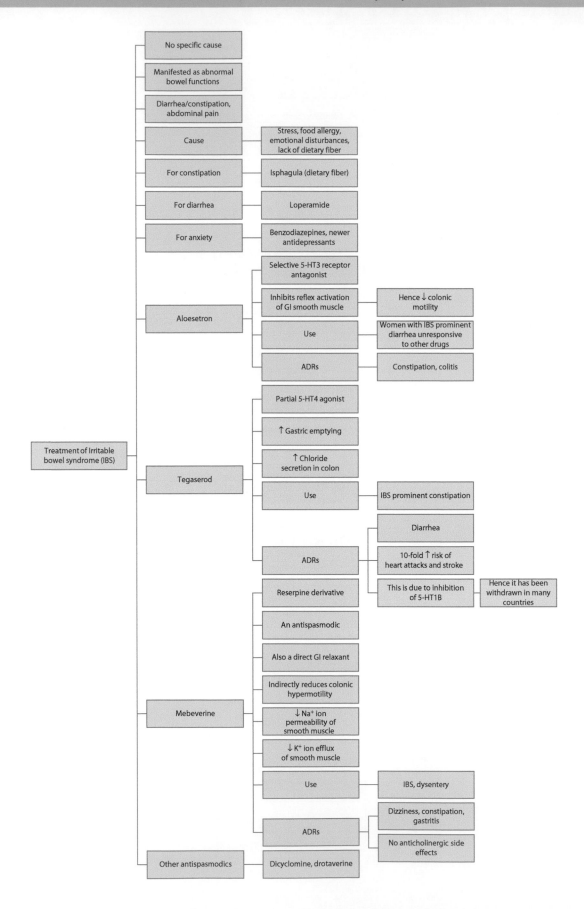

46.9 INFLAMMATORY BOWEL DISEASES (IBD) AND TREATMENT

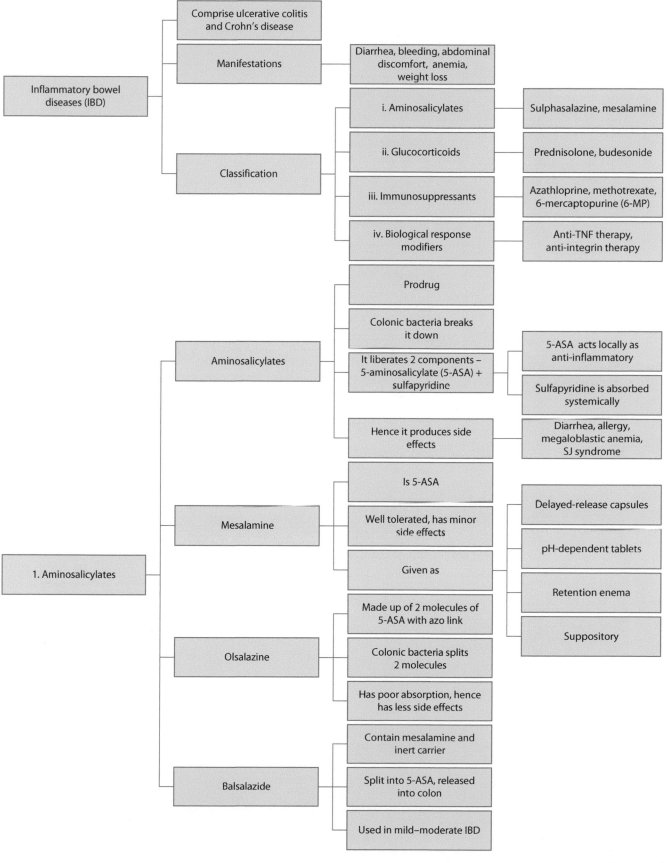

46.9 INFLAMMATORY BOWEL DISEASES (IBD) AND TREATMENT (Continued)

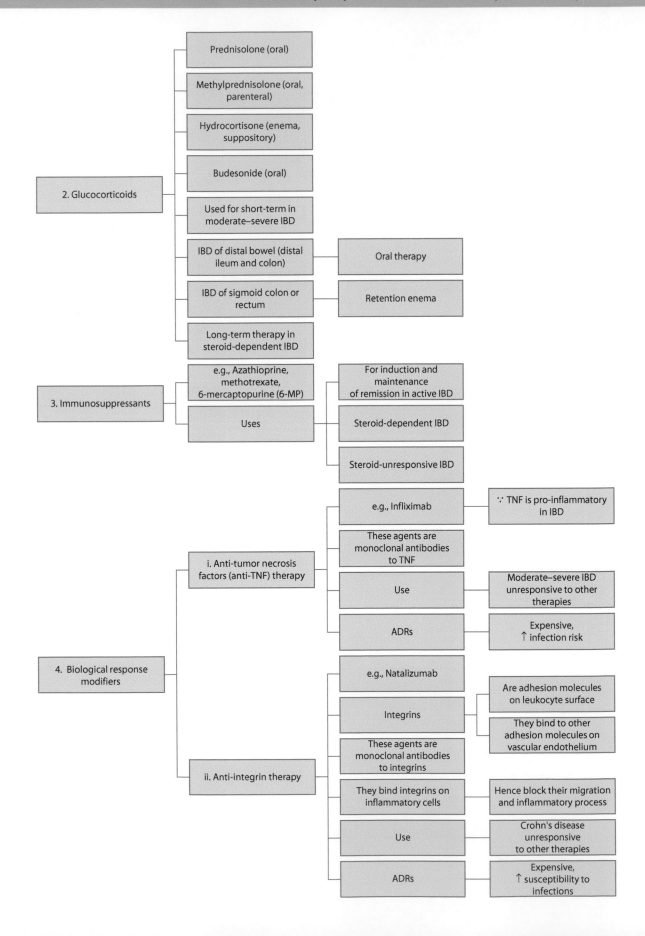

2. Glucocorticoids
- Prednisolone (oral)
- Methylprednisolone (oral, parenteral)
- Hydrocortisone (enema, suppository)
- Budesonide (oral)
- Used for short-term in moderate–severe IBD
- IBD of distal bowel (distal ileum and colon) → Oral therapy
- IBD of sigmoid colon or rectum → Retention enema
- Long-term therapy in steroid-dependent IBD

3. Immunosuppressants
- e.g., Azathioprine, methotrexate, 6-mercaptopurine (6-MP)
- Uses
  - For induction and maintenance of remission in active IBD
  - Steroid-dependent IBD
  - Steroid-unresponsive IBD

4. Biological response modifiers

i. Anti-tumor necrosis factors (anti-TNF) therapy
- e.g., Infliximab → ∵ TNF is pro-inflammatory in IBD
- These agents are monoclonal antibodies to TNF
- Use → Moderate–severe IBD unresponsive to other therapies
- ADRs → Expensive, ↑ infection risk

ii. Anti-integrin therapy
- e.g., Natalizumab
- Integrins
  - Are adhesion molecules on leukocyte surface
  - They bind to other adhesion molecules on vascular endothelium
- These agents are monoclonal antibodies to integrins
- They bind integrins on inflammatory cells → Hence block their migration and inflammatory process
- Use → Crohn's disease unresponsive to other therapies
- ADRs → Expensive, ↑ susceptibility to infections

Drug treatment of diarrhea

47.1 PRINCIPLES OF DIARRHEA TREATMENT AND ORS

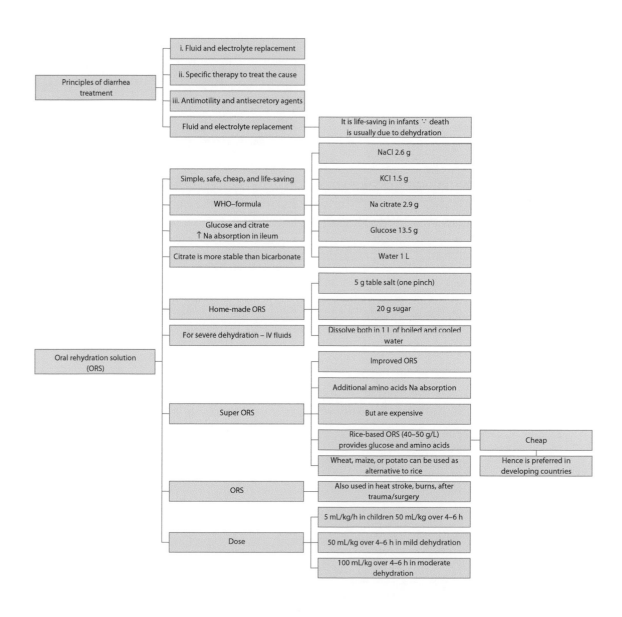

47.2 SPECIFIC THERAPY

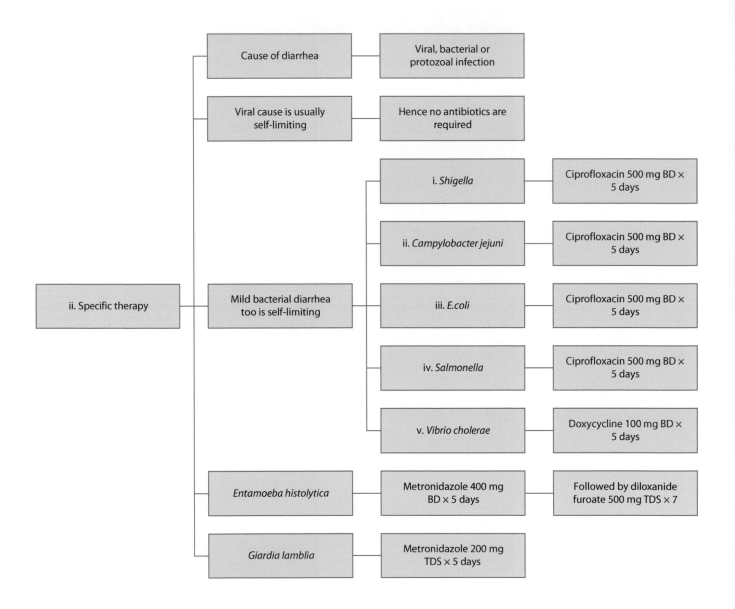

47.3 ANTIMOTILITY AND ANTISECRETORY AGENTS AND ADSORBANTS

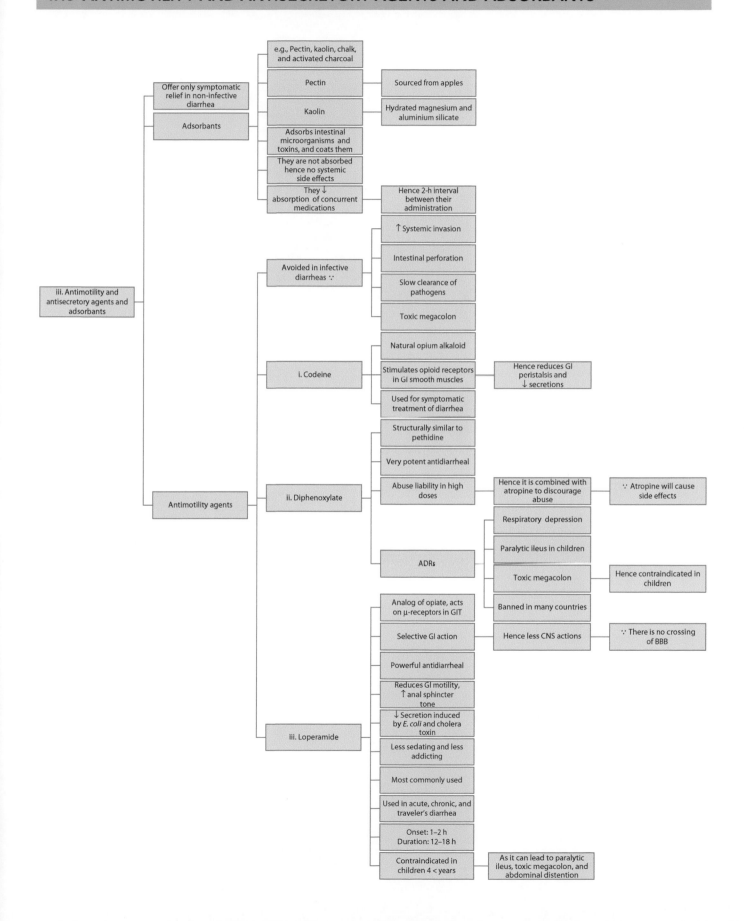

47.4 ANTISECRETORY AGENTS AND PROBIOTICS

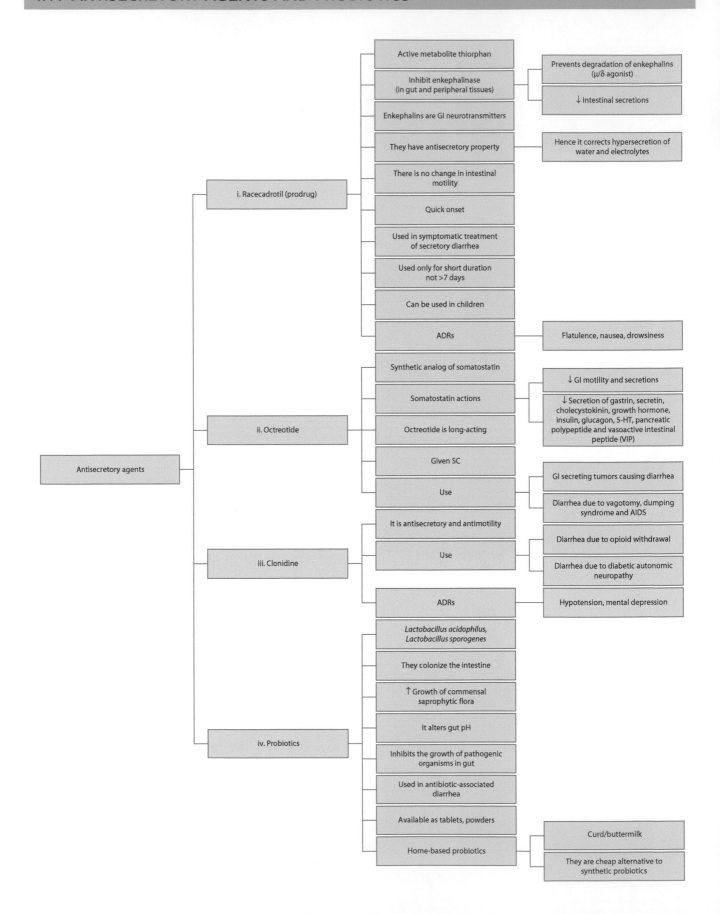

47.5 ANTISPASMODICS

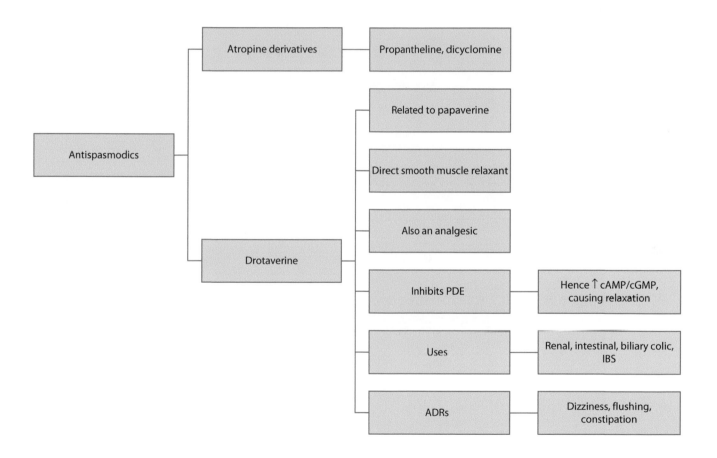

PART IX

Endocrine pharmacology

Hypothalamic and pituitary hormones

48.1 HYPOTHALAMIC AND PITUITARY HORMONES – TYPES, MODES, AND MECHANISM OF ACTION

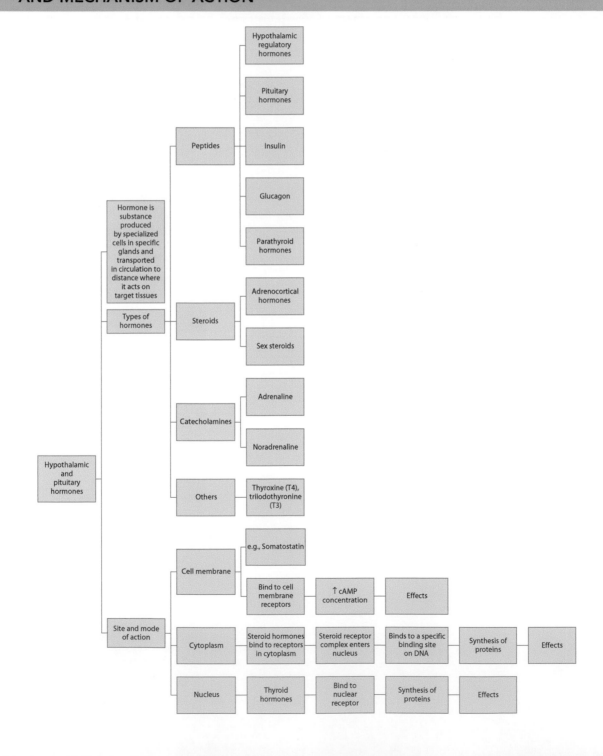

48.2 HYPOTHALAMIC HORMONES

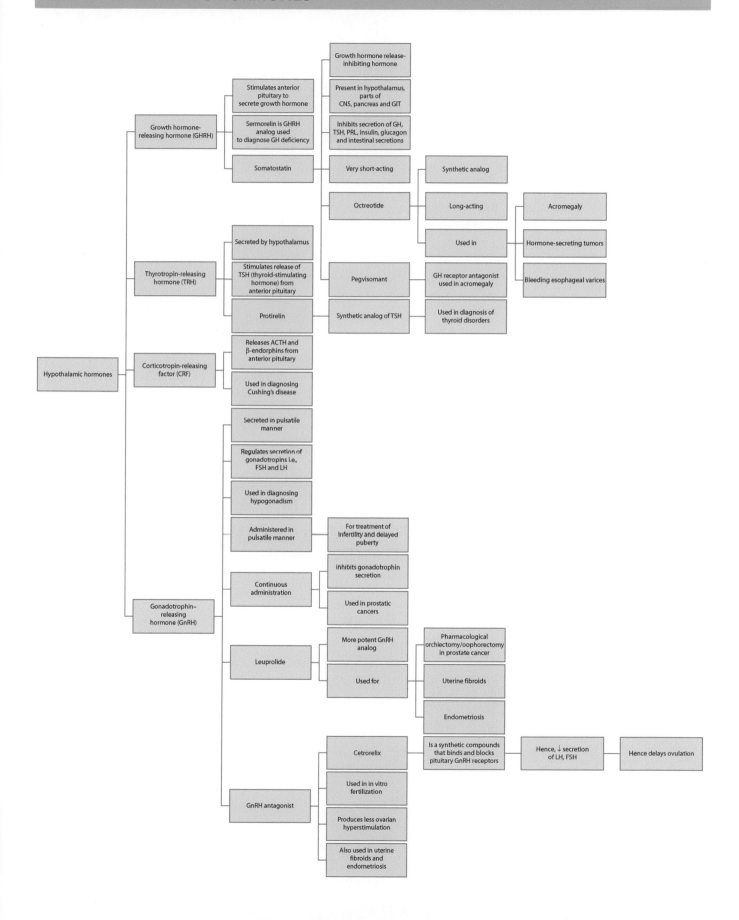

- **Hypothalamic hormones**
  - **Growth hormone-releasing hormone (GHRH)**
    - Stimulates anterior pituitary to secrete growth hormone
      - Growth hormone release-inhibiting hormone
    - Sermorelin is GHRH analog used to diagnose GH deficiency
      - Present in hypothalamus, parts of CNS, pancreas and GIT
    - Somatostatin
      - Inhibits secretion of GH, TSH, PRL, insulin, glucagon and intestinal secretions
      - Very short-acting
    - Octreotide
      - Synthetic analog
      - Long-acting
        - Acromegaly
      - Used in
        - Hormone-secreting tumors
        - Bleeding esophageal varices
    - Pegvisomant
      - GH receptor antagonist used in acromegaly
  - **Thyrotropin-releasing hormone (TRH)**
    - Secreted by hypothalamus
    - Stimulates release of TSH (thyroid-stimulating hormone) from anterior pituitary
    - Protirelin
      - Synthetic analog of TSH
        - Used in diagnosis of thyroid disorders
  - **Corticotropin-releasing factor (CRF)**
    - Releases ACTH and β-endorphins from anterior pituitary
    - Used in diagnosing Cushing's disease
  - **Gonadotrophin–releasing hormone (GnRH)**
    - Secreted in pulsatile manner
    - Regulates secretion of gonadotropins i.e., FSH and LH
    - Used in diagnosing hypogonadism
    - Administered in pulsatile manner
      - For treatment of infertility and delayed puberty
    - Continuous administration
      - Inhibits gonadotrophin secretion
      - Used in prostatic cancers
    - Leuprolide
      - More potent GnRH analog
        - Pharmacological orchiectomy/oophorectomy in prostate cancer
      - Used for
        - Uterine fibroids
        - Endometriosis
    - GnRH antagonist
      - Cetrorelix
        - Is a synthetic compounds that binds and blocks pituitary GnRH receptors
          - Hence, ↓ secretion of LH, FSH
            - Hence delays ovulation
      - Used in in vitro fertilization
      - Produces less ovarian hyperstimulation
      - Also used in uterine fibroids and endometriosis

48.3 ANTERIOR PITUITARY HORMONES

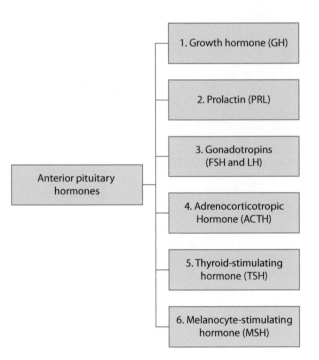

48.4 GROWTH HORMONE (SOMATOTROPHIN)

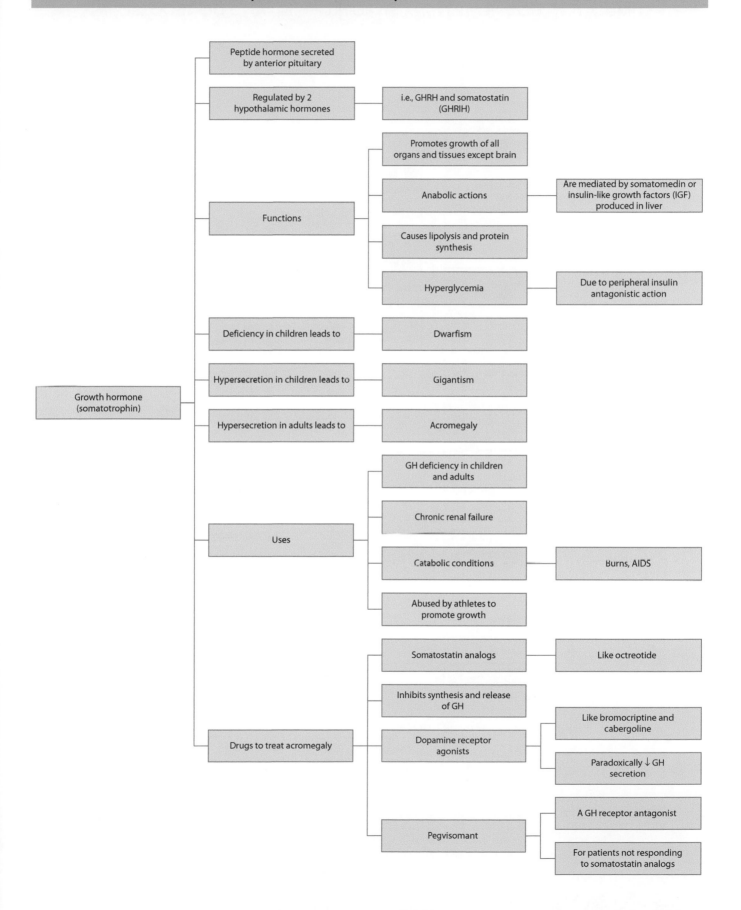

48.5 CORTICOTROPIN (ADRENOCORTICOTROPIC HORMONE – ACTH), THYROID-STIMULATING HORMONE (TSH, THYROTROPHIN), AND GONADOTROPINS

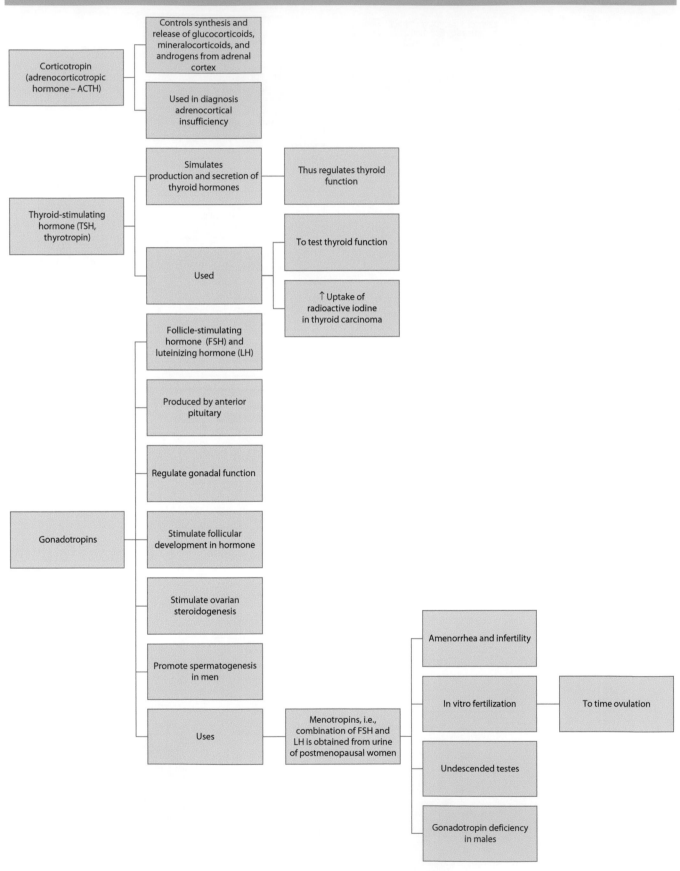

Corticotropin (adrenocorticotropic hormone – ACTH)
- Controls synthesis and release of glucocorticoids, mineralocorticoids, and androgens from adrenal cortex
- Used in diagnosis adrenocortical insufficiency

Thyroid-stimulating hormone (TSH, thyrotropin)
- Simulates production and secretion of thyroid hormones
  - Thus regulates thyroid function
- Used
  - To test thyroid function
  - ↑ Uptake of radioactive iodine in thyroid carcinoma

Gonadotropins
- Follicle-stimulating hormone (FSH) and luteinizing hormone (LH)
- Produced by anterior pituitary
- Regulate gonadal function
- Stimulate follicular development in hormone
- Stimulate ovarian steroidogenesis
- Promote spermatogenesis in men
- Uses
  - Menotropins, i.e., combination of FSH and LH is obtained from urine of postmenopausal women
    - Amenorrhea and infertility
    - In vitro fertilization
      - To time ovulation
    - Undescended testes
    - Gonadotropin deficiency in males

48.6 PROLACTIN

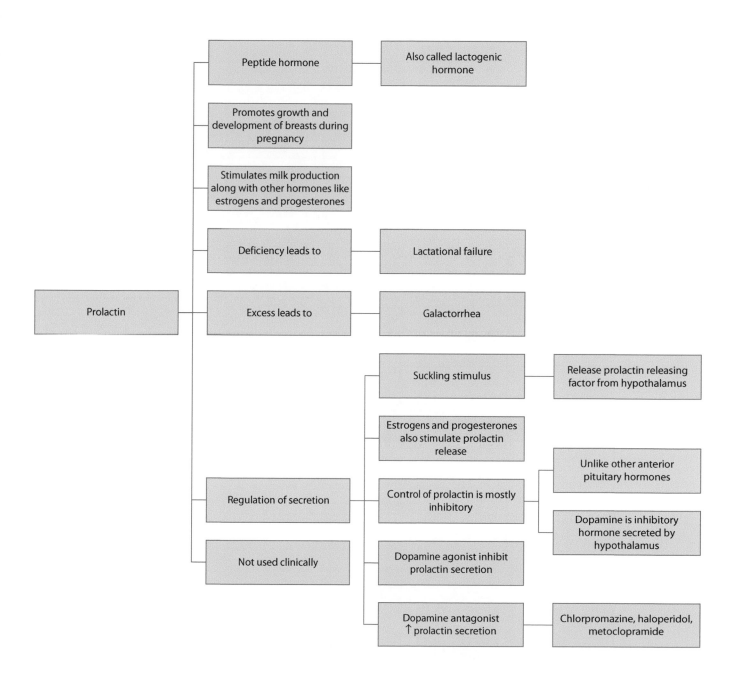

48.7 HYPERPROLACTEMIA AND DOPAMINE RECEPTOR AGONISTS

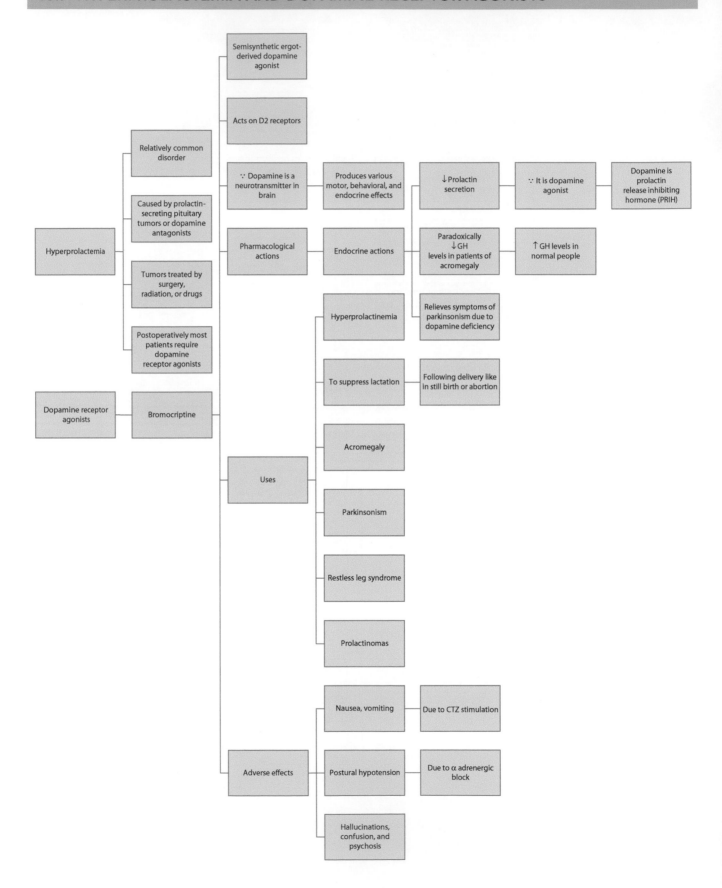

Hyperprolactemia
- Relatively common disorder
- Caused by prolactin-secreting pituitary tumors or dopamine antagonists
- Tumors treated by surgery, radiation, or drugs
- Postoperatively most patients require dopamine receptor agonists

Dopamine receptor agonists → Bromocriptine
- Semisynthetic ergot-derived dopamine agonist
- Acts on D2 receptors
- Pharmacological actions
  - ∵ Dopamine is a neurotransmitter in brain → Produces various motor, behavioral, and endocrine effects → ↓ Prolactin secretion → ∵ It is dopamine agonist → Dopamine is prolactin release inhibiting hormone (PRIH)
  - Endocrine actions → Paradoxically ↓ GH levels in patients of acromegaly → ↑ GH levels in normal people
- Uses
  - Hyperprolactinemia → Relieves symptoms of parkinsonism due to dopamine deficiency
  - To suppress lactation → Following delivery like in still birth or abortion
  - Acromegaly
  - Parkinsonism
  - Restless leg syndrome
  - Prolactinomas
- Adverse effects
  - Nausea, vomiting → Due to CTZ stimulation
  - Postural hypotension → Due to α adrenergic block
  - Hallucinations, confusion, and psychosis

49

Thyroid hormones and antithyroid agents

49.1 THYROID HORMONES – REGULATION AND SYNTHESIS

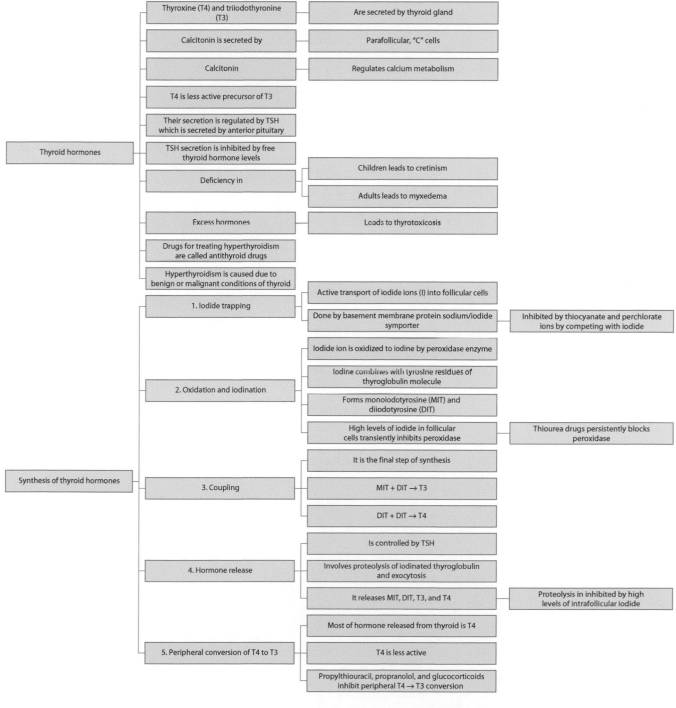

Thyroid hormones

- Thyroxine (T4) and triiodothyronine (T3) → Are secreted by thyroid gland
- Calcitonin is secreted by → Parafollicular, "C" cells
- Calcitonin → Regulates calcium metabolism
- T4 is less active precursor of T3
- Their secretion is regulated by TSH which is secreted by anterior pituitary
- TSH secretion is inhibited by free thyroid hormone levels
- Deficiency in
  - Children leads to cretinism
  - Adults leads to myxedema
- Excess hormones → Leads to thyrotoxicosis
- Drugs for treating hyperthyroidism are called antithyroid drugs
- Hyperthyroidism is caused due to benign or malignant conditions of thyroid

Synthesis of thyroid hormones

- 1. Iodide trapping
  - Active transport of iodide ions (I) into follicular cells
  - Done by basement membrane protein sodium/iodide symporter → Inhibited by thiocyanate and perchlorate ions by competing with iodide
- 2. Oxidation and iodination
  - Iodide ion is oxidized to iodine by peroxidase enzyme
  - Iodine combines with tyrosine residues of thyroglobulin molecule
  - Forms monoiodotyrosine (MIT) and diiodotyrosine (DIT)
  - High levels of iodide in follicular cells transiently inhibits peroxidase → Thiourea drugs persistently blocks peroxidase
- 3. Coupling
  - It is the final step of synthesis
  - MIT + DIT → T3
  - DIT + DIT → T4
- 4. Hormone release
  - Is controlled by TSH
  - Involves proteolysis of iodinated thyroglobulin and exocytosis
  - It releases MIT, DIT, T3, and T4 → Proteolysis in inhibited by high levels of intrafollicular iodide
- 5. Peripheral conversion of T4 to T3
  - Most of hormone released from thyroid is T4
  - T4 is less active
  - Propylthiouracil, propranolol, and glucocorticoids inhibit peripheral T4 → T3 conversion

49.2 MECHANISM OF ACTION, PREPARATIONS, AND THERAPEUTIC USES

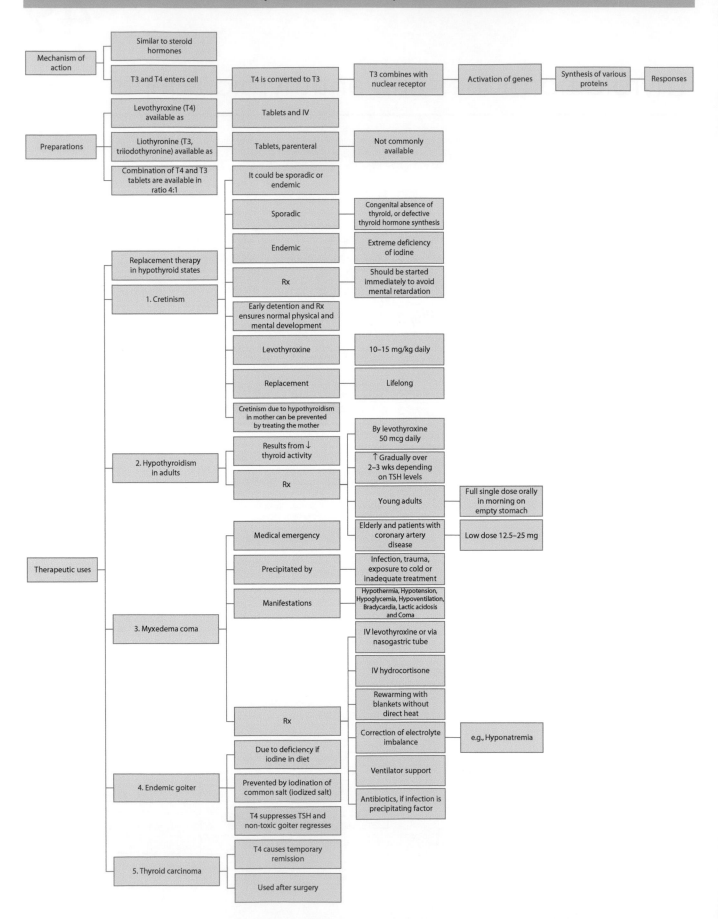

49.3 HYPERTHYROIDISM AND CLASSIFICATION OF ANTITHYROID DRUGS

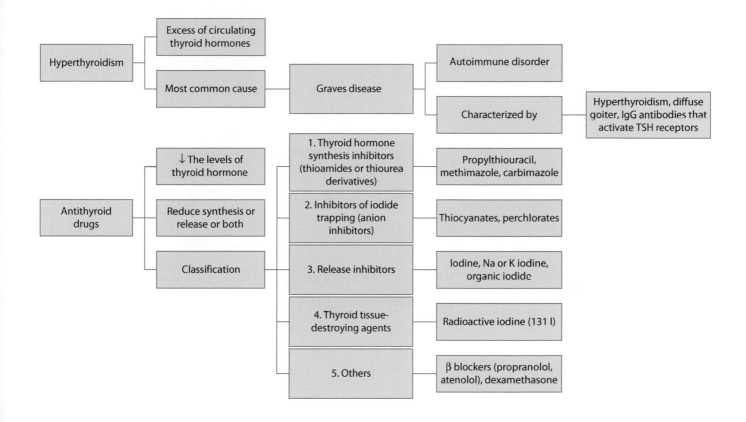

49.4 THIOAMIDES (THIOUREA DERIVATIVES)

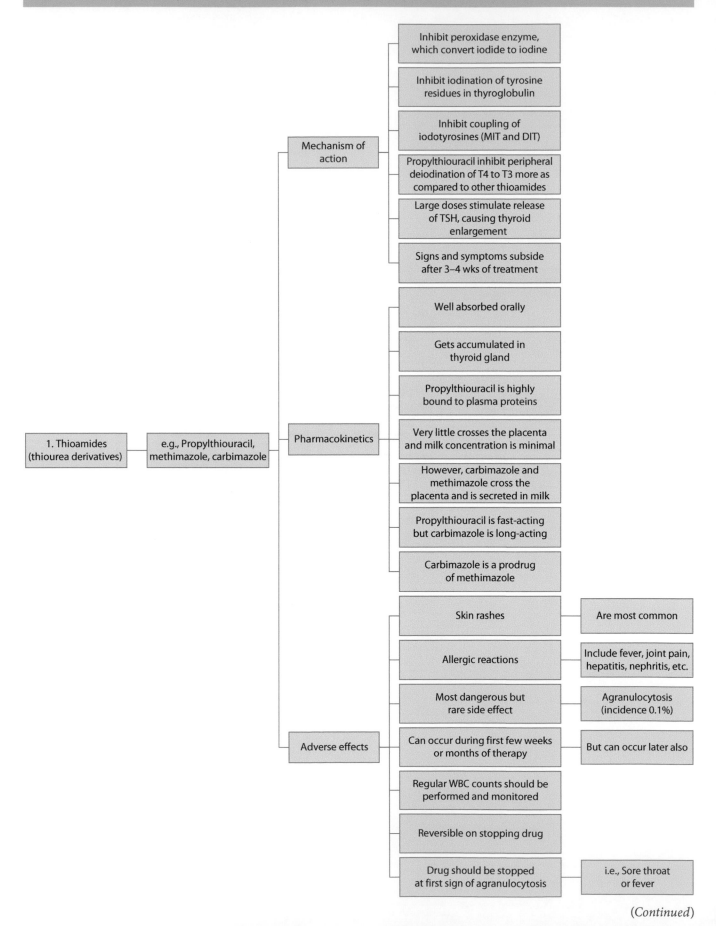

(Continued)

49.4 THIOAMIDES (THIOUREA DERIVATIVES) – USES (Continued)

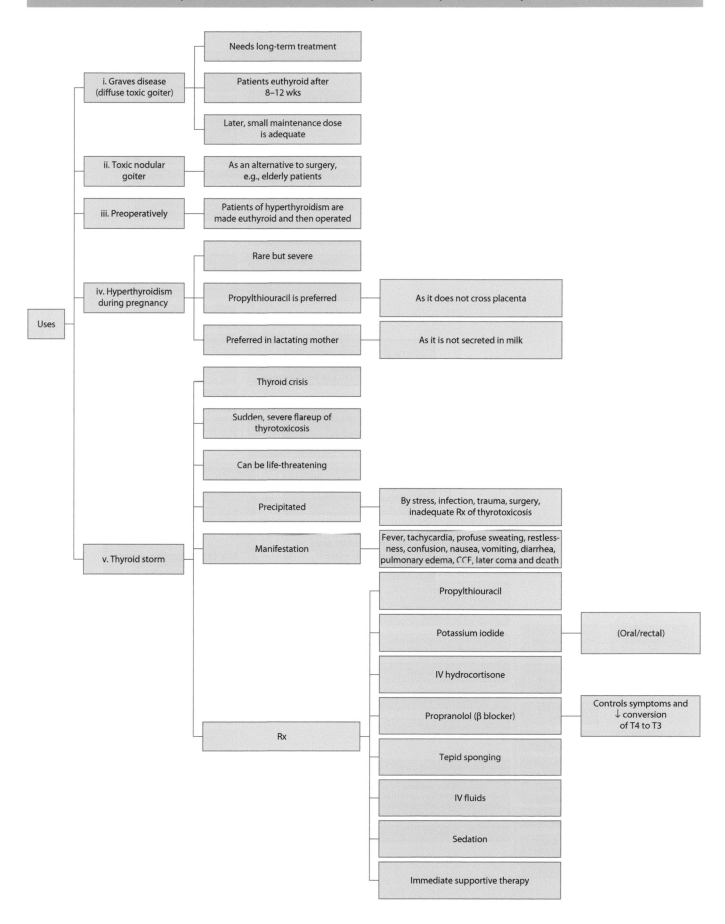

Uses

i. Graves disease (diffuse toxic goiter)
- Needs long-term treatment
- Patients euthyroid after 8–12 wks
- Later, small maintenance dose is adequate

ii. Toxic nodular goiter
- As an alternative to surgery, e.g., elderly patients

iii. Preoperatively
- Patients of hyperthyroidism are made euthyroid and then operated

iv. Hyperthyroidism during pregnancy
- Rare but severe
- Propylthiouracil is preferred — As it does not cross placenta
- Preferred in lactating mother — As it is not secreted in milk

v. Thyroid storm
- Thyroid crisis
- Sudden, severe flareup of thyrotoxicosis
- Can be life-threatening
- Precipitated — By stress, infection, trauma, surgery, inadequate Rx of thyrotoxicosis
- Manifestation — Fever, tachycardia, profuse sweating, restlessness, confusion, nausea, vomiting, diarrhea, pulmonary edema, CCF, later coma and death
- Rx
  - Propylthiouracil
  - Potassium iodide — (Oral/rectal)
  - IV hydrocortisone
  - Propranolol (β blocker) — Controls symptoms and ↓ conversion of T4 to T3
  - Tepid sponging
  - IV fluids
  - Sedation
  - Immediate supportive therapy

49.7 RADIOACTIVE IODINE (^{131}I)

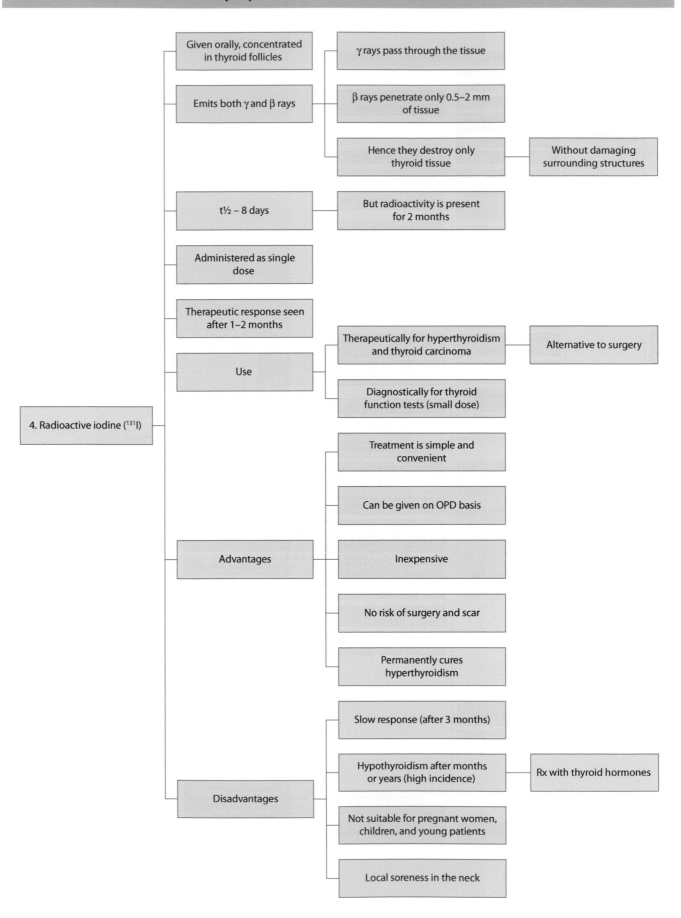

49.8 MANAGEMENT OF THYROTOXIC CRISIS (THYROID STORM)

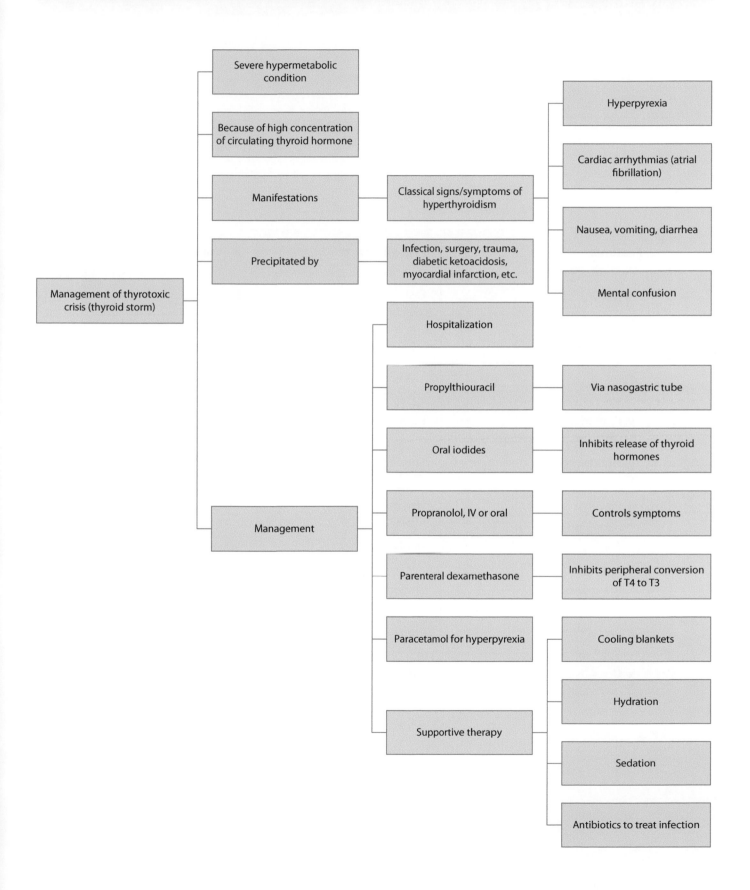

49.9 DIFFERENCES BETWEEN PROPYLTHIOURACIL AND METHIMAZOLE (CARBIMAZOLE)

Features	Propylthiouracil	Methimazole
i. Onset	Fast	Slow
ii. Potency	Less	More
iii. t½	1–2 h	6 h
iv. Protein binding	High	Low
v. Duration of action	Short (4–8 h)	Long (12–24 h)
vi. Placenta transfer	Negligible	Easy
vii. Secretion in milk	Negligible	Significant
viii. Pregnancy	Preferred	Not Preferred
ix. Lactation	Preferred	Not Preferred
x. Dose	Tid – qid	Od – bid

50

Estrogen, progestins, and hormonal contraceptives

50.1 ESTROGENS – TYPES AND MECHANISM OF ACTION

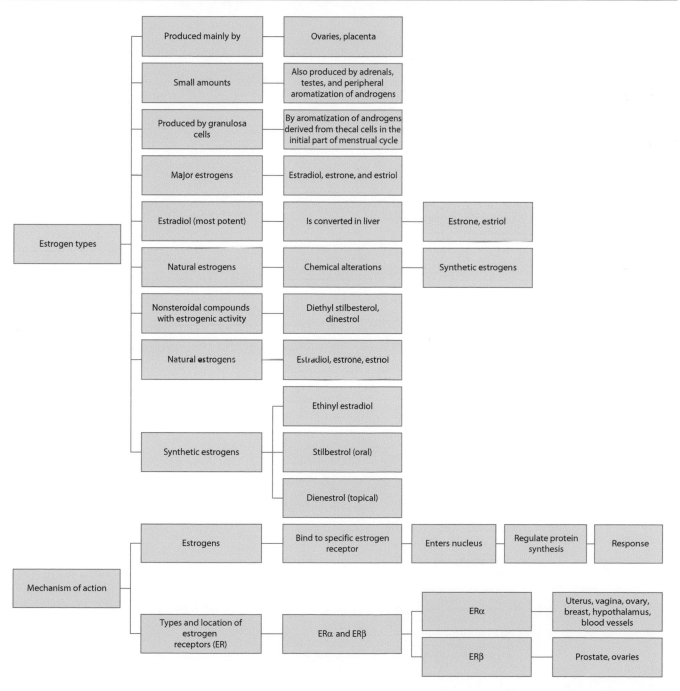

50.2 ACTIONS AND PHARMACOKINETICS

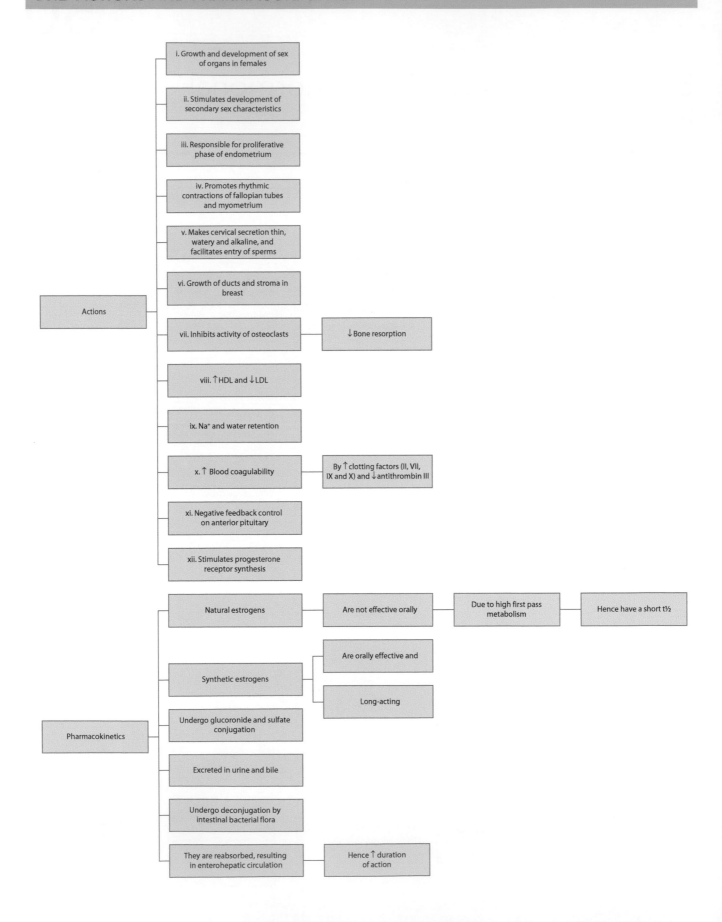

Actions

i. Growth and development of sex of organs in females

ii. Stimulates development of secondary sex characteristics

iii. Responsible for proliferative phase of endometrium

iv. Promotes rhythmic contractions of fallopian tubes and myometrium

v. Makes cervical secretion thin, watery and alkaline, and facilitates entry of sperms

vi. Growth of ducts and stroma in breast

vii. Inhibits activity of osteoclasts → ↓ Bone resorption

viii. ↑ HDL and ↓ LDL

ix. Na⁺ and water retention

x. ↑ Blood coagulability → By ↑ clotting factors (II, VII, IX and X) and ↓ antithrombin III

xi. Negative feedback control on anterior pituitary

xii. Stimulates progesterone receptor synthesis

Pharmacokinetics

Natural estrogens → Are not effective orally → Due to high first pass metabolism → Hence have a short t½

Synthetic estrogens → Are orally effective and / Long-acting

Undergo glucoronide and sulfate conjugation

Excreted in urine and bile

Undergo deconjugation by intestinal bacterial flora

They are reabsorbed, resulting in enterohepatic circulation → Hence ↑ duration of action

50.3 USES, ADRs, AND PREPARATIONS

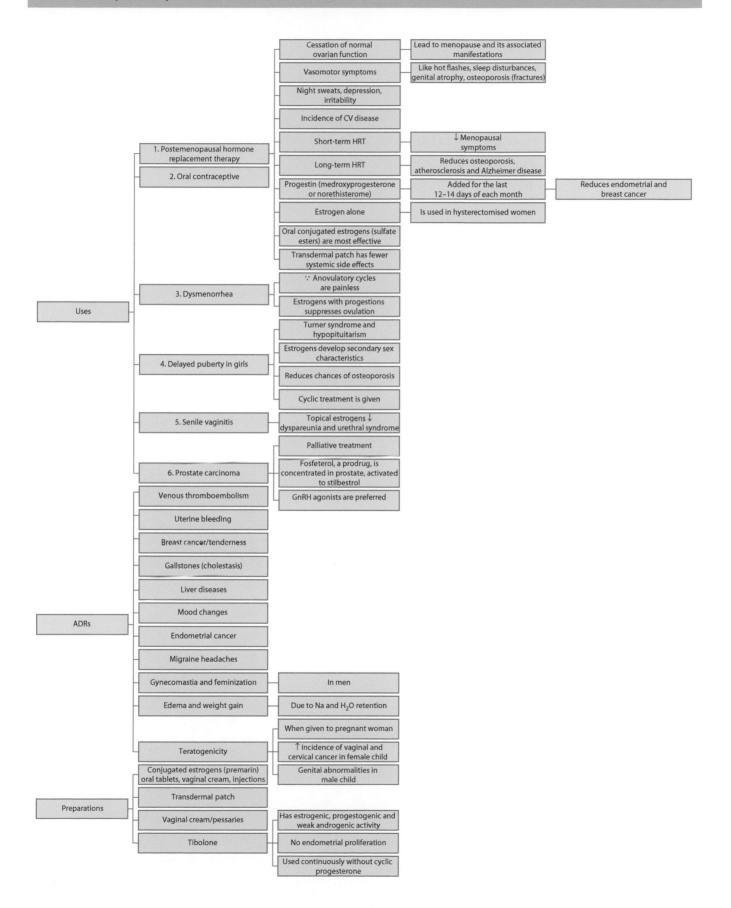

50.4 ANTIESTROGENS

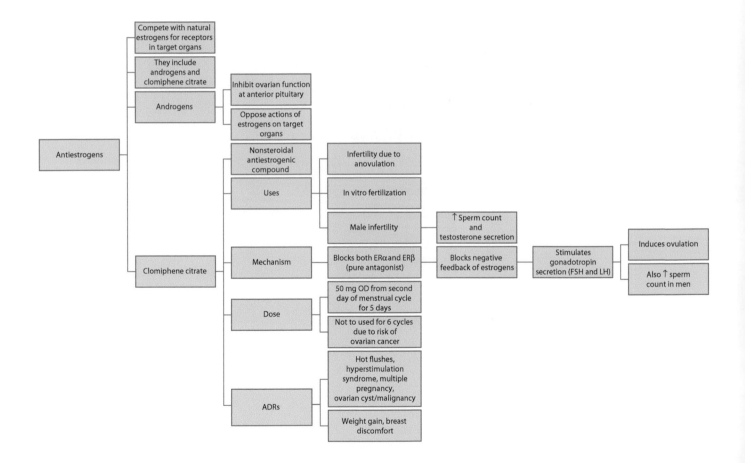

50.5 SELECTIVE ESTROGEN RECEPTOR MODULATORS (SERMs) AND ESTROGEN SYNTHESIS INHIBITORS

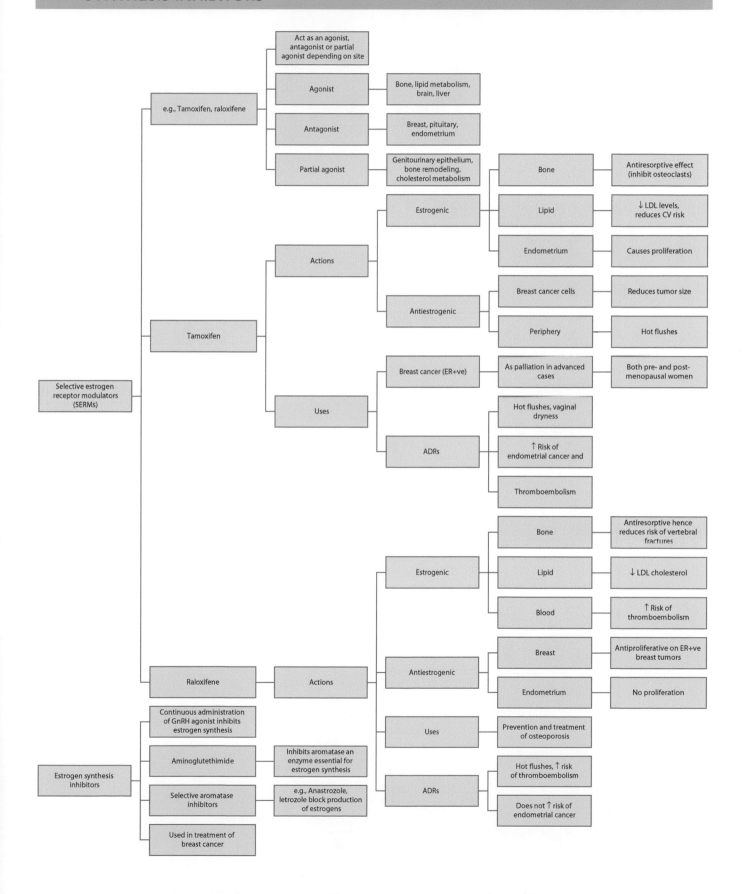

50.6 PROGESTINS – TYPES, ACTIONS, AND PHARMACOKINETICS

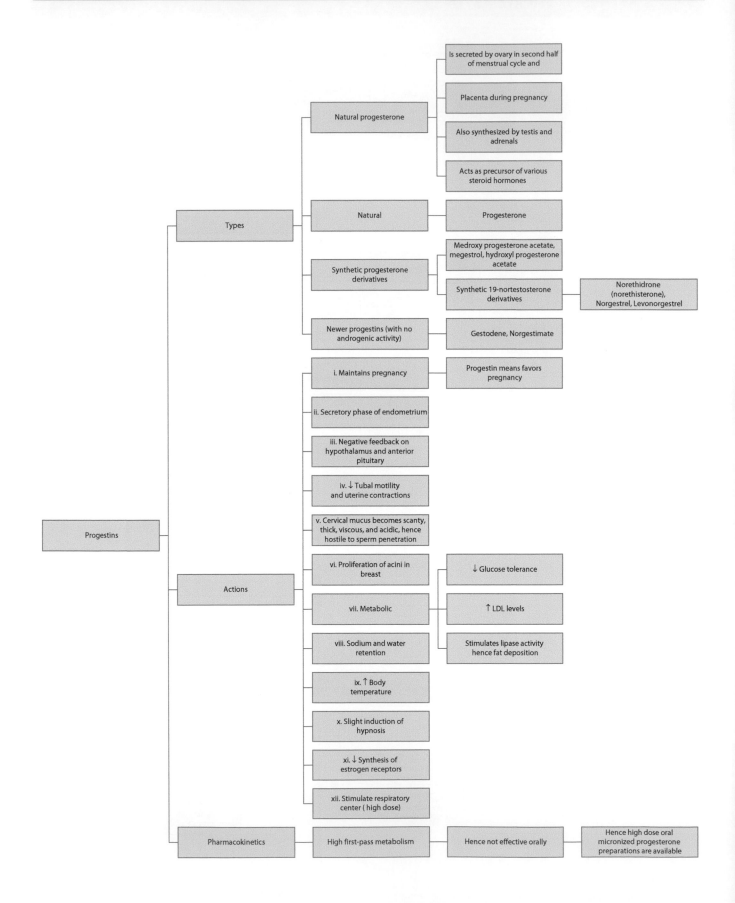

Progestins

Types

Natural progesterone
- Is secreted by ovary in second half of menstrual cycle and
- Placenta during pregnancy
- Also synthesized by testis and adrenals
- Acts as precursor of various steroid hormones

Natural — Progesterone

Synthetic progesterone derivatives
- Medroxy progesterone acetate, megestrol, hydroxyl progesterone acetate
- Synthetic 19-nortestosterone derivatives — Norethidrone (norethisterone), Norgestrel, Levonorgestrel

Newer progestins (with no androgenic activity) — Gestodene, Norgestimate

Actions

i. Maintains pregnancy — Progestin means favors pregnancy

ii. Secretory phase of endometrium

iii. Negative feedback on hypothalamus and anterior pituitary

iv. ↓ Tubal motility and uterine contractions

v. Cervical mucus becomes scanty, thick, viscous, and acidic, hence hostile to sperm penetration

vi. Proliferation of acini in breast

vii. Metabolic
- ↓ Glucose tolerance
- ↑ LDL levels
- Stimulates lipase activity hence fat deposition

viii. Sodium and water retention

ix. ↑ Body temperature

x. Slight induction of hypnosis

xi. ↓ Synthesis of estrogen receptors

xii. Stimulate respiratory center (high dose)

Pharmacokinetics — High first-pass metabolism — Hence not effective orally — Hence high dose oral micronized progesterone preparations are available

50.7 USES AND ADRs OF PROGESTINS

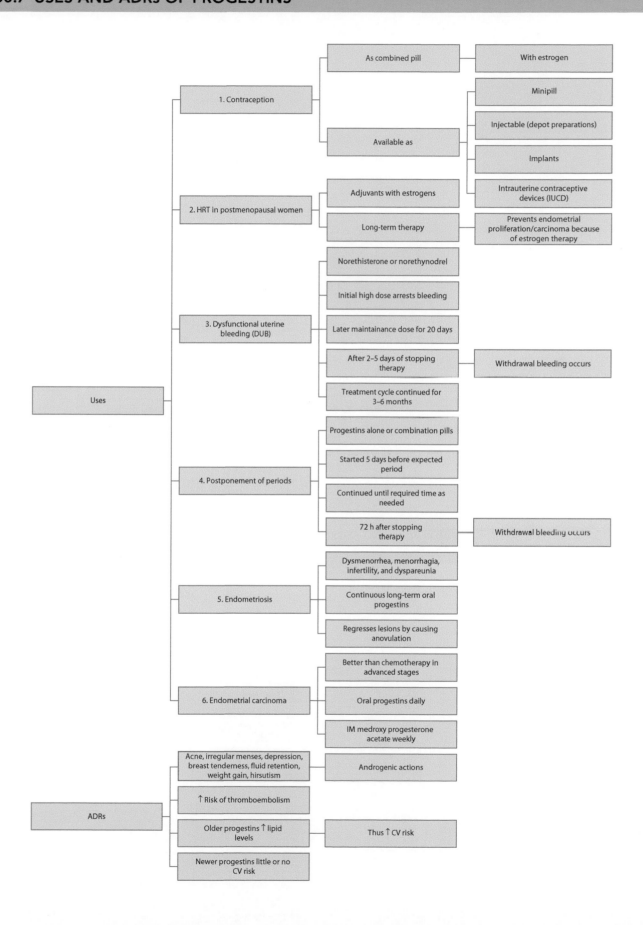

50.8 ANTIPROGESTINS

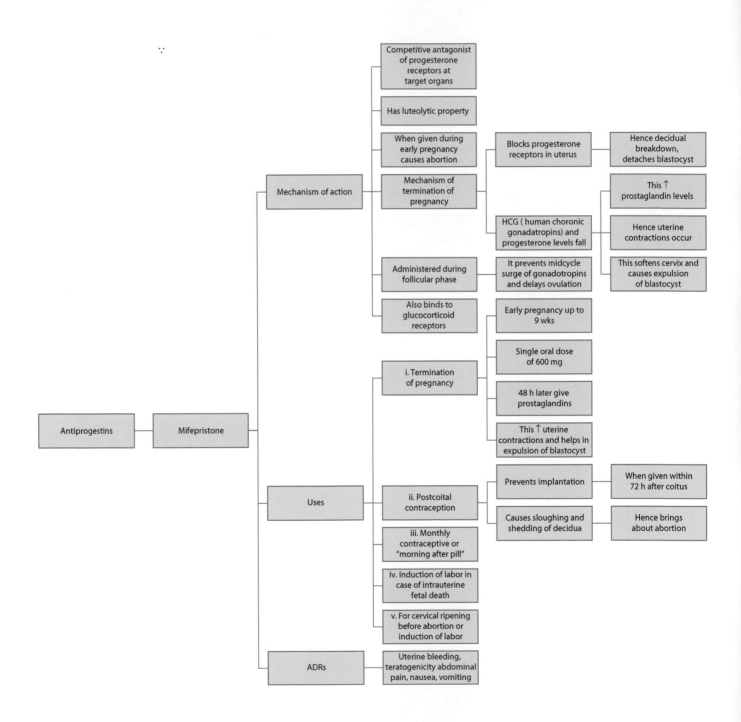

50.9 DRUG TREATMENT OF MENOPAUSAL SYMPTOMS

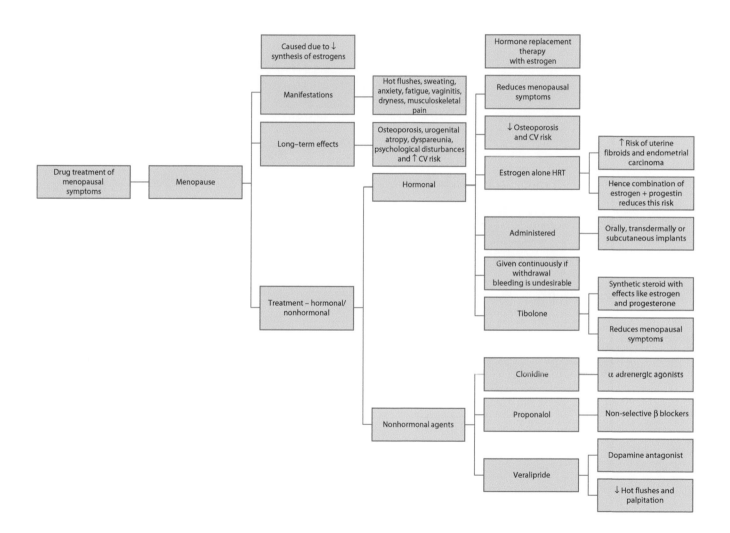

50.10 TYPES OF HORMONAL CONTRACEPTIVES

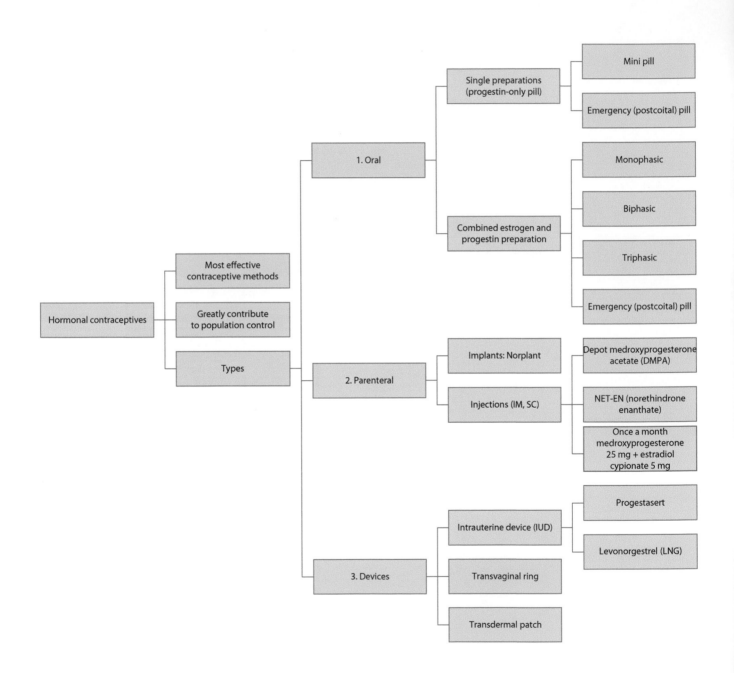

50.11 COMBINED ESTROGEN (E) AND PROGESTIN (P) PREPARATIONS

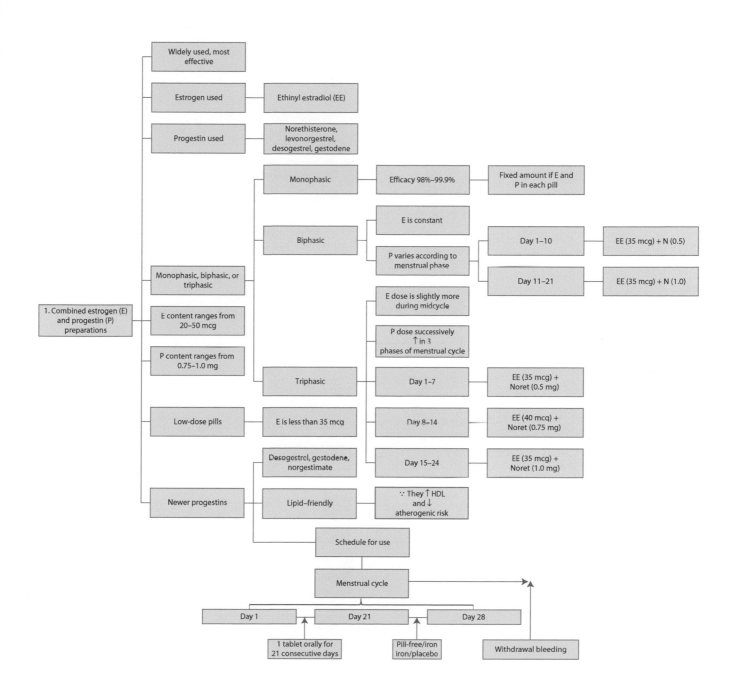

50.12 BENEFITS OF HORMONAL CONTRACEPTION AND CONTRAINDICATIONS

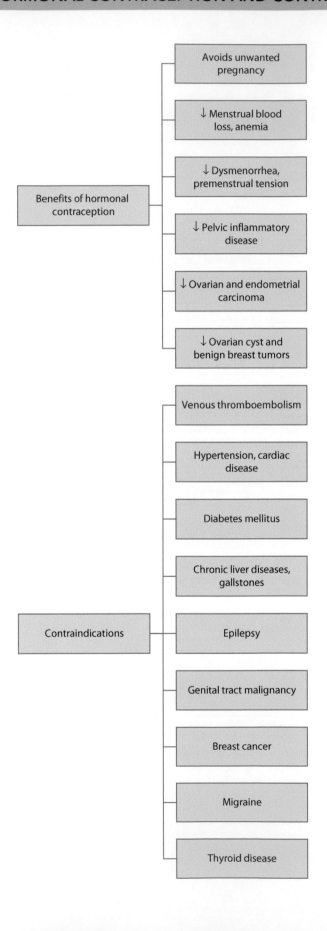

50.13 SINGLE PREPARATIONS AND POSTCOITAL (EMERGENCY CONTRACEPTION) PILL

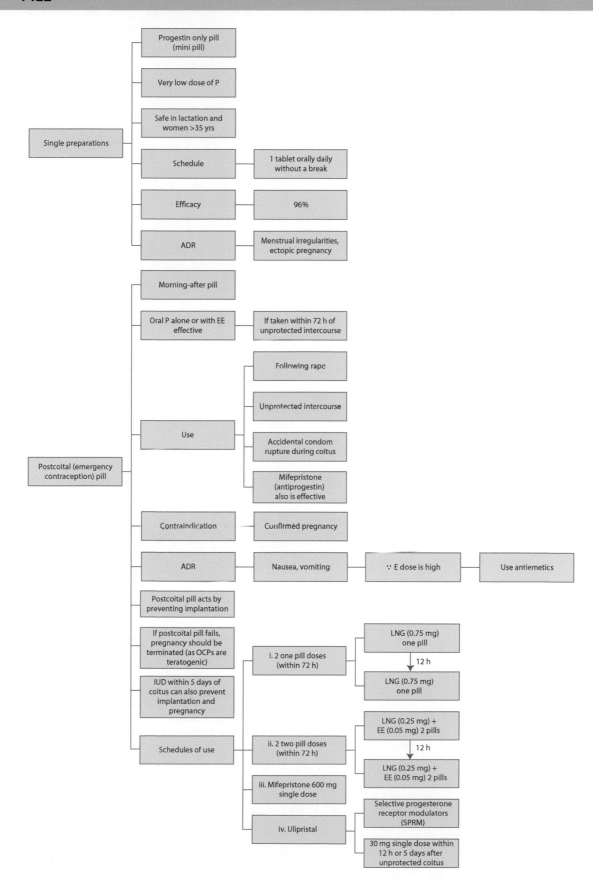

50.14 PARENTERAL CONTRACEPTIVES

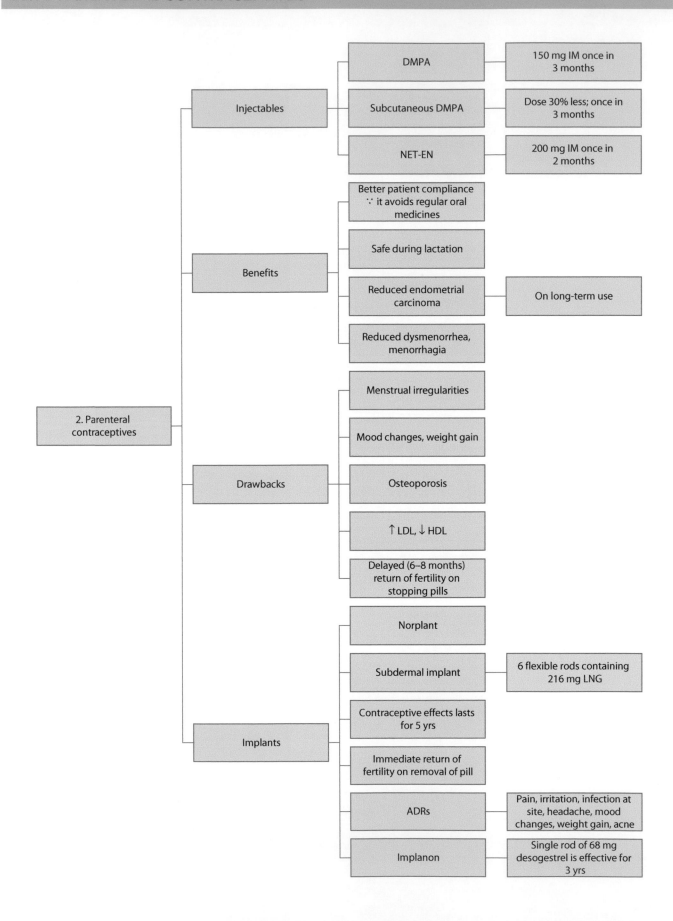

50.15 DEVICES AND MECHANISM OF ACTION OF CONTRACEPTIVES

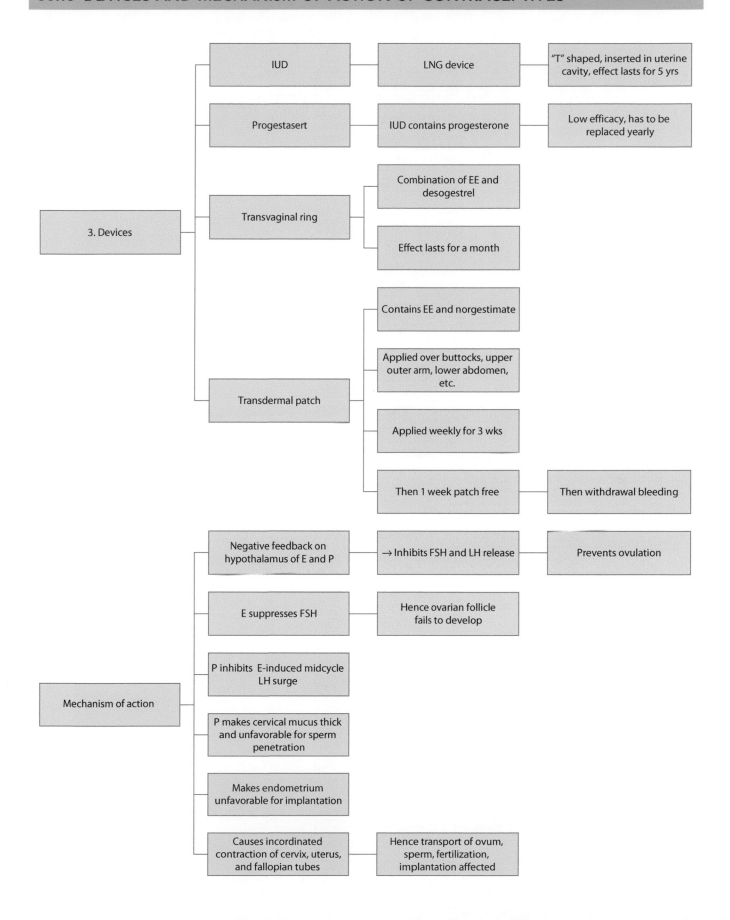

3. Devices

- IUD
  - LNG device
    - "T" shaped, inserted in uterine cavity, effect lasts for 5 yrs
- Progestasert
  - IUD contains progesterone
    - Low efficacy, has to be replaced yearly
- Transvaginal ring
  - Combination of EE and desogestrel
  - Effect lasts for a month
- Transdermal patch
  - Contains EE and norgestimate
  - Applied over buttocks, upper outer arm, lower abdomen, etc.
  - Applied weekly for 3 wks
  - Then 1 week patch free
    - Then withdrawal bleeding

Mechanism of action

- Negative feedback on hypothalamus of E and P
  - → Inhibits FSH and LH release
    - Prevents ovulation
- E suppresses FSH
  - Hence ovarian follicle fails to develop
- P inhibits E-induced midcycle LH surge
- P makes cervical mucus thick and unfavorable for sperm penetration
- Makes endometrium unfavorable for implantation
- Causes incordinated contraction of cervix, uterus, and fallopian tubes
  - Hence transport of ovum, sperm, fertilization, implantation affected

50.16 ADVERSE EFFECTS, DRUG-INTERACTIONS, AND CENTCHROMAN

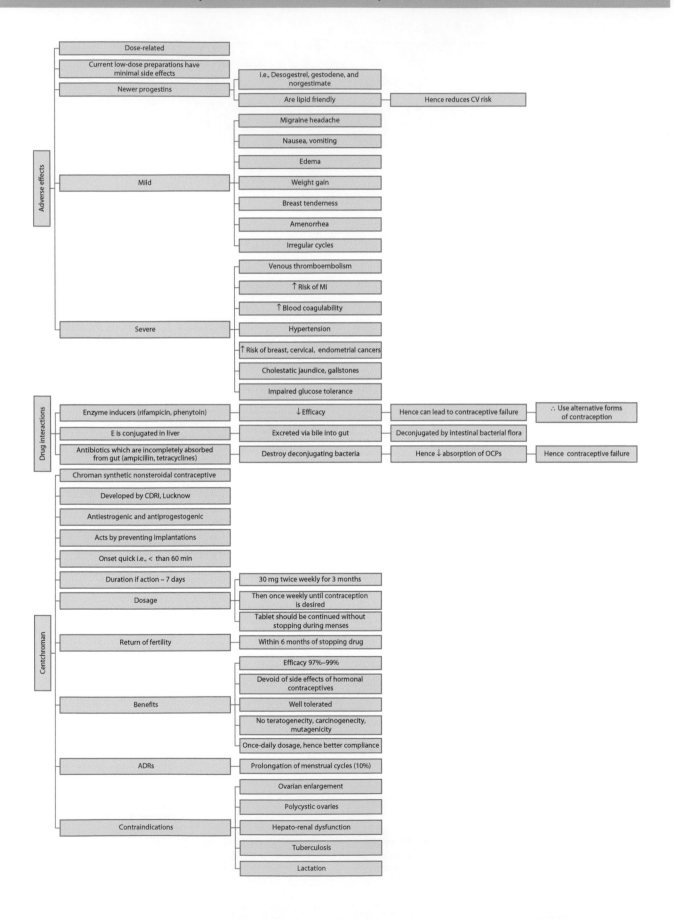

Adverse effects

- Dose-related
- Current low-dose preparations have minimal side effects
- Newer progestins
  - i.e., Desogestrel, gestodene, and norgestimate
  - Are lipid friendly → Hence reduces CV risk
- Mild
  - Migraine headache
  - Nausea, vomiting
  - Edema
  - Weight gain
  - Breast tenderness
  - Amenorrhea
  - Irregular cycles
- Severe
  - Venous thromboembolism
  - ↑ Risk of MI
  - ↑ Blood coagulability
  - Hypertension
  - ↑ Risk of breast, cervical, endometrial cancers
  - Cholestatic jaundice, gallstones
  - Impaired glucose tolerance

Drug interactions

- Enzyme inducers (rifampicin, phenytoin) → ↓ Efficacy → Hence can lead to contraceptive failure → ∴ Use alternative forms of contraception
- E is conjugated in liver → Excreted via bile into gut → Deconjugated by intestinal bacterial flora
- Antibiotics which are incompletely absorbed from gut (ampicillin, tetracyclines) → Destroy deconjugating bacteria → Hence ↓ absorption of OCPs → Hence contraceptive failure

Centchroman

- Chroman synthetic nonsteroidal contraceptive
- Developed by CDRI, Lucknow
- Antiestrogenic and antiprogestogenic
- Acts by preventing implantations
- Onset quick i.e., < than 60 min
- Duration if action – 7 days
- Dosage
  - 30 mg twice weekly for 3 months
  - Then once weekly until contraception is desired
  - Tablet should be continued without stopping during menses
- Return of fertility
  - Within 6 months of stopping drug
- Benefits
  - Efficacy 97%–99%
  - Devoid of side effects of hormonal contraceptives
  - Well tolerated
  - No teratogenecity, carcinogenecity, mutagenicity
  - Once-daily dosage, hence better compliance
- ADRs
  - Prolongation of menstrual cycles (10%)
- Contraindications
  - Ovarian enlargement
  - Polycystic ovaries
  - Hepato-renal dysfunction
  - Tuberculosis
  - Lactation

Androgens and anabolic steroids

51.1 ANDROGENS – PHYSIOLOGY, CLASSIFICATION, ACTIONS, AND MECHANISM OF ACTION

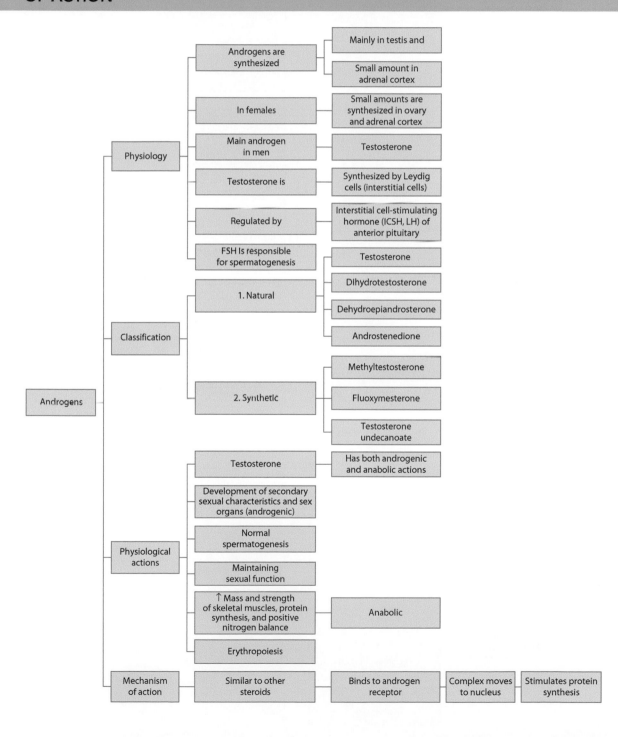

51.2 THERAPEUTIC USES, ADVERSE EFFECTS, AND PRECAUTIONS AND CONTRAINDICATIONS

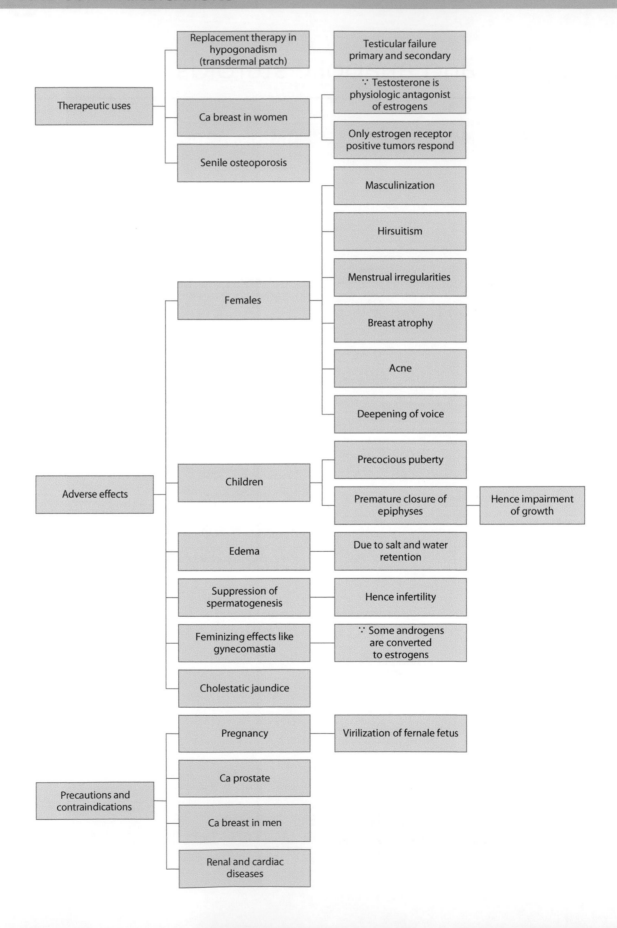

51.3 ANABOLIC STEROIDS

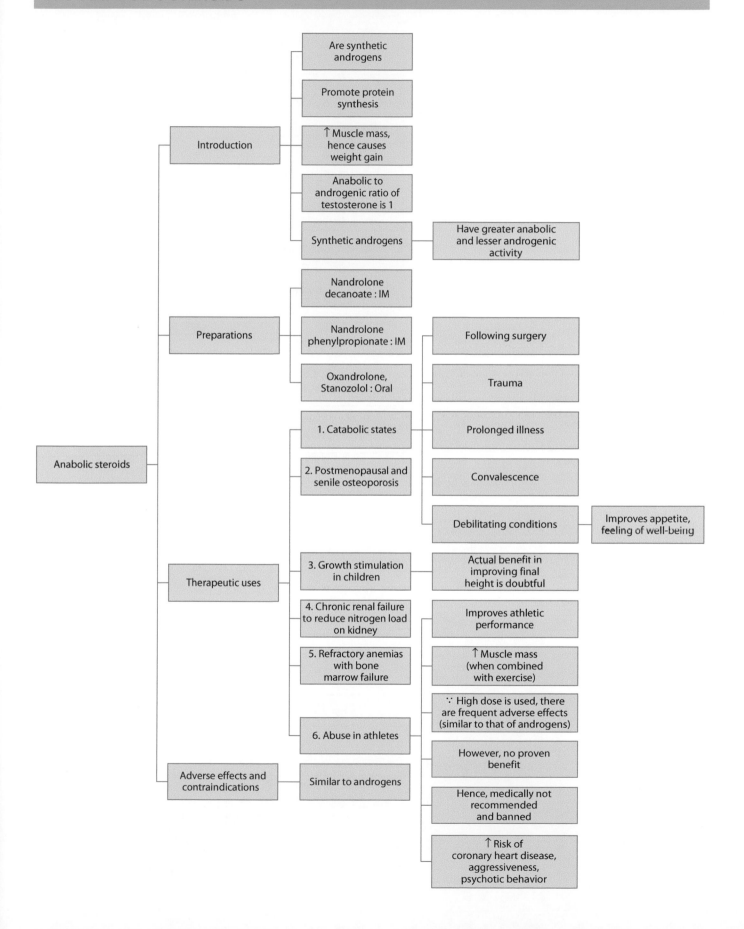

51.4 ANTIANDROGENS

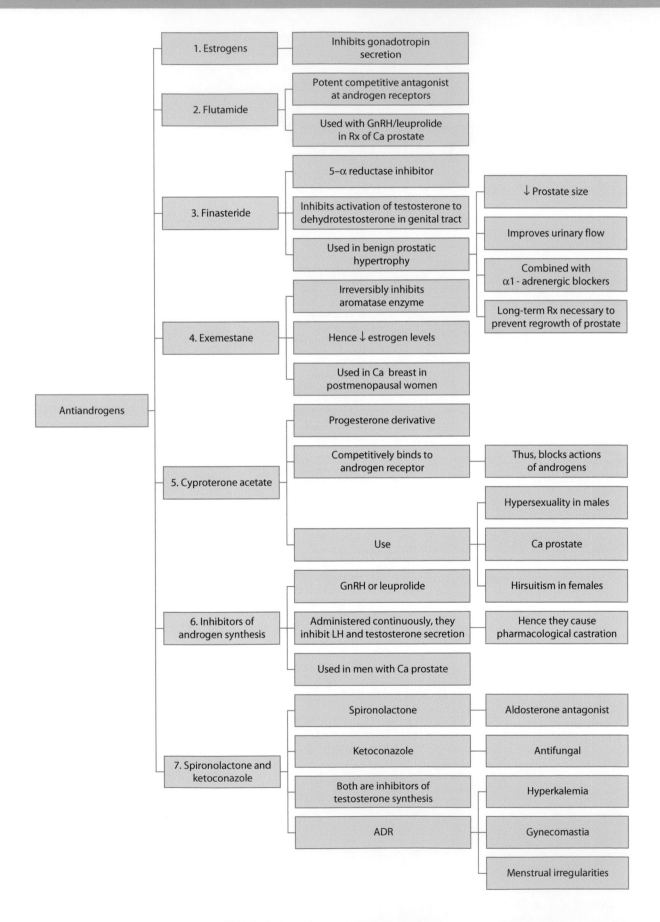

51.5 MALE CONTRACEPTIVES AND DRUGS FOR MALE SEXUAL DYSFUNCTION (ERECTILE DYSFUNCTION/IMPOTENCE)

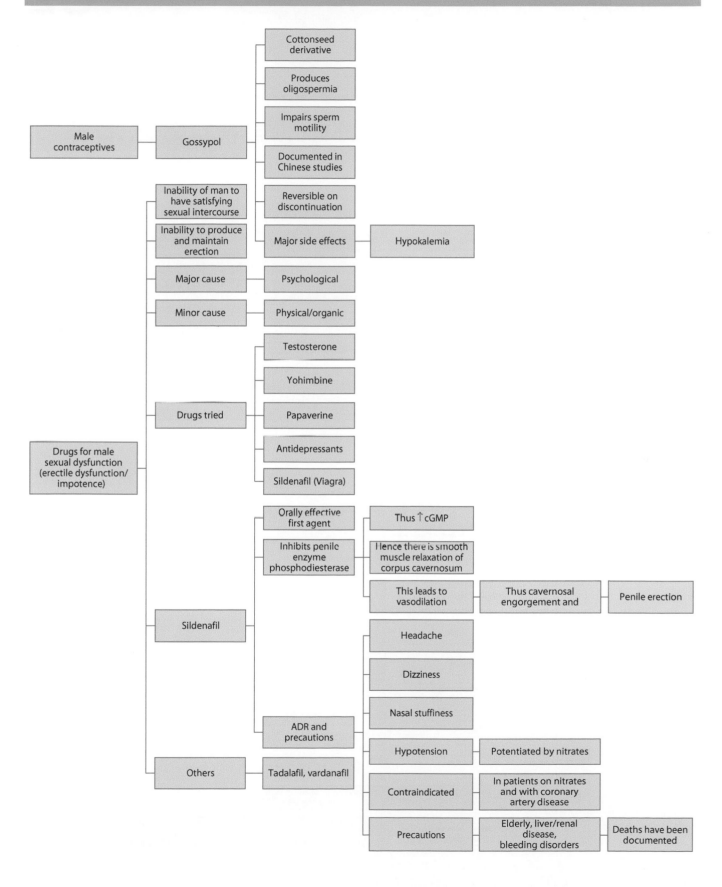

Corticosteroids

52

52.1 CORTICOSTEROIDS – INTRODUCTION, STRUCTURE SYNTHESIS, AND RELEASE

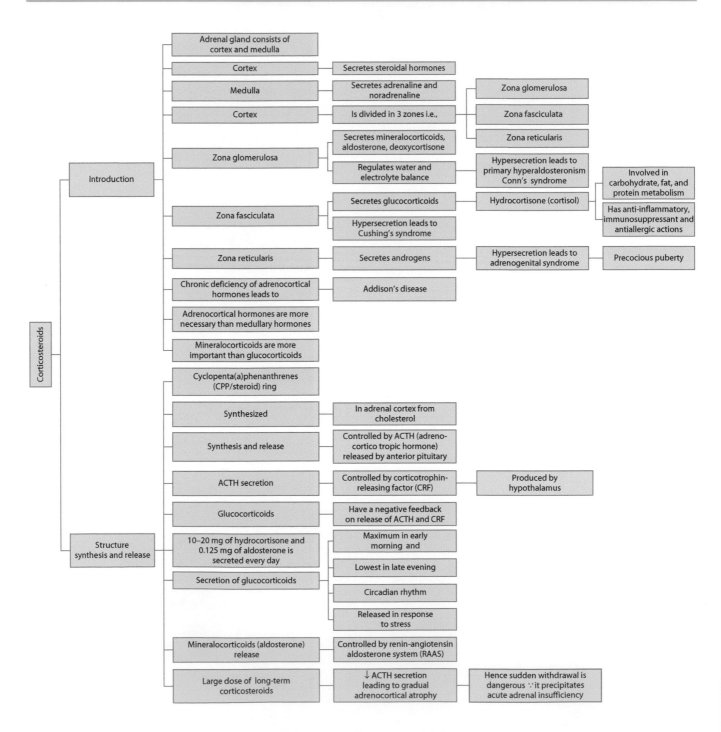

52.2 MECHANISM OF ACTION AND PHARMACOKINETICS

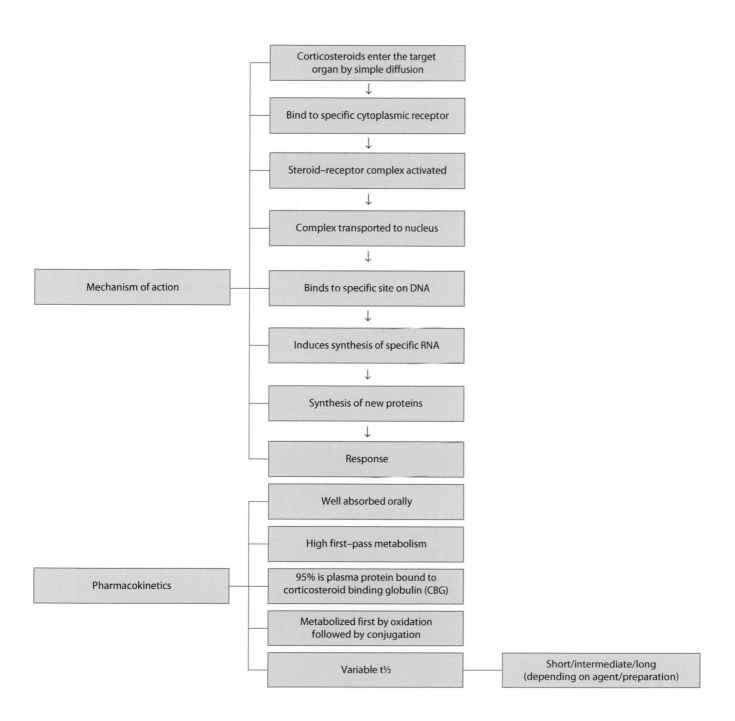

52.3 GLUCOCORTICOID ACTIONS

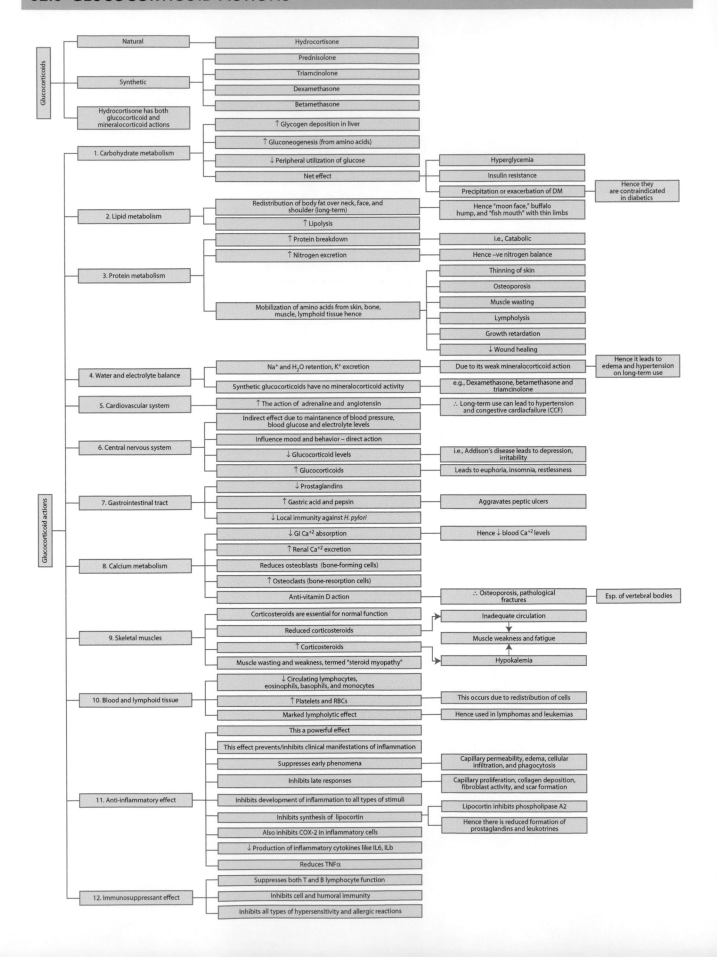

52.4 THERAPEUTIC USES

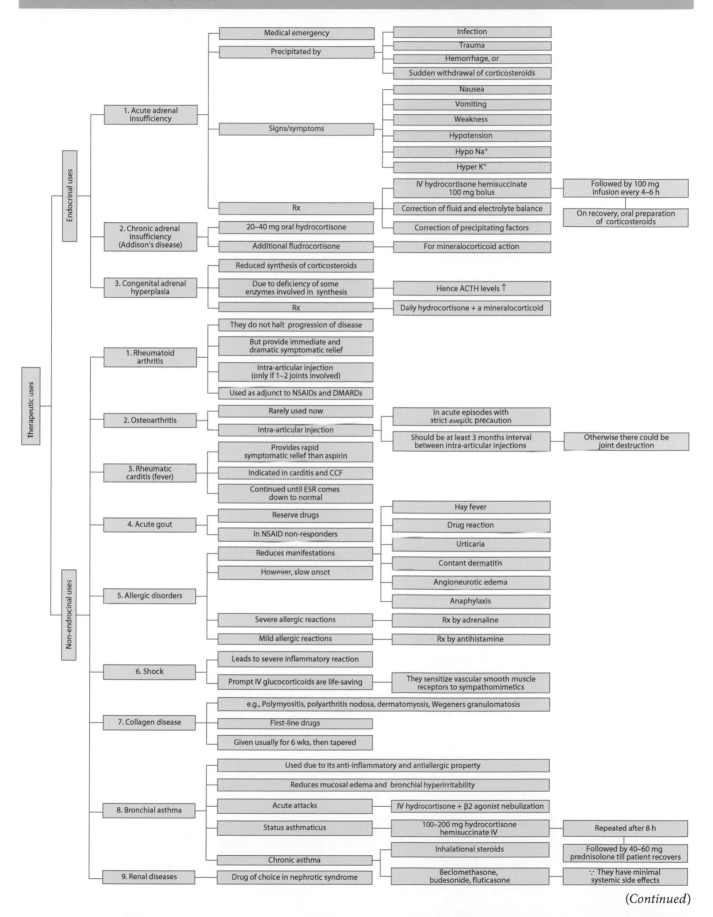

(Continued)

52.4 THERAPEUTIC USES (Continued)

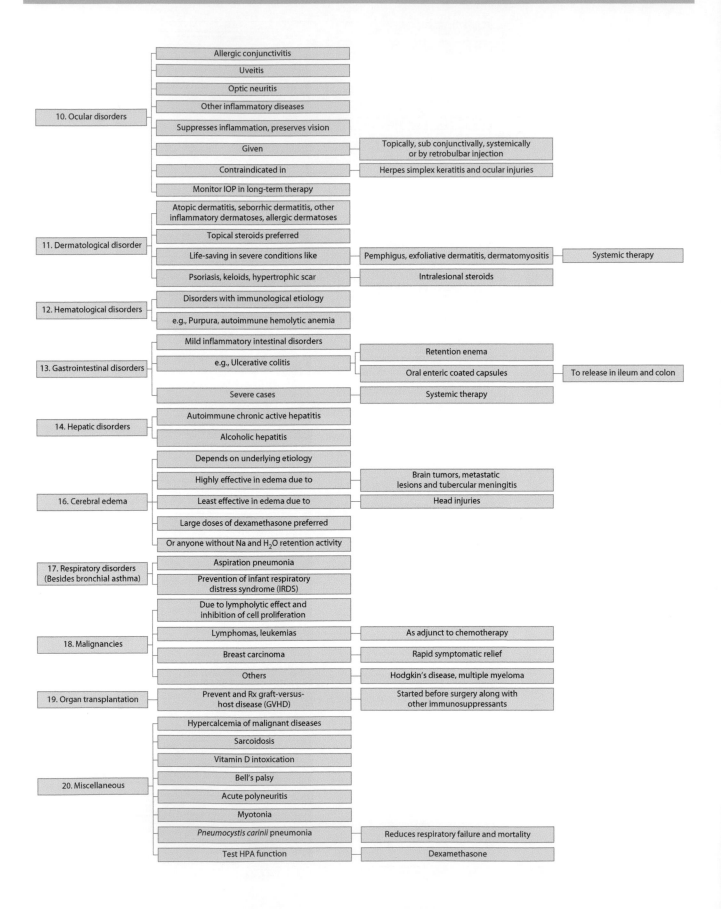

10. Ocular disorders
- Allergic conjunctivitis
- Uveitis
- Optic neuritis
- Other inflammatory diseases
- Suppresses inflammation, preserves vision
- Given — Topically, sub conjunctivally, systemically or by retrobulbar injection
- Contraindicated in — Herpes simplex keratitis and ocular injuries
- Monitor IOP in long-term therapy

11. Dermatological disorder
- Atopic dermatitis, seborrhic dermatitis, other inflammatory dermatoses, allergic dermatoses
- Topical steroids preferred
- Life-saving in severe conditions like — Pemphigus, exfoliative dermatitis, dermatomyositis — Systemic therapy
- Psoriasis, keloids, hypertrophic scar — Intralesional steroids

12. Hematological disorders
- Disorders with immunological etiology
- e.g., Purpura, autoimmune hemolytic anemia

13. Gastrointestinal disorders
- Mild inflammatory intestinal disorders
- e.g., Ulcerative colitis
  - Retention enema
  - Oral enteric coated capsules — To release in ileum and colon
- Severe cases — Systemic therapy

14. Hepatic disorders
- Autoimmune chronic active hepatitis
- Alcoholic hepatitis

16. Cerebral edema
- Depends on underlying etiology
- Highly effective in edema due to — Brain tumors, metastatic lesions and tubercular meningitis
- Least effective in edema due to — Head injuries
- Large doses of dexamethasone preferred
- Or anyone without Na and H_2O retention activity

17. Respiratory disorders (Besides bronchial asthma)
- Aspiration pneumonia
- Prevention of infant respiratory distress syndrome (IRDS)

18. Malignancies
- Due to lympholytic effect and inhibition of cell proliferation
- Lymphomas, leukemias — As adjunct to chemotherapy
- Breast carcinoma — Rapid symptomatic relief
- Others — Hodgkin's disease, multiple myeloma

19. Organ transplantation
- Prevent and Rx graft-versus-host disease (GVHD) — Started before surgery along with other immunosuppressants

20. Miscellaneous
- Hypercalcemia of malignant diseases
- Sarcoidosis
- Vitamin D intoxication
- Bell's palsy
- Acute polyneuritis
- Myotonia
- *Pneumocystis carinii* pneumonia — Reduces respiratory failure and mortality
- Test HPA function — Dexamethasone

52.5 ADVERSE EFFECTS

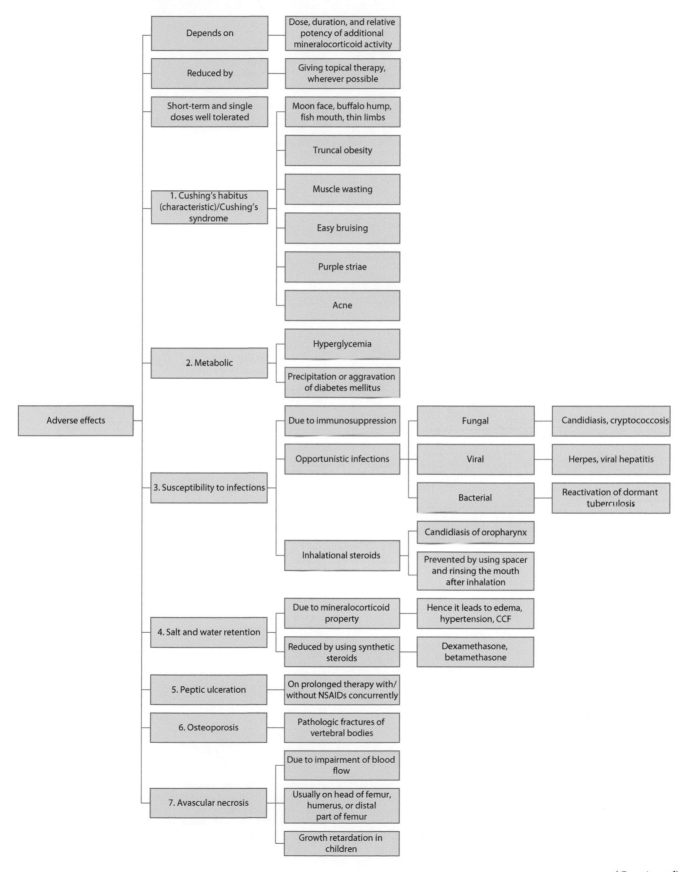

(Continued)

52.5 ADVERSE EFFECTS (Continued)

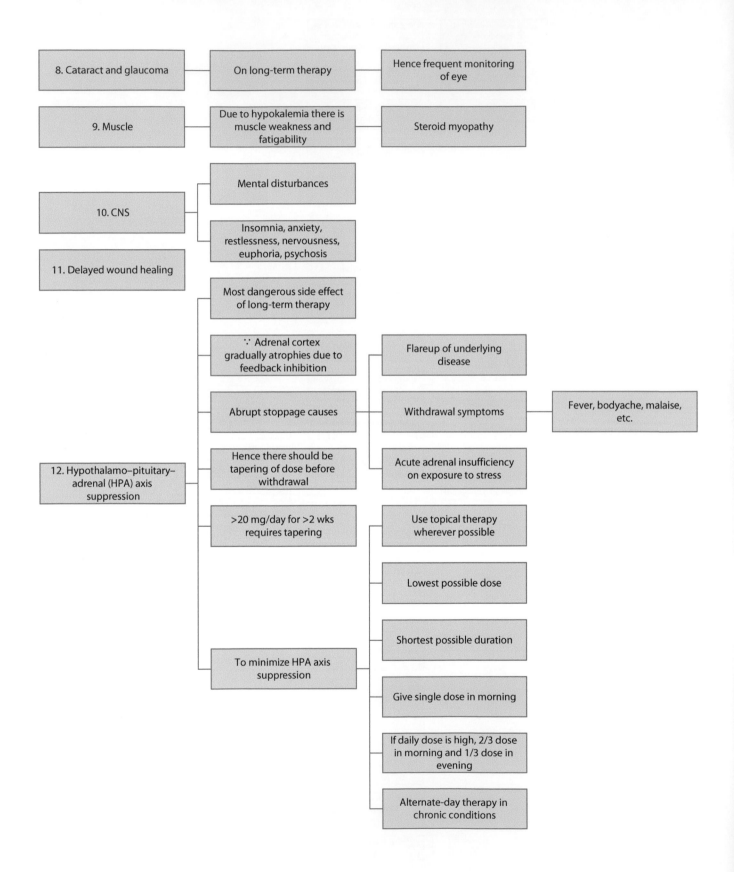

8. Cataract and glaucoma — On long-term therapy — Hence frequent monitoring of eye

9. Muscle — Due to hypokalemia there is muscle weakness and fatigability — Steroid myopathy

10. CNS
- Mental disturbances
- Insomnia, anxiety, restlessness, nervousness, euphoria, psychosis

11. Delayed wound healing

12. Hypothalamo–pituitary–adrenal (HPA) axis suppression
- Most dangerous side effect of long-term therapy
- ∵ Adrenal cortex gradually atrophies due to feedback inhibition
- Abrupt stoppage causes
  - Flareup of underlying disease
  - Withdrawal symptoms — Fever, bodyache, malaise, etc.
  - Acute adrenal insufficiency on exposure to stress
- Hence there should be tapering of dose before withdrawal
- >20 mg/day for >2 wks requires tapering
- To minimize HPA axis suppression
  - Use topical therapy wherever possible
  - Lowest possible dose
  - Shortest possible duration
  - Give single dose in morning
  - If daily dose is high, 2/3 dose in morning and 1/3 dose in evening
  - Alternate-day therapy in chronic conditions

52.6 CONTRAINDICATIONS

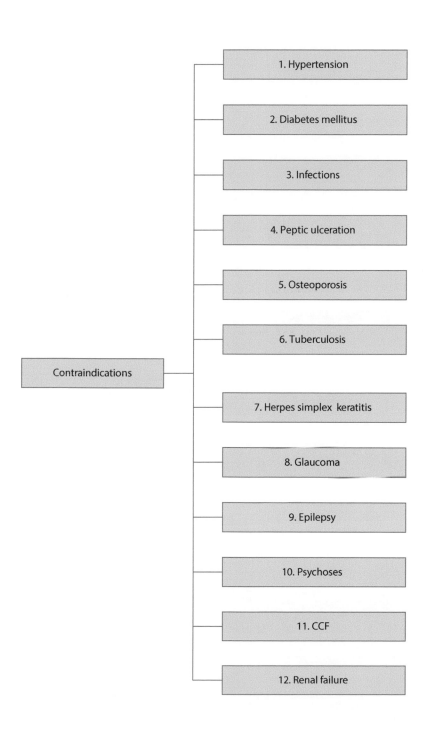

52.7 PREPARATIONS AND CLASSIFICATIONS

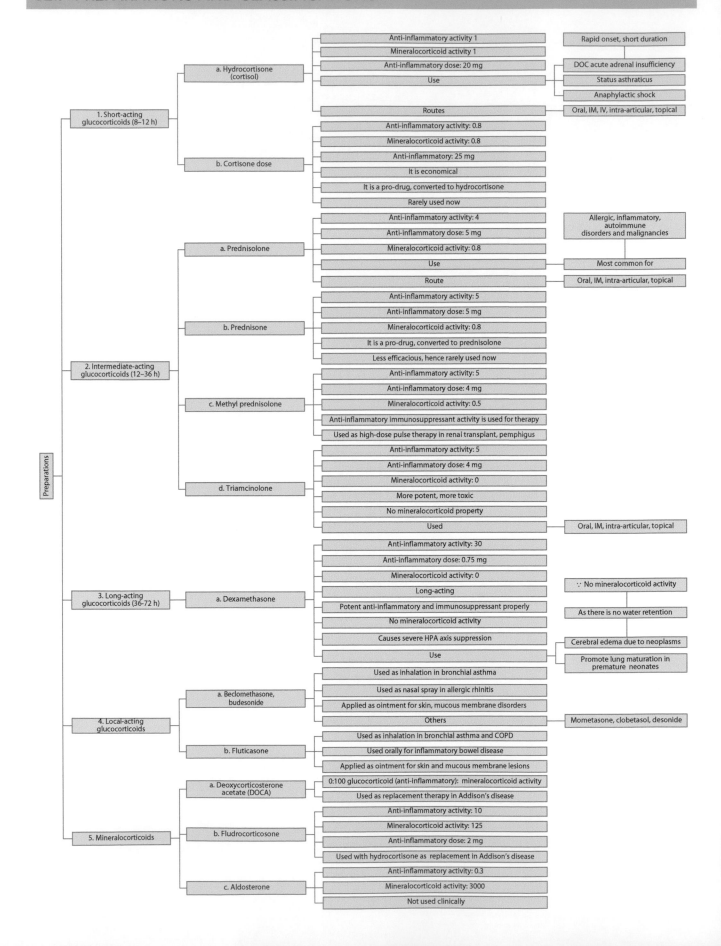

53

Insulin and oral antidiabetic agents

53.1 INSULIN REGULATION AND GLUCOSE TRANSPORTERS (GLUT)

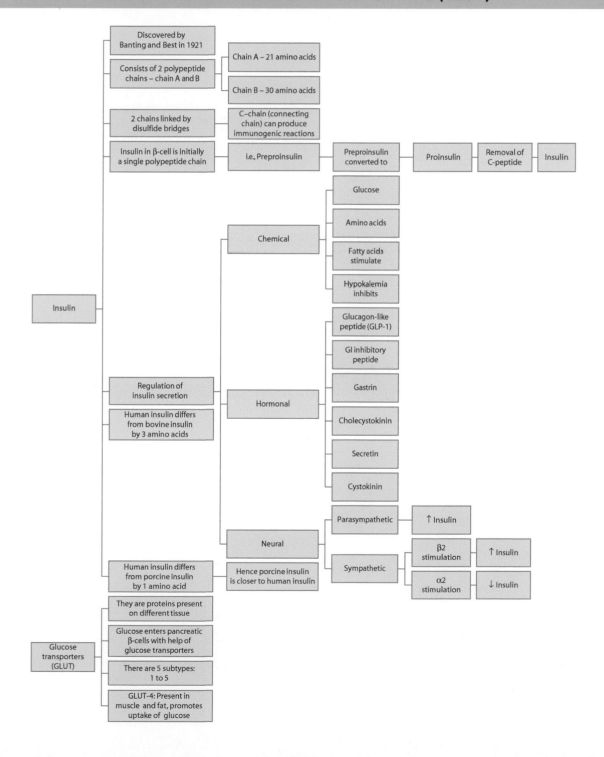

479

53.2 ACTIONS OF INSULIN AND MECHANISM OF ACTION

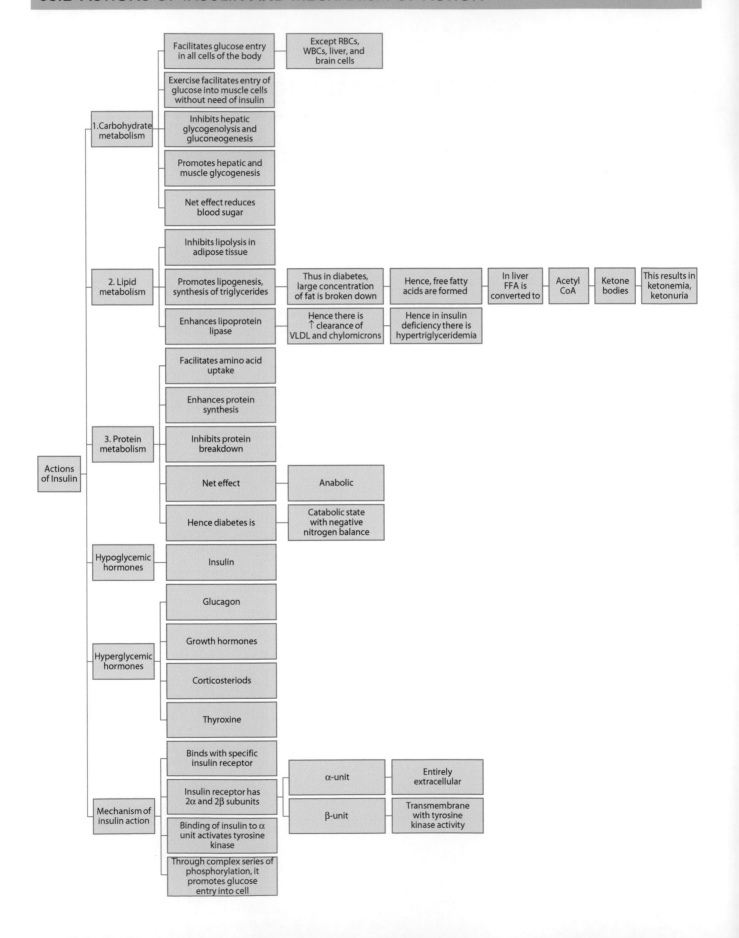

53.3 PHARMACOKINETICS AND PREPARATIONS

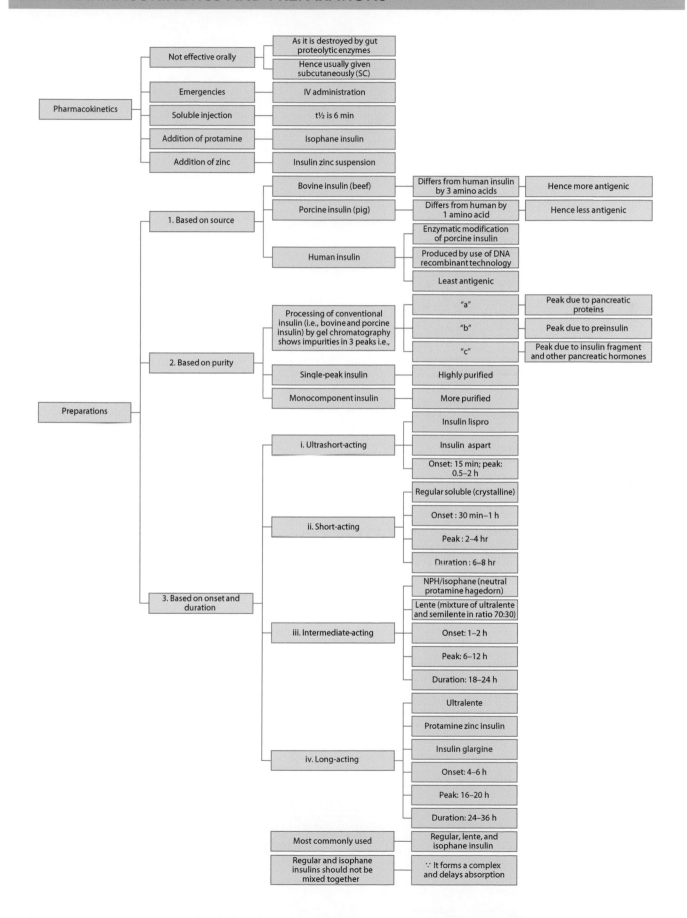

53.4 UNITAGE AND DOSAGE, HUMAN INSULINS, AND INSULIN ANALOGS

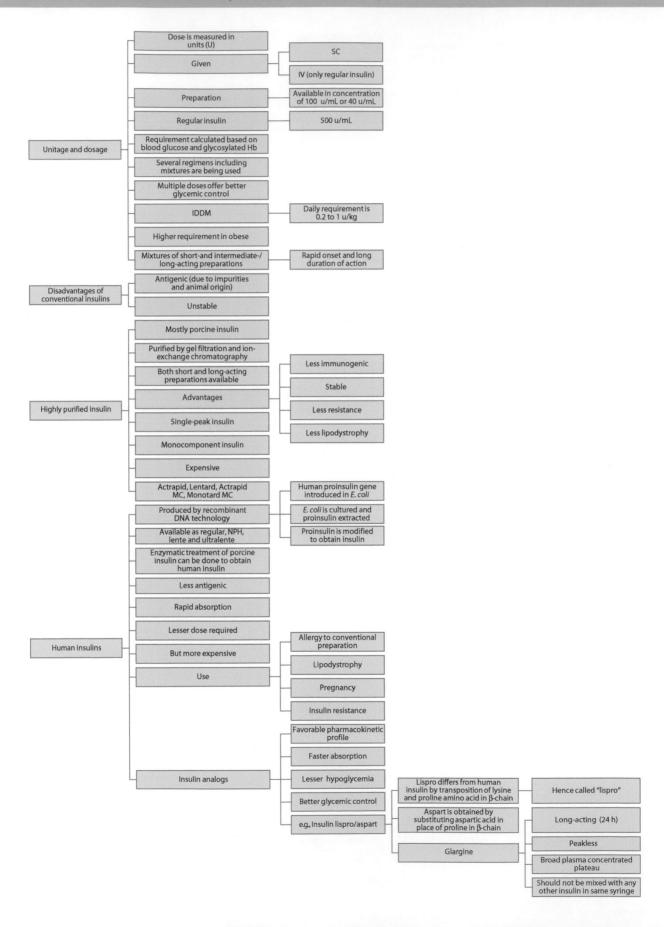

Unitage and dosage
- Dose is measured in units (U)
- Given
  - SC
  - IV (only regular insulin)
- Preparation
  - Available in concentration of 100 u/mL or 40 u/mL
- Regular insulin
  - 500 u/mL
- Requirement calculated based on blood glucose and glycosylated Hb
- Several regimens including mixtures are being used
- Multiple doses offer better glycemic control
- IDDM
  - Daily requirement is 0.2 to 1 u/kg
- Higher requirement in obese
- Mixtures of short- and intermediate-/long-acting preparations
  - Rapid onset and long duration of action

Disadvantages of conventional insulins
- Antigenic (due to impurities and animal origin)
- Unstable

Highly purified insulin
- Mostly porcine insulin
- Purified by gel filtration and ion-exchange chromatography
- Both short and long-acting preparations available
- Advantages
  - Less immunogenic
  - Stable
  - Less resistance
  - Less lipodystrophy
- Single-peak insulin
- Monocomponent insulin
- Expensive
- Actrapid, Lentard, Actrapid MC, Monotard MC

Human insulins
- Produced by recombinant DNA technology
  - Human proinsulin gene introduced in *E. coli*
  - *E. coli* is cultured and proinsulin extracted
  - Proinsulin is modified to obtain insulin
- Available as regular, NPH, lente and ultralente
- Enzymatic treatment of porcine insulin can be done to obtain human insulin
- Less antigenic
- Rapid absorption
- Lesser dose required
- But more expensive
- Use
  - Allergy to conventional preparation
  - Lipodystrophy
  - Pregnancy
  - Insulin resistance
- Insulin analogs
  - Favorable pharmacokinetic profile
  - Faster absorption
  - Lesser hypoglycemia
  - Better glycemic control
  - e.g., Insulin lispro/aspart
    - Lispro differs from human insulin by transposition of lysine and proline amino acid in β-chain
      - Hence called "lispro"
    - Aspart is obtained by substituting aspartic acid in place of proline in β-chain
    - Glargine
      - Long-acting (24 h)
      - Peakless
      - Broad plasma concentrated plateau
      - Should not be mixed with any other insulin in same syringe

53.5 INSULIN DEVICES AND USE OF INSULIN

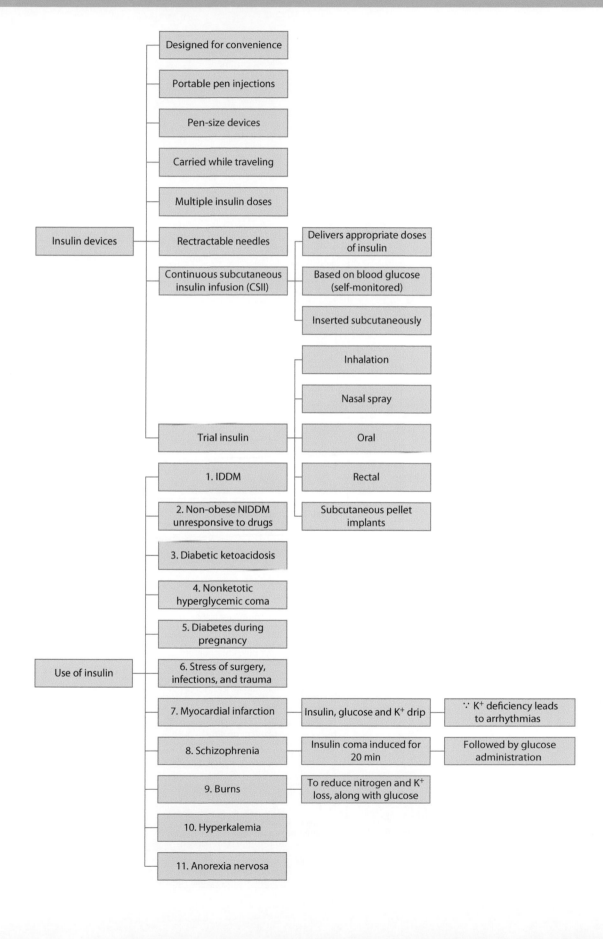

53.6 ADVERSE EFFECTS AND DRUG INTERACTIONS

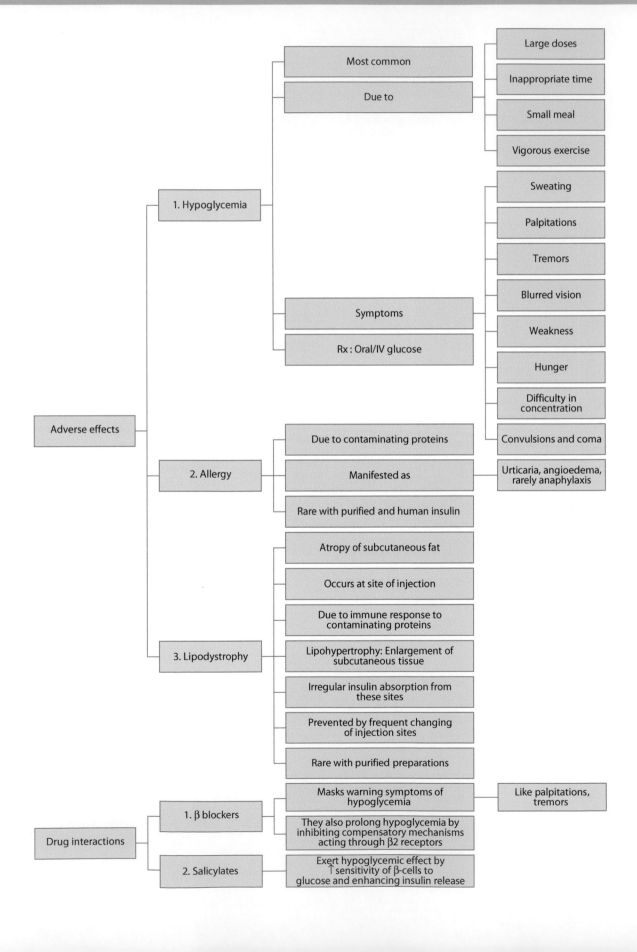

53.7 ORAL ANTIDIABETIC AGENTS – CLASSIFICATION

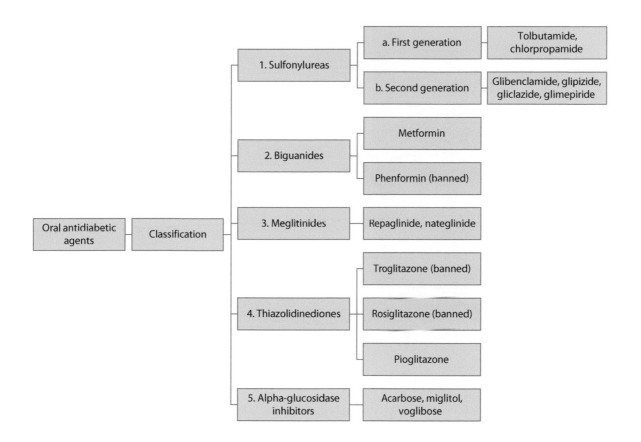

53.8 SULFONYLUREAS

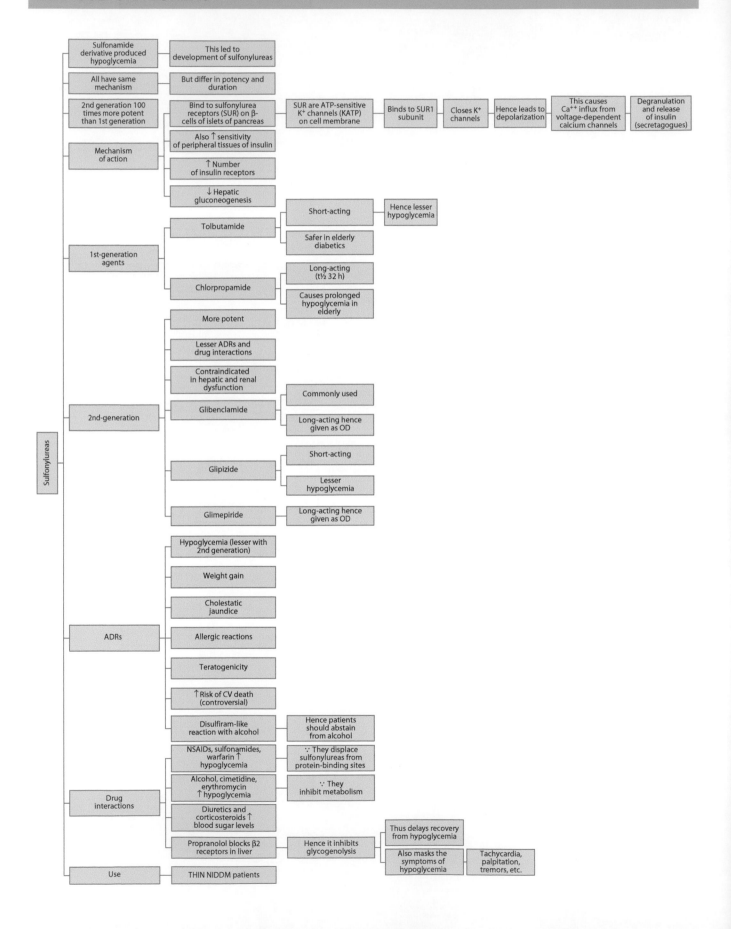

53.9 BIGUANIDES AND MEGLITINIDE ANALOGS

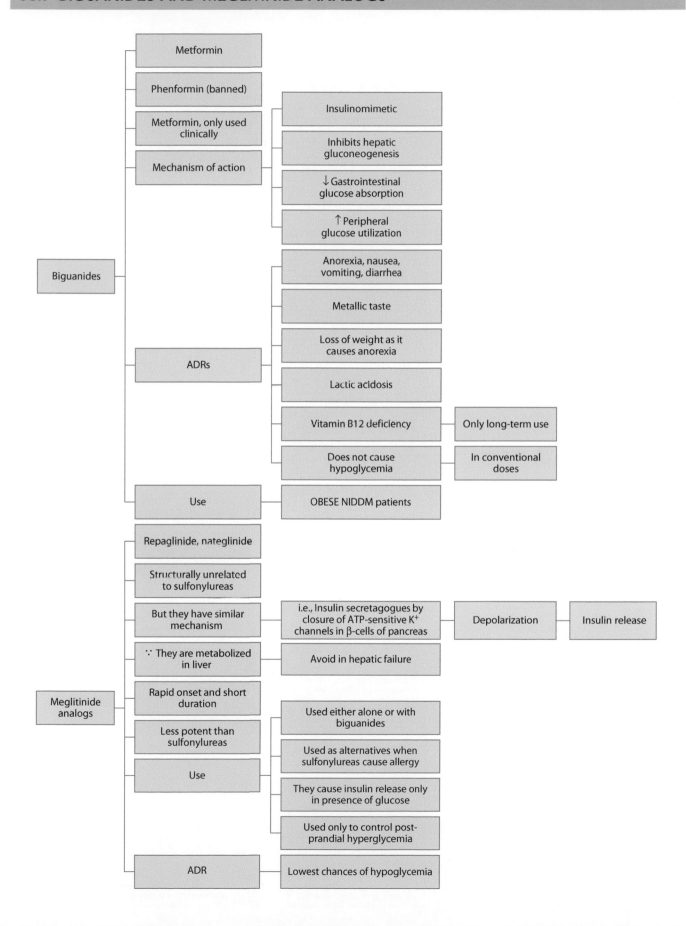

53.10 THIAZOLIDINEDIONES (TZD) AND ALPHA-GLUCOSIDASE INHIBITOR

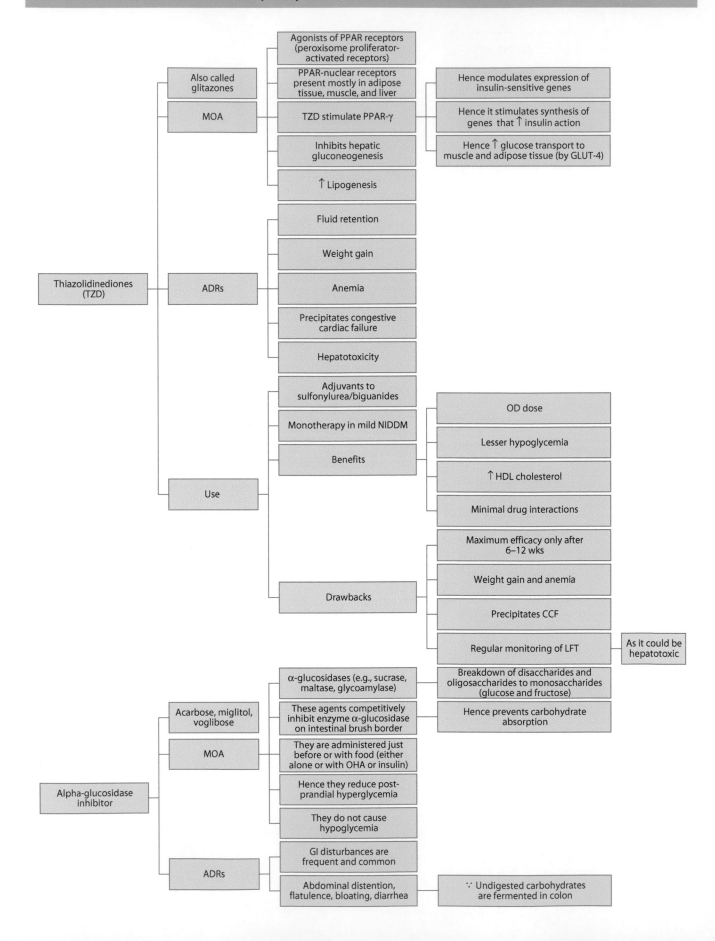

53.11 NEW DRUGS FOR DIABETES MELLITUS

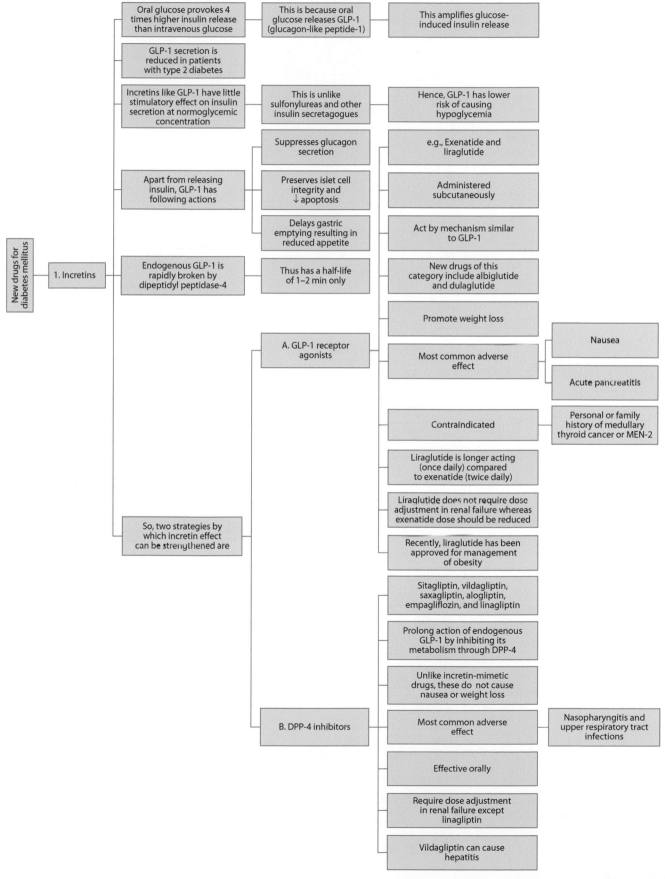

(Continued)

53.11 NEW DRUGS FOR DIABETES MELLITUS (Continued)

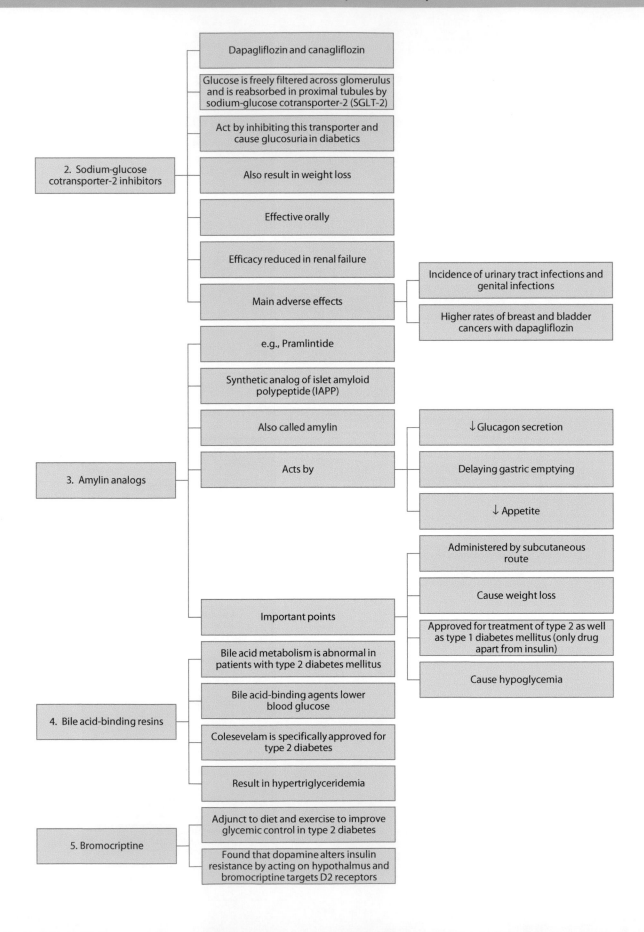

2. Sodium-glucose cotransporter-2 inhibitors
- Dapagliflozin and canagliflozin
- Glucose is freely filtered across glomerulus and is reabsorbed in proximal tubules by sodium-glucose cotransporter-2 (SGLT-2)
- Act by inhibiting this transporter and cause glucosuria in diabetics
- Also result in weight loss
- Effective orally
- Efficacy reduced in renal failure
- Main adverse effects
  - Incidence of urinary tract infections and genital infections
  - Higher rates of breast and bladder cancers with dapagliflozin

3. Amylin analogs
- e.g., Pramlintide
- Synthetic analog of islet amyloid polypeptide (IAPP)
- Also called amylin
- Acts by
  - ↓ Glucagon secretion
  - Delaying gastric emptying
  - ↓ Appetite
- Important points
  - Administered by subcutaneous route
  - Cause weight loss
  - Approved for treatment of type 2 as well as type 1 diabetes mellitus (only drug apart from insulin)
  - Cause hypoglycemia

4. Bile acid-binding resins
- Bile acid metabolism is abnormal in patients with type 2 diabetes mellitus
- Bile acid-binding agents lower blood glucose
- Colesevelam is specifically approved for type 2 diabetes
- Result in hypertriglyceridemia

5. Bromocriptine
- Adjunct to diet and exercise to improve glycemic control in type 2 diabetes
- Found that dopamine alters insulin resistance by acting on hypothalmus and bromocriptine targets D2 receptors

Agents affecting calcium balance

54.1 CALCIUM PREPARATIONS AND USES

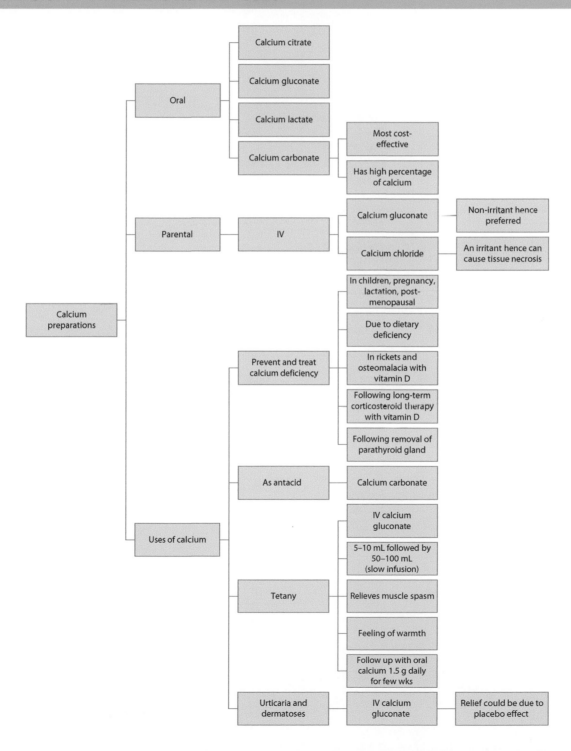

54.2 PARATHYROID HORMONE (PTH)

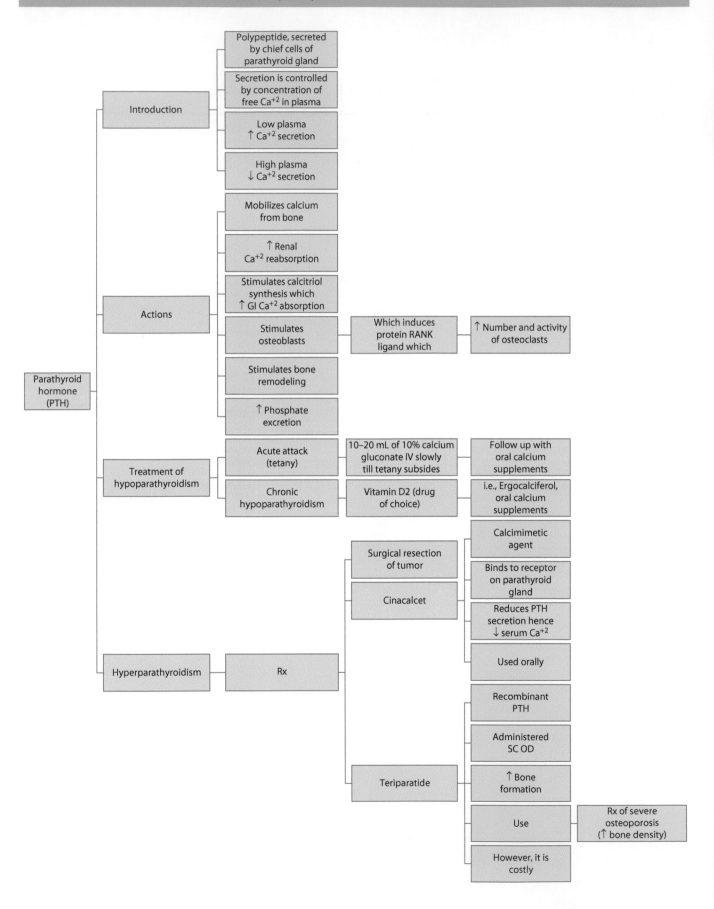

Parathyroid hormone (PTH)

Introduction
- Polypeptide, secreted by chief cells of parathyroid gland
- Secretion is controlled by concentration of free Ca^{+2} in plasma
- Low plasma ↑ Ca^{+2} secretion
- High plasma ↓ Ca^{+2} secretion

Actions
- Mobilizes calcium from bone
- ↑ Renal Ca^{+2} reabsorption
- Stimulates calcitriol synthesis which ↑ GI Ca^{+2} absorption
- Stimulates osteoblasts → Which induces protein RANK ligand which → ↑ Number and activity of osteoclasts
- Stimulates bone remodeling
- ↑ Phosphate excretion

Treatment of hypoparathyroidism
- Acute attack (tetany) → 10–20 mL of 10% calcium gluconate IV slowly till tetany subsides → Follow up with oral calcium supplements
- Chronic hypoparathyroidism → Vitamin D2 (drug of choice) → i.e., Ergocalciferol, oral calcium supplements

Hyperparathyroidism → Rx
- Surgical resection of tumor
- Cinacalcet
  - Calcimimetic agent
  - Binds to receptor on parathyroid gland
  - Reduces PTH secretion hence ↓ serum Ca^{+2}
  - Used orally
- Teriparatide
  - Recombinant PTH
  - Administered SC OD
  - ↑ Bone formation
  - Use → Rx of severe osteoporosis (↑ bone density)
  - However, it is costly

54.3 CALCITONIN

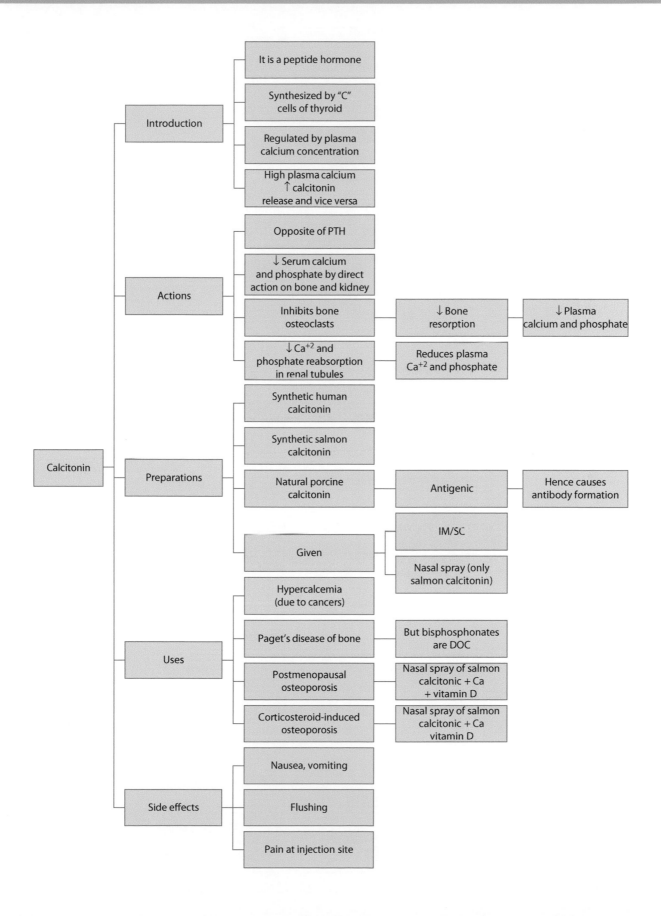

54.4 VITAMIN D

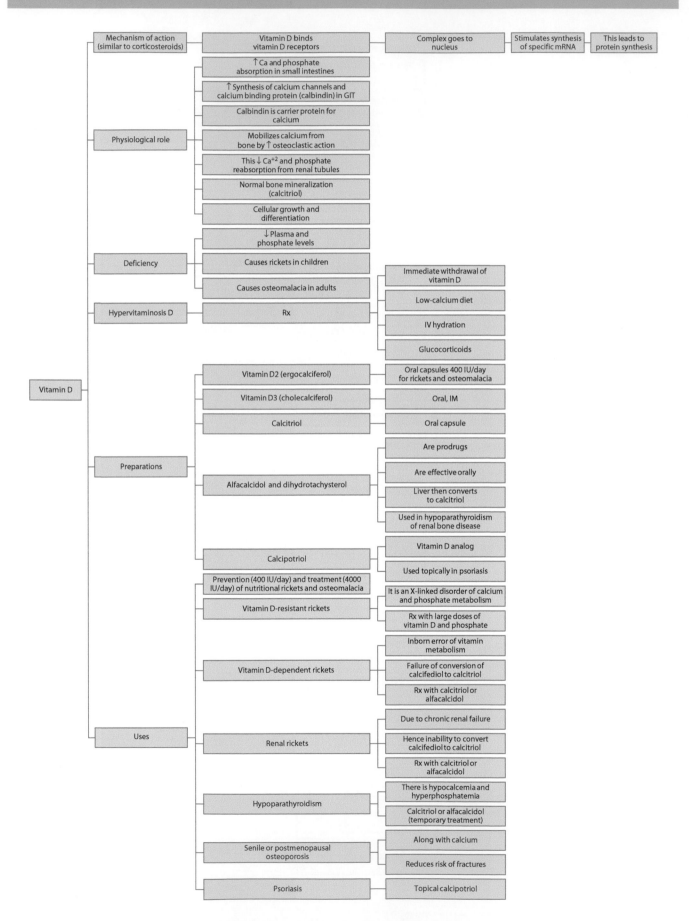

Mechanism of action (similar to corticosteroids): Vitamin D binds vitamin D receptors → Complex goes to nucleus → Stimulates synthesis of specific mRNA → This leads to protein synthesis

Physiological role:
- ↑ Ca and phosphate absorption in small intestines
- ↑ Synthesis of calcium channels and calcium binding protein (calbindin) in GIT
- Calbindin is carrier protein for calcium
- Mobilizes calcium from bone by ↑ osteoclastic action
- This ↓ Ca⁺² and phosphate reabsorption from renal tubules
- Normal bone mineralization (calcitriol)
- Cellular growth and differentiation

Deficiency:
- ↓ Plasma and phosphate levels
- Causes rickets in children
- Causes osteomalacia in adults

Hypervitaminosis D:
- Rx:
  - Immediate withdrawal of vitamin D
  - Low-calcium diet
  - IV hydration
  - Glucocorticoids

Preparations:
- Vitamin D2 (ergocalciferol): Oral capsules 400 IU/day for rickets and osteomalacia
- Vitamin D3 (cholecalciferol): Oral, IM
- Calcitriol: Oral capsule
- Alfacalcidol and dihydrotachysterol:
  - Are prodrugs
  - Are effective orally
  - Liver then converts to calcitriol
  - Used in hypoparathyroidism of renal bone disease
- Calcipotriol:
  - Vitamin D analog
  - Used topically in psoriasis

Uses:
- Prevention (400 IU/day) and treatment (4000 IU/day) of nutritional rickets and osteomalacia
- Vitamin D-resistant rickets:
  - It is an X-linked disorder of calcium and phosphate metabolism
  - Rx with large doses of vitamin D and phosphate
- Vitamin D-dependent rickets:
  - Inborn error of vitamin metabolism
  - Failure of conversion of calcifediol to calcitriol
  - Rx with calcitriol or alfacalcidol
- Renal rickets:
  - Due to chronic renal failure
  - Hence inability to convert calcifediol to calcitriol
  - Rx with calcitriol or alfacalcidol
- Hypoparathyroidism:
  - There is hypocalcemia and hyperphosphatemia
  - Calcitriol or alfacalcidol (temporary treatment)
- Senile or postmenopausal osteoporosis:
  - Along with calcium
  - Reduces risk of fractures
- Psoriasis:
  - Topical calcipotriol

54.5 BISPHOSPHONATES

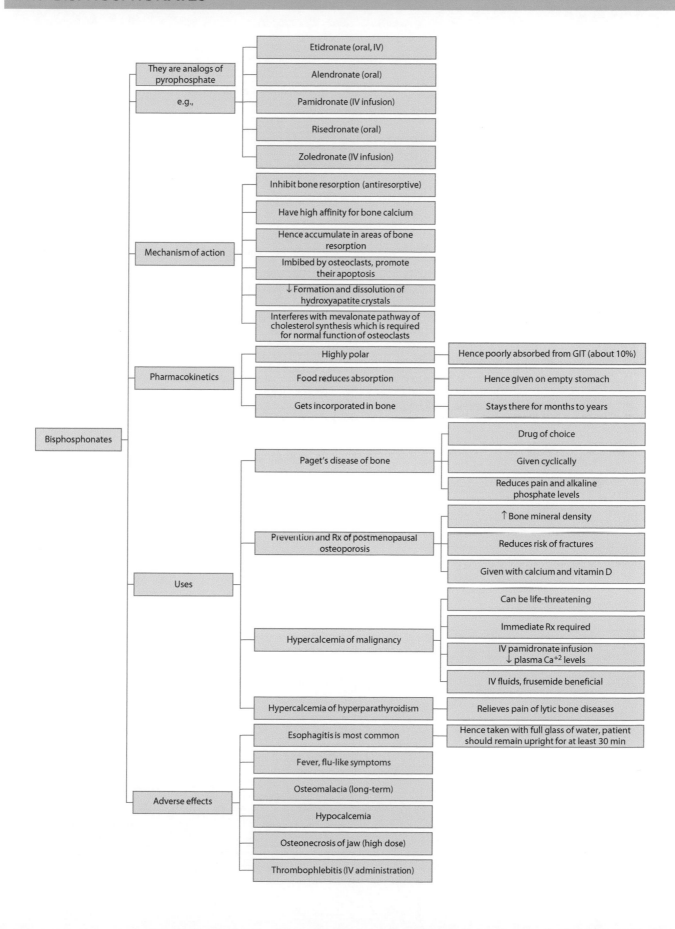

Bisphosphonates

They are analogs of pyrophosphate

e.g.,
- Etidronate (oral, IV)
- Alendronate (oral)
- Pamidronate (IV infusion)
- Risedronate (oral)
- Zoledronate (IV infusion)

Mechanism of action
- Inhibit bone resorption (antiresorptive)
- Have high affinity for bone calcium
- Hence accumulate in areas of bone resorption
- Imbibed by osteoclasts, promote their apoptosis
- ↓ Formation and dissolution of hydroxyapatite crystals
- Interferes with mevalonate pathway of cholesterol synthesis which is required for normal function of osteoclasts

Pharmacokinetics
- Highly polar → Hence poorly absorbed from GIT (about 10%)
- Food reduces absorption → Hence given on empty stomach
- Gets incorporated in bone → Stays there for months to years

Uses
- Paget's disease of bone
  - Drug of choice
  - Given cyclically
  - Reduces pain and alkaline phosphate levels
- Prevention and Rx of postmenopausal osteoporosis
  - ↑ Bone mineral density
  - Reduces risk of fractures
  - Given with calcium and vitamin D
- Hypercalcemia of malignancy
  - Can be life-threatening
  - Immediate Rx required
  - IV pamidronate infusion ↓ plasma Ca^{+2} levels
  - IV fluids, frusemide beneficial
- Hypercalcemia of hyperparathyroidism → Relieves pain of lytic bone diseases

Adverse effects
- Esophagitis is most common → Hence taken with full glass of water, patient should remain upright for at least 30 min
- Fever, flu-like symptoms
- Osteomalacia (long-term)
- Hypocalcemia
- Osteonecrosis of jaw (high dose)
- Thrombophlebitis (IV administration)

54.6 PREVENTION AND TREATMENT OF OSTEOPOROSIS, AND DRUGS OF ABUSE IN SPORTS

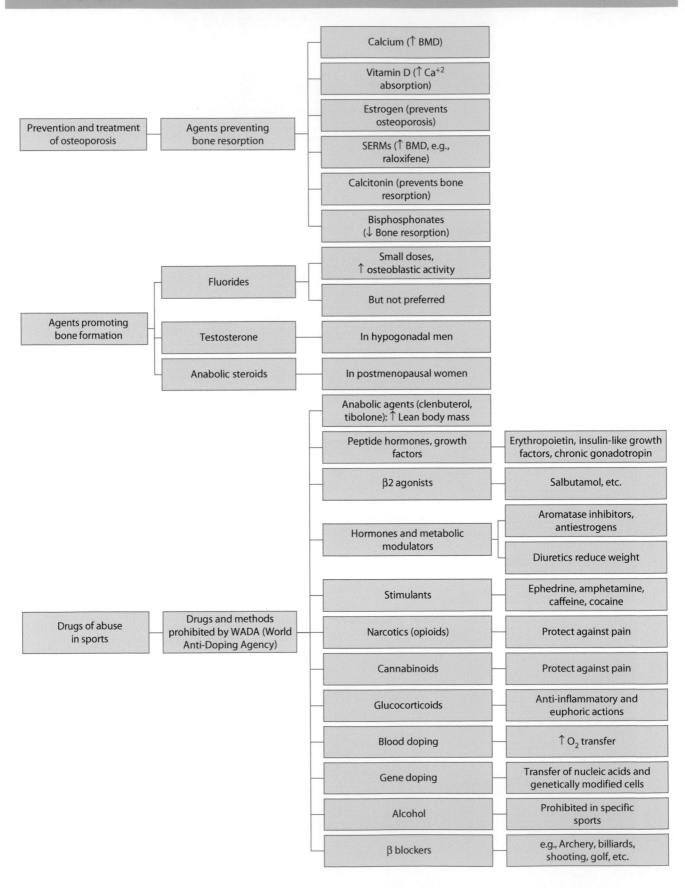

Drugs acting on uterus

55.1 UTERINE STIMULANTS

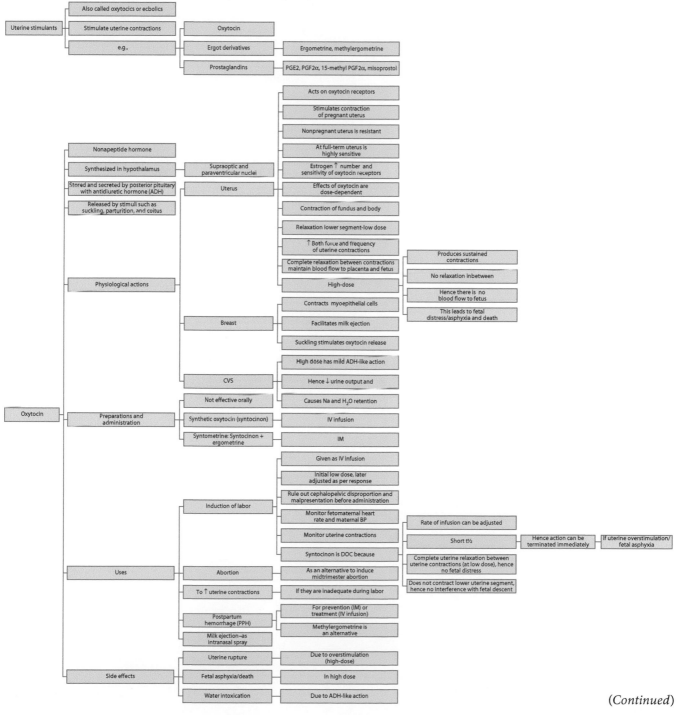

- **Uterine stimulants**
  - Also called oxytocics or ecbolics
  - Stimulate uterine contractions
  - e.g.,
    - Oxytocin
    - Ergot derivatives → Ergometrine, methylergometrine
    - Prostaglandins → PGE2, PGF2α, 15-methyl PGF2α, misoprostol

- **Oxytocin**
  - Nonapeptide hormone
  - Synthesized in hypothalamus
  - Stored and secreted by posterior pituitary with antidiuretic hormone (ADH)
  - Released by stimuli such as suckling, parturition, and coitus
  - **Physiological actions**
    - Supraoptic and paraventricular nuclei
    - Uterus
      - Acts on oxytocin receptors
      - Stimulates contraction of pregnant uterus
      - Nonpregnant uterus is resistant
      - At full-term uterus is highly sensitive
      - Estrogen ↑ number and sensitivity of oxytocin receptors
      - Effects of oxytocin are dose-dependent
      - Contraction of fundus and body
      - Relaxation lower segment-low dose
      - ↑ Both force and frequency of uterine contractions
      - Complete relaxation between contractions maintain blood flow to placenta and fetus
      - High-dose
        - Produces sustained contractions
        - No relaxation inbetween
        - Hence there is no blood flow to fetus
        - This leads to fetal distress/asphyxia and death
    - Breast
      - Contracts myoepithelial cells
      - Facilitates milk ejection
      - Suckling stimulates oxytocin release
    - CVS
      - High dose has mild ADH-like action
      - Hence ↓ urine output and
      - Causes Na and H_2O retention
  - **Preparations and administration**
    - Not effective orally
    - Synthetic oxytocin (syntocinon) → IV infusion
    - Syntometrine: Syntocinon + ergometrine → IM
  - **Uses**
    - Induction of labor
      - Given as IV infusion
      - Initial low dose, later adjusted as per response
      - Rule out cephalopelvic disproportion and malpresentation before administration
      - Monitor fetomaternal heart rate and maternal BP
      - Monitor uterine contractions
        - Rate of infusion can be adjusted
        - Short t½ → Hence action can be terminated immediately → If uterine overstimulation/fetal asphyxia
      - Syntocinon is DOC because
        - Complete uterine relaxation between uterine contractions (at low dose), hence no fetal distress
        - Does not contract lower uterine segment, hence no interference with fetal descent
    - Abortion → As an alternative to induce midtrimester abortion
    - To ↑ uterine contractions → If they are inadequate during labor
    - Postpartum hemorrhage (PPH)
      - For prevention (IM) or treatment (IV infusion)
      - Methylergometrine is an alternative
    - Milk ejection–as intranasal spray
  - **Side effects**
    - Uterine rupture → Due to overstimulation (high-dose)
    - Fetal asphyxia/death → In high dose
    - Water intoxication → Due to ADH-like action

(Continued)

55.1 UTERINE STIMULANTS (Continued)

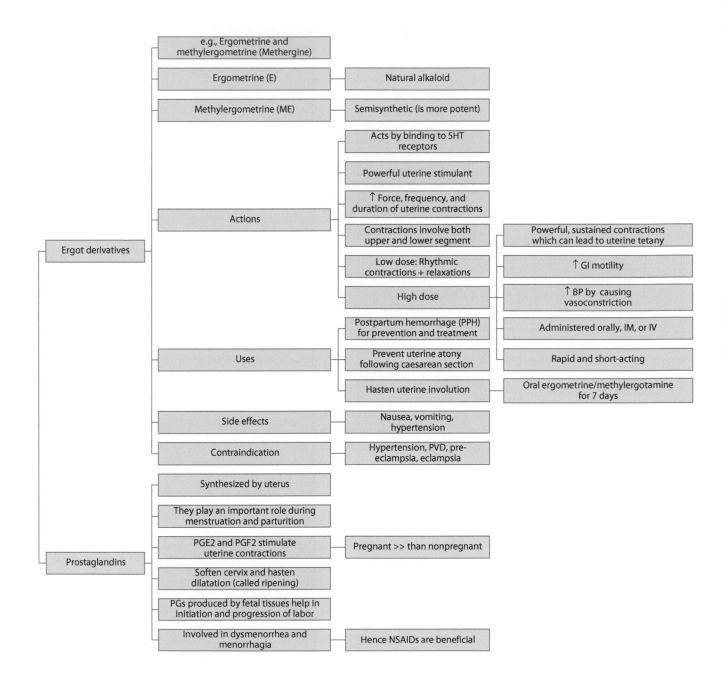

Ergot derivatives

- e.g., Ergometrine and methylergometrine (Methergine)
- Ergometrine (E) — Natural alkaloid
- Methylergometrine (ME) — Semisynthetic (is more potent)
- Actions
  - Acts by binding to 5HT receptors
  - Powerful uterine stimulant
  - ↑ Force, frequency, and duration of uterine contractions
  - Contractions involve both upper and lower segment — Powerful, sustained contractions which can lead to uterine tetany
  - Low dose: Rhythmic contractions + relaxations — ↑ GI motility
  - High dose — ↑ BP by causing vasoconstriction
- Uses
  - Postpartum hemorrhage (PPH) for prevention and treatment — Administered orally, IM, or IV
  - Prevent uterine atony following caesarean section — Rapid and short-acting
  - Hasten uterine involution — Oral ergometrine/methylergotamine for 7 days
- Side effects — Nausea, vomiting, hypertension
- Contraindication — Hypertension, PVD, pre-eclampsia, eclampsia

Prostaglandins

- Synthesized by uterus
- They play an important role during menstruation and parturition
- PGE2 and PGF2 stimulate uterine contractions — Pregnant >> than nonpregnant
- Soften cervix and hasten dilatation (called ripening)
- PGs produced by fetal tissues help in initiation and progression of labor
- Involved in dysmenorrhea and menorrhagia — Hence NSAIDs are beneficial

(Continued)

55.1 UTERINE STIMULANTS (Continued)

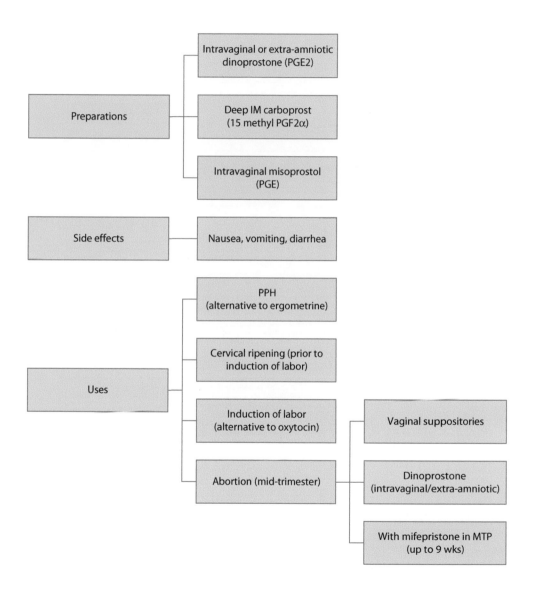

55.2 UTERINE RELAXANTS (TOCOLYTICS)

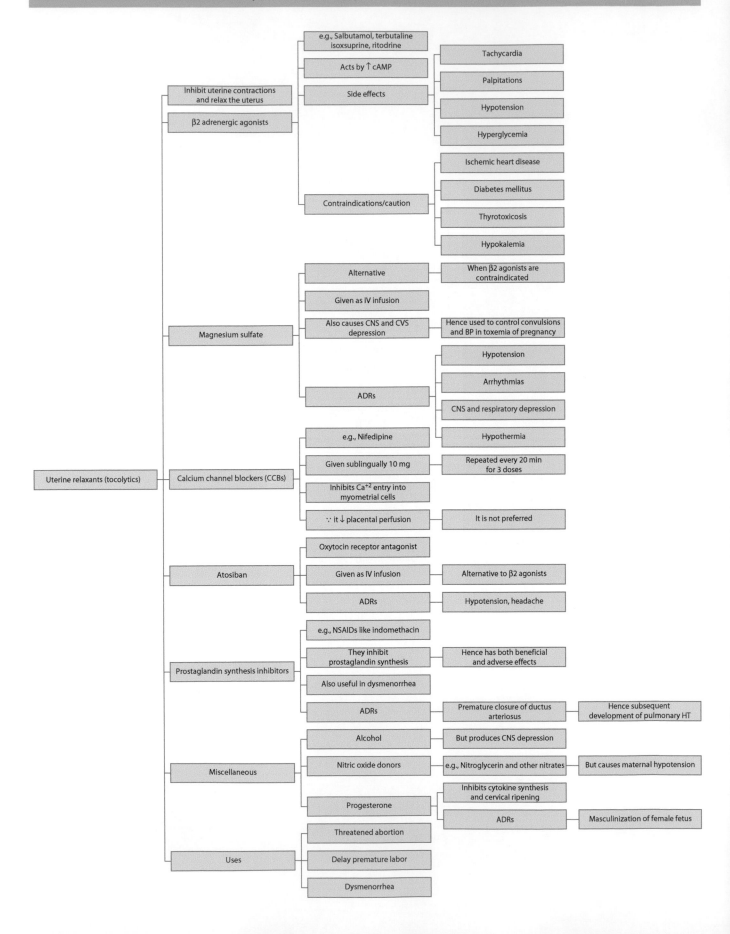

55.3 DIFFERENCES BETWEEN OXYTOCIN AND ERGOMETRINE

Oxytocin	Ergometrine
1. Synthetic (commercial)	Natural
2. Peptide	Alkaloid
3. Acts on oxytocin receptors	5-HT receptors
4. Endogenous	Exogenous
5. Only IV	Oral, IM and IV
6. Short duration t½ 15 min	Long duration t½ 2 h
7. Contracts body & fundus	Contracts whole uterus
8. Relaxes lower segment	No relaxation
9. Induces labor, milk ejection	PPH, uterine involution

PART X

Chemotherapy

General chemotherapy

56.1 DEFINITIONS AND CLASSIFICATIONS

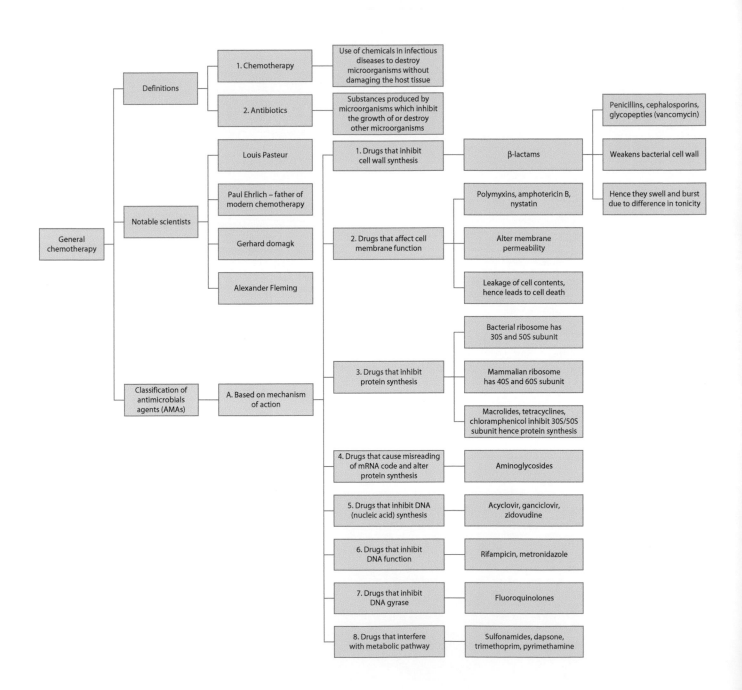

56.2 CLASSIFICATIONS

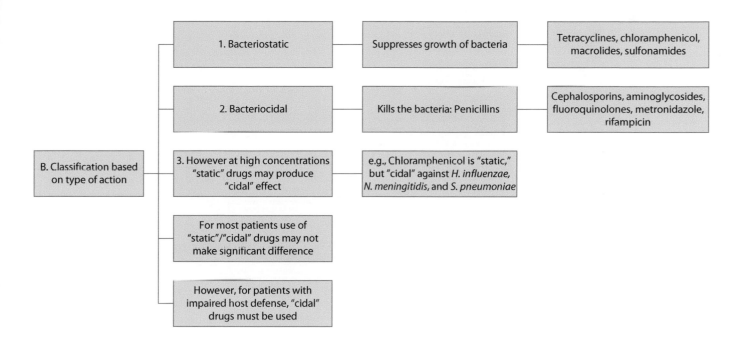

56.3 CLASSIFICATION, FACTORS INFLUENCING SUCCESSFUL CHEMOTHERAPY, AND ANTIMICROBIAL RESISTANCE

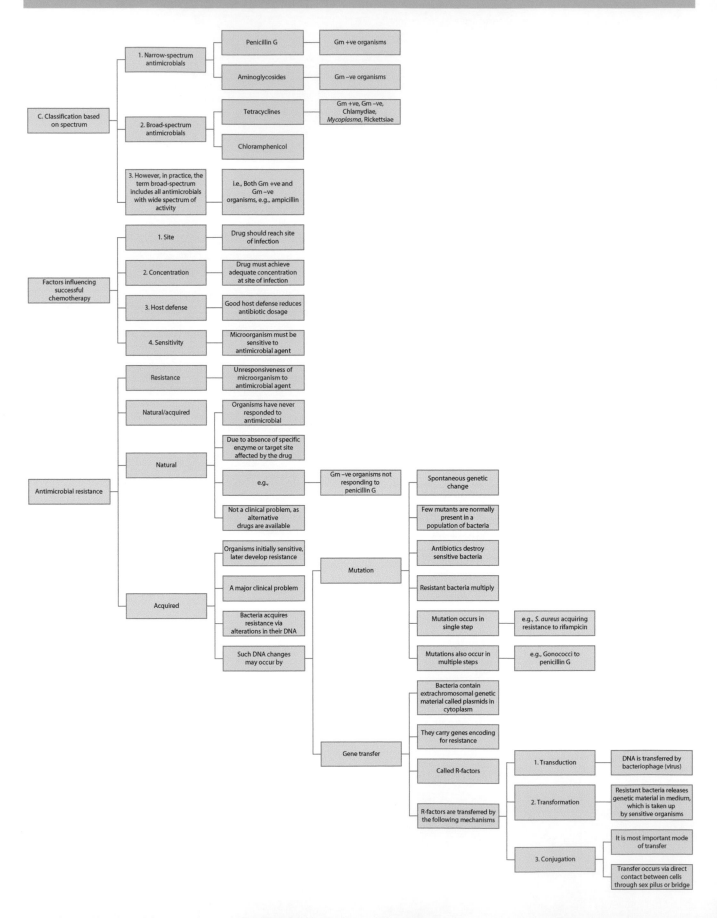

56.4 ANTIMICROBIAL RESISTANCE

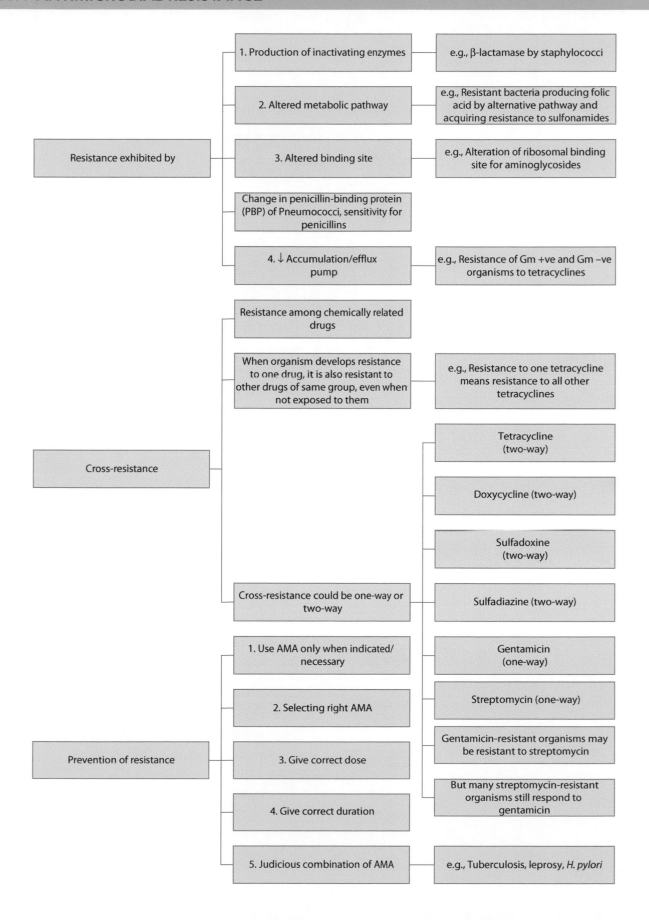

56.5 SELECTION OF APPROPRIATE AMA

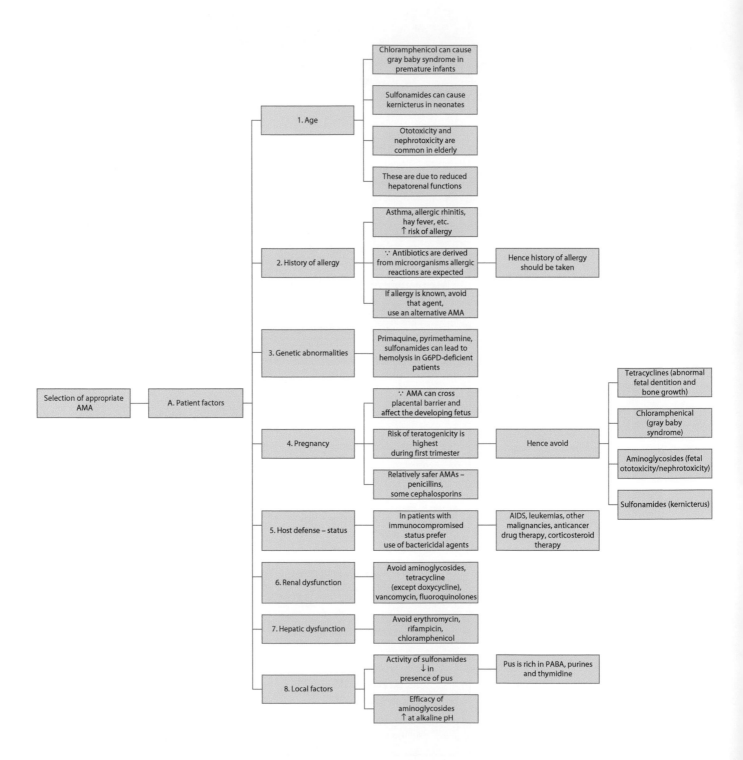

(Continued)

56.5 SELECTION OF APPROPRIATE AMA (Continued)

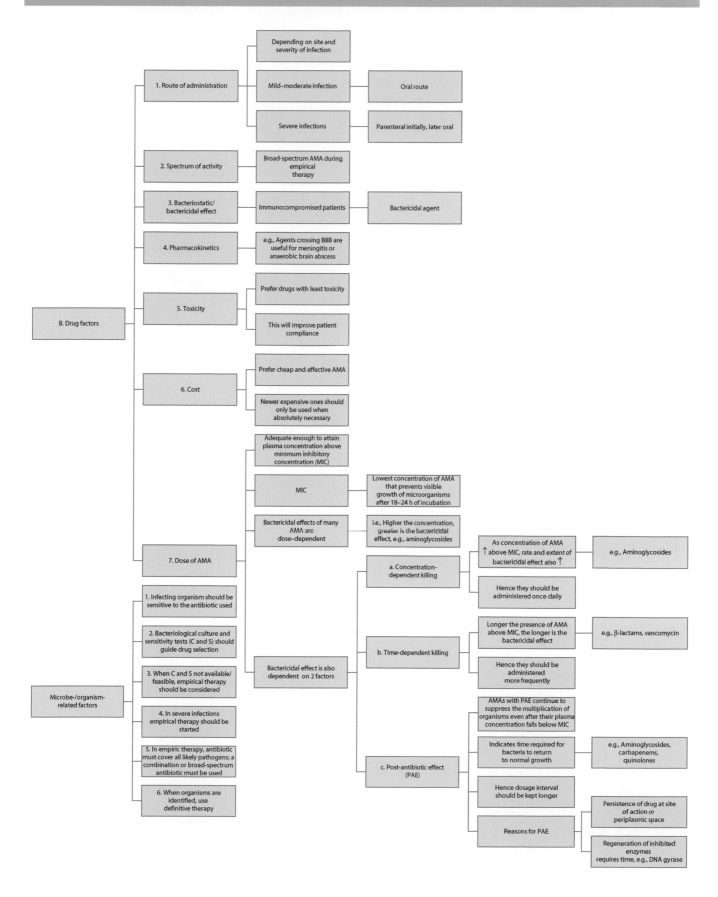

56.6 AMA COMBINATIONS

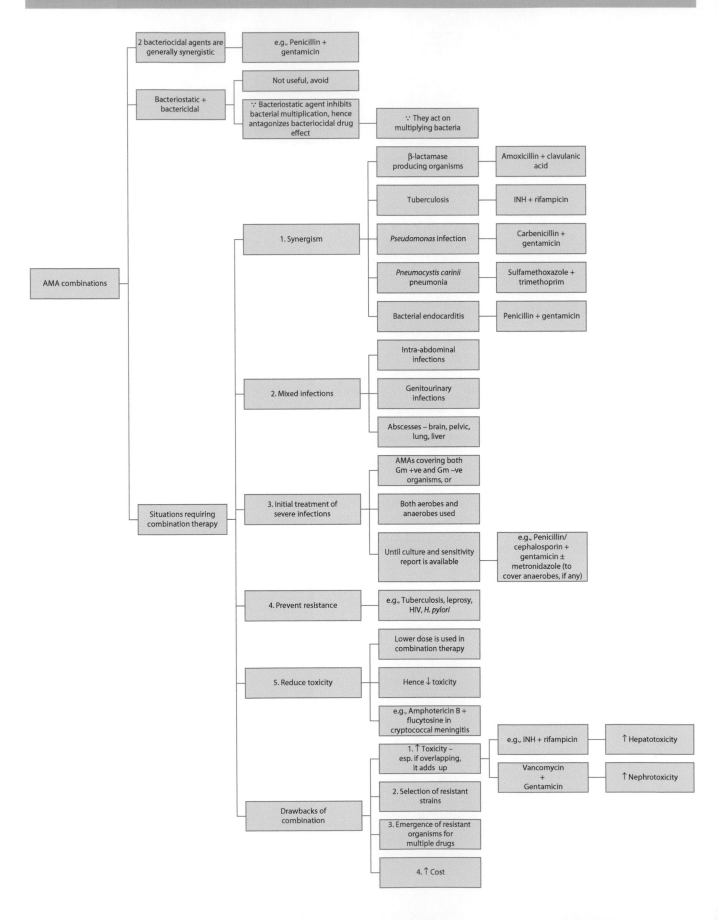

- 2 bacteriocidal agents are generally synergistic
  - e.g., Penicillin + gentamicin
- Bacteriostatic + bactericidal
  - Not useful, avoid
  - ∵ Bacteriostatic agent inhibits bacterial multiplication, hence antagonizes bacteriocidal drug effect
    - ∵ They act on multiplying bacteria

AMA combinations

- Situations requiring combination therapy
  - 1. Synergism
    - β-lactamase producing organisms → Amoxicillin + clavulanic acid
    - Tuberculosis → INH + rifampicin
    - *Pseudomonas* infection → Carbenicillin + gentamicin
    - *Pneumocystis carinii* pneumonia → Sulfamethoxazole + trimethoprim
    - Bacterial endocarditis → Penicillin + gentamicin
  - 2. Mixed infections
    - Intra-abdominal infections
    - Genitourinary infections
    - Abscesses – brain, pelvic, lung, liver
  - 3. Initial treatment of severe infections
    - AMAs covering both Gm +ve and Gm –ve organisms, or
    - Both aerobes and anaerobes used
    - Until culture and sensitivity report is available
      - e.g., Penicillin/ cephalosporin + gentamicin ± metronidazole (to cover anaerobes, if any)
  - 4. Prevent resistance
    - e.g., Tuberculosis, leprosy, HIV, *H. pylori*
  - 5. Reduce toxicity
    - Lower dose is used in combination therapy
    - Hence ↓ toxicity
    - e.g., Amphotericin B + flucytosine in cryptococcal meningitis
  - Drawbacks of combination
    - 1. ↑ Toxicity – esp. if overlapping, it adds up
      - e.g., INH + rifampicin → ↑ Hepatotoxicity
      - Vancomycin + Gentamicin → ↑ Nephrotoxicity
    - 2. Selection of resistant strains
    - 3. Emergence of resistant organisms for multiple drugs
    - 4. ↑ Cost

56.7 CHEMOPROPHYLAXIS

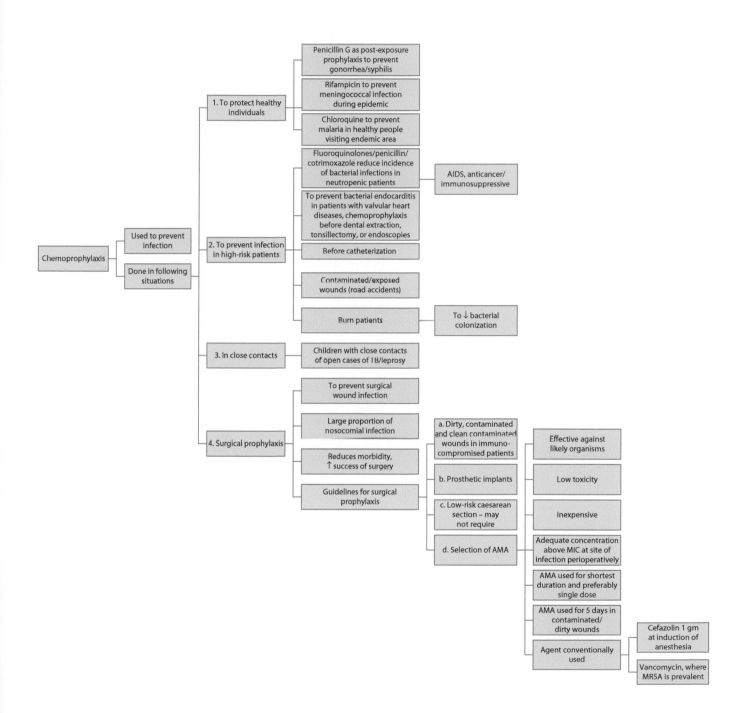

56.8 SUPERINFECTION (SUPRAINFECTION)

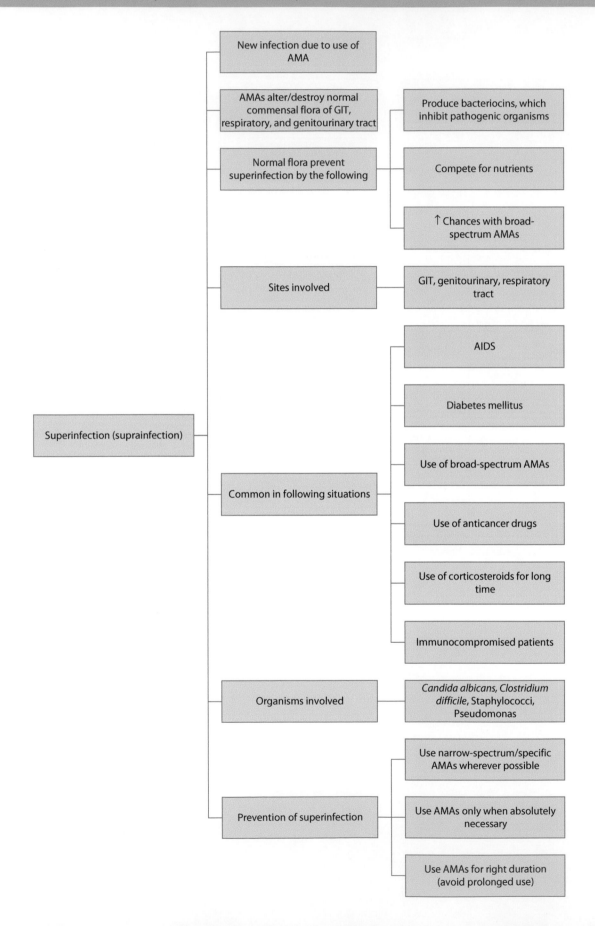

57

Beta-lactam antibiotics

57.1 PENICILLINS

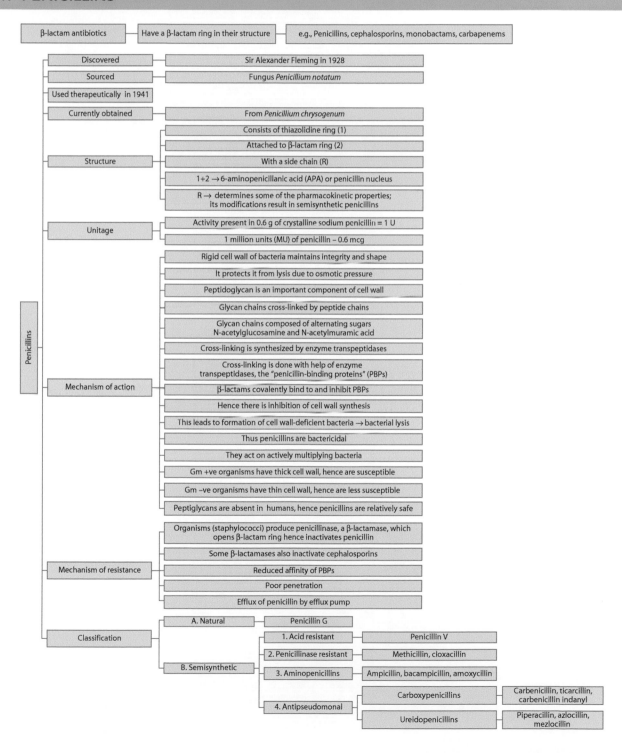

| β-lactam antibiotics | Have a β-lactam ring in their structure | e.g., Penicillins, cephalosporins, monobactams, carbapenems |

Penicillins

- **Discovered** — Sir Alexander Fleming in 1928
- **Sourced** — Fungus *Penicillium notatum*
- **Used therapeutically in 1941**
- **Currently obtained** — From *Penicillium chrysogenum*
- **Structure**
  - Consists of thiazolidine ring (1)
  - Attached to β-lactam ring (2)
  - With a side chain (R)
  - 1+2 → 6-aminopenicillanic acid (APA) or penicillin nucleus
  - R → determines some of the pharmacokinetic properties; its modifications result in semisynthetic penicillins
- **Unitage**
  - Activity present in 0.6 g of crystalline sodium penicillin = 1 U
  - 1 million units (MU) of penicillin – 0.6 mcg
- **Mechanism of action**
  - Rigid cell wall of bacteria maintains integrity and shape
  - It protects it from lysis due to osmotic pressure
  - Peptidoglycan is an important component of cell wall
  - Glycan chains cross-linked by peptide chains
  - Glycan chains composed of alternating sugars N-acetylglucosamine and N-acetylmuramic acid
  - Cross-linking is synthesized by enzyme transpeptidases
  - Cross-linking is done with help of enzyme transpeptidases, the "penicillin-binding proteins" (PBPs)
  - β-lactams covalently bind to and inhibit PBPs
  - Hence there is inhibition of cell wall synthesis
  - This leads to formation of cell wall-deficient bacteria → bacterial lysis
  - Thus penicillins are bactericidal
  - They act on actively multiplying bacteria
  - Gm +ve organisms have thick cell wall, hence are susceptible
  - Gm –ve organisms have thin cell wall, hence are less susceptible
  - Peptiglycans are absent in humans, hence penicillins are relatively safe
- **Mechanism of resistance**
  - Organisms (staphylococci) produce penicillinase, a β-lactamase, which opens β-lactam ring hence inactivates penicillin
  - Some β-lactamases also inactivate cephalosporins
  - Reduced affinity of PBPs
  - Poor penetration
  - Efflux of penicillin by efflux pump
- **Classification**
  - **A. Natural** — Penicillin G
  - **B. Semisynthetic**
    - 1. Acid resistant — Penicillin V
    - 2. Penicillinase resistant — Methicillin, cloxacillin
    - 3. Aminopenicillins — Ampicillin, bacampicillin, amoxycillin
    - 4. Antipseudomonal
      - Carboxypenicillins — Carbenicillin, ticarcillin, carbenicillin indanyl
      - Ureidopenicillins — Piperacillin, azlocillin, mezlocillin

57.2 NATURAL PENICILLINS

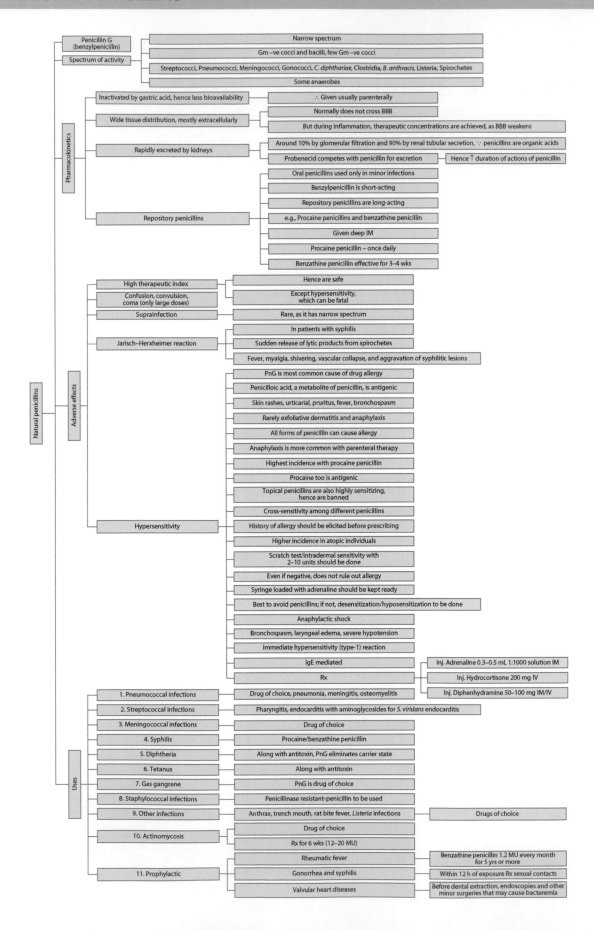

Natural penicillins

Penicillin G (benzylpenicillin)

Spectrum of activity
- Narrow spectrum
- Gm –ve cocci and bacilli, few Gm –ve cocci
- Streptococci, Pneumococci, Meningococci, Gonococci, *C. diphthariae*, Clostridia, *B. anthracis*, Listeria, Spirochetes
- Some anaerobes

Pharmacokinetics
- Inactivated by gastric acid, hence less bioavailability
  - ∴ Given usually parenterally
- Wide tissue distribution, mostly extracellularly
  - Normally does not cross BBB
  - But during inflammation, therapeutic concentrations are achieved, as BBB weakens
- Rapidly excreted by kidneys
  - Around 10% by glomerular filtration and 90% by renal tubular secretion, ∵ penicillins are organic acids
  - Probenecid competes with penicillin for excretion — Hence ↑ duration of actions of penicillin
- Repository penicillins
  - Oral penicillins used only in minor infections
  - Benzylpenicillin is short-acting
  - Repository penicillins are long-acting
  - e.g., Procaine penicillins and benzathine penicillin
  - Given deep IM
  - Procaine penicillin – once daily
  - Benzathine penicillin effective for 3–4 wks

Adverse effects
- High therapeutic index
  - Hence are safe
  - Except hypersensitivity, which can be fatal
- Confusion, convulsion, coma (only large doses)
- Suprainfection
  - Rare, as it has narrow spectrum
- Jarisch–Herxheimer reaction
  - In patients with syphilis
  - Sudden release of lytic products from spirochetes
  - Fever, myalgia, shivering, vascular collapse, and aggravation of syphilitic lesions
- Hypersensitivity
  - PnG is most common cause of drug allergy
  - Penicilloic acid, a metabolite of penicillin, is antigenic
  - Skin rashes, urticarial, pruritus, fever, bronchospasm
  - Rarely exfoliative dermatitis and anaphylaxis
  - All forms of penicillin can cause allergy
  - Anaphylaxis is more common with parenteral therapy
  - Highest incidence with procaine penicillin
  - Procaine too is antigenic
  - Topical penicillins are also highly sensitizing, hence are banned
  - Cross-sensitivity among different penicillins
  - History of allergy should be elicited before prescribing
  - Higher incidence in atopic individuals
  - Scratch test/intradermal sensitivity with 2–10 units should be done
  - Even if negative, does not rule out allergy
  - Syringe loaded with adrenaline should be kept ready
  - Best to avoid penicillins; if not, desensitization/hyposensitization to be done
  - Anaphylactic shock
  - Bronchospasm, laryngeal edema, severe hypotension
  - Immediate hypersensitivity (type-1) reaction
  - IgE mediated
  - Rx
    - Inj. Adrenaline 0.3–0.5 mL 1:1000 solution IM
    - Inj. Hydrocortisone 200 mg IV
    - Inj. Diphenhydramine 50–100 mg IM/IV

Uses
1. Pneumococcal infections — Drug of choice, pneumonia, meningitis, osteomyelitis
2. Streptococcal infections — Pharyngitis, endocarditis with aminoglycosides for *S. viridans* endocarditis
3. Meningococcal infections — Drug of choice
4. Syphilis — Procaine/benzathine penicillin
5. Diphtheria — Along with antitoxin, PnG eliminates carrier state
6. Tetanus — Along with antitoxin
7. Gas gangrene — PnG is drug of choice
8. Staphylococcal infections — Penicillinase resistant-penicillin to be used
9. Other infections — Anthrax, trench mouth, rat bite fever, *Listeria* infections — Drugs of choice
10. Actinomycosis
    - Drug of choice
    - Rx for 6 wks (12–20 MU)
11. Prophylactic
    - Rheumatic fever — Benzathine penicillin 1.2 MU every month for 5 yrs or more
    - Gonorrhea and syphilis — Within 12 h of exposure Rx sexual contacts
    - Valvular heart diseases — Before dental extraction, endoscopies and other minor surgeries that may cause bacteremia

57.3 SEMISYNTHETIC PENICILLINS

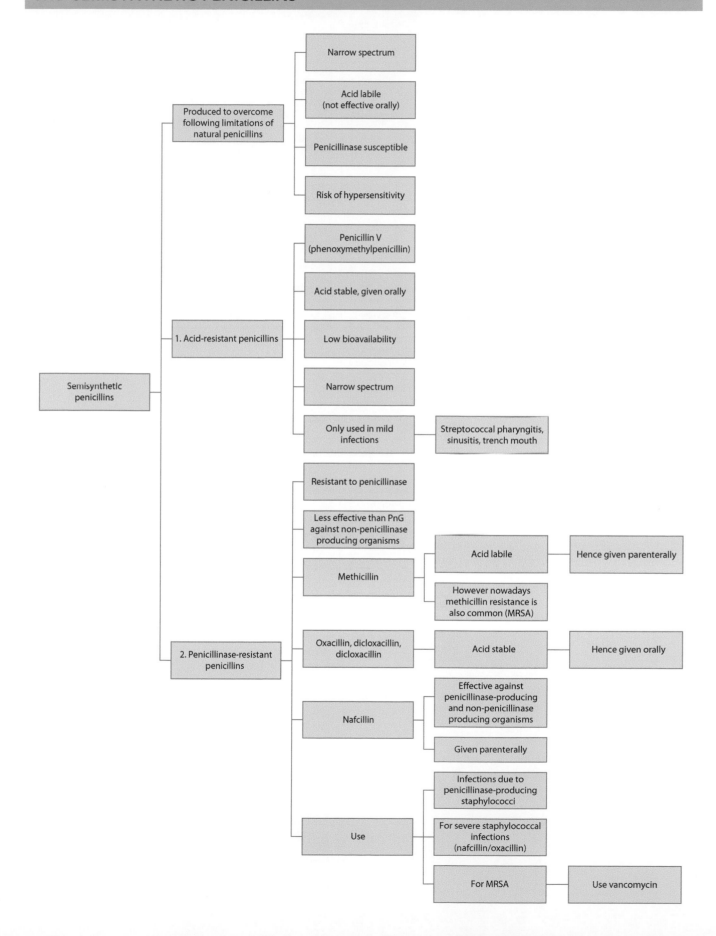

57.4 AMINOPENICILLIN

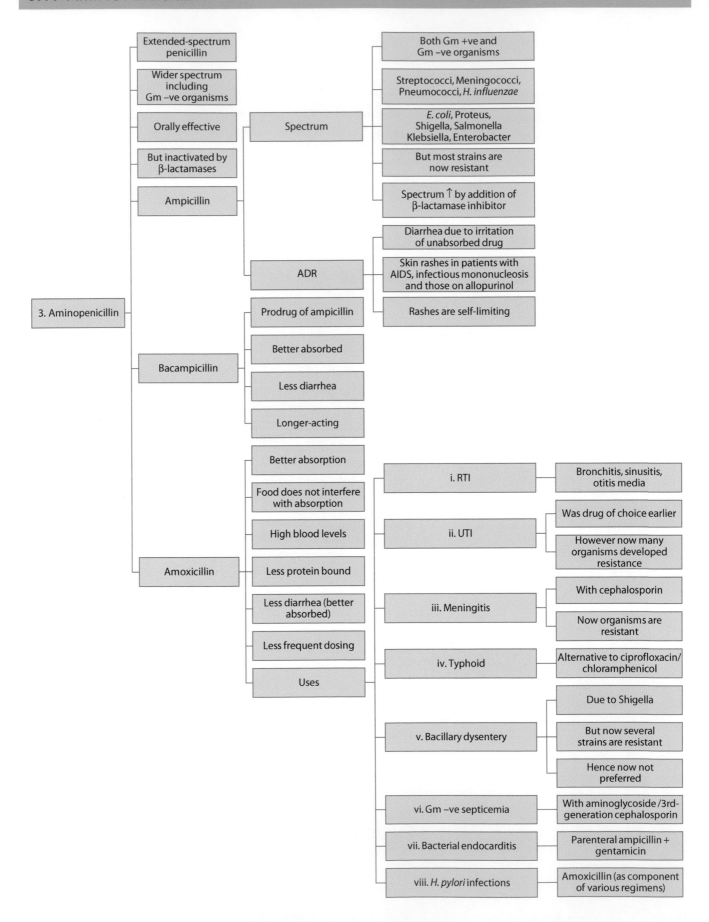

57.5 ANTIPSEUDOMONAL PENICILLINS

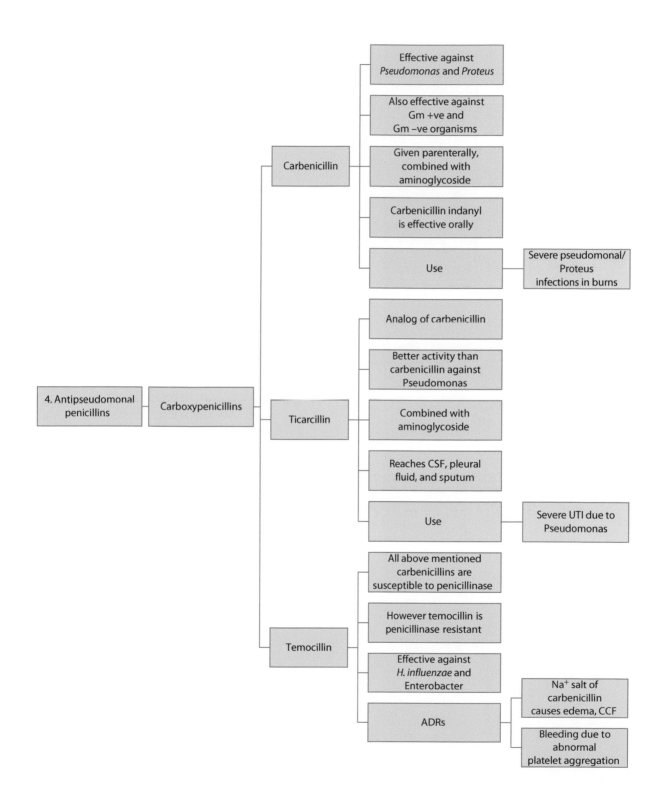

57.6 UREIDOPENICILLINS AND AMIDINOPENICILLINS

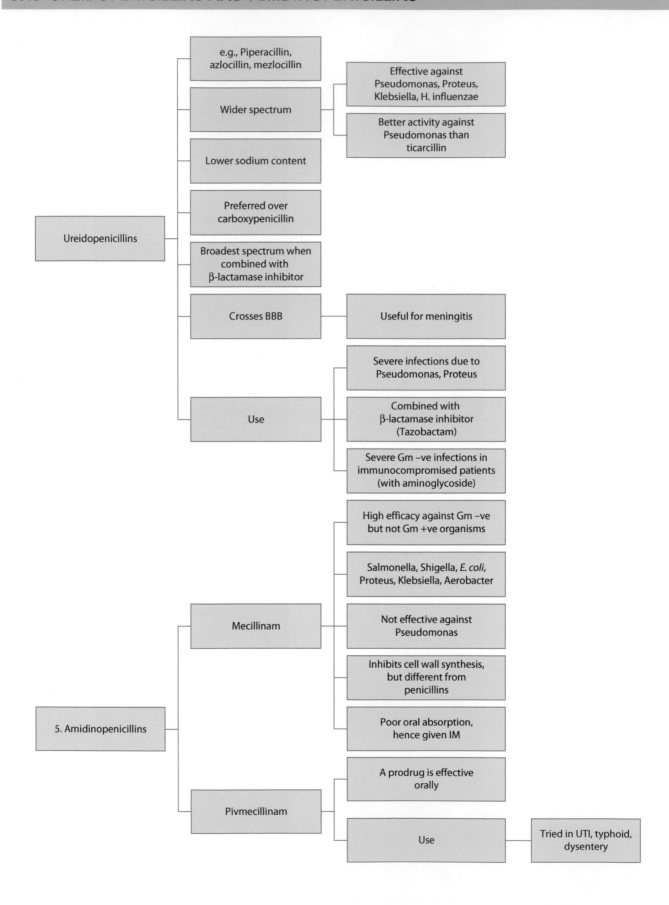

Ureidopenicillins

- e.g., Piperacillin, azlocillin, mezlocillin
- Wider spectrum
  - Effective against Pseudomonas, Proteus, Klebsiella, H. influenzae
  - Better activity against Pseudomonas than ticarcillin
- Lower sodium content
- Preferred over carboxypenicillin
- Broadest spectrum when combined with β-lactamase inhibitor
- Crosses BBB
  - Useful for meningitis
- Use
  - Severe infections due to Pseudomonas, Proteus
  - Combined with β-lactamase inhibitor (Tazobactam)
  - Severe Gm –ve infections in immunocompromised patients (with aminoglycoside)

5. Amidinopenicillins

- Mecillinam
  - High efficacy against Gm –ve but not Gm +ve organisms
  - Salmonella, Shigella, E. coli, Proteus, Klebsiella, Aerobacter
  - Not effective against Pseudomonas
  - Inhibits cell wall synthesis, but different from penicillins
  - Poor oral absorption, hence given IM
- Pivmecillinam
  - A prodrug is effective orally
  - Use
    - Tried in UTI, typhoid, dysentery

57.7 β-LACTAMASE INHIBITORS

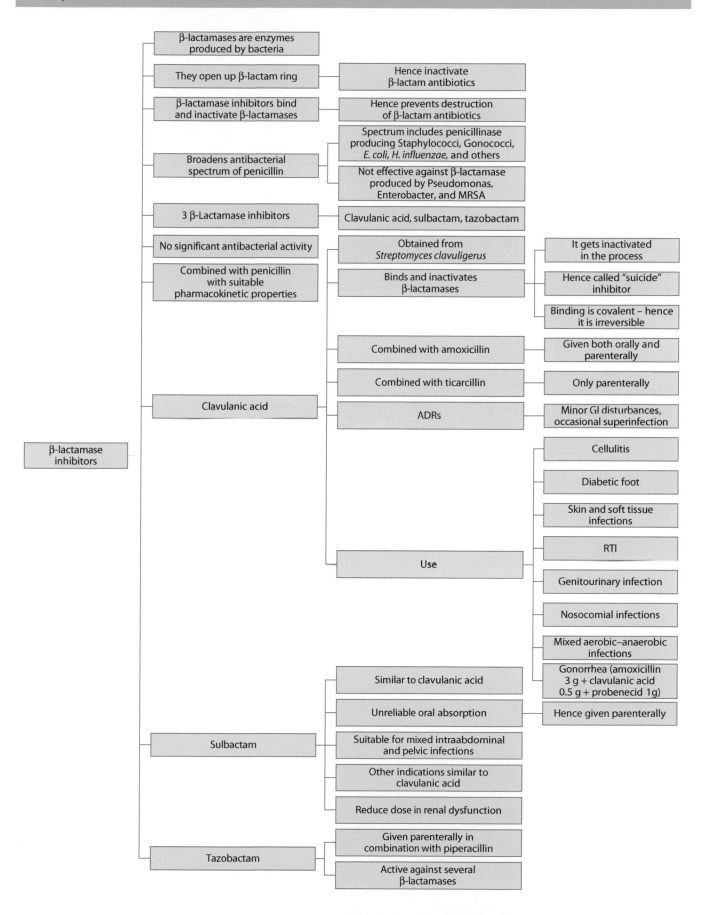

57.8 CEPHALOSPORINS

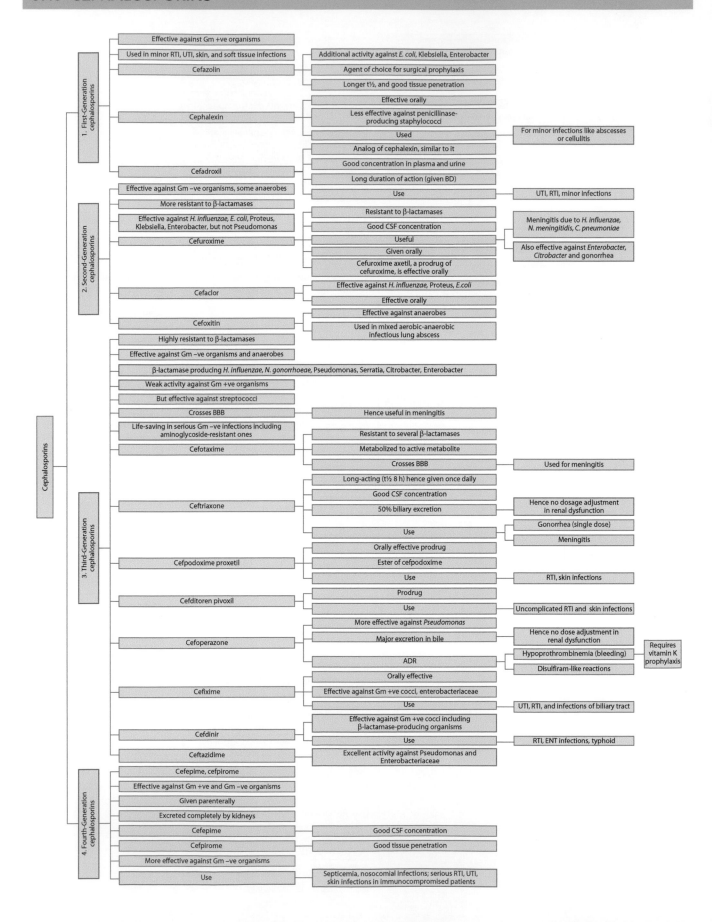

57.9 CEPHALOSPORINS – ADRs AND USE

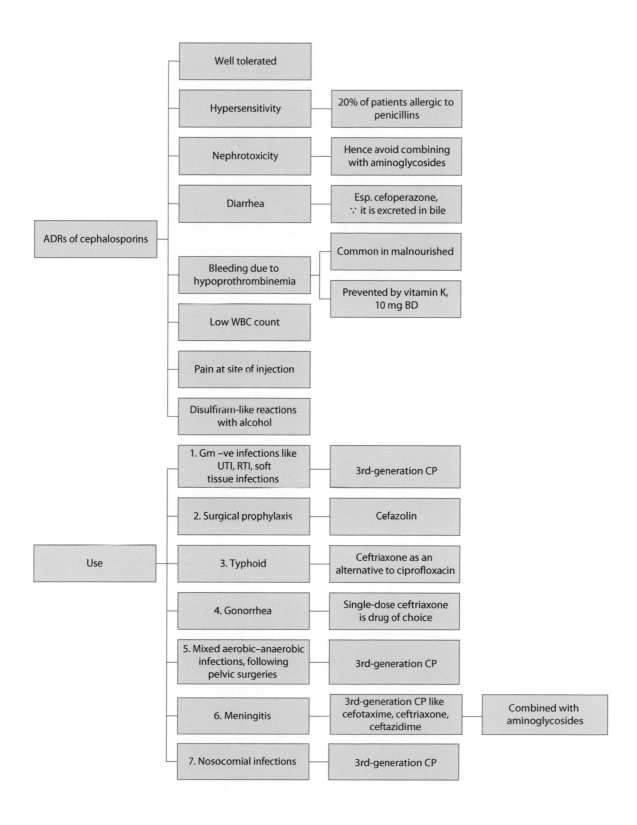

57.10 CARBAPENEMS

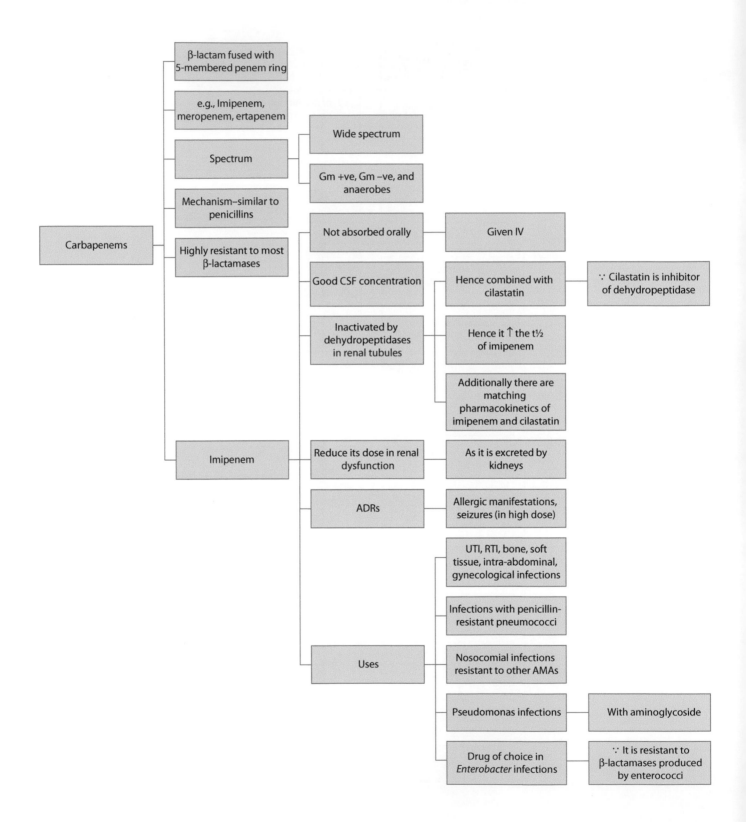

(Continued)

57.10 CARBAPENEMS (Continued)

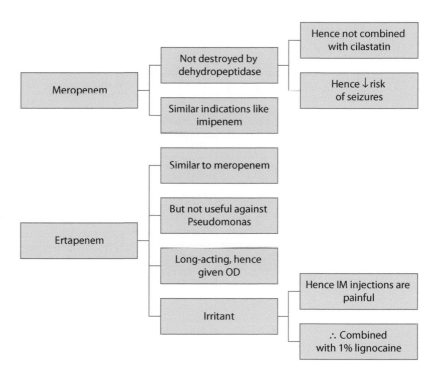

57.11 CARBACEPHEMS AND MONOBACTAMS

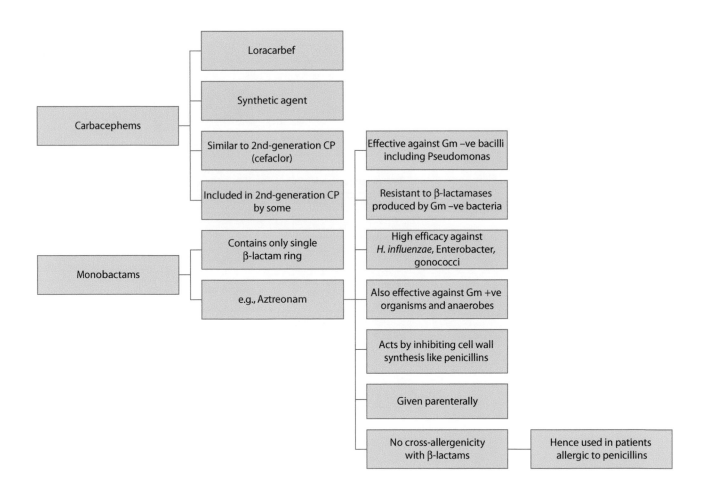

Sulfonamides

58.1 SULFONAMIDES – INTRODUCTION, CLASSIFICATION, SPECTRUM, MECHANISM OF ACTION, AND RESISTANCE

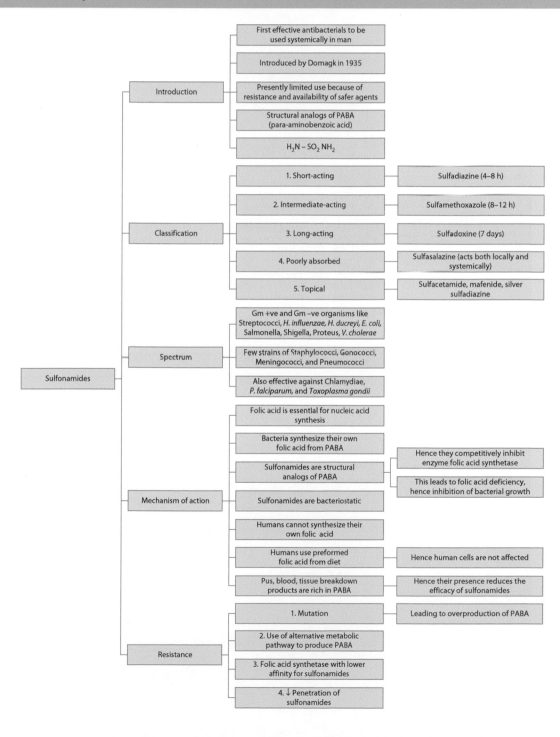

Sulfonamides

Introduction
- First effective antibacterials to be used systemically in man
- Introduced by Domagk in 1935
- Presently limited use because of resistance and availability of safer agents
- Structural analogs of PABA (para-aminobenzoic acid)
- $H_2N - SO_2 NH_2$

Classification
- 1. Short-acting → Sulfadiazine (4–8 h)
- 2. Intermediate-acting → Sulfamethoxazole (8–12 h)
- 3. Long-acting → Sulfadoxine (7 days)
- 4. Poorly absorbed → Sulfasalazine (acts both locally and systemically)
- 5. Topical → Sulfacetamide, mafenide, silver sulfadiazine

Spectrum
- Gm +ve and Gm –ve organisms like Streptococci, *H. influenzae*, *H. ducreyi*, *E. coli*, Salmonella, Shigella, Proteus, *V. cholerae*
- Few strains of Staphylococci, Gonococci, Meningococci, and Pneumococci
- Also effective against Chlamydiae, *P. falciparum*, and *Toxoplasma gondii*

Mechanism of action
- Folic acid is essential for nucleic acid synthesis
- Bacteria synthesize their own folic acid from PABA
- Sulfonamides are structural analogs of PABA
  - Hence they competitively inhibit enzyme folic acid synthetase
  - This leads to folic acid deficiency, hence inhibition of bacterial growth
- Sulfonamides are bacteriostatic
- Humans cannot synthesize their own folic acid
- Humans use preformed folic acid from diet → Hence human cells are not affected
- Pus, blood, tissue breakdown products are rich in PABA → Hence their presence reduces the efficacy of sulfonamides

Resistance
- 1. Mutation → Leading to overproduction of PABA
- 2. Use of alternative metabolic pathway to produce PABA
- 3. Folic acid synthetase with lower affinity for sulfonamides
- 4. ↓ Penetration of sulfonamides

58.2 SULFONAMIDES – PHARMACOKINETICS, ADVERSE EFFECTS, AND USES

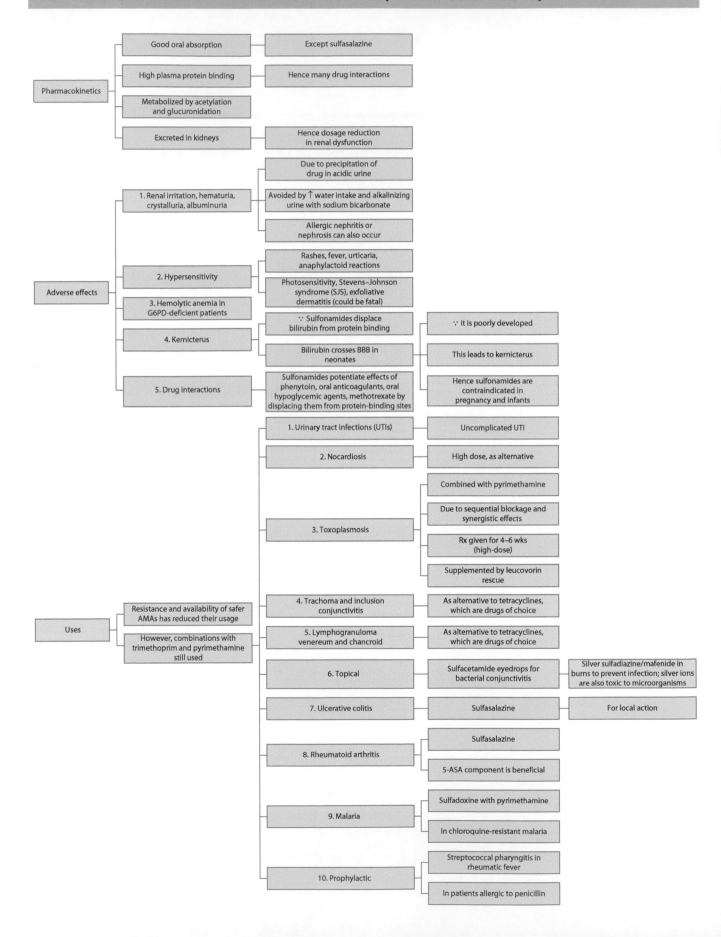

Pharmacokinetics
- Good oral absorption — Except sulfasalazine
- High plasma protein binding — Hence many drug interactions
- Metabolized by acetylation and glucuronidation
- Excreted in kidneys — Hence dosage reduction in renal dysfunction

Adverse effects
- 1. Renal irritation, hematuria, crystalluria, albuminuria
  - Due to precipitation of drug in acidic urine
  - Avoided by ↑ water intake and alkalinizing urine with sodium bicarbonate
  - Allergic nephritis or nephrosis can also occur
- 2. Hypersensitivity
  - Rashes, fever, urticaria, anaphylactoid reactions
  - Photosensitivity, Stevens–Johnson syndrome (SJS), exfoliative dermatitis (could be fatal)
- 3. Hemolytic anemia in G6PD-deficient patients
- 4. Kernicterus
  - ∵ Sulfonamides displace bilirubin from protein binding — ∵ It is poorly developed
  - Bilirubin crosses BBB in neonates — This leads to kernicterus
- 5. Drug interactions
  - Sulfonamides potentiate effects of phenytoin, oral anticoagulants, oral hypoglycemic agents, methotrexate by displacing them from protein-binding sites — Hence sulfonamides are contraindicated in pregnancy and infants

Uses
- Resistance and availability of safer AMAs has reduced their usage
- However, combinations with trimethoprim and pyrimethamine still used
  - 1. Urinary tract infections (UTIs) — Uncomplicated UTI
  - 2. Nocardiosis — High dose, as alternative
  - 3. Toxoplasmosis
    - Combined with pyrimethamine
    - Due to sequential blockage and synergistic effects
    - Rx given for 4–6 wks (high-dose)
    - Supplemented by leucovorin rescue
  - 4. Trachoma and inclusion conjunctivitis — As alternative to tetracyclines, which are drugs of choice
  - 5. Lymphogranuloma venereum and chancroid — As alternative to tetracyclines, which are drugs of choice
  - 6. Topical — Sulfacetamide eyedrops for bacterial conjunctivitis — Silver sulfadiazine/mafenide in burns to prevent infection; silver ions are also toxic to microorganisms
  - 7. Ulcerative colitis — Sulfasalazine — For local action
  - 8. Rheumatoid arthritis
    - Sulfasalazine
    - 5-ASA component is beneficial
  - 9. Malaria
    - Sulfadoxine with pyrimethamine
    - In chloroquine-resistant malaria
  - 10. Prophylactic
    - Streptococcal pharyngitis in rheumatic fever
    - In patients allergic to penicillin

58.3 COTRIMOXAZOLE

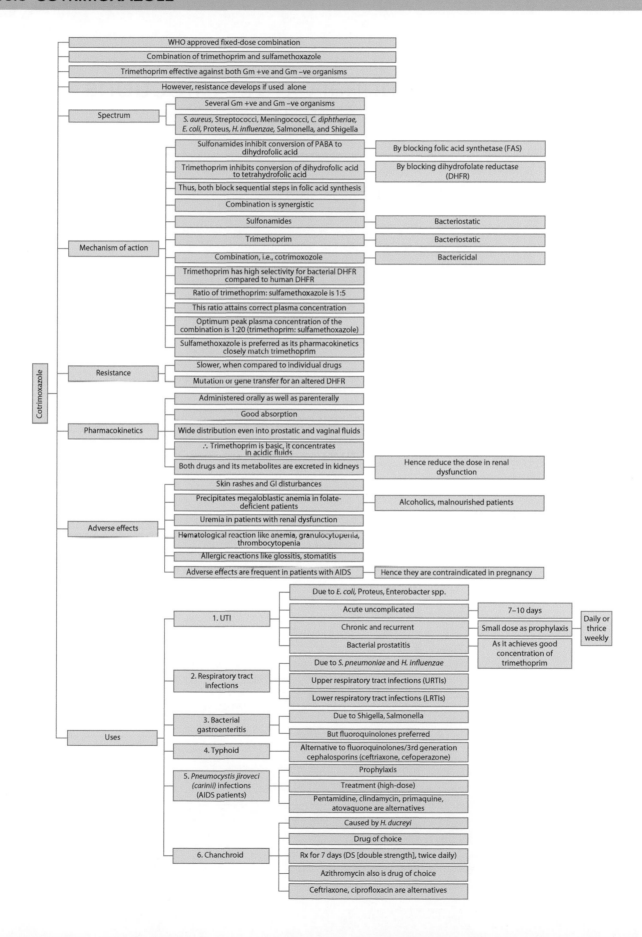

59

Chemotherapy of urinary tract infections and sexually transmitted diseases

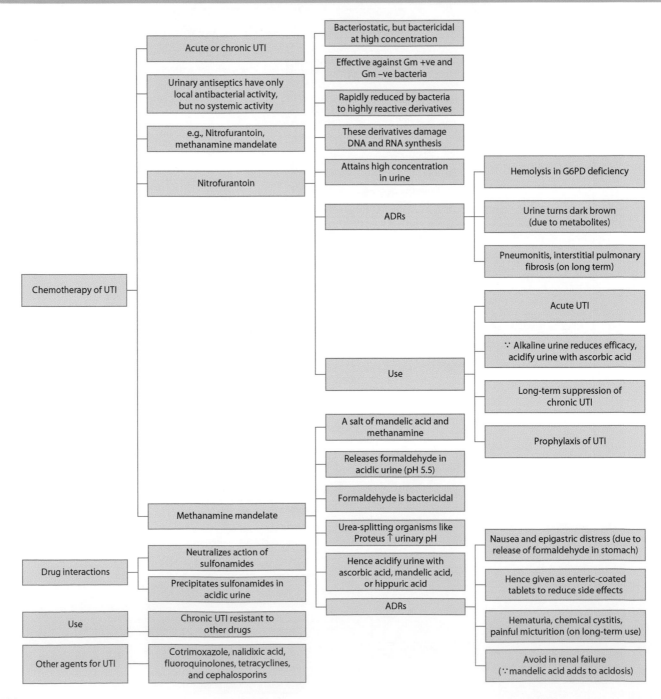

59.2 URINARY ANALGESICS

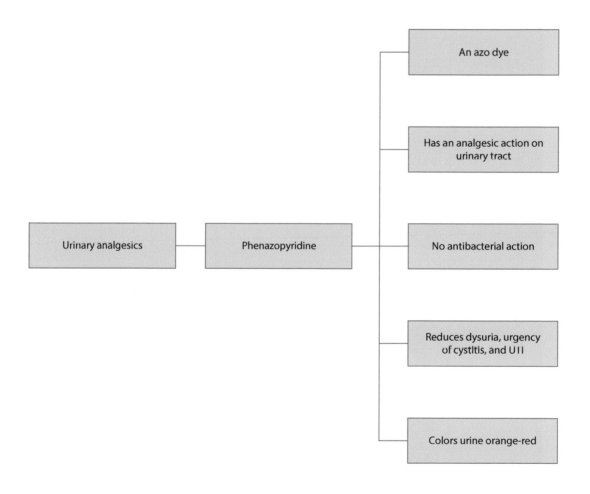

59.3 CHEMOTHERAPY OF SEXUALLY TRANSMITTED DISEASES

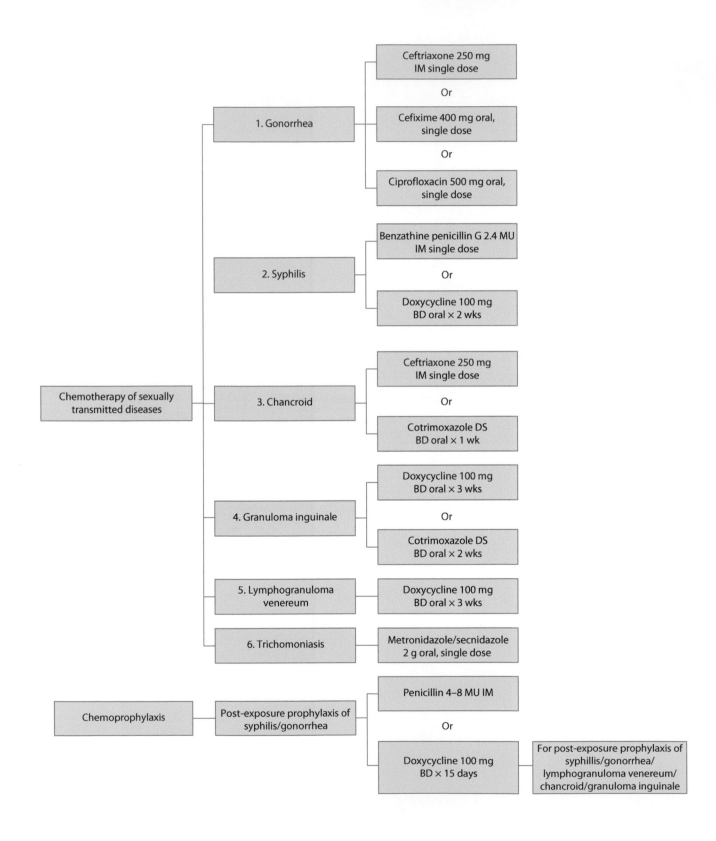

60

Quinolones

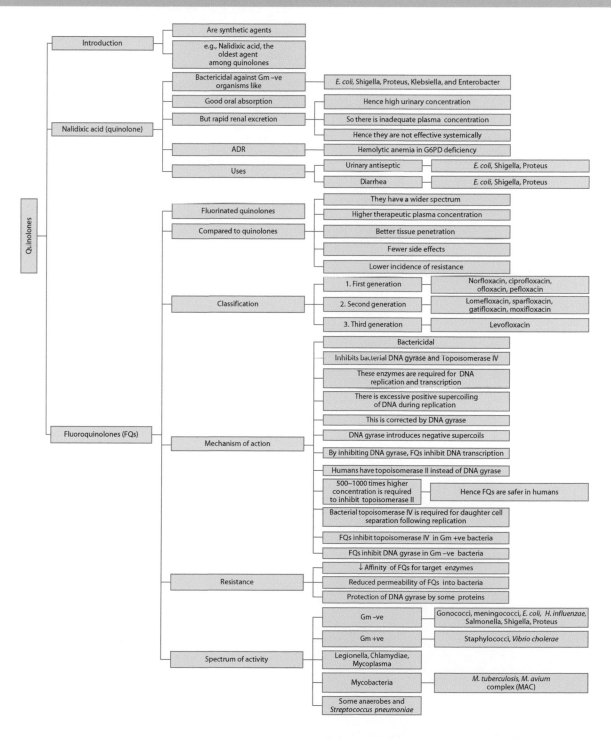

60.2 INDIVIDUAL AGENTS

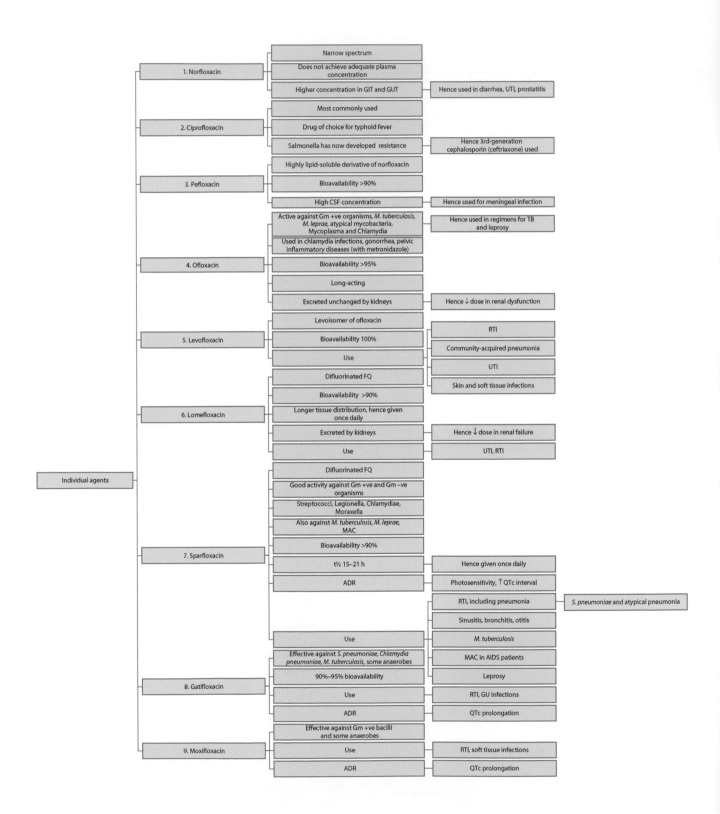

61

Macrolides

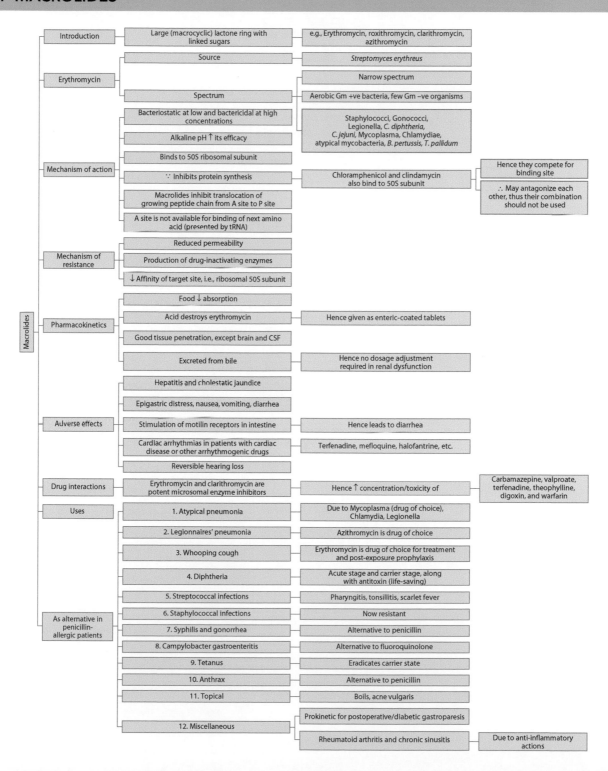

Introduction	Large (macrocyclic) lactone ring with linked sugars	e.g., Erythromycin, roxithromycin, clarithromycin, azithromycin
Erythromycin	Source	*Streptomyces erythreus*
	Spectrum	Narrow spectrum
		Aerobic Gm +ve bacteria, few Gm –ve organisms
Mechanism of action	Bacteriostatic at low and bactericidal at high concentrations	Staphylococci, Gonococci, Legionella, C. diphtheria, C. jejuni, Mycoplasma, Chlamydiae, atypical mycobacteria, B. pertussis, T. pallidum
	Alkaline pH ↑ its efficacy	
	Binds to 50S ribosomal subunit	
	∴ Inhibits protein synthesis	Chloramphenicol and clindamycin also bind to 50S subunit → Hence they compete for binding site; ∴ May antagonize each other, thus their combination should not be used
	Macrolides inhibit translocation of growing peptide chain from A site to P site	
	A site is not available for binding of next amino acid (presented by tRNA)	
Mechanism of resistance	Reduced permeability	
	Production of drug-inactivating enzymes	
	↓ Affinity of target site, i.e., ribosomal 50S subunit	
Pharmacokinetics	Food ↓ absorption	
	Acid destroys erythromycin	Hence given as enteric-coated tablets
	Good tissue penetration, except brain and CSF	
	Excreted from bile	Hence no dosage adjustment required in renal dysfunction
Adverse effects	Hepatitis and cholestatic jaundice	
	Epigastric distress, nausea, vomiting, diarrhea	
	Stimulation of motilin receptors in intestine	Hence leads to diarrhea
	Cardiac arrhythmias in patients with cardiac disease or other arrhythmogenic drugs	Terfenadine, mefloquine, halofantrine, etc.
	Reversible hearing loss	
Drug interactions	Erythromycin and clarithromycin are potent microsomal enzyme inhibitors	Hence ↑ concentration/toxicity of → Carbamazepine, valproate, terfenadine, theophylline, digoxin, and warfarin
Uses	1. Atypical pneumonia	Due to Mycoplasma (drug of choice), Chlamydia, Legionella
	2. Legionnaires' pneumonia	Azithromycin is drug of choice
	3. Whooping cough	Erythromycin is drug of choice for treatment and post-exposure prophylaxis
	4. Diphtheria	Acute stage and carrier stage, along with antitoxin (life-saving)
As alternative in penicillin-allergic patients	5. Streptococcal infections	Pharyngitis, tonsillitis, scarlet fever
	6. Staphylococcal infections	Now resistant
	7. Syphilis and gonorrhea	Alternative to penicillin
	8. Campylobacter gastroenteritis	Alternative to fluoroquinolone
	9. Tetanus	Eradicates carrier state
	10. Anthrax	Alternative to penicillin
	11. Topical	Boils, acne vulgaris
	12. Miscellaneous	Prokinetic for postoperative/diabetic gastroparesis
		Rheumatoid arthritis and chronic sinusitis → Due to anti-inflammatory actions

533

61.2 INDIVIDUAL MACROLIDES AND COMPARISON

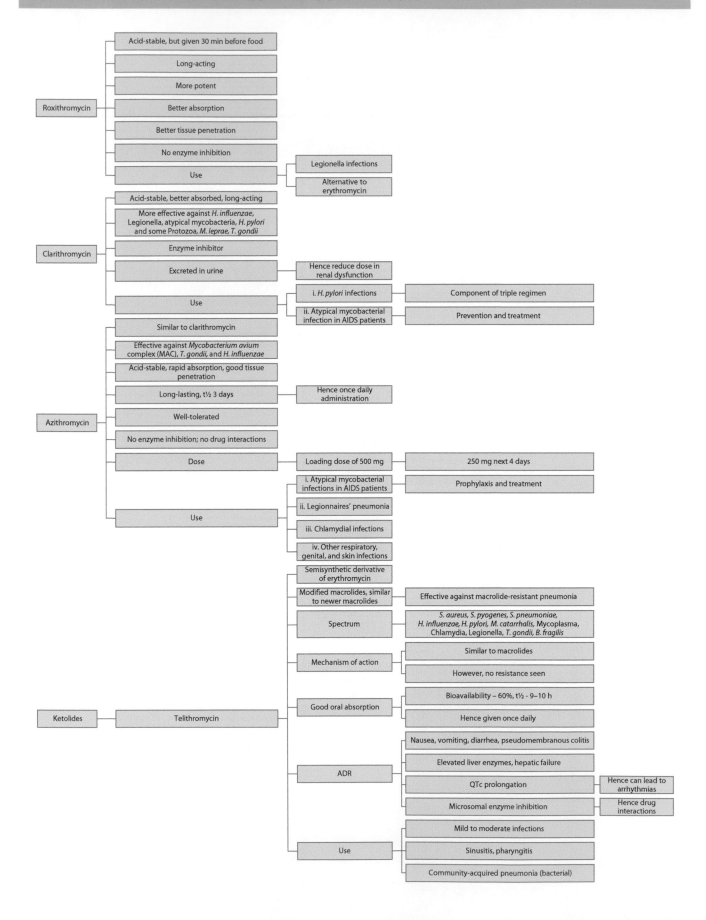

Roxithromycin
- Acid-stable, but given 30 min before food
- Long-acting
- More potent
- Better absorption
- Better tissue penetration
- No enzyme inhibition
- Use
  - Legionella infections
  - Alternative to erythromycin

Clarithromycin
- Acid-stable, better absorbed, long-acting
- More effective against *H. influenzae*, Legionella, atypical mycobacteria, *H. pylori* and some Protozoa, *M. leprae*, *T. gondii*
- Enzyme inhibitor
- Excreted in urine
  - Hence reduce dose in renal dysfunction
- Use
  - i. *H. pylori* infections — Component of triple regimen
  - ii. Atypical mycobacterial infection in AIDS patients — Prevention and treatment

Azithromycin
- Similar to clarithromycin
- Effective against *Mycobacterium avium* complex (MAC), *T. gondii*, and *H. influenzae*
- Acid-stable, rapid absorption, good tissue penetration
- Long-lasting, t½ 3 days
  - Hence once daily administration
- Well-tolerated
- No enzyme inhibition; no drug interactions
- Dose
  - Loading dose of 500 mg — 250 mg next 4 days
- Use
  - i. Atypical mycobacterial infections in AIDS patients — Prophylaxis and treatment
  - ii. Legionnaires' pneumonia
  - iii. Chlamydial infections
  - iv. Other respiratory, genital, and skin infections

Ketolides — **Telithromycin**
- Semisynthetic derivative of erythromycin
- Modified macrolides, similar to newer macrolides — Effective against macrolide-resistant pneumonia
- Spectrum — *S. aureus, S. pyogenes, S. pneumoniae, H. influenzae, H. pylori, M. catarrhalis*, Mycoplasma, Chlamydia, Legionella, *T. gondii, B. fragilis*
- Mechanism of action
  - Similar to macrolides
  - However, no resistance seen
- Good oral absorption
  - Bioavailability – 60%, t½ - 9–10 h
  - Hence given once daily
- ADR
  - Nausea, vomiting, diarrhea, pseudomembranous colitis
  - Elevated liver enzymes, hepatic failure
  - QTc prolongation — Hence can lead to arrhythmias
  - Microsomal enzyme inhibition — Hence drug interactions
- Use
  - Mild to moderate infections
  - Sinusitis, pharyngitis
  - Community-acquired pneumonia (bacterial)

Broad-spectrum antibiotics – Tetracyclines and chloramphenicol

62.1 TETRACYCLINES – INTRODUCTION, CLASSIFICATION, AND MECHANISM OF ACTION

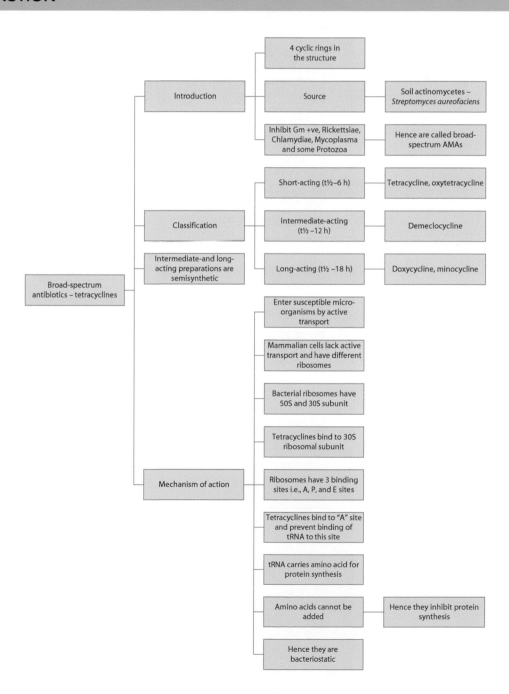

62.2 SPECTRUM OF ACTIVITY AND RESISTANCE

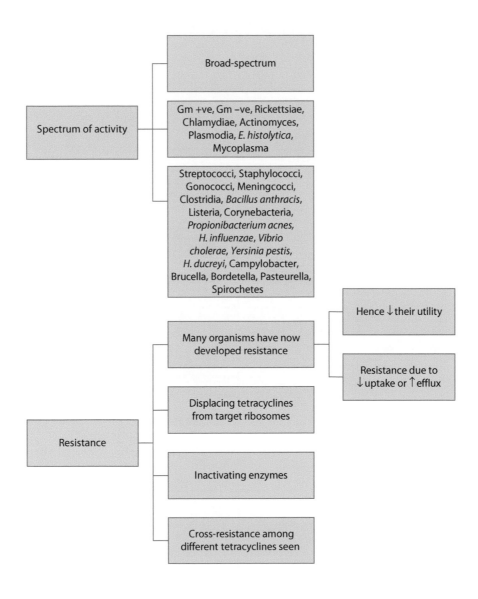

62.3 PHARMACOKINETICS AND ADMINISTRATION

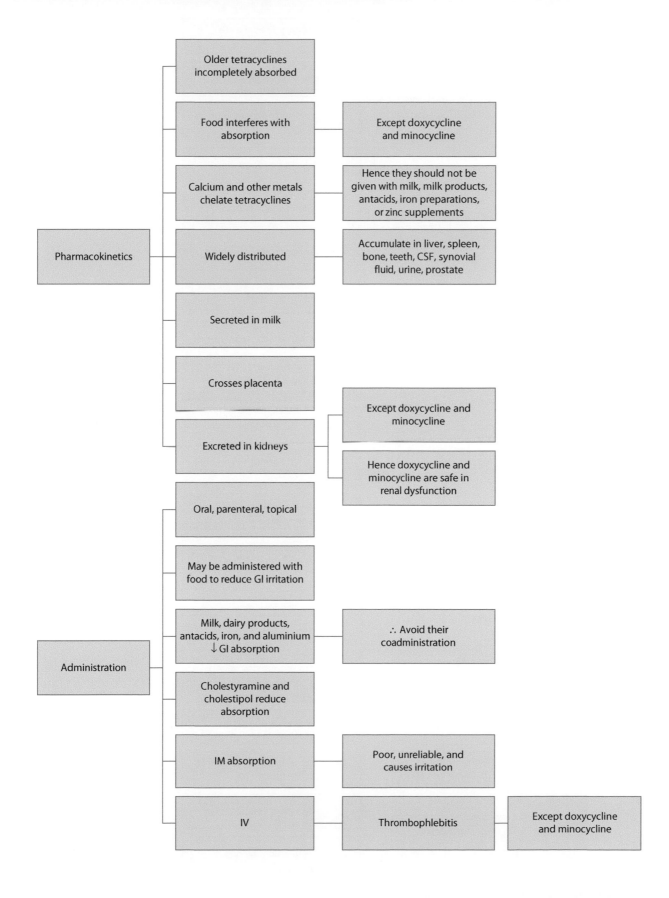

62.4 ADVERSE EFFECTS

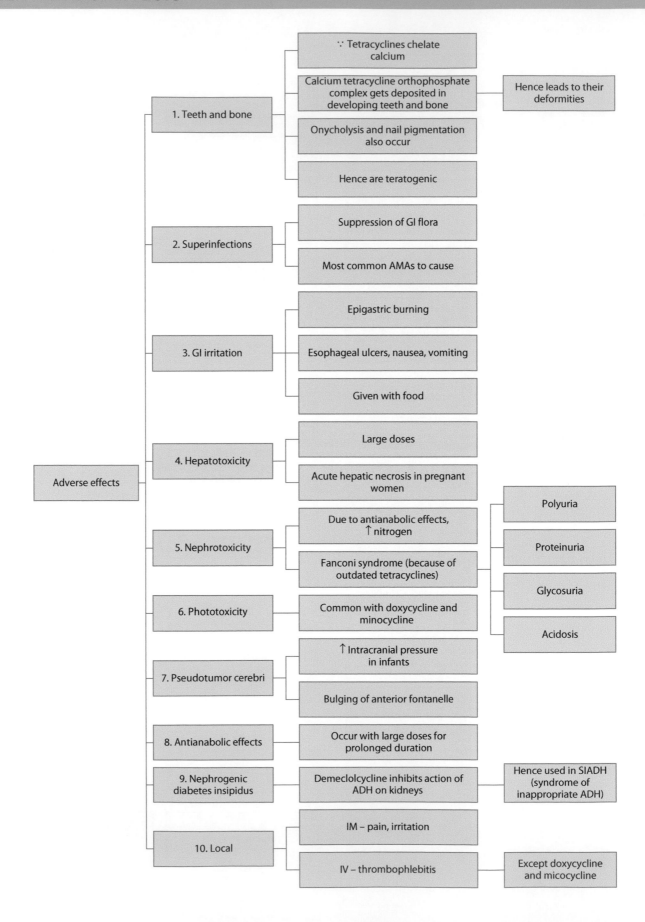

62.5 USES

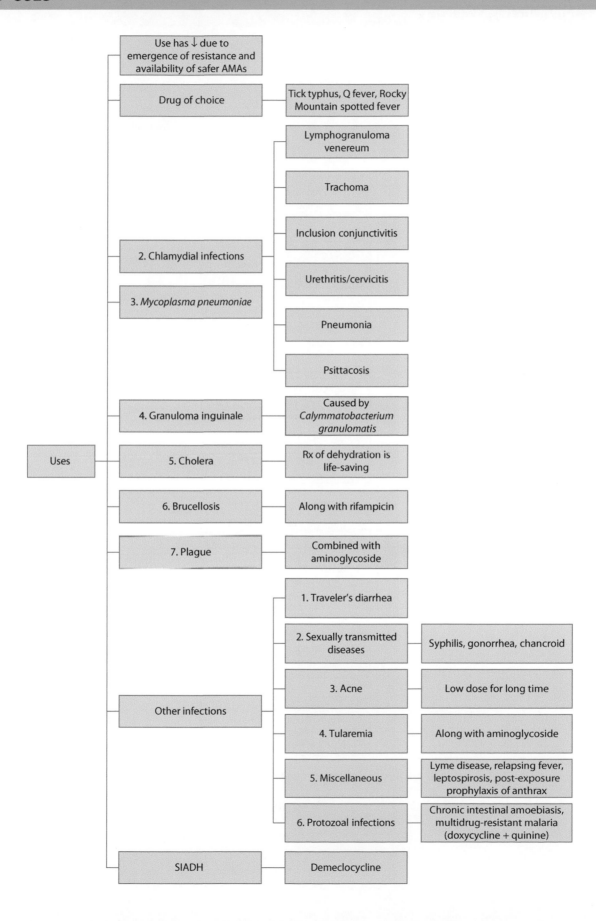

62.6 CONTRAINDICATIONS AND ADVANTAGES/FEATURES OF DOXYCYLINE AND MINOCYCLINE

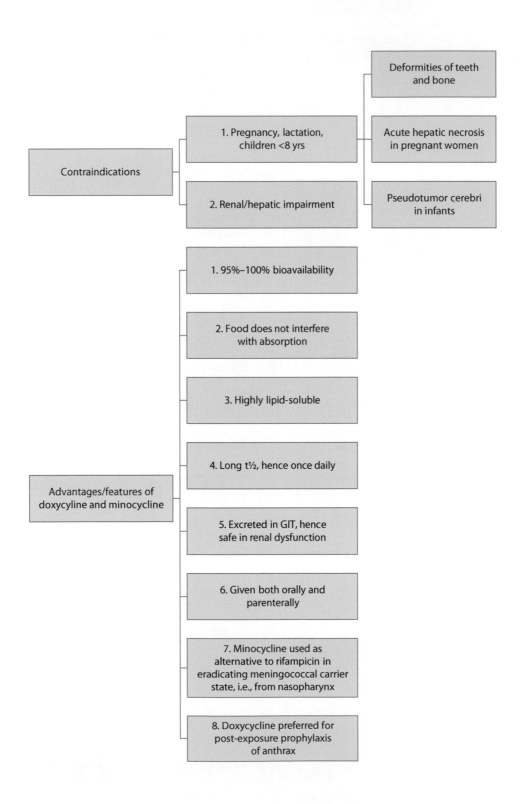

Contraindications

1. Pregnancy, lactation, children <8 yrs

2. Renal/hepatic impairment

Deformities of teeth and bone

Acute hepatic necrosis in pregnant women

Pseudotumor cerebri in infants

Advantages/features of doxycyline and minocycline

1. 95%–100% bioavailability

2. Food does not interfere with absorption

3. Highly lipid-soluble

4. Long t½, hence once daily

5. Excreted in GIT, hence safe in renal dysfunction

6. Given both orally and parenterally

7. Minocycline used as alternative to rifampicin in eradicating meningococcal carrier state, i.e., from nasopharynx

8. Doxycycline preferred for post-exposure prophylaxis of anthrax

62.7 COMPARE/CONTRAST – TETRACYCLINE vs. DOXYCYCLINE

	Tetracycline	Doxycycline
1. Source	Semisynthetic	Semisynthetic
2. GI absorption	Incomplete	Complete
3. Bioavailability	75%	95%
4. t½	8–10 h	18–24 h
5. Lipid solubility	Low	High
6. Dosing	QID	OD
7. Excretion	Kidney	GIT
8. Safety in renal impairment	Not safe	Safe
9. GI flora	High suppression	Low suppression
10. Phototoxicity	Low	High

62.8 CHLORAMPHENICOL – MECHANISM OF ACTION, SPECTRUM OF ACTIVITY, MECHANISM OF RESISTANCE, AND PHARMACOKINETICS

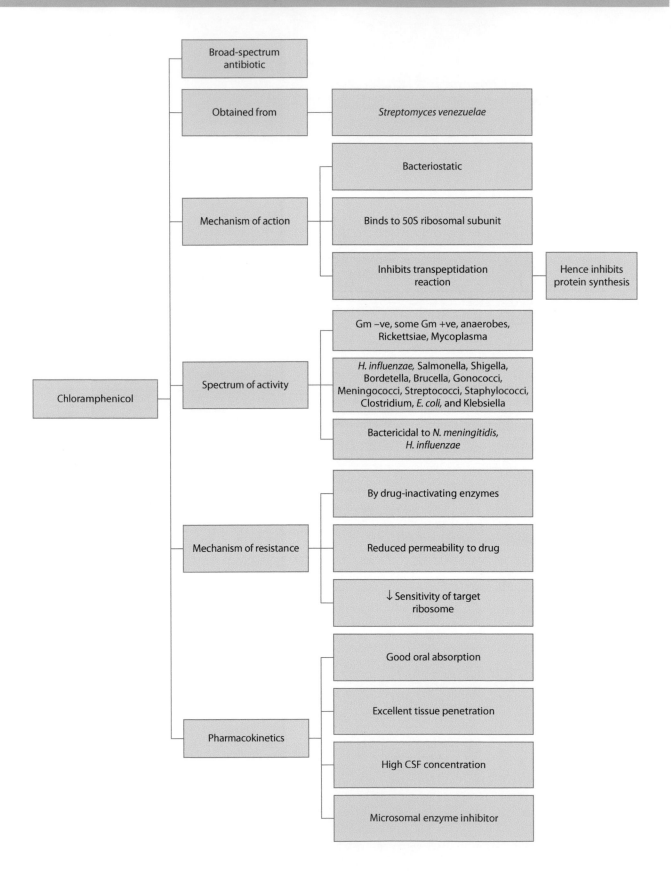

62.9 ADVERSE EFFECTS, DRUG INTERACTIONS, AND USES

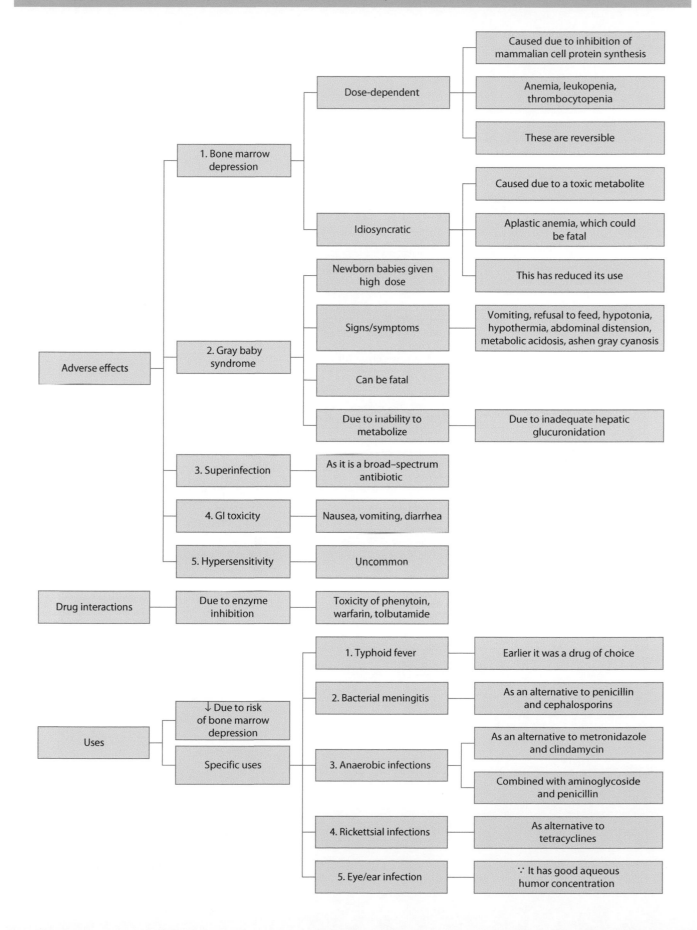

62.10 TIGECYCLINE

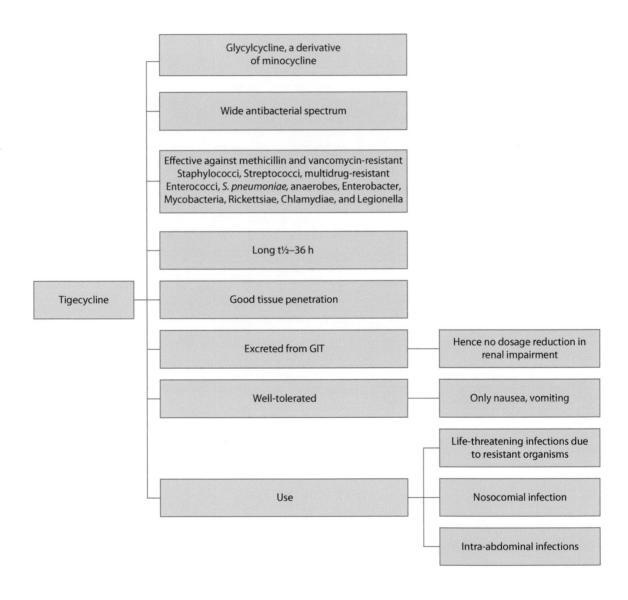

Aminoglycosides

63

63.1 INTRODUCTION AND COMMON PROPERTIES

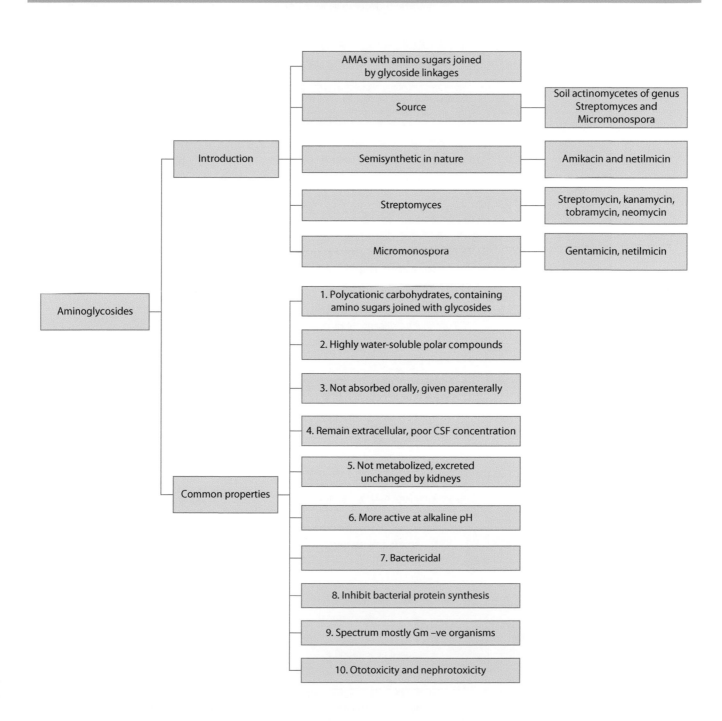

63.2 SPECTRUM, MECHANISM OF ACTION, AND MECHANISM OF RESISTANCE

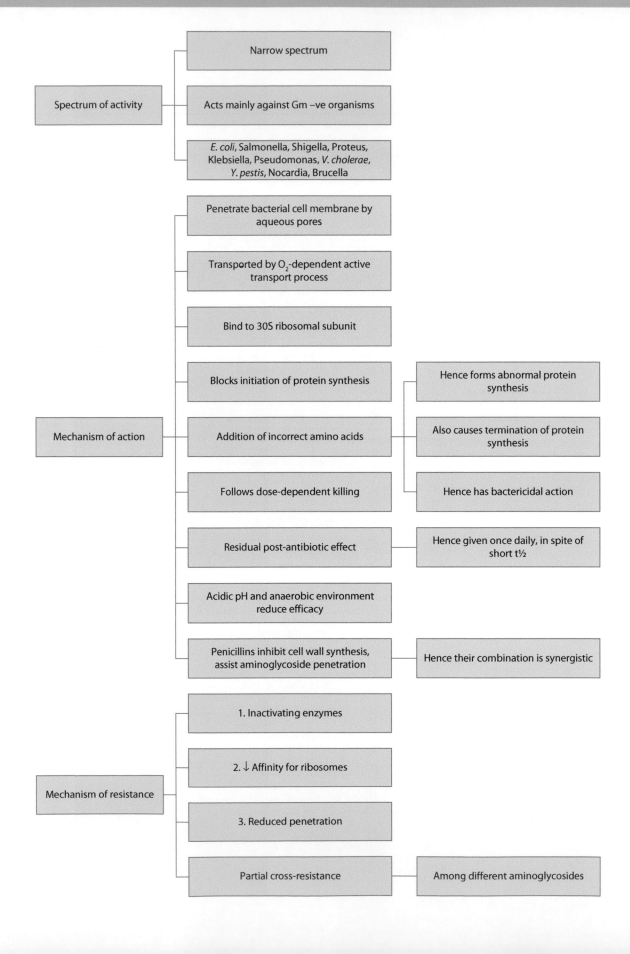

63.3 PHARMACOKINETICS AND ADRs

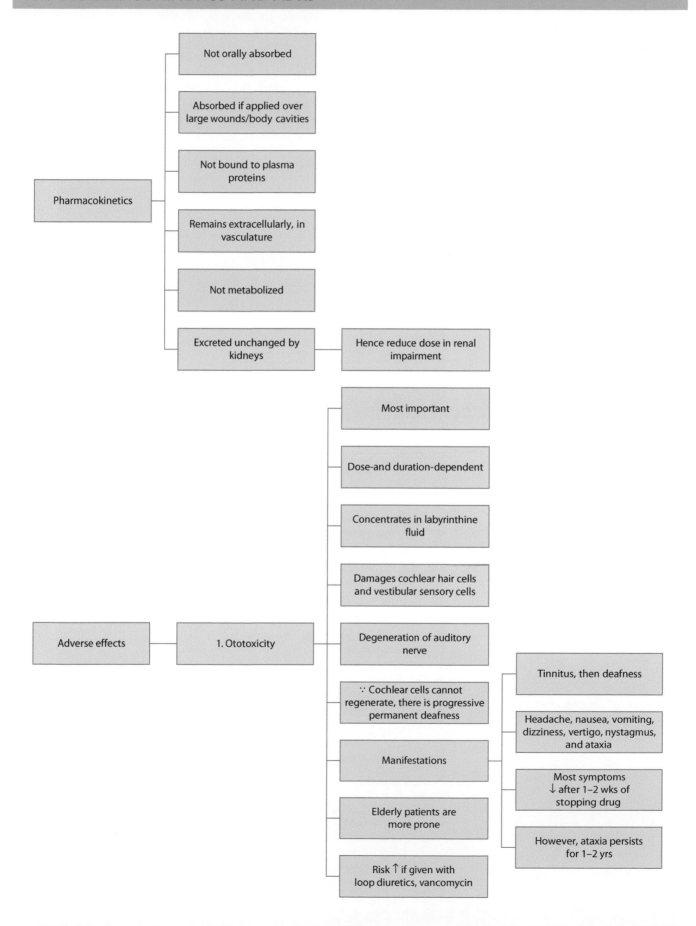

63.4 ADRs AND PRECAUTIONS

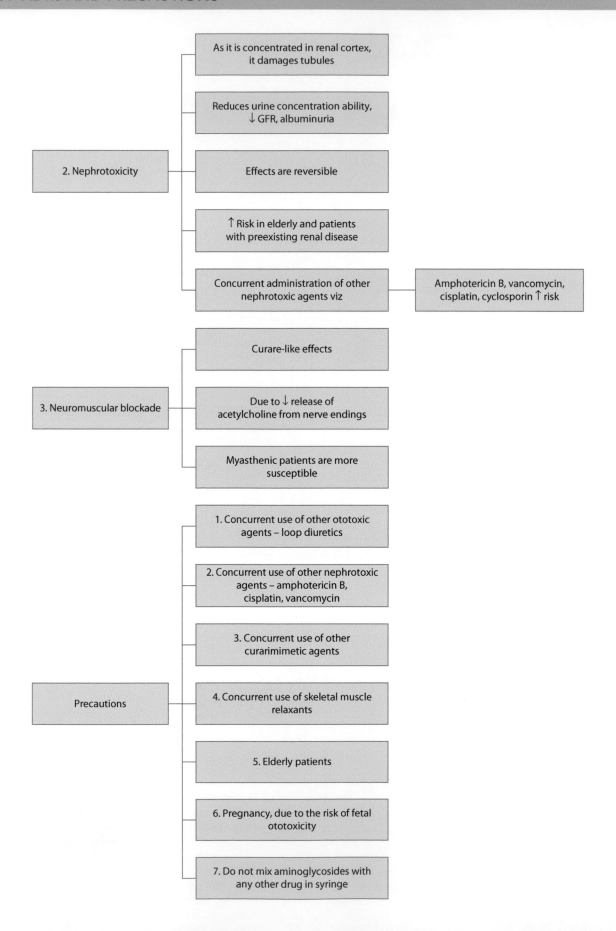

2. Nephrotoxicity
- As it is concentrated in renal cortex, it damages tubules
- Reduces urine concentration ability, ↓ GFR, albuminuria
- Effects are reversible
- ↑ Risk in elderly and patients with preexisting renal disease
- Concurrent administration of other nephrotoxic agents viz → Amphotericin B, vancomycin, cisplatin, cyclosporin ↑ risk

3. Neuromuscular blockade
- Curare-like effects
- Due to ↓ release of acetylcholine from nerve endings
- Myasthenic patients are more susceptible

Precautions
- 1. Concurrent use of other ototoxic agents – loop diuretics
- 2. Concurrent use of other nephrotoxic agents – amphotericin B, cisplatin, vancomycin
- 3. Concurrent use of other curarimimetic agents
- 4. Concurrent use of skeletal muscle relaxants
- 5. Elderly patients
- 6. Pregnancy, due to the risk of fetal ototoxicity
- 7. Do not mix aminoglycosides with any other drug in syringe

63.5 USES OF GENTAMICIN

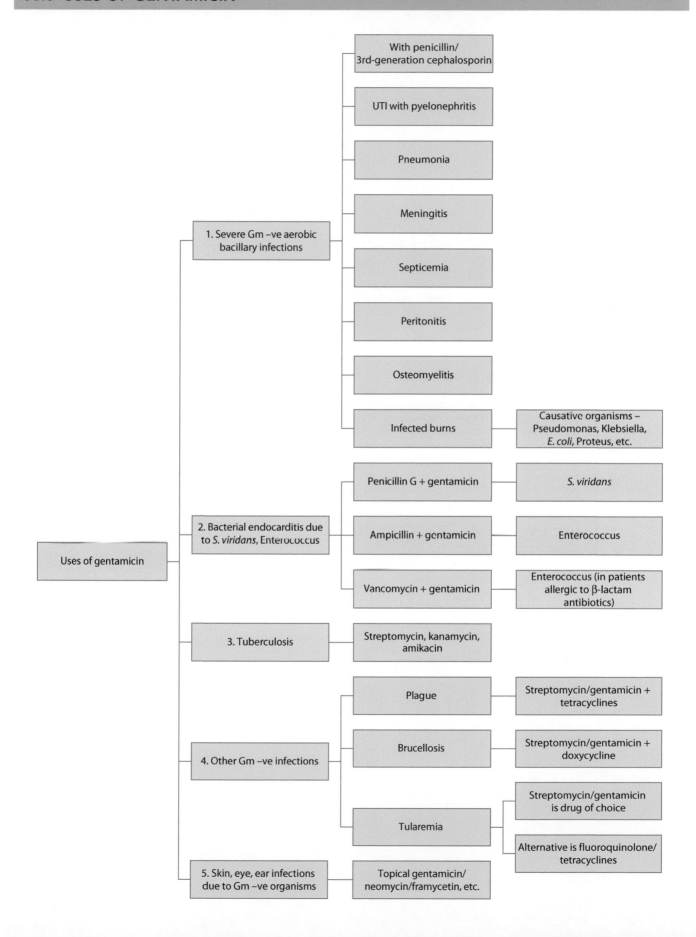

63.6 OTHER AMINOGLYCOSIDES

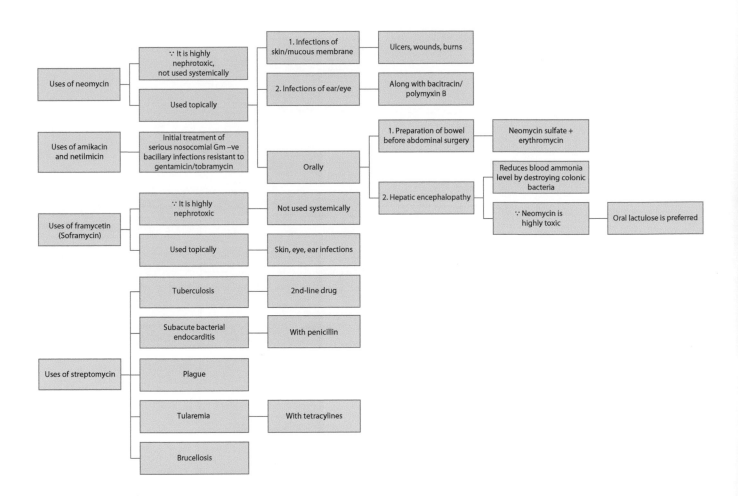

64

Miscellaneous antibiotics

64.1 LINCOSAMIDES, GLYCOPEPTIDES, AND TEICOPLANIN

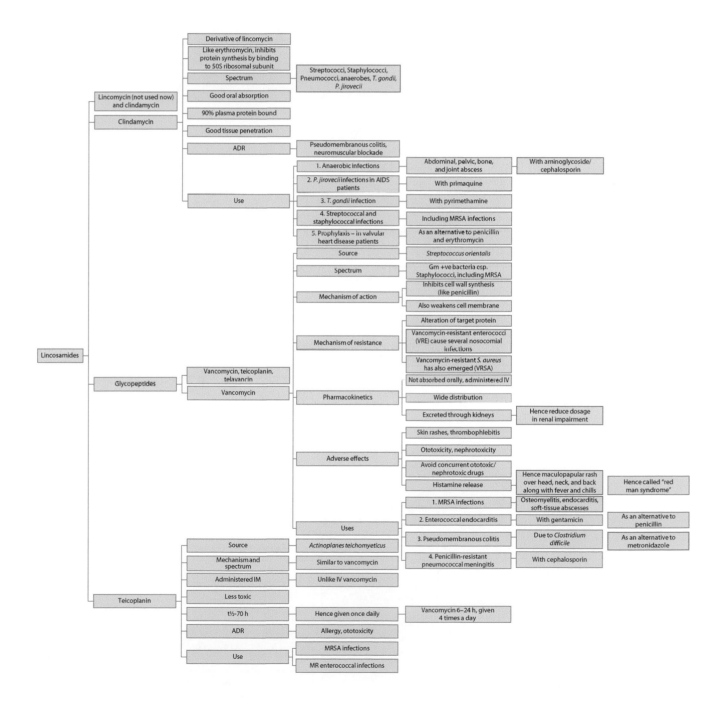

64.2 POLYPEPTIDE ANTIBIOTICS

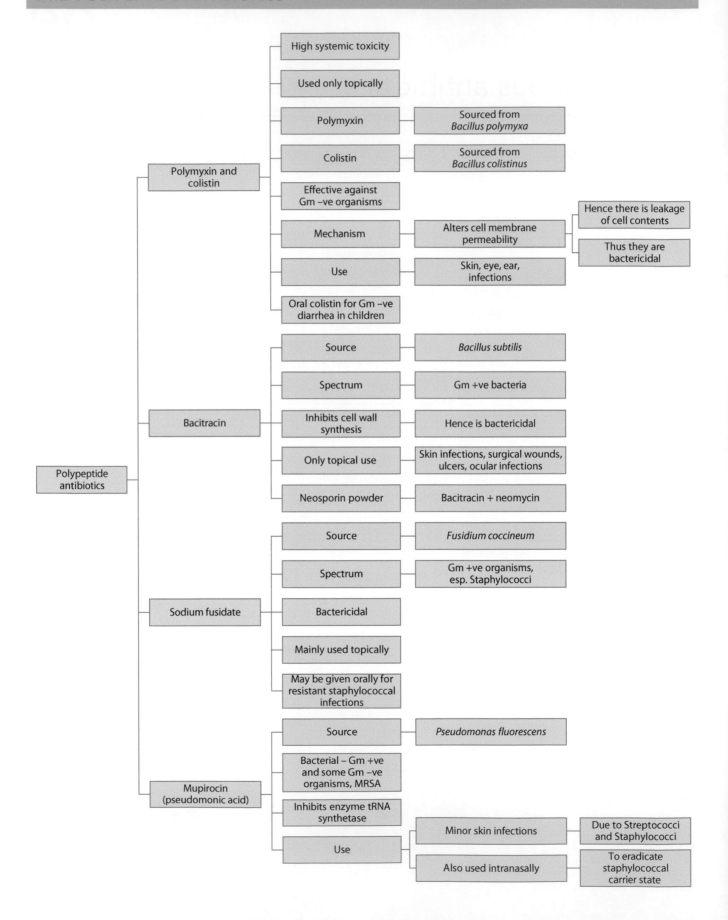

64.3 FOSFOMYCIN, STREPTOGRAMINS, OXAZOLIDINONES, AND DAPTOMYCIN

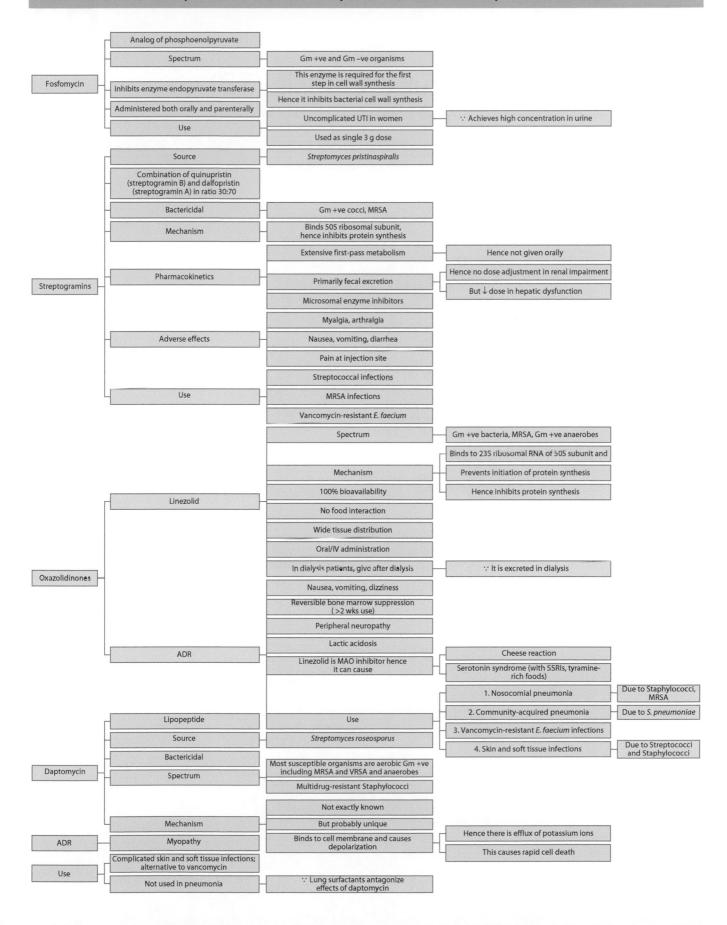

Chemotherapy of tuberculosis (TB)

65.1 INTRODUCTION AND CLASSIFICATION

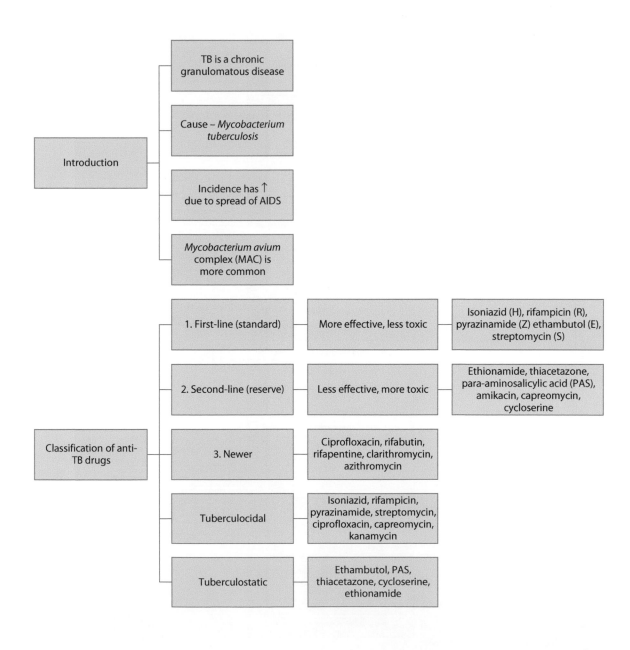

65.2 FIRST-LINE DRUGS – ISONIAZID

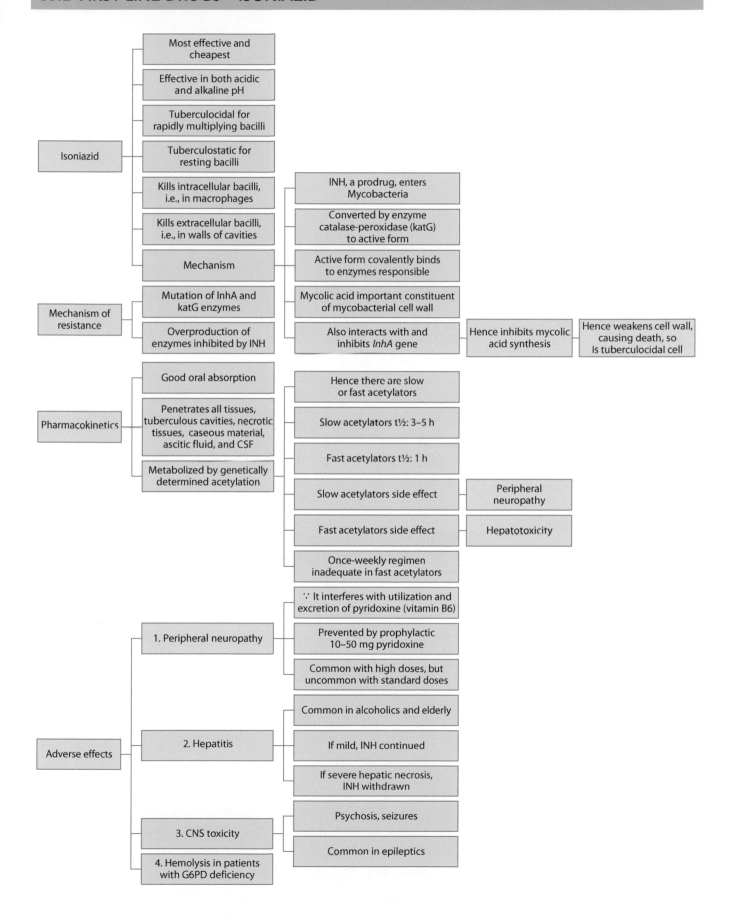

Isoniazid
- Most effective and cheapest
- Effective in both acidic and alkaline pH
- Tuberculocidal for rapidly multiplying bacilli
- Tuberculostatic for resting bacilli
- Kills intracellular bacilli, i.e., in macrophages
- Kills extracellular bacilli, i.e., in walls of cavities
- Mechanism
  - INH, a prodrug, enters Mycobacteria
  - Converted by enzyme catalase-peroxidase (katG) to active form
  - Active form covalently binds to enzymes responsible
  - Mycolic acid important constituent of mycobacterial cell wall
  - Also interacts with and inhibits *InhA* gene → Hence inhibits mycolic acid synthesis → Hence weakens cell wall, causing death, so Is tuberculocidal cell

Mechanism of resistance
- Mutation of InhA and katG enzymes
- Overproduction of enzymes inhibited by INH

Pharmacokinetics
- Good oral absorption
- Penetrates all tissues, tuberculous cavities, necrotic tissues, caseous material, ascitic fluid, and CSF
- Metabolized by genetically determined acetylation
  - Hence there are slow or fast acetylators
  - Slow acetylators t½: 3–5 h
  - Fast acetylators t½: 1 h
  - Slow acetylators side effect → Peripheral neuropathy
  - Fast acetylators side effect → Hepatotoxicity
  - Once-weekly regimen inadequate in fast acetylators

Adverse effects
- 1. Peripheral neuropathy
  - ∵ It interferes with utilization and excretion of pyridoxine (vitamin B6)
  - Prevented by prophylactic 10–50 mg pyridoxine
  - Common with high doses, but uncommon with standard doses
- 2. Hepatitis
  - Common in alcoholics and elderly
  - If mild, INH continued
  - If severe hepatic necrosis, INH withdrawn
- 3. CNS toxicity
  - Psychosis, seizures
  - Common in epileptics
- 4. Hemolysis in patients with G6PD deficiency

65.3 RIFAMPICIN (RIFAMPIN)

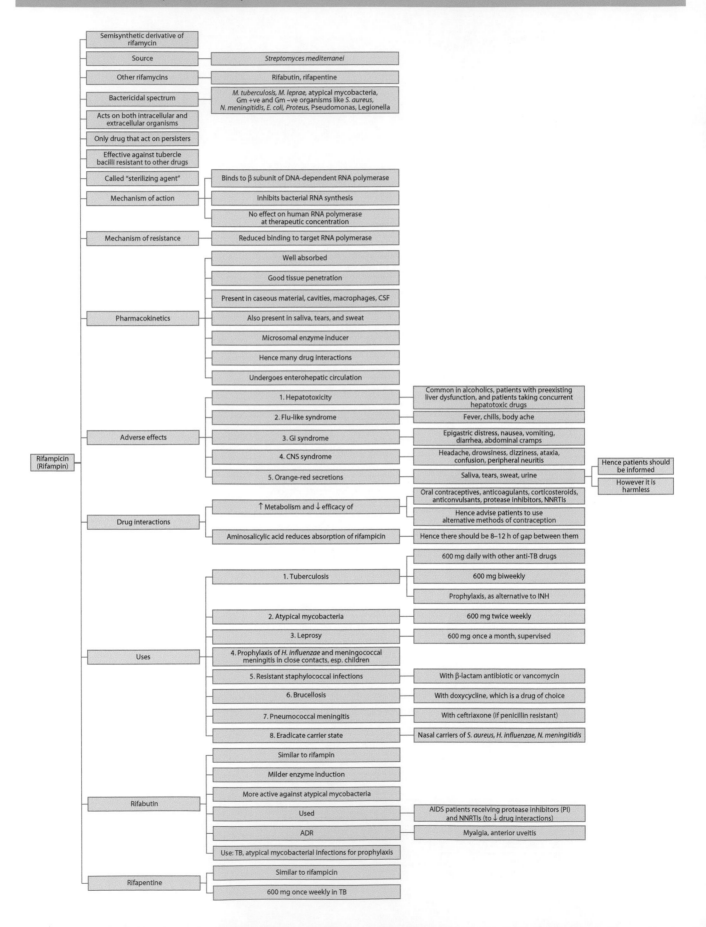

65.4 PYRAZINAMIDE, ETHAMBUTOL, AND STREPTOMYCIN

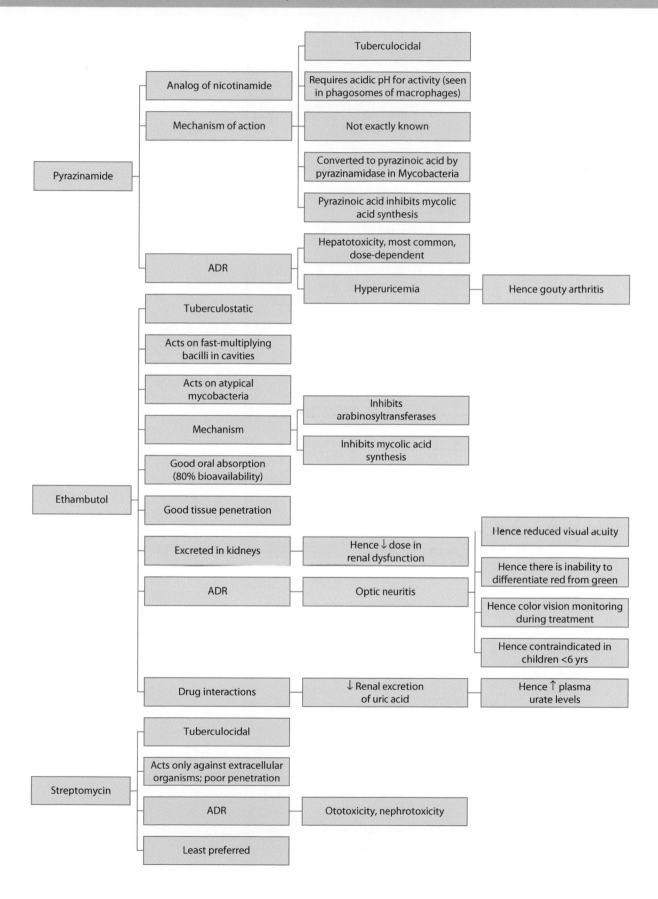

65.5 SECOND-LINE DRUGS

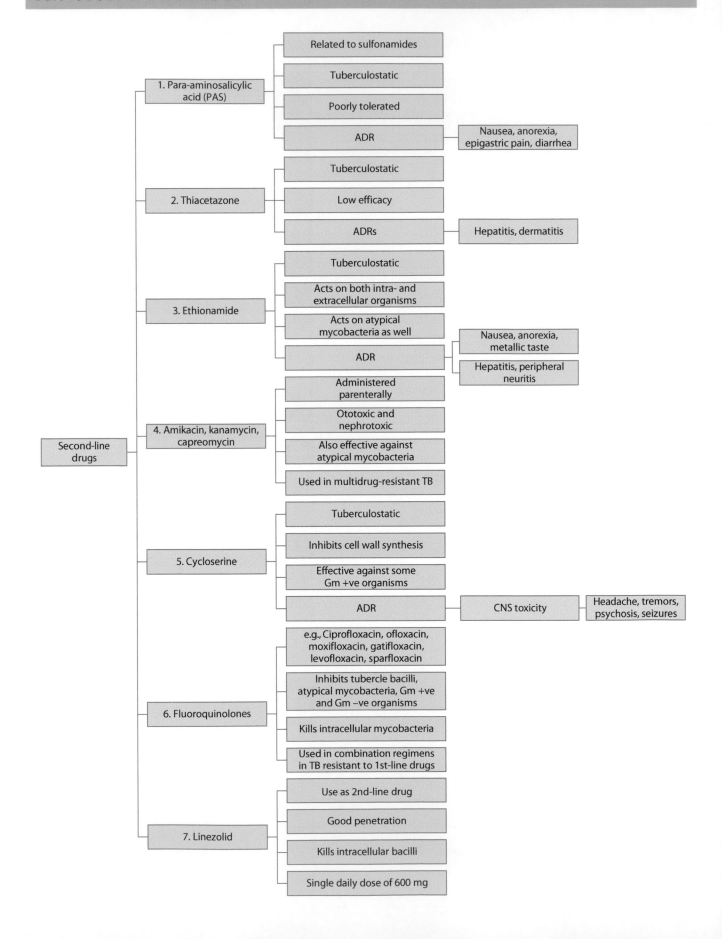

Second-line drugs

1. Para-aminosalicylic acid (PAS)
- Related to sulfonamides
- Tuberculostatic
- Poorly tolerated
- ADR — Nausea, anorexia, epigastric pain, diarrhea

2. Thiacetazone
- Tuberculostatic
- Low efficacy
- ADRs — Hepatitis, dermatitis

3. Ethionamide
- Tuberculostatic
- Acts on both intra- and extracellular organisms
- Acts on atypical mycobacteria as well
- ADR
  - Nausea, anorexia, metallic taste
  - Hepatitis, peripheral neuritis

4. Amikacin, kanamycin, capreomycin
- Administered parenterally
- Ototoxic and nephrotoxic
- Also effective against atypical mycobacteria
- Used in multidrug-resistant TB

5. Cycloserine
- Tuberculostatic
- Inhibits cell wall synthesis
- Effective against some Gm +ve organisms
- ADR — CNS toxicity — Headache, tremors, psychosis, seizures

6. Fluoroquinolones
- e.g., Ciprofloxacin, ofloxacin, moxifloxacin, gatifloxacin, levofloxacin, sparfloxacin
- Inhibits tubercle bacilli, atypical mycobacteria, Gm +ve and Gm –ve organisms
- Kills intracellular mycobacteria
- Used in combination regimens in TB resistant to 1st-line drugs

7. Linezolid
- Use as 2nd-line drug
- Good penetration
- Kills intracellular bacilli
- Single daily dose of 600 mg

65.6 TREATMENT OF TUBERCULOSIS – OBJECTIVES AND REGIMENS

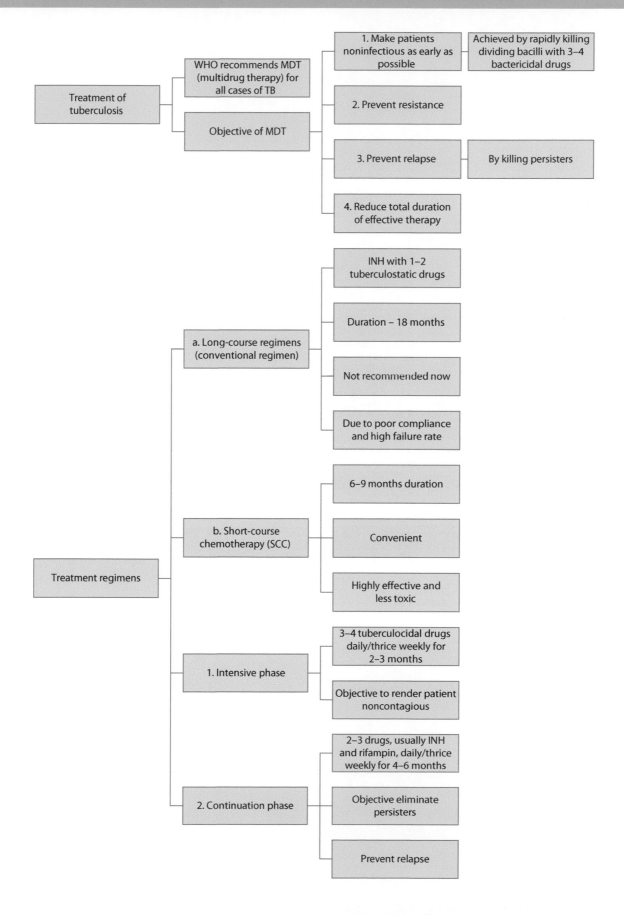

65.7 DOSES OF COMMONLY USED ANTI-TB DRUGS

Recommended dosage	Daily mg/kg	50 kg	Thrice weekly mg/kg	50 kg
1. Isoniazid (H)	5 (4–6)	300 mg	10 (8–12)	600 mg
2. Rifampicin (R)	10 (8–12)	600 mg	10 (8–12)	600 mg
3. Pyrazinamide (Z)	25 (20–30)	1500 mg	35 (35–40)	2000 mg
4. Ethambutol (E)	15 (15–20)	1000 mg	30 (20–30)	1000 mg
5. Streptomycin (S)	15 (12–18)	1000 mg	15 (12–18)	1000 mg

65.8 WHO GUIDELINES FOR TB TREATMENT

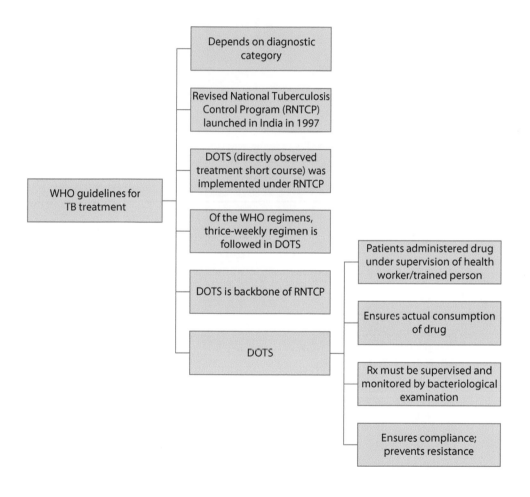

65.9 DOTS, TB TREATMENT REGIMENS

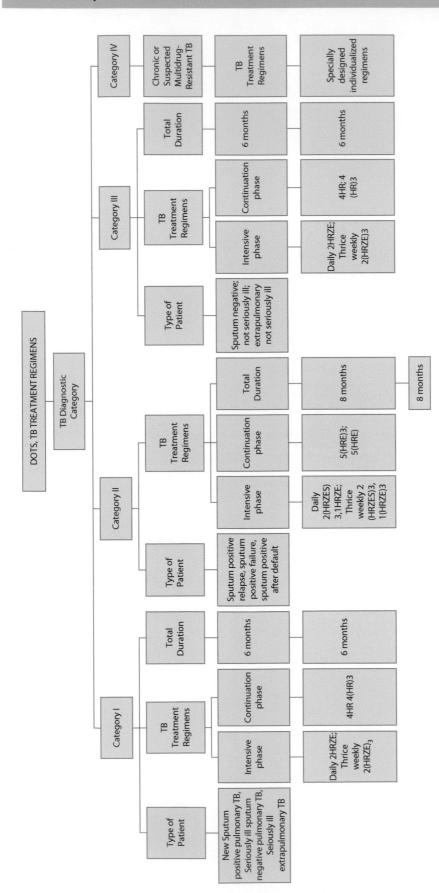

- Prefix before number indicates months of treatment
- Subscript after regimen indicates number of doses per week
- No subscript means regimen is given daily
- H - isoniazid, R - rifampicin, Z - pyrazinamide, E - ethambutol, S - streptomycin
- HRZ are given orally
- S is given IM

65.10 MULTIDRUG-RESISTANT TUBERCULOSIS (MDR-TB), TB IN HIV PATIENTS, TB IN PREGNANCY, CHEMOPROPHYLAXIS OF TB, ROLE OF GLUCOCORTICOIDS IN TB, AND DRUGS FOR *MYCOBACTERIUM AVIUM* COMPLEX (MAC)

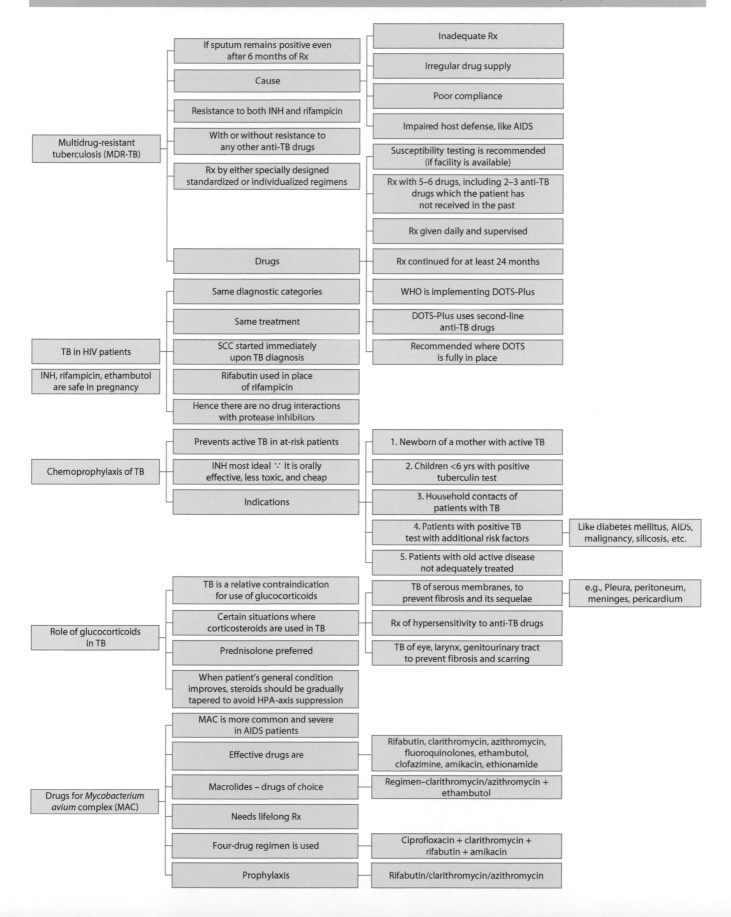

Chemotherapy of leprosy

66.1 DRUGS USED IN LEPROSY

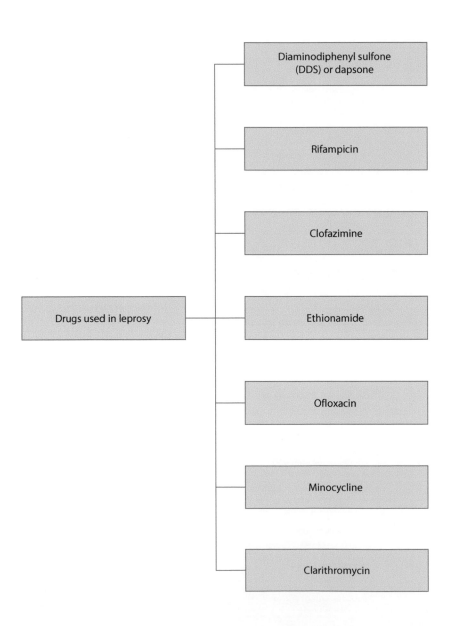

66.2 DAPSONE (DDS), RIFAMPICIN, CLOFAZIMINE, ETHIONAMIDE, AND NEWER AGENTS

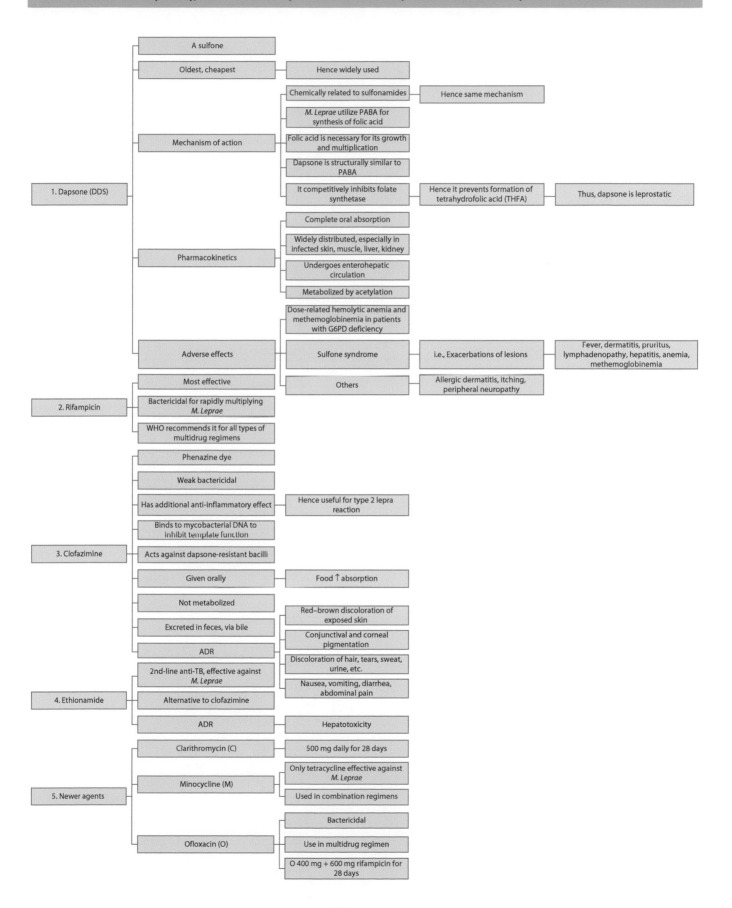

66.3 TREATMENT OF LEPROSY AND LEPRA REACTIONS

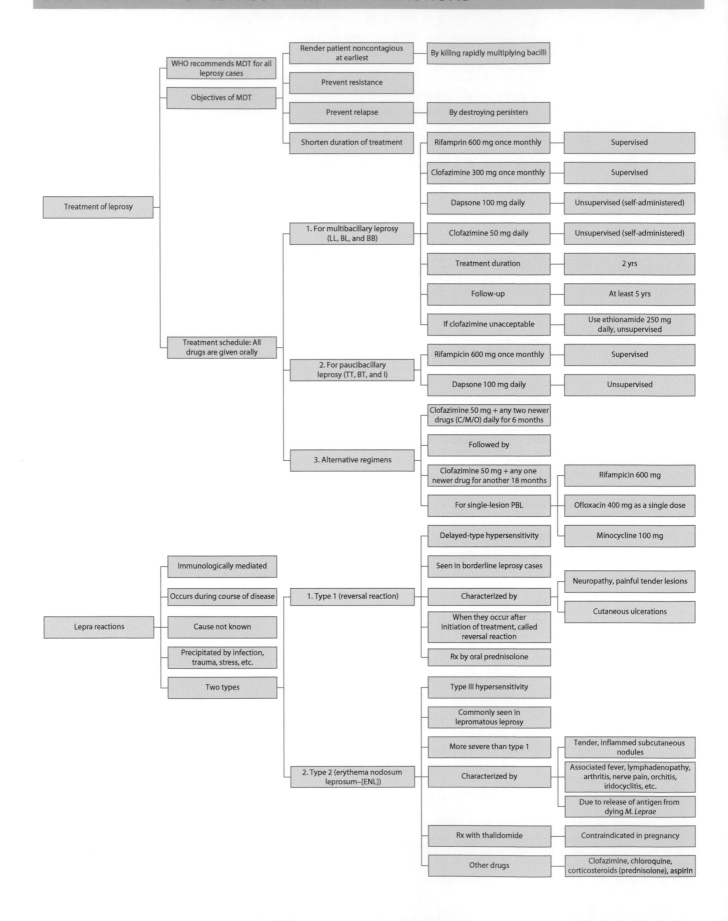

Chemotherapy of malaria

67.1 CLASSIFICATION OF ANTIMALARIALS

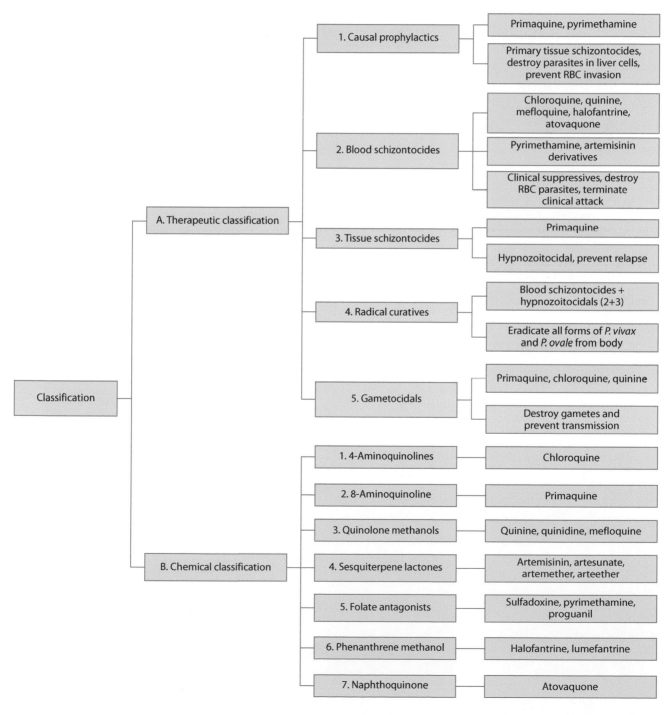

67.2 CHLOROQUINE – MECHANISM OF ACTION AND RESISTANCE

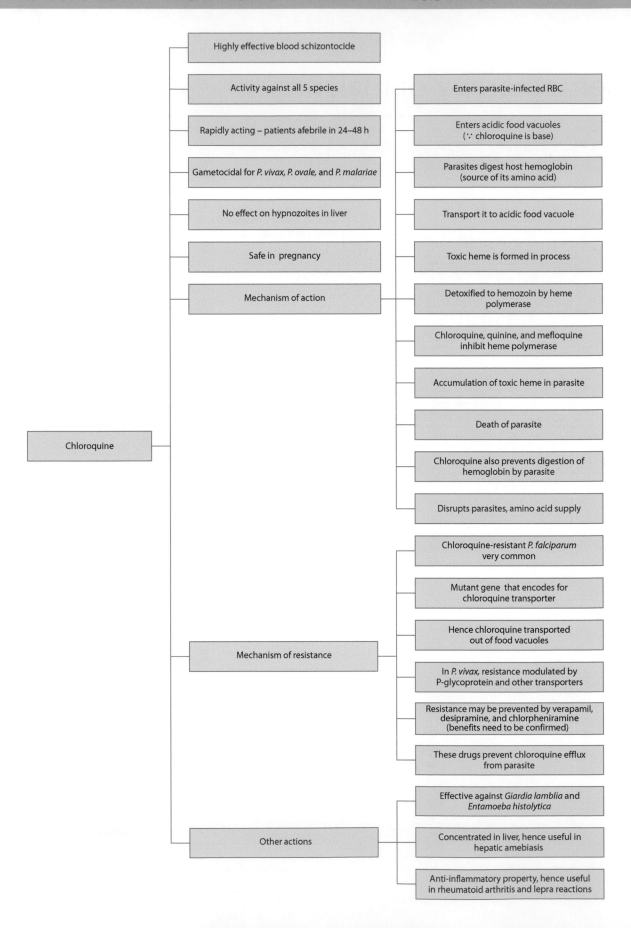

Chloroquine

- Highly effective blood schizontocide
- Activity against all 5 species
- Rapidly acting – patients afebrile in 24–48 h
- Gametocidal for *P. vivax, P. ovale,* and *P. malariae*
- No effect on hypnozoites in liver
- Safe in pregnancy
- Mechanism of action
  - Enters parasite-infected RBC
  - Enters acidic food vacuoles (∵ chloroquine is base)
  - Parasites digest host hemoglobin (source of its amino acid)
  - Transport it to acidic food vacuole
  - Toxic heme is formed in process
  - Detoxified to hemozoin by heme polymerase
  - Chloroquine, quinine, and mefloquine inhibit heme polymerase
  - Accumulation of toxic heme in parasite
  - Death of parasite
  - Chloroquine also prevents digestion of hemoglobin by parasite
  - Disrupts parasites, amino acid supply
- Mechanism of resistance
  - Chloroquine-resistant *P. falciparum* very common
  - Mutant gene that encodes for chloroquine transporter
  - Hence chloroquine transported out of food vacuoles
  - In *P. vivax*, resistance modulated by P-glycoprotein and other transporters
  - Resistance may be prevented by verapamil, desipramine, and chlorpheniramine (benefits need to be confirmed)
  - These drugs prevent chloroquine efflux from parasite
- Other actions
  - Effective against *Giardia lamblia* and *Entamoeba histolytica*
  - Concentrated in liver, hence useful in hepatic amebiasis
  - Anti-inflammatory property, hence useful in rheumatoid arthritis and lepra reactions

67.3 PHARMACOKINETICS AND ADVERSE EFFECTS

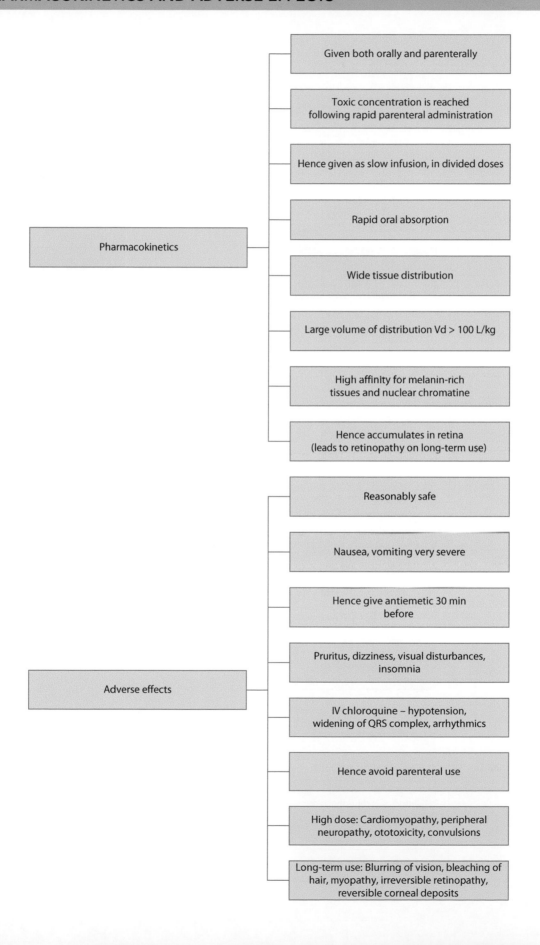

Pharmacokinetics

- Given both orally and parenterally
- Toxic concentration is reached following rapid parenteral administration
- Hence given as slow infusion, in divided doses
- Rapid oral absorption
- Wide tissue distribution
- Large volume of distribution Vd > 100 L/kg
- High affinity for melanin-rich tissues and nuclear chromatine
- Hence accumulates in retina (leads to retinopathy on long-term use)

Adverse effects

- Reasonably safe
- Nausea, vomiting very severe
- Hence give antiemetic 30 min before
- Pruritus, dizziness, visual disturbances, insomnia
- IV chloroquine – hypotension, widening of QRS complex, arrhythmics
- Hence avoid parenteral use
- High dose: Cardiomyopathy, peripheral neuropathy, ototoxicity, convulsions
- Long-term use: Blurring of vision, bleaching of hair, myopathy, irreversible retinopathy, reversible corneal deposits

67.4 USES

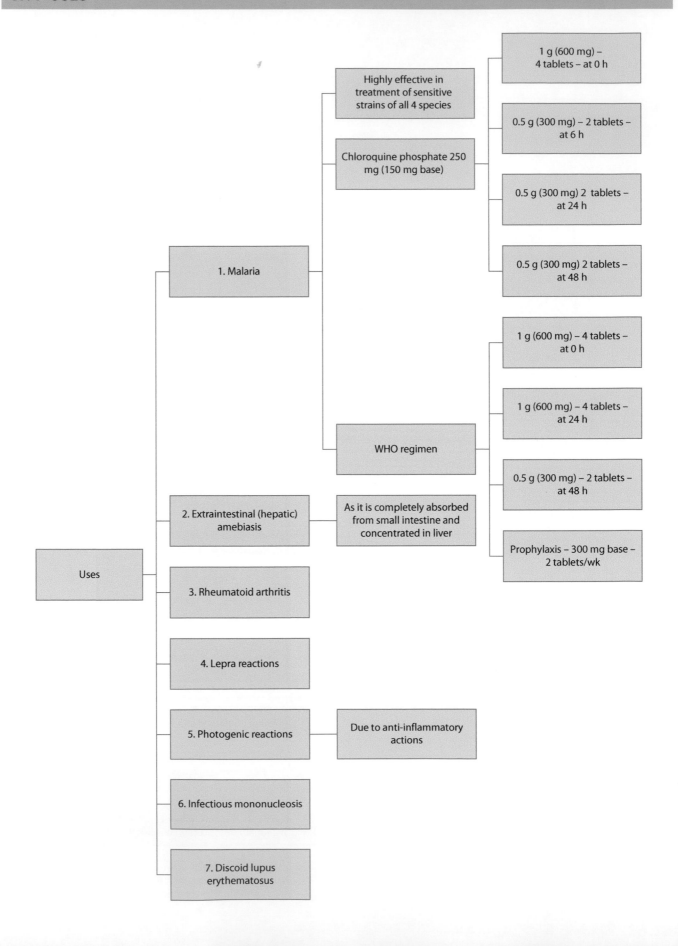

67.5 PRECAUTIONS AND CONTRAINDICATIONS

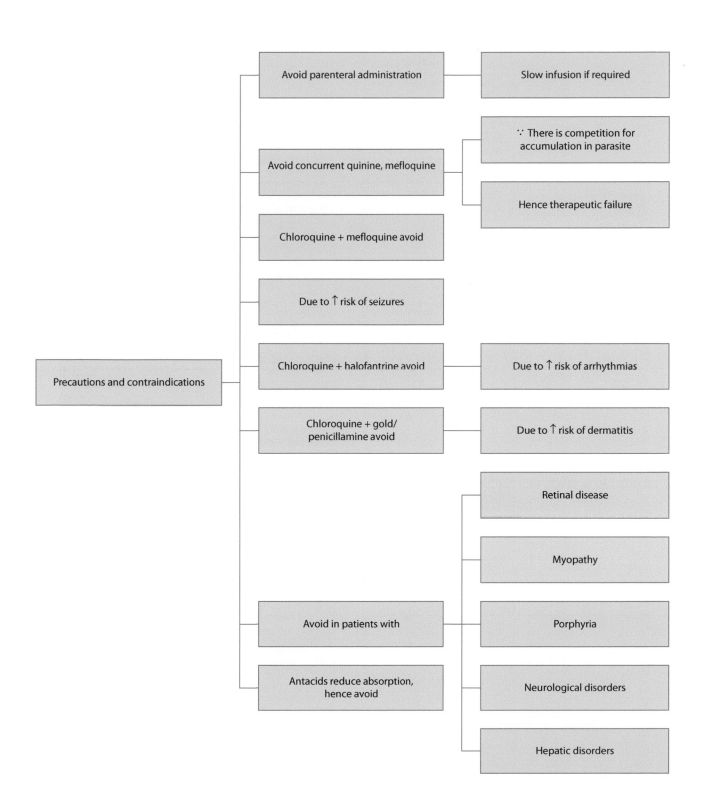

67.6 MEFLOQUINE AND HALOFANTRINE

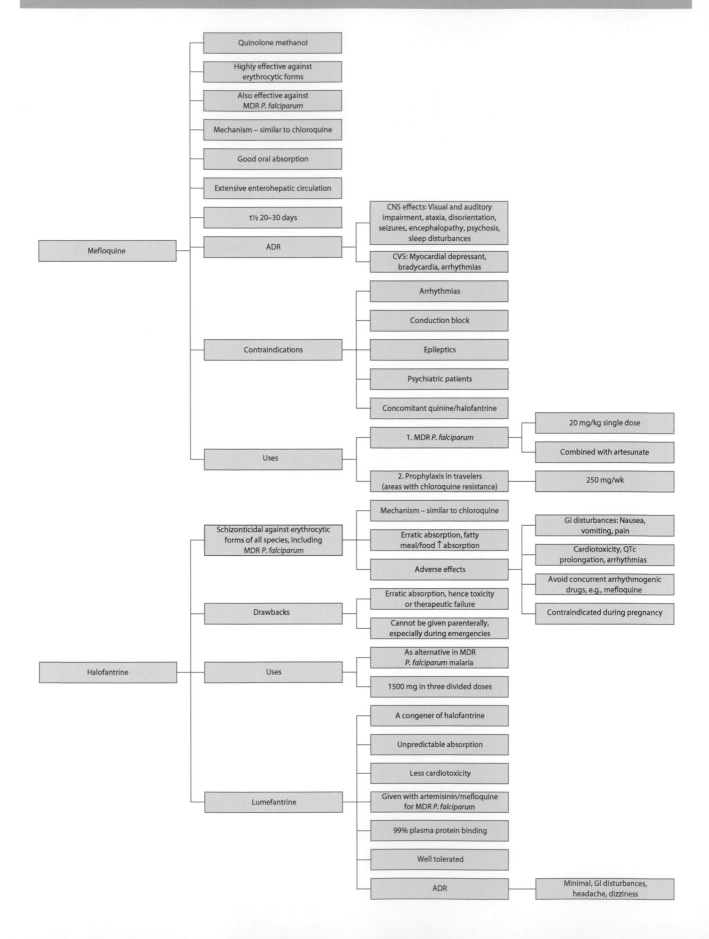

67.7 PRIMAQUINE

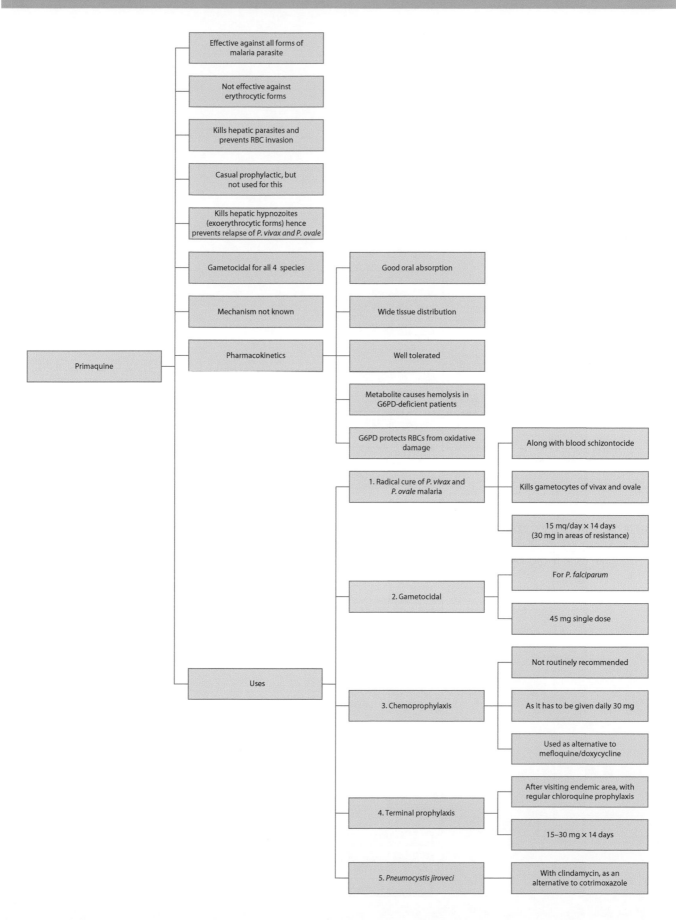

67.8 QUININE

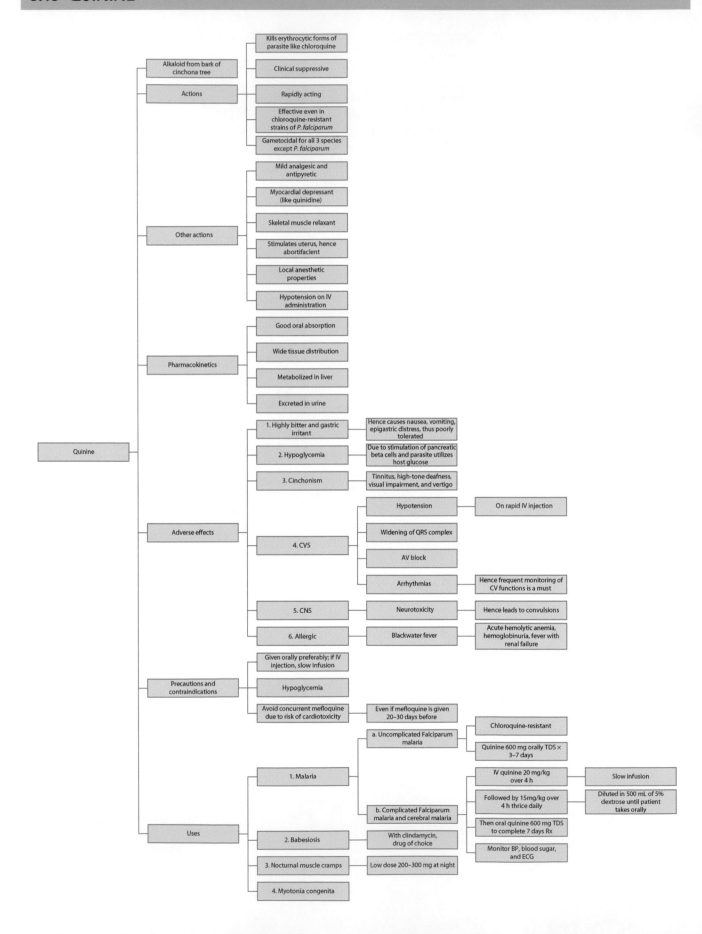

67.9 FOLATE ANTAGONIST – PYRIMETHAMINE

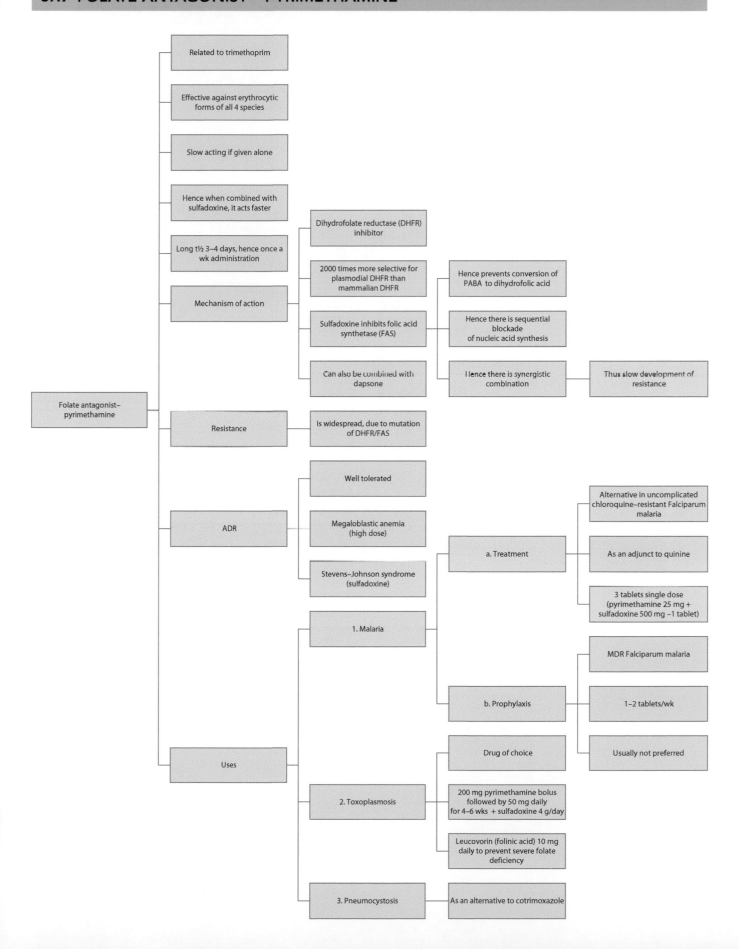

Folate antagonist–pyrimethamine

- Related to trimethoprim
- Effective against erythrocytic forms of all 4 species
- Slow acting if given alone
- Hence when combined with sulfadoxine, it acts faster
- Long t½ 3–4 days, hence once a wk administration
- Mechanism of action
  - Dihydrofolate reductase (DHFR) inhibitor
  - 2000 times more selective for plasmodial DHFR than mammalian DHFR
    - Hence prevents conversion of PABA to dihydrofolic acid
  - Sulfadoxine inhibits folic acid synthetase (FAS)
    - Hence there is sequential blockade of nucleic acid synthesis
  - Can also be combined with dapsone
    - Hence there is synergistic combination
      - Thus slow development of resistance
- Resistance
  - Is widespread, due to mutation of DHFR/FAS
- ADR
  - Well tolerated
  - Megaloblastic anemia (high dose)
  - Stevens–Johnson syndrome (sulfadoxine)
- Uses
  - 1. Malaria
    - a. Treatment
      - Alternative in uncomplicated chloroquine–resistant Falciparum malaria
      - As an adjunct to quinine
      - 3 tablets single dose (pyrimethamine 25 mg + sulfadoxine 500 mg –1 tablet)
    - b. Prophylaxis
      - MDR Falciparum malaria
      - 1–2 tablets/wk
      - Usually not preferred
  - 2. Toxoplasmosis
    - Drug of choice
    - 200 mg pyrimethamine bolus followed by 50 mg daily for 4–6 wks + sulfadoxine 4 g/day
    - Leucovorin (folinic acid) 10 mg daily to prevent severe folate deficiency
  - 3. Pneumocystosis
    - As an alternative to cotrimoxazole

67.10 PROGUANIL (CHLOROGUANIDE) AND ATOVAQUONE

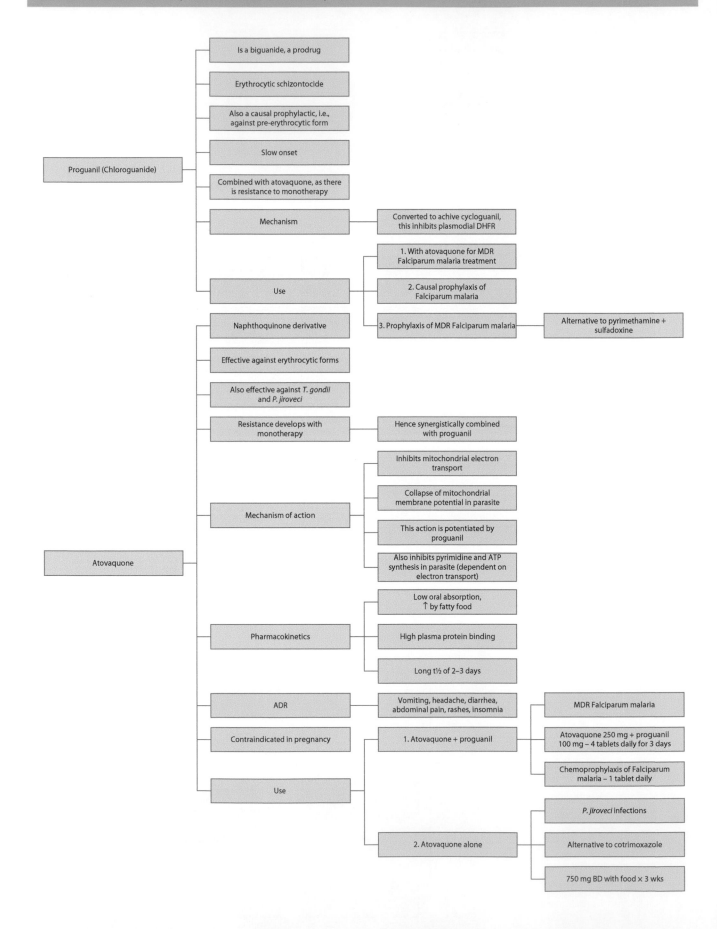

Proguanil (Chloroguanide)
- Is a biguanide, a prodrug
- Erythrocytic schizontocide
- Also a causal prophylactic, i.e., against pre-erythrocytic form
- Slow onset
- Combined with atovaquone, as there is resistance to monotherapy
- Mechanism
  - Converted to achive cycloguanil, this inhibits plasmodial DHFR
- Use
  - 1. With atovaquone for MDR Falciparum malaria treatment
  - 2. Causal prophylaxis of Falciparum malaria
  - 3. Prophylaxis of MDR Falciparum malaria
    - Alternative to pyrimethamine + sulfadoxine

Atovaquone
- Naphthoquinone derivative
- Effective against erythrocytic forms
- Also effective against *T. gondii* and *P. jiroveci*
- Resistance develops with monotherapy
  - Hence synergistically combined with proguanil
- Mechanism of action
  - Inhibits mitochondrial electron transport
  - Collapse of mitochondrial membrane potential in parasite
  - This action is potentiated by proguanil
  - Also inhibits pyrimidine and ATP synthesis in parasite (dependent on electron transport)
- Pharmacokinetics
  - Low oral absorption, ↑ by fatty food
  - High plasma protein binding
  - Long t½ of 2–3 days
- ADR
  - Vomiting, headache, diarrhea, abdominal pain, rashes, insomnia
- Contraindicated in pregnancy
- Use
  - 1. Atovaquone + proguanil
    - MDR Falciparum malaria
    - Atovaquone 250 mg + proguanil 100 mg – 4 tablets daily for 3 days
    - Chemoprophylaxis of Falciparum malaria – 1 tablet daily
  - 2. Atovaquone alone
    - *P. jiroveci* infections
    - Alternative to cotrimoxazole
    - 750 mg BD with food × 3 wks

67.11 ARTEMISININ AND DERIVATIVES

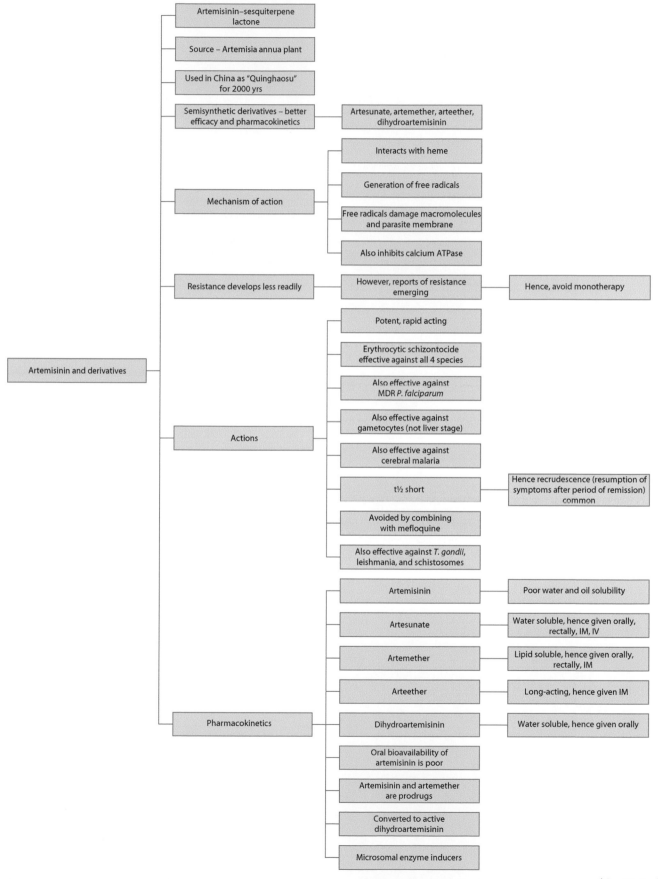

(Continued)

67.11 ARTEMISININ AND DERIVATIVES (Continued)

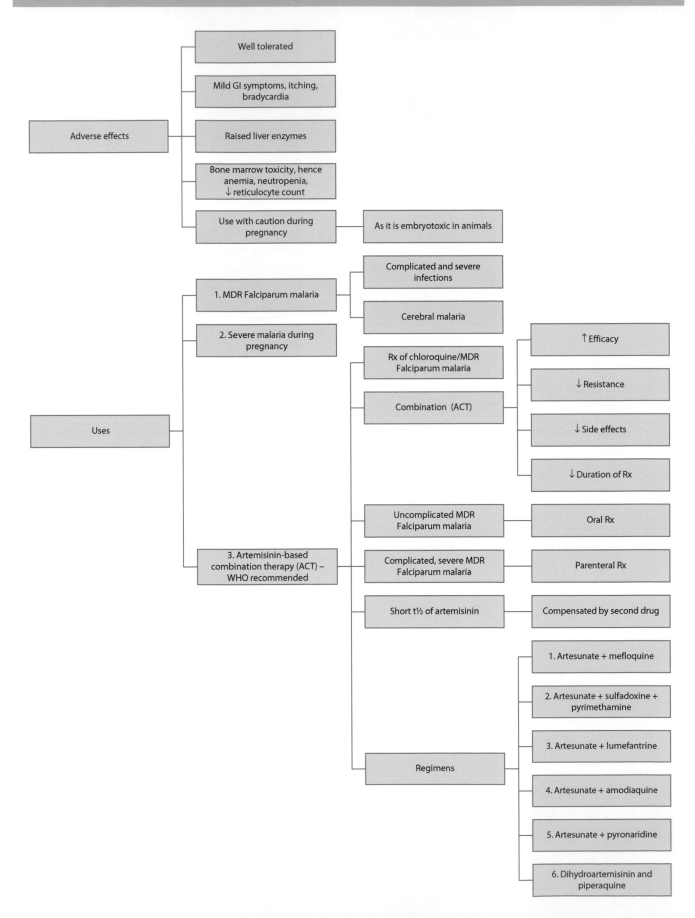

Adverse effects
- Well tolerated
- Mild GI symptoms, itching, bradycardia
- Raised liver enzymes
- Bone marrow toxicity, hence anemia, neutropenia, ↓ reticulocyte count
- Use with caution during pregnancy → As it is embryotoxic in animals

Uses
1. MDR Falciparum malaria
   - Complicated and severe infections
   - Cerebral malaria
2. Severe malaria during pregnancy
3. Artemisinin-based combination therapy (ACT) – WHO recommended
   - Rx of chloroquine/MDR Falciparum malaria
   - Combination (ACT)
     - ↑ Efficacy
     - ↓ Resistance
     - ↓ Side effects
     - ↓ Duration of Rx
   - Uncomplicated MDR Falciparum malaria → Oral Rx
   - Complicated, severe MDR Falciparum malaria → Parenteral Rx
   - Short t½ of artemisinin → Compensated by second drug
   - Regimens
     1. Artesunate + mefloquine
     2. Artesunate + sulfadoxine + pyrimethamine
     3. Artesunate + lumefantrine
     4. Artesunate + amodiaquine
     5. Artesunate + pyronaridine
     6. Dihydroartemisinin and piperaquine

67.12 REGIMENS FOR MALARIA CHEMOPROPHYLAXIS

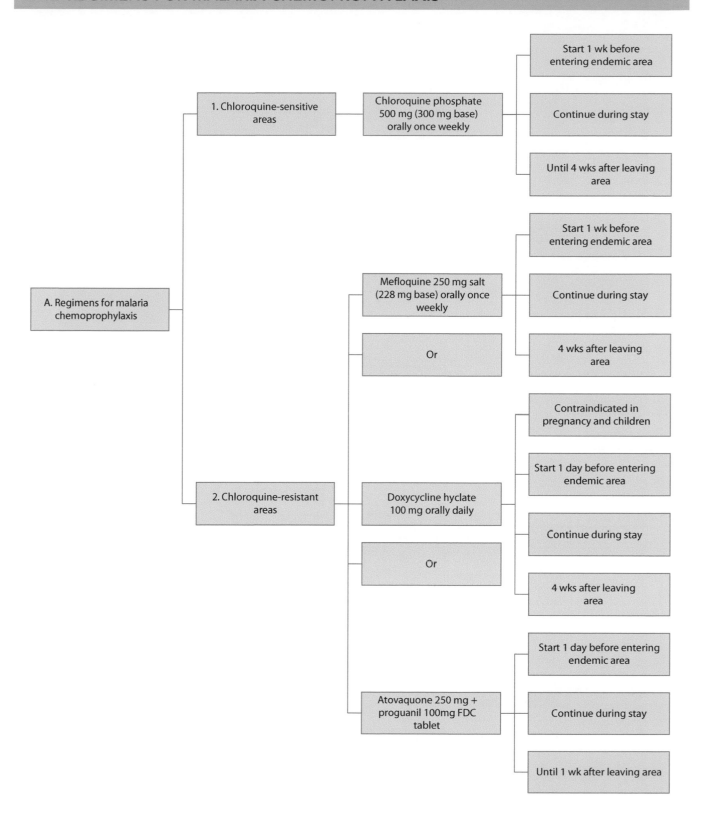

67.13 REGIMENS FOR MALARIA TREATMENT

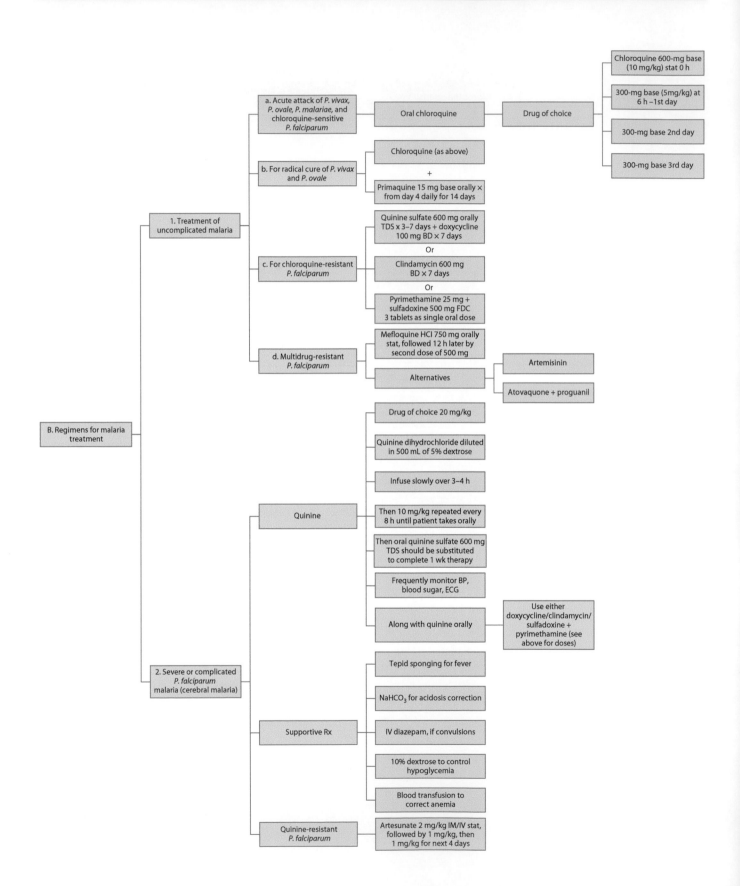

Drugs for amebiasis/pneumocystosis/leishmaniasis/trypanosomiasis

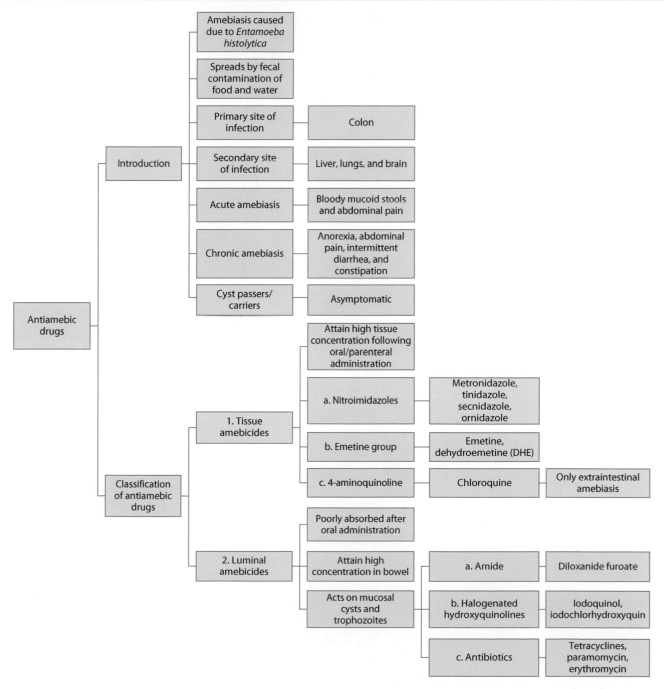

68.2 METRONIDAZOLE (MTZ)

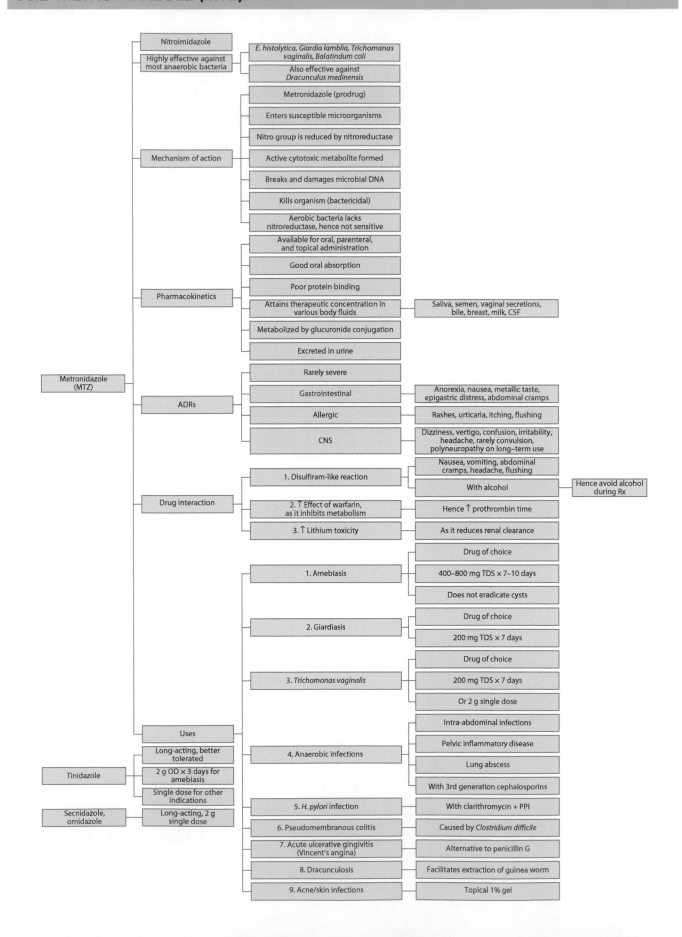

Metronidazole (MTZ)

- **Nitroimidazole**
- **Highly effective against most anaerobic bacteria**
  - *E. histolytica, Giardia lamblia, Trichomanas vaginalis, Balatindum coli*
  - Also effective against *Dracunculus medinensis*
- **Mechanism of action**
  - Metronidazole (prodrug)
  - Enters susceptible microorganisms
  - Nitro group is reduced by nitroreductase
  - Active cytotoxic metabolite formed
  - Breaks and damages microbial DNA
  - Kills organism (bactericidal)
  - Aerobic bacteria lacks nitroreductase, hence not sensitive
- **Pharmacokinetics**
  - Available for oral, parenteral, and topical administration
  - Good oral absorption
  - Poor protein binding
  - Attains therapeutic concentration in various body fluids
    - Saliva, semen, vaginal secretions, bile, breast, milk, CSF
  - Metabolized by glucuronide conjugation
  - Excreted in urine
- **ADRs**
  - Rarely severe
  - Gastrointestinal
    - Anorexia, nausea, metallic taste, epigastric distress, abdominal cramps
  - Allergic
    - Rashes, urticaria, itching, flushing
  - CNS
    - Dizziness, vertigo, confusion, irritability, headache, rarely convulsion, polyneuropathy on long–term use
- **Drug interaction**
  - 1. Disulfiram-like reaction
    - Nausea, vomiting, abdominal cramps, headache, flushing
    - With alcohol — Hence avoid alcohol during Rx
  - 2. ↑ Effect of warfarin, as it inhibits metabolism
    - Hence ↑ prothrombin time
  - 3. ↑ Lithium toxicity
    - As it reduces renal clearance
- **Uses**
  - 1. Amebiasis
    - Drug of choice
    - 400–800 mg TDS × 7–10 days
    - Does not eradicate cysts
  - 2. Giardiasis
    - Drug of choice
    - 200 mg TDS × 7 days
  - 3. *Trichomonas vaginalis*
    - Drug of choice
    - 200 mg TDS × 7 days
    - Or 2 g single dose
  - 4. Anaerobic infections
    - Intra-abdominal infections
    - Pelvic inflammatory disease
    - Lung abscess
    - With 3rd generation cephalosporins
  - 5. *H. pylori* infection
    - With clarithromycin + PPI
  - 6. Pseudomembranous colitis
    - Caused by *Clostridium difficile*
  - 7. Acute ulcerative gingivitis (Vincent's angina)
    - Alternative to penicillin G
  - 8. Dracunculosis
    - Facilitates extraction of guinea worm
  - 9. Acne/skin infections
    - Topical 1% gel

Tinidazole
- Long-acting, better tolerated
- 2 g OD × 3 days for amebiasis
- Single dose for other indications

Secnidazole, ornidazole
- Long-acting, 2 g single dose

68.3 EMETINE AND DEHYDROEMETINE, DILOXANIDE FUROATE (DF)

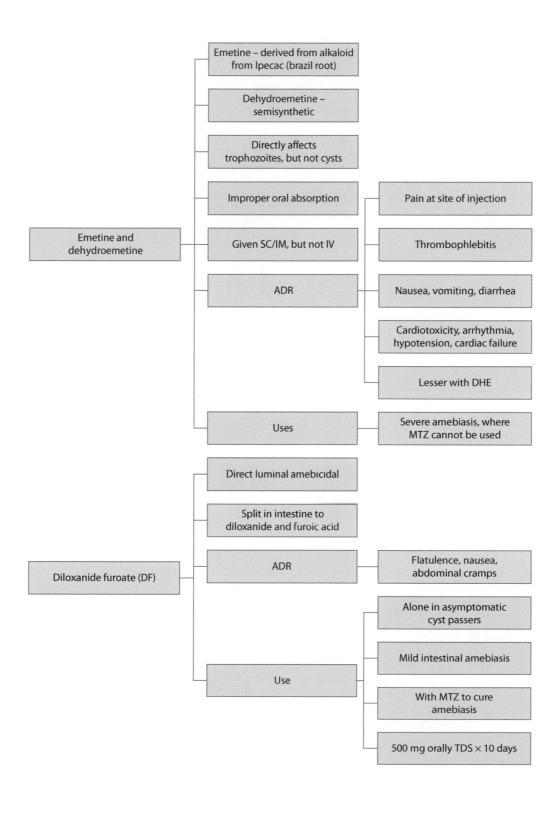

Emetine and dehydroemetine
- Emetine – derived from alkaloid from Ipecac (brazil root)
- Dehydroemetine – semisynthetic
- Directly affects trophozoites, but not cysts
- Improper oral absorption
- Given SC/IM, but not IV
- ADR
  - Pain at site of injection
  - Thrombophlebitis
  - Nausea, vomiting, diarrhea
  - Cardiotoxicity, arrhythmia, hypotension, cardiac failure
  - Lesser with DHE
- Uses
  - Severe amebiasis, where MTZ cannot be used

Diloxanide furoate (DF)
- Direct luminal amebicidal
- Split in intestine to diloxanide and furoic acid
- ADR
  - Flatulence, nausea, abdominal cramps
- Use
  - Alone in asymptomatic cyst passers
  - Mild intestinal amebiasis
  - With MTZ to cure amebiasis
  - 500 mg orally TDS × 10 days

68.4 NITAZOXANIDE, IODOQUINOL, AND QUINIODOCHLOR

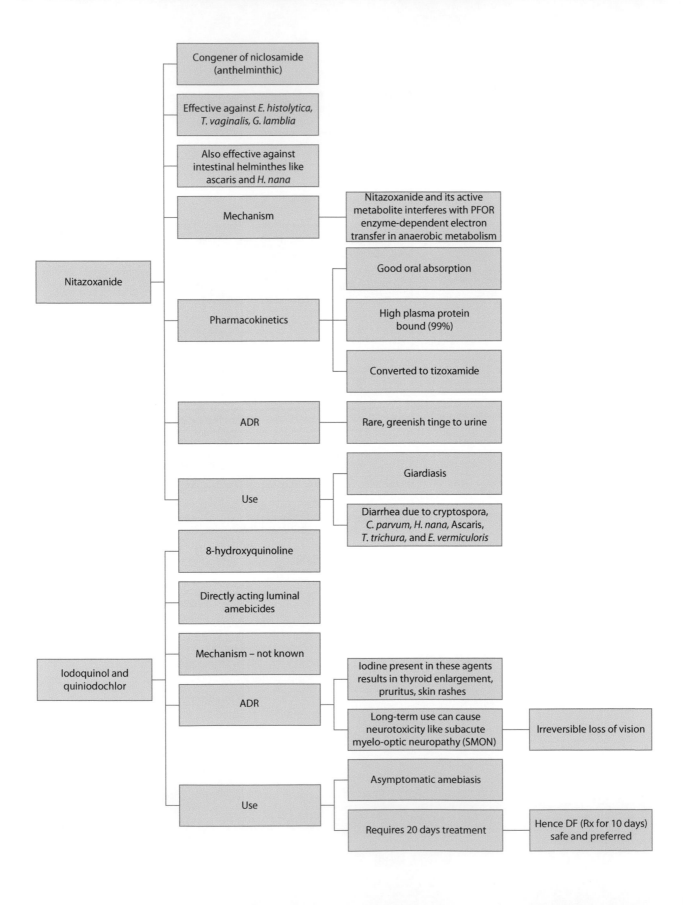

68.5 PAROMOMYCIN, TETRACYCLINE, AND CHLOROQUINE

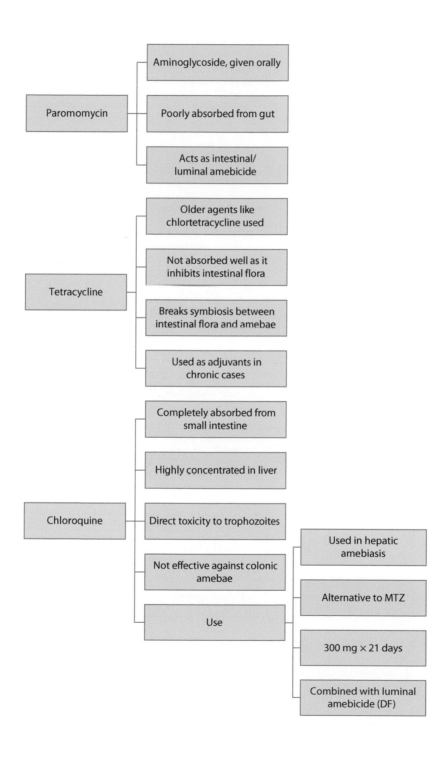

68.6 TREATMENT OF AMEBIASIS, TREATMENT OF PNEUMOCYSTOSIS

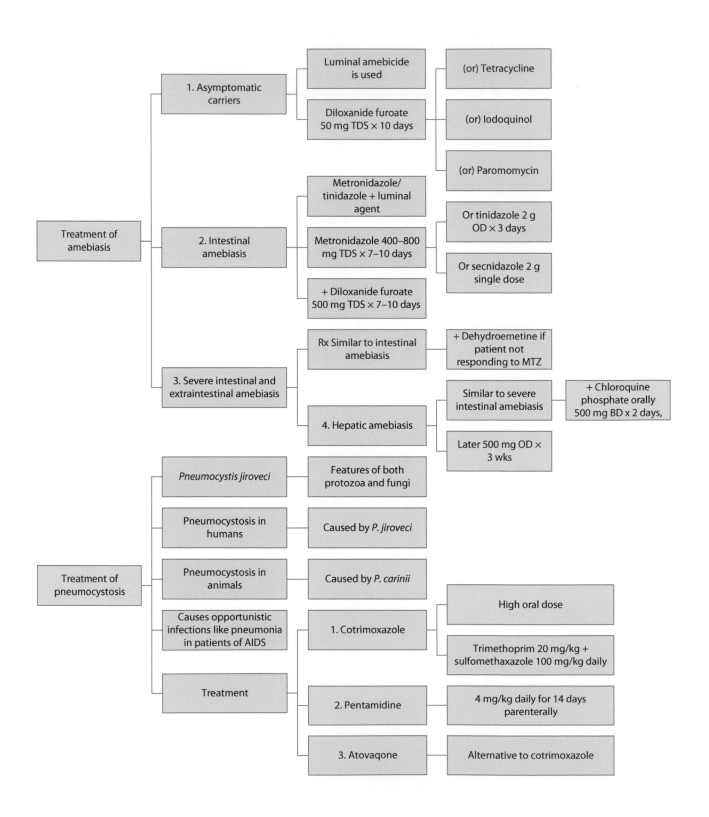

68.7 TREATMENT OF LEISHMANIASIS

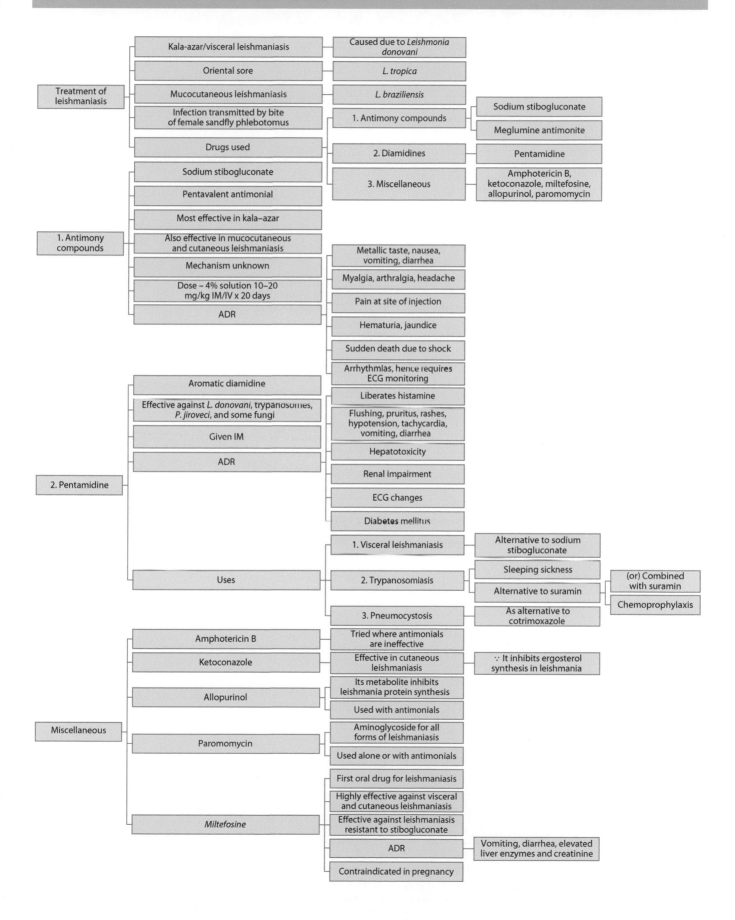

Treatment of leishmaniasis
- Kala-azar/visceral leishmaniasis — Caused due to *Leishmonia donovani*
- Oriental sore — *L. tropica*
- Mucocutaneous leishmaniasis — *L. braziliensis*
- Infection transmitted by bite of female sandfly phlebotomus
- Drugs used
  - 1. Antimony compounds — Sodium stibogluconate; Meglumine antimonite
  - 2. Diamidines — Pentamidine
  - 3. Miscellaneous — Amphotericin B, ketoconazole, miltefosine, allopurinol, paromomycin

1. Antimony compounds
- Sodium stibogluconate
- Pentavalent antimonial
- Most effective in kala–azar
- Also effective in mucocutaneous and cutaneous leishmaniasis
- Mechanism unknown
- Dose – 4% solution 10–20 mg/kg IM/IV x 20 days
- ADR
  - Metallic taste, nausea, vomiting, diarrhea
  - Myalgia, arthralgia, headache
  - Pain at site of injection
  - Hematuria, jaundice
  - Sudden death due to shock
  - Arrhythmias, hence requires ECG monitoring

2. Pentamidine
- Aromatic diamidine
- Effective against *L. donovani*, trypanosomes, *P. jiroveci*, and some fungi
- Given IM
- ADR
  - Liberates histamine
  - Flushing, pruritus, rashes, hypotension, tachycardia, vomiting, diarrhea
  - Hepatotoxicity
  - Renal impairment
  - ECG changes
  - Diabetes mellitus
- Uses
  - 1. Visceral leishmaniasis — Alternative to sodium stibogluconate
  - 2. Trypanosomiasis — Sleeping sickness; Alternative to suramin — (or) Combined with suramin; Chemoprophylaxis
  - 3. Pneumocystosis — As alternative to cotrimoxazole

Miscellaneous
- Amphotericin B — Tried where antimonials are ineffective
- Ketoconazole — Effective in cutaneous leishmaniasis — ∵ It inhibits ergosterol synthesis in leishmania
- Allopurinol — Its metabolite inhibits leishmania protein synthesis; Used with antimonials
- Paromomycin — Aminoglycoside for all forms of leishmaniasis; Used alone or with antimonials
- *Miltefosine*
  - First oral drug for leishmaniasis
  - Highly effective against visceral and cutaneous leishmaniasis
  - Effective against leishmaniasis resistant to stibogluconate
  - ADR — Vomiting, diarrhea, elevated liver enzymes and creatinine
  - Contraindicated in pregnancy

68.8 DRUGS FOR DERMAL LEISHMANIASIS (ORIENTAL SORE), TREATMENT OF TRYPANOSOMIASIS

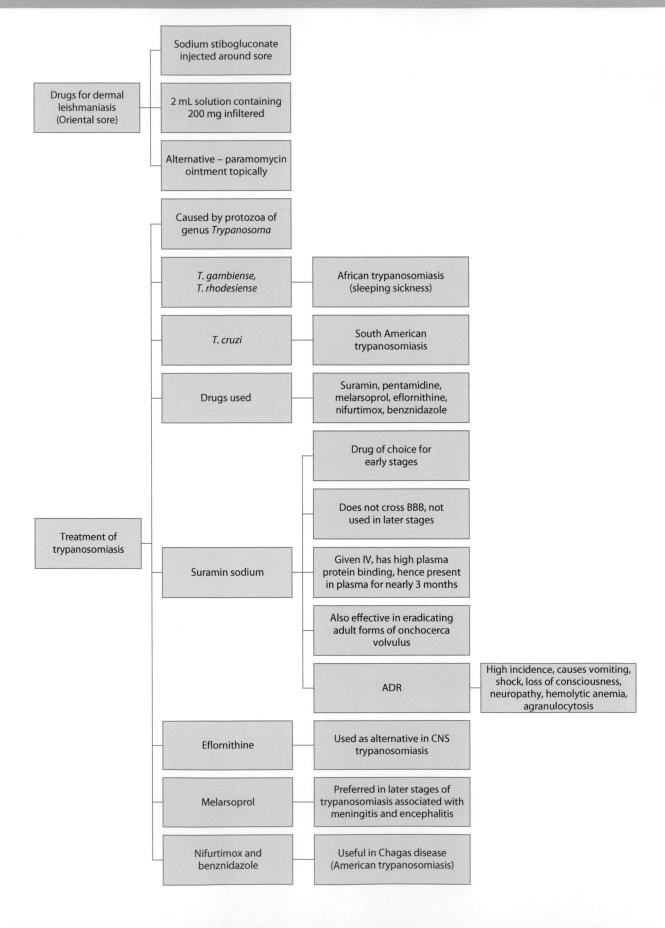

Antiviral drugs

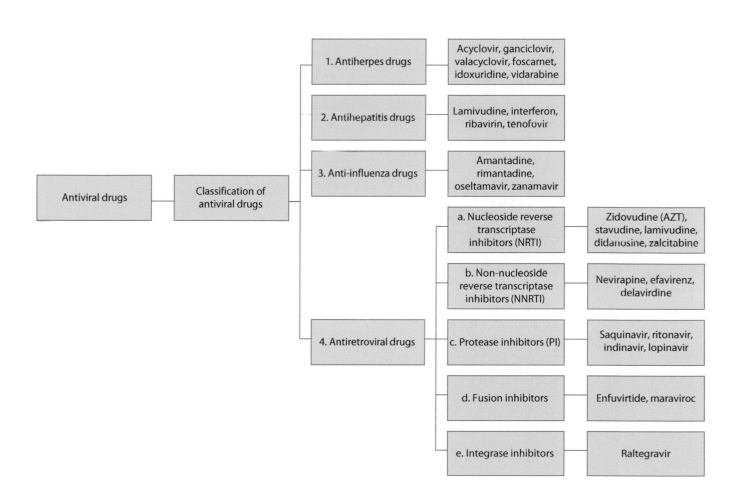

69.2 ANTIHERPES AGENT – ACYCLOVIR

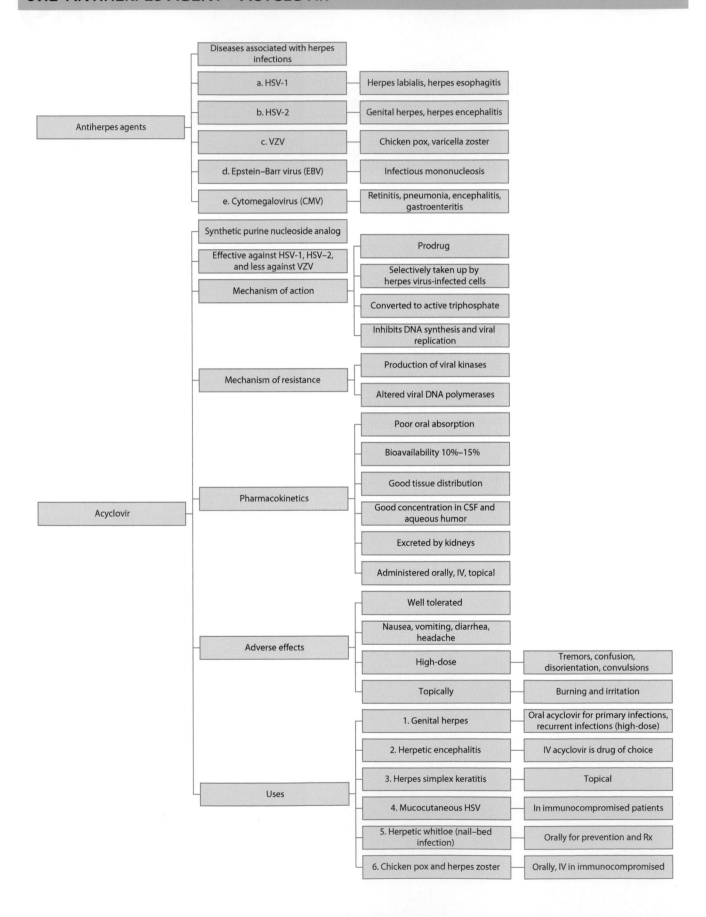

69.3 OTHER ANTIHERPES DRUGS

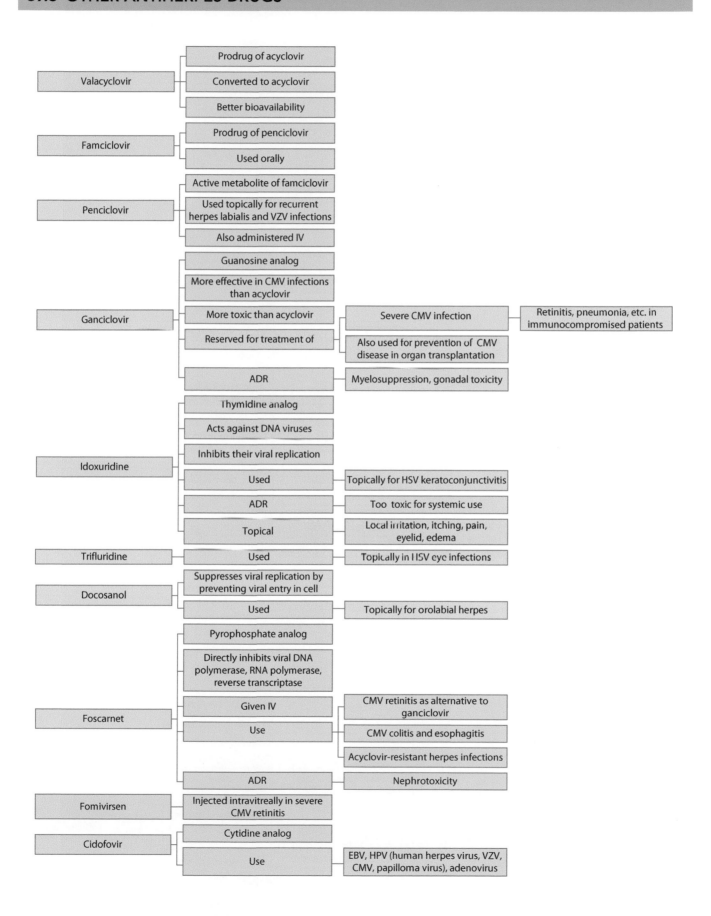

Valacyclovir
- Prodrug of acyclovir
- Converted to acyclovir
- Better bioavailability

Famciclovir
- Prodrug of penciclovir
- Used orally

Penciclovir
- Active metabolite of famciclovir
- Used topically for recurrent herpes labialis and VZV infections
- Also administered IV

Ganciclovir
- Guanosine analog
- More effective in CMV infections than acyclovir
- More toxic than acyclovir
- Reserved for treatment of
  - Severe CMV infection → Retinitis, pneumonia, etc. in immunocompromised patients
  - Also used for prevention of CMV disease in organ transplantation
- ADR → Myelosuppression, gonadal toxicity

Idoxuridine
- Thymidine analog
- Acts against DNA viruses
- Inhibits their viral replication
- Used → Topically for HSV keratoconjunctivitis
- ADR → Too toxic for systemic use
- Topical → Local irritation, itching, pain, eyelid, edema

Trifluridine
- Used → Topically in HSV eye infections

Docosanol
- Suppresses viral replication by preventing viral entry in cell
- Used → Topically for orolabial herpes

Foscarnet
- Pyrophosphate analog
- Directly inhibits viral DNA polymerase, RNA polymerase, reverse transcriptase
- Given IV
- Use
  - CMV retinitis as alternative to ganciclovir
  - CMV colitis and esophagitis
  - Acyclovir-resistant herpes infections
- ADR → Nephrotoxicity

Fomivirsen
- Injected intravitreally in severe CMV retinitis

Cidofovir
- Cytidine analog
- Use → EBV, HPV (human herpes virus, VZV, CMV, papilloma virus), adenovirus

69.4 ANTIINFLUENZA VIRUS AGENTS

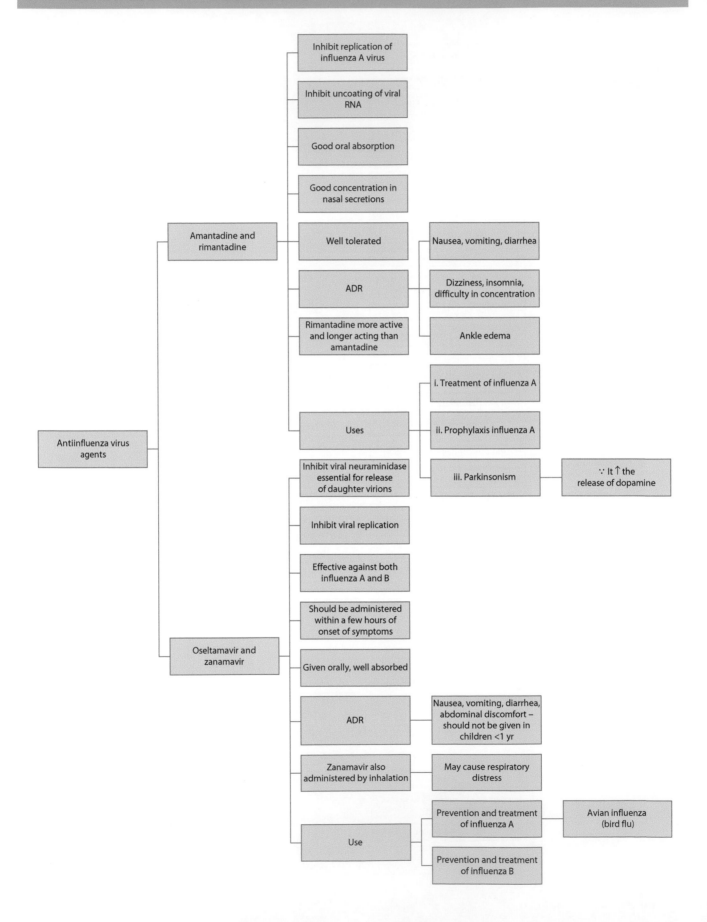

69.5 ANTIHEPATITIS DRUGS

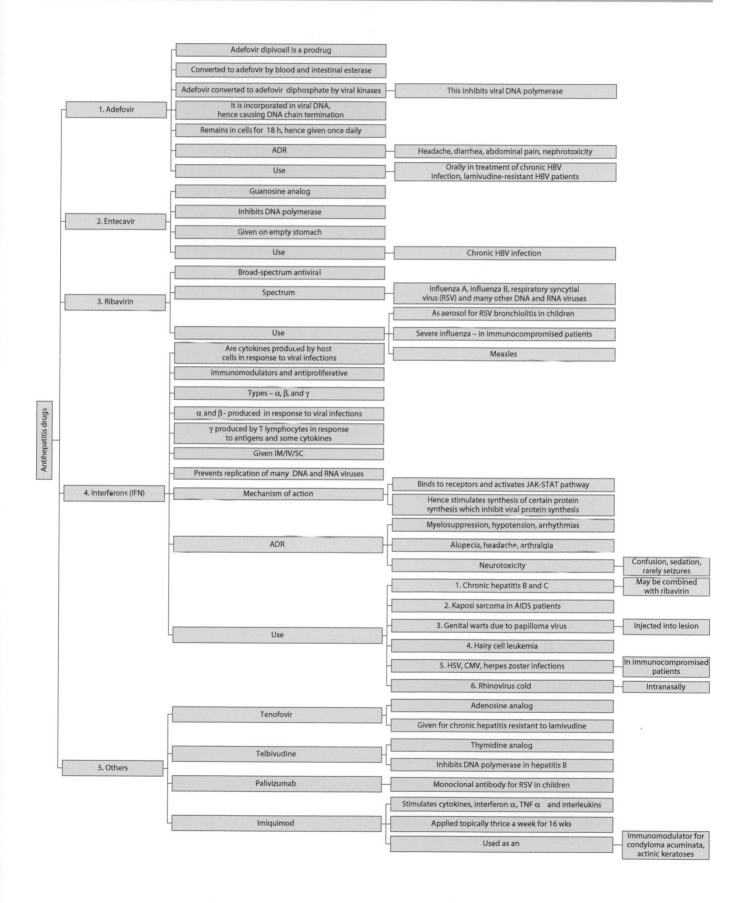

Antihepatitis drugs

1. Adefovir
- Adefovir dipivoxil is a prodrug
- Converted to adefovir by blood and intestinal esterase
- Adefovir converted to adefovir diphosphate by viral kinases → This inhibits viral DNA polymerase
- It is incorporated in viral DNA, hence causing DNA chain termination
- Remains in cells for 18 h, hence given once daily
- ADR → Headache, diarrhea, abdominal pain, nephrotoxicity
- Use → Orally in treatment of chronic HBV infection, lamivudine-resistant HBV patients

2. Entecavir
- Guanosine analog
- Inhibits DNA polymerase
- Given on empty stomach
- Use → Chronic HBV infection

3. Ribavirin
- Broad-spectrum antiviral
- Spectrum → Influenza A, influenza B, respiratory syncytial virus (RSV) and many other DNA and RNA viruses
- Use →
  - As aerosol for RSV bronchiolitis in children
  - Severe influenza – in immunocompromised patients
  - Measles

4. Interferons (IFN)
- Are cytokines produced by host cells in response to viral infections
- Immunomodulators and antiproliferative
- Types – α, β, and γ
- α and β - produced in response to viral infections
- γ produced by T lymphocytes in response to antigens and some cytokines
- Given IM/IV/SC
- Prevents replication of many DNA and RNA viruses
- Mechanism of action →
  - Binds to receptors and activates JAK-STAT pathway
  - Hence stimulates synthesis of certain protein synthesis which inhibit viral protein synthesis
- ADR →
  - Myelosuppression, hypotension, arrhythmias
  - Alopecia, headache, arthralgia
  - Neurotoxicity → Confusion, sedation, rarely seizures
- Use →
  1. Chronic hepatitis B and C → May be combined with ribavirin
  2. Kaposi sarcoma in AIDS patients
  3. Genital warts due to papilloma virus → Injected into lesion
  4. Hairy cell leukemia
  5. HSV, CMV, herpes zoster infections → In immunocompromised patients
  6. Rhinovirus cold → Intranasally

5. Others
- Tenofovir
  - Adenosine analog
  - Given for chronic hepatitis resistant to lamivudine
- Telbivudine
  - Thymidine analog
  - Inhibits DNA polymerase in hepatitis B
- Palivizumab
  - Monoclonal antibody for RSV in children
- Imiquimod
  - Stimulates cytokines, interferon α, TNF α and interleukins
  - Applied topically thrice a week for 16 wks
  - Used as an → Immunomodulator for condyloma acuminata, actinic keratoses

69.6 ANTIRETROVIRAL DRUGS – INTRODUCTION AND CLASSIFICATION

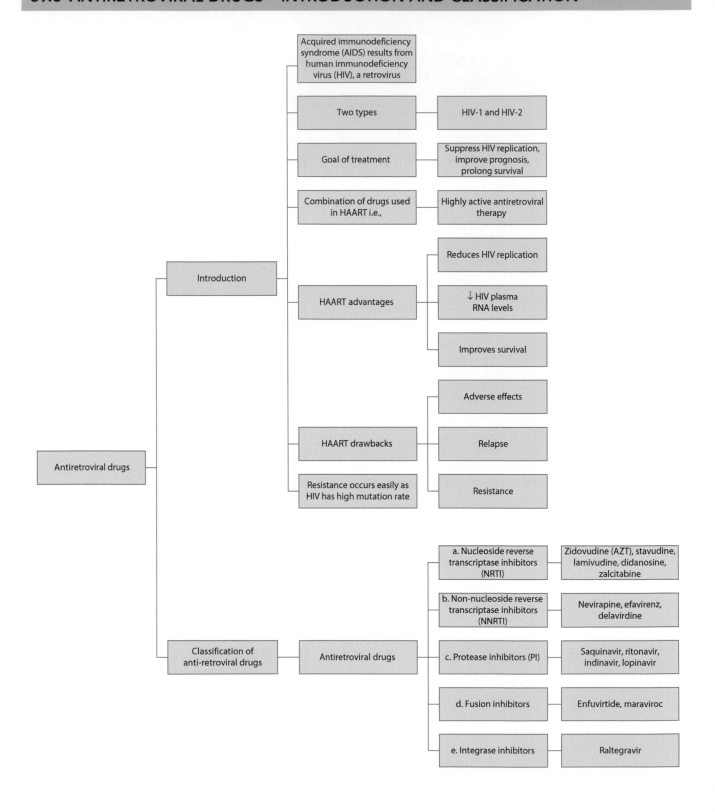

69.7 NUCLEOSIDE REVERSE TRANSCRIPTION INHIBITORS (NRTIs)

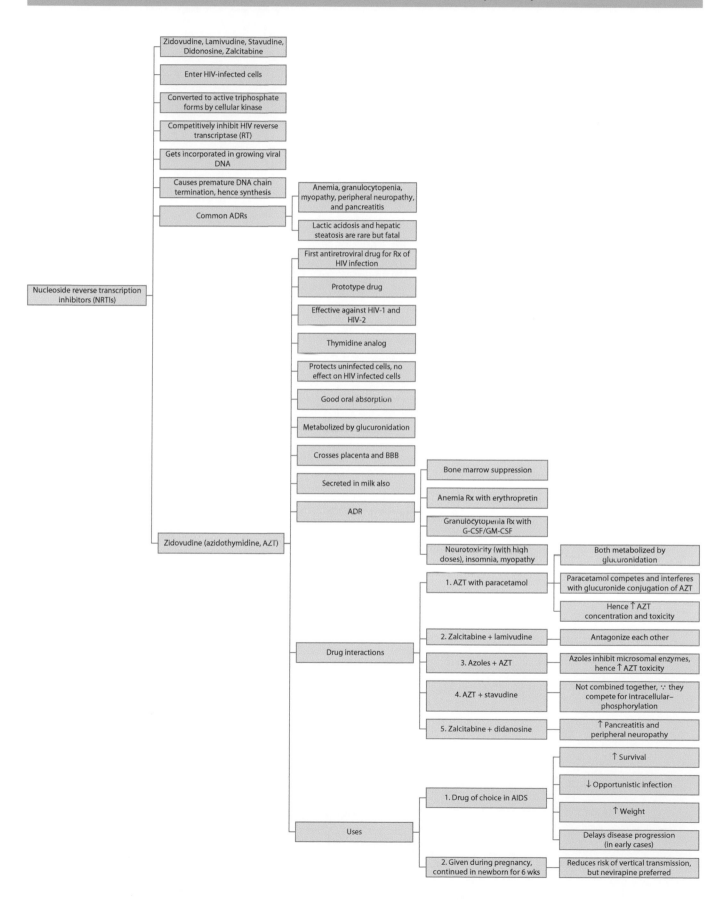

69.8 OTHER NRTIs

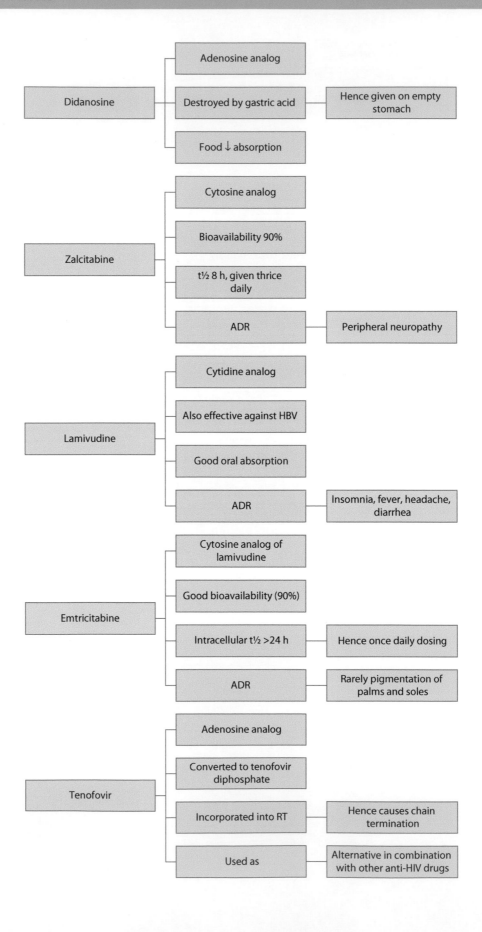

Didanosine
- Adenosine analog
- Destroyed by gastric acid → Hence given on empty stomach
- Food ↓ absorption

Zalcitabine
- Cytosine analog
- Bioavailability 90%
- t½ 8 h, given thrice daily
- ADR → Peripheral neuropathy

Lamivudine
- Cytidine analog
- Also effective against HBV
- Good oral absorption
- ADR → Insomnia, fever, headache, diarrhea

Emtricitabine
- Cytosine analog of lamivudine
- Good bioavailability (90%)
- Intracellular t½ >24 h → Hence once daily dosing
- ADR → Rarely pigmentation of palms and soles

Tenofovir
- Adenosine analog
- Converted to tenofovir diphosphate
- Incorporated into RT → Hence causes chain termination
- Used as → Alternative in combination with other anti-HIV drugs

69.9 PROTEASE INHIBITORS (PIs)

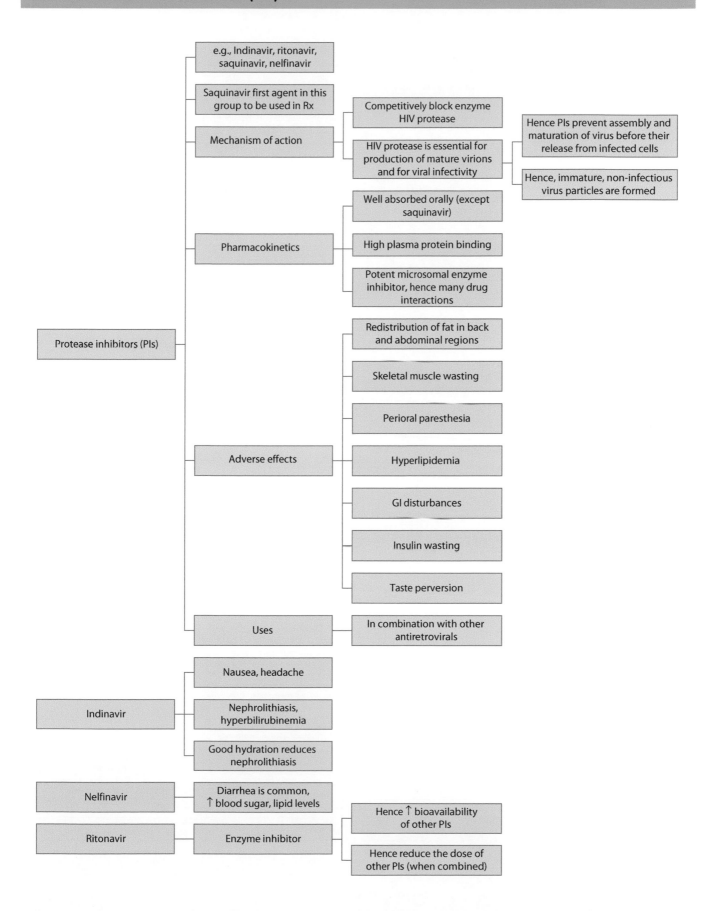

Protease inhibitors (PIs)

- e.g., Indinavir, ritonavir, saquinavir, nelfinavir
- Saquinavir first agent in this group to be used in Rx
- Mechanism of action
  - Competitively block enzyme HIV protease
  - HIV protease is essential for production of mature virions and for viral infectivity
    - Hence PIs prevent assembly and maturation of virus before their release from infected cells
    - Hence, immature, non-infectious virus particles are formed
- Pharmacokinetics
  - Well absorbed orally (except saquinavir)
  - High plasma protein binding
  - Potent microsomal enzyme inhibitor, hence many drug interactions
- Adverse effects
  - Redistribution of fat in back and abdominal regions
  - Skeletal muscle wasting
  - Perioral paresthesia
  - Hyperlipidemia
  - GI disturbances
  - Insulin wasting
  - Taste perversion
- Uses
  - In combination with other antiretrovirals

Indinavir

- Nausea, headache
- Nephrolithiasis, hyperbilirubinemia
- Good hydration reduces nephrolithiasis

Nelfinavir

- Diarrhea is common, ↑ blood sugar, lipid levels

Ritonavir

- Enzyme inhibitor
  - Hence ↑ bioavailability of other PIs
  - Hence reduce the dose of other PIs (when combined)

69.10 NON-NUCLEOSIDE REVERSE TRANSCRIPTASE INHIBITORS (NNRTIs)

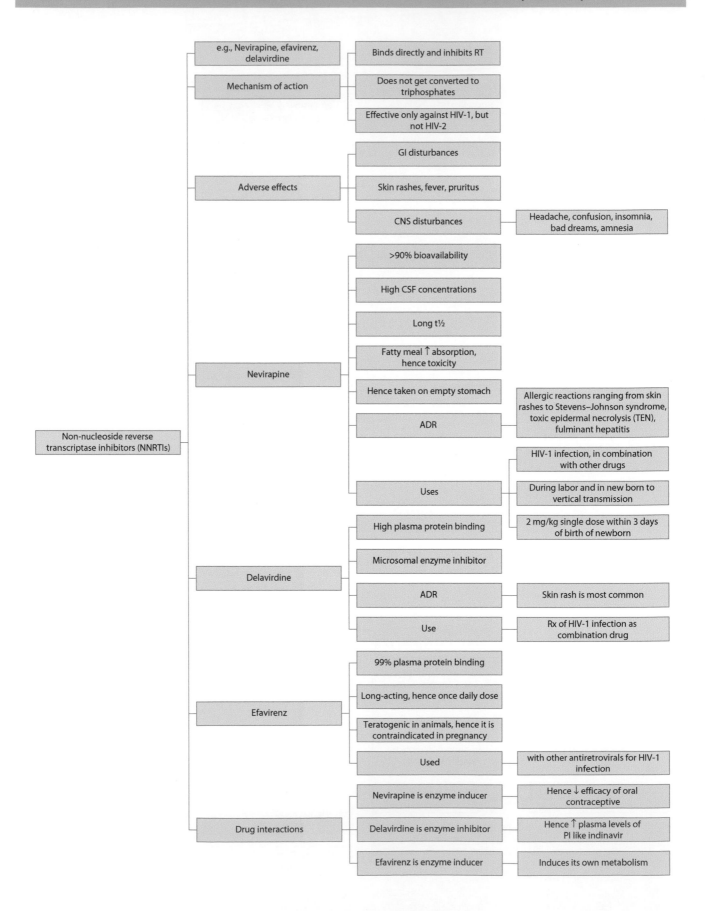

Non-nucleoside reverse transcriptase inhibitors (NNRTIs)

- e.g., Nevirapine, efavirenz, delavirdine
- Mechanism of action
  - Binds directly and inhibits RT
  - Does not get converted to triphosphates
  - Effective only against HIV-1, but not HIV-2
- Adverse effects
  - GI disturbances
  - Skin rashes, fever, pruritus
  - CNS disturbances — Headache, confusion, insomnia, bad dreams, amnesia
- Nevirapine
  - >90% bioavailability
  - High CSF concentrations
  - Long t½
  - Fatty meal ↑ absorption, hence toxicity
  - Hence taken on empty stomach
  - ADR — Allergic reactions ranging from skin rashes to Stevens–Johnson syndrome, toxic epidermal necrolysis (TEN), fulminant hepatitis
  - Uses
    - HIV-1 infection, in combination with other drugs
    - During labor and in new born to vertical transmission
    - 2 mg/kg single dose within 3 days of birth of newborn
- Delavirdine
  - High plasma protein binding
  - Microsomal enzyme inhibitor
  - ADR — Skin rash is most common
  - Use — Rx of HIV-1 infection as combination drug
- Efavirenz
  - 99% plasma protein binding
  - Long-acting, hence once daily dose
  - Teratogenic in animals, hence it is contraindicated in pregnancy
  - Used — with other antiretrovirals for HIV-1 infection
- Drug interactions
  - Nevirapine is enzyme inducer — Hence ↓ efficacy of oral contraceptive
  - Delavirdine is enzyme inhibitor — Hence ↑ plasma levels of PI like indinavir
  - Efavirenz is enzyme inducer — Induces its own metabolism

69.11 ENTRY INHIBITOR

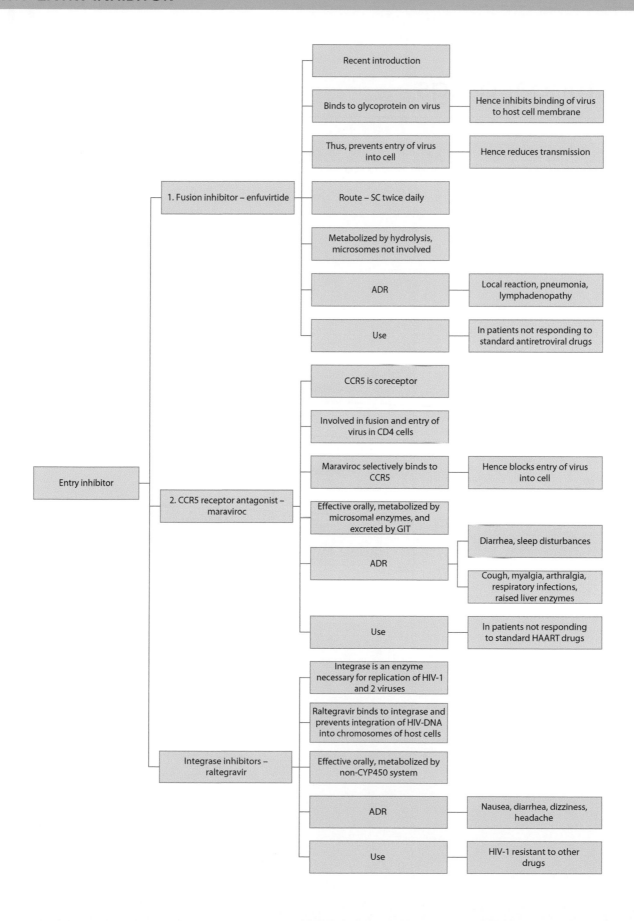

Entry inhibitor

1. Fusion inhibitor – enfuvirtide
- Recent introduction
- Binds to glycoprotein on virus → Hence inhibits binding of virus to host cell membrane
- Thus, prevents entry of virus into cell → Hence reduces transmission
- Route – SC twice daily
- Metabolized by hydrolysis, microsomes not involved
- ADR → Local reaction, pneumonia, lymphadenopathy
- Use → In patients not responding to standard antiretroviral drugs

2. CCR5 receptor antagonist – maraviroc
- CCR5 is coreceptor
- Involved in fusion and entry of virus in CD4 cells
- Maraviroc selectively binds to CCR5 → Hence blocks entry of virus into cell
- Effective orally, metabolized by microsomal enzymes, and excreted by GIT
- ADR → Diarrhea, sleep disturbances
- ADR → Cough, myalgia, arthralgia, respiratory infections, raised liver enzymes
- Use → In patients not responding to standard HAART drugs

Integrase inhibitors – raltegravir
- Integrase is an enzyme necessary for replication of HIV-1 and 2 viruses
- Raltegravir binds to integrase and prevents integration of HIV-DNA into chromosomes of host cells
- Effective orally, metabolized by non-CYP450 system
- ADR → Nausea, diarrhea, dizziness, headache
- Use → HIV-1 resistant to other drugs

70

Antifungal drugs

70.1 CLASSIFICATION OF ANTIFUNGAL DRUGS

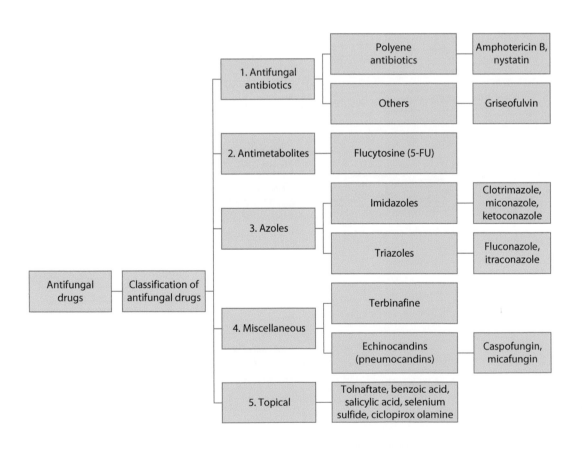

70.2 ANTIFUNGAL ANTIBIOTICS – AMPHOTERICIN B (AMB)

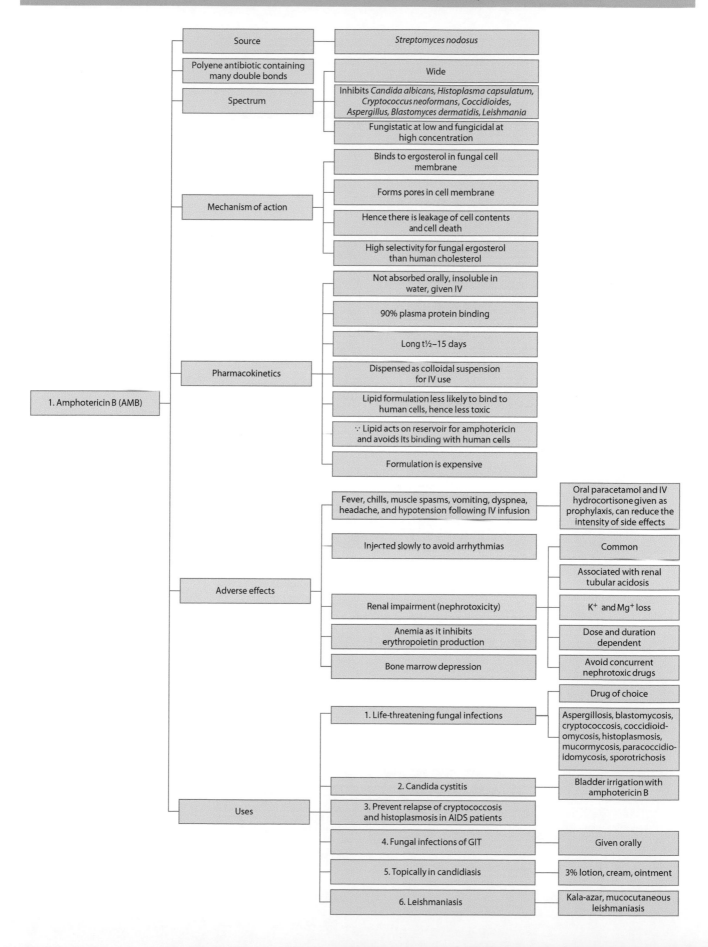

1. Amphotericin B (AMB)

- **Source** → *Streptomyces nodosus*
- **Polyene antibiotic containing many double bonds**
- **Spectrum**
  - Wide
  - Inhibits *Candida albicans, Histoplasma capsulatum, Cryptococcus neoformans, Coccidioides, Aspergillus, Blastomyces dermatidis, Leishmania*
  - Fungistatic at low and fungicidal at high concentration
- **Mechanism of action**
  - Binds to ergosterol in fungal cell membrane
  - Forms pores in cell membrane
  - Hence there is leakage of cell contents and cell death
  - High selectivity for fungal ergosterol than human cholesterol
- **Pharmacokinetics**
  - Not absorbed orally, insoluble in water, given IV
  - 90% plasma protein binding
  - Long t½–15 days
  - Dispensed as colloidal suspension for IV use
  - Lipid formulation less likely to bind to human cells, hence less toxic
  - ∴ Lipid acts on reservoir for amphotericin and avoids Its binding with human cells
  - Formulation is expensive
- **Adverse effects**
  - Fever, chills, muscle spasms, vomiting, dyspnea, headache, and hypotension following IV infusion
    - Oral paracetamol and IV hydrocortisone given as prophylaxis, can reduce the intensity of side effects
  - Injected slowly to avoid arrhythmias
  - Renal impairment (nephrotoxicity)
    - Common
    - Associated with renal tubular acidosis
    - K⁺ and Mg⁺ loss
    - Dose and duration dependent
    - Avoid concurrent nephrotoxic drugs
  - Anemia as it inhibits erythropoietin production
  - Bone marrow depression
- **Uses**
  - 1. Life-threatening fungal infections
    - Drug of choice
    - Aspergillosis, blastomycosis, cryptococcosis, coccidioidomycosis, histoplasmosis, mucormycosis, paracoccidioidomycosis, sporotrichosis
  - 2. Candida cystitis
    - Bladder irrigation with amphotericin B
  - 3. Prevent relapse of cryptococcosis and histoplasmosis in AIDS patients
  - 4. Fungal infections of GIT
    - Given orally
  - 5. Topically in candidiasis
    - 3% lotion, cream, ointment
  - 6. Leishmaniasis
    - Kala-azar, mucocutaneous leishmaniasis

70.3 NYSTATIN, GRISEOFULVIN

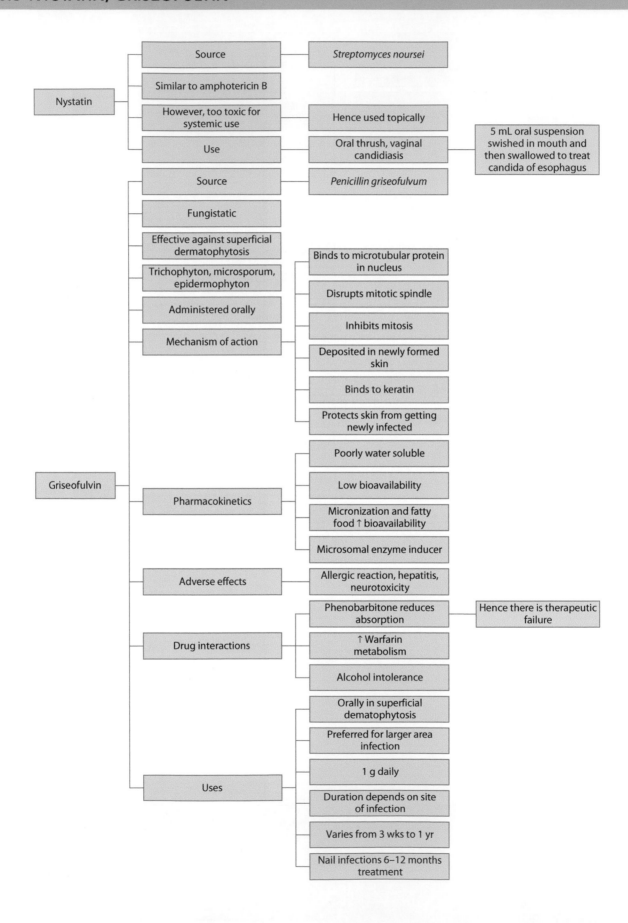

Nystatin
- Source → *Streptomyces noursei*
- Similar to amphotericin B
- However, too toxic for systemic use → Hence used topically
- Use → Oral thrush, vaginal candidiasis → 5 mL oral suspension swished in mouth and then swallowed to treat candida of esophagus

Griseofulvin
- Source → *Penicillin griseofulvum*
- Fungistatic
- Effective against superficial dermatophytosis
- Trichophyton, microsporum, epidermophyton
- Administered orally
- Mechanism of action
  - Binds to microtubular protein in nucleus
  - Disrupts mitotic spindle
  - Inhibits mitosis
  - Deposited in newly formed skin
  - Binds to keratin
  - Protects skin from getting newly infected
- Pharmacokinetics
  - Poorly water soluble
  - Low bioavailability
  - Micronization and fatty food ↑ bioavailability
  - Microsomal enzyme inducer
- Adverse effects → Allergic reaction, hepatitis, neurotoxicity
- Drug interactions
  - Phenobarbitone reduces absorption → Hence there is therapeutic failure
  - ↑ Warfarin metabolism
  - Alcohol intolerance
- Uses
  - Orally in superficial dematophytosis
  - Preferred for larger area infection
  - 1 g daily
  - Duration depends on site of infection
  - Varies from 3 wks to 1 yr
  - Nail infections 6–12 months treatment

70.4 ANTIMETABOLITES

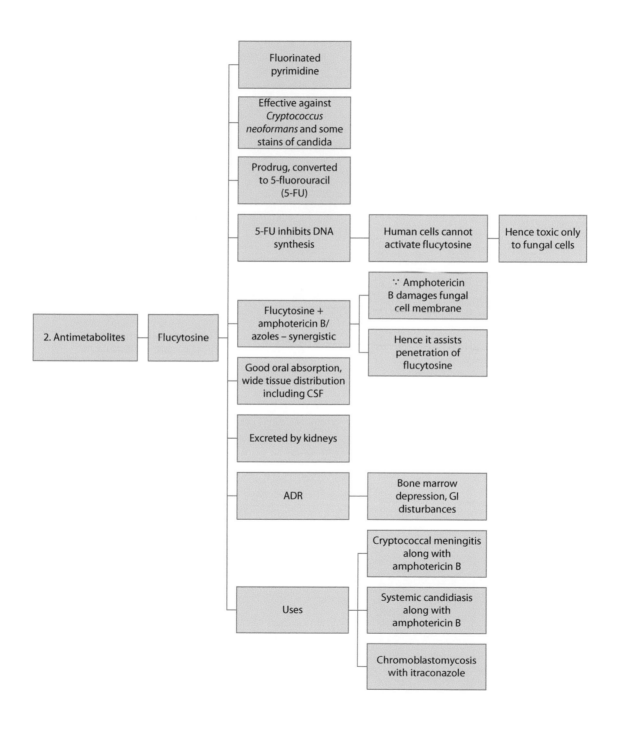

70.5 AZOLES

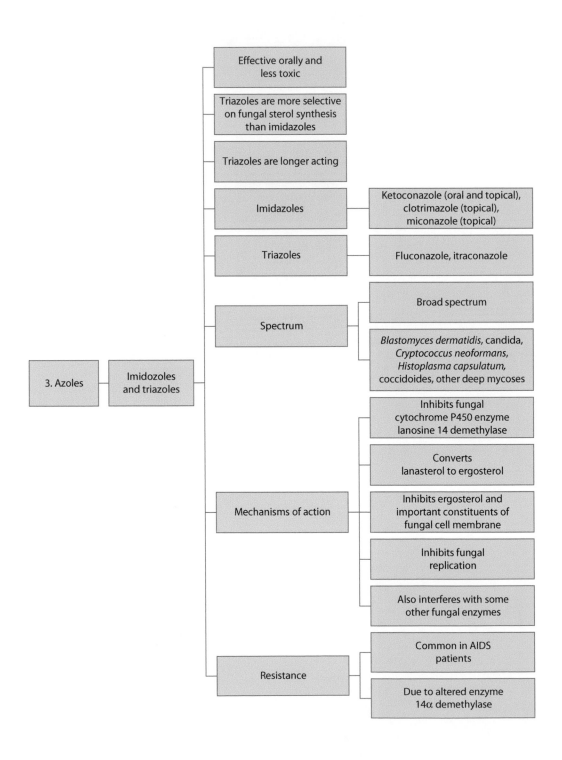

70.6 KETOCONAZOLE

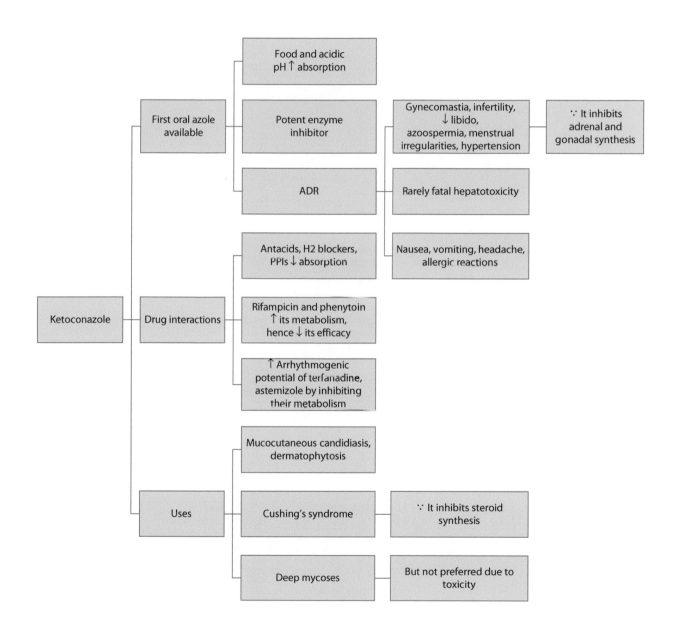

70.7 FLUCONAZOLE

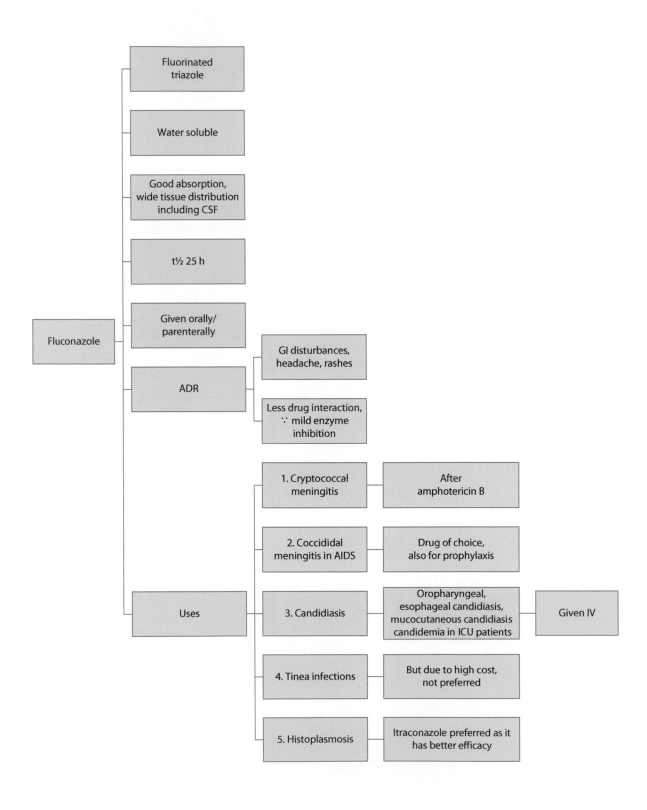

70.8 ITRACONAZOLE

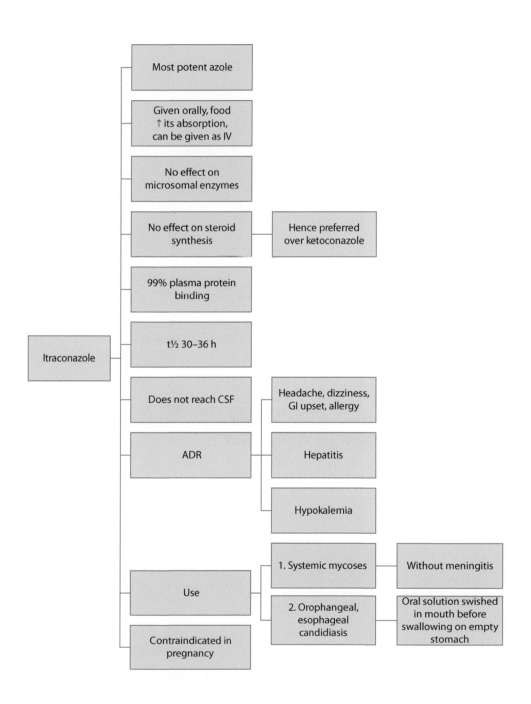

70.9 TOPICAL AZOLES

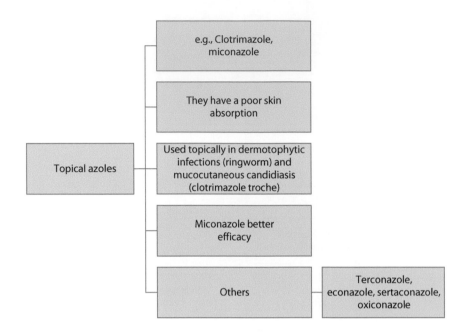

Topical azoles
- e.g., Clotrimazole, miconazole
- They have a poor skin absorption
- Used topically in dermotophytic infections (ringworm) and mucocutaneous candidiasis (clotrimazole troche)
- Miconazole better efficacy
- Others → Terconazole, econazole, sertaconazole, oxiconazole

70.10 MISCELLANEOUS – TERBINAFINE

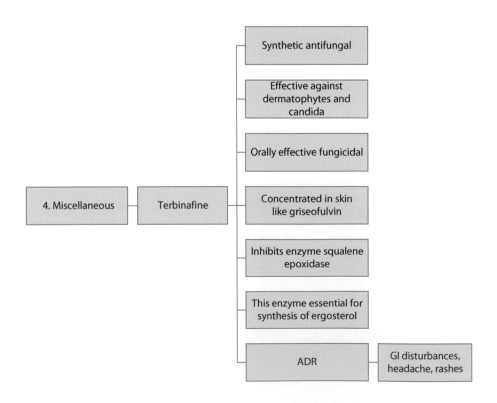

4. Miscellaneous → Terbinafine
- Synthetic antifungal
- Effective against dermatophytes and candida
- Orally effective fungicidal
- Concentrated in skin like griseofulvin
- Inhibits enzyme squalene epoxidase
- This enzyme essential for synthesis of ergosterol
- ADR → GI disturbances, headache, rashes

70.11 ECHINOCANDINS OR PNEUMOCANDINS

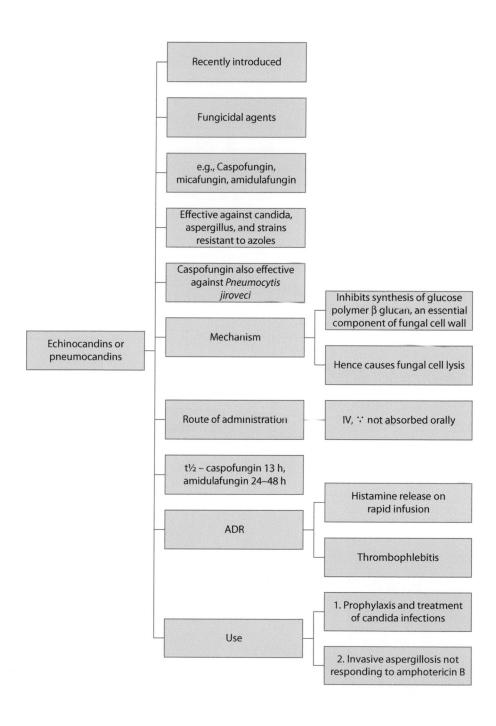

70.12 TOPICAL ANTIFUNGALS AND NEWER AGENTS

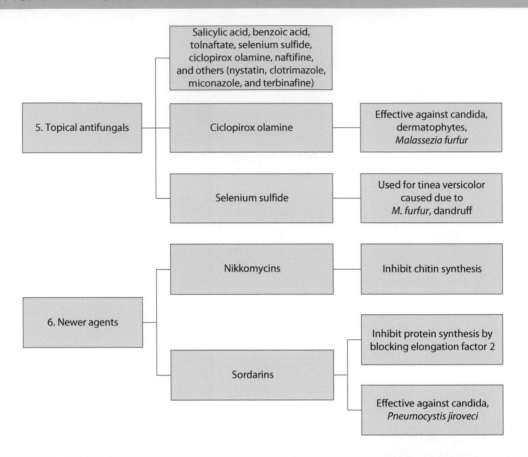

5. Topical antifungals
- Salicylic acid, benzoic acid, tolnaftate, selenium sulfide, ciclopirox olamine, naftifine, and others (nystatin, clotrimazole, miconazole, and terbinafine)
- Ciclopirox olamine — Effective against candida, dermatophytes, *Malassezia furfur*
- Selenium sulfide — Used for tinea versicolor caused due to *M. furfur*, dandruff

6. Newer agents
- Nikkomycins — Inhibit chitin synthesis
- Sordarins — Inhibit protein synthesis by blocking elongation factor 2 — Effective against candida, *Pneumocystis jiroveci*

70.13 DRUGS USED IN SUPERFICIAL MYCOSES

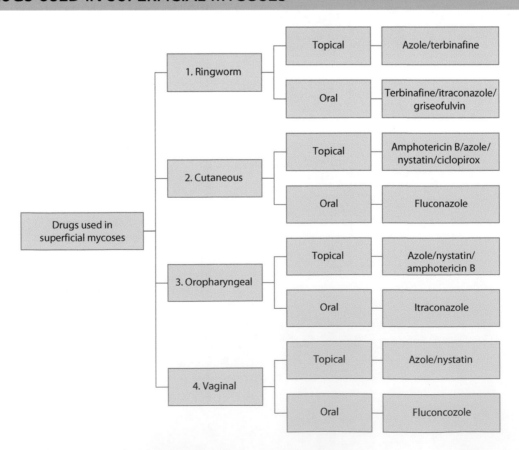

Drugs used in superficial mycoses

1. Ringworm
- Topical — Azole/terbinafine
- Oral — Terbinafine/itraconazole/griseofulvin

2. Cutaneous
- Topical — Amphotericin B/azole/nystatin/ciclopirox
- Oral — Fluconazole

3. Oropharyngeal
- Topical — Azole/nystatin/amphotericin B
- Oral — Itraconazole

4. Vaginal
- Topical — Azole/nystatin
- Oral — Fluconcozole

70.14 DRUGS FOR SYSTEMIC FUNGAL INFECTIONS

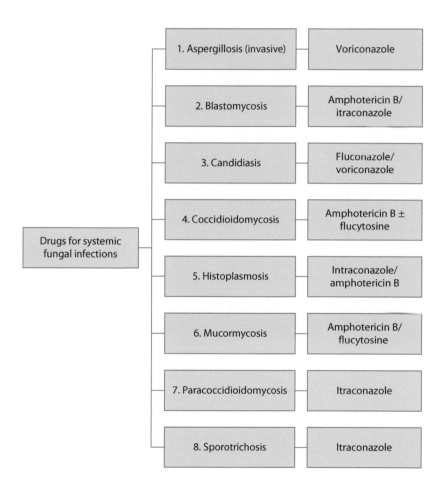

Anthelmintics

71.1 MEBENDAZOLE

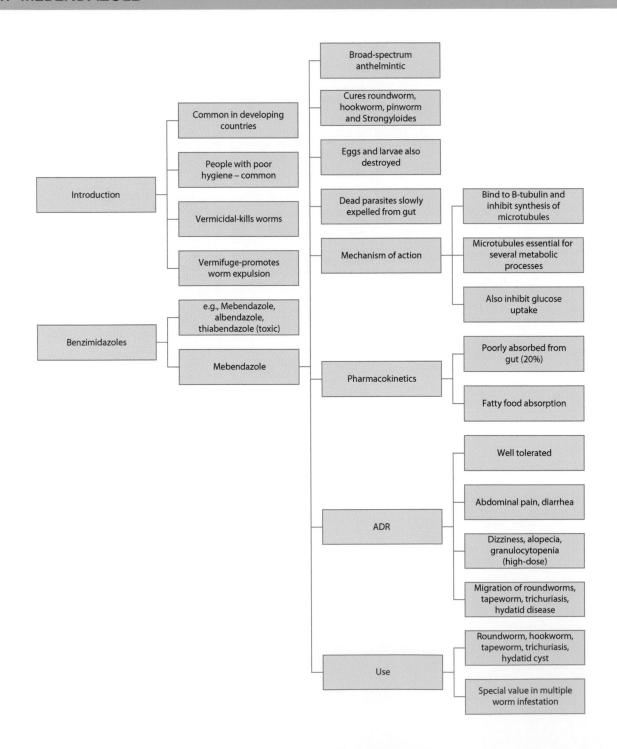

71.2 ALBENDAZOLE, PYRANTEL PAMOATE, PIPERAZINE CITRATE

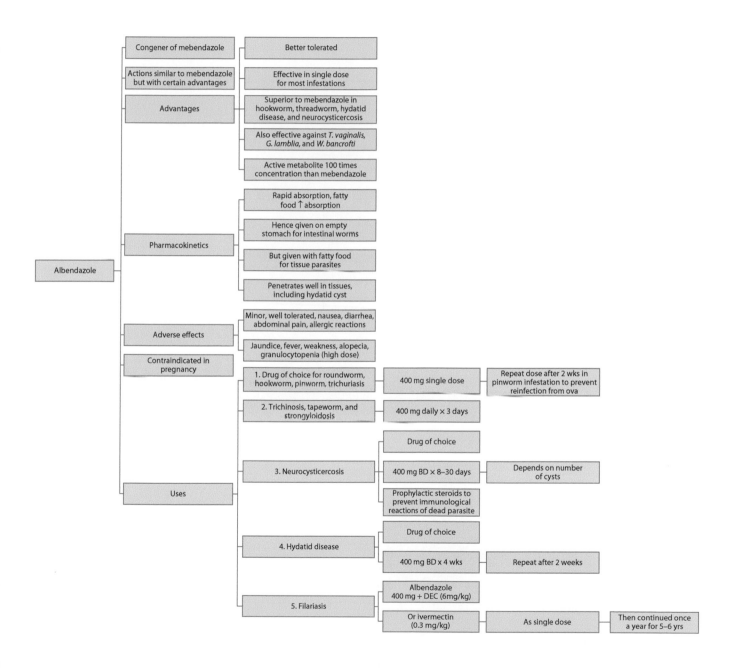

Albendazole
- Congener of mebendazole — Better tolerated
- Actions similar to mebendazole but with certain advantages
  - Advantages
    - Effective in single dose for most infestations
    - Superior to mebendazole in hookworm, threadworm, hydatid disease, and neurocysticercosis
    - Also effective against *T. vaginalis*, *G. lamblia*, and *W. bancrofti*
    - Active metabolite 100 times concentration than mebendazole
  - Pharmacokinetics
    - Rapid absorption, fatty food ↑ absorption
    - Hence given on empty stomach for intestinal worms
    - But given with fatty food for tissue parasites
    - Penetrates well in tissues, including hydatid cyst
  - Adverse effects
    - Minor, well tolerated, nausea, diarrhea, abdominal pain, allergic reactions
    - Jaundice, fever, weakness, alopecia, granulocytopenia (high dose)
- Contraindicated in pregnancy
- Uses
  1. Drug of choice for roundworm, hookworm, pinworm, trichuriasis — 400 mg single dose — Repeat dose after 2 wks in pinworm infestation to prevent reinfection from ova
  2. Trichinosis, tapeworm, and strongyloidosis — 400 mg daily × 3 days
  3. Neurocysticercosis
     - Drug of choice
     - 400 mg BD × 8–30 days — Depends on number of cysts
     - Prophylactic steroids to prevent immunological reactions of dead parasite
  4. Hydatid disease
     - Drug of choice
     - 400 mg BD × 4 wks — Repeat after 2 weeks
  5. Filariasis
     - Albendazole 400 mg + DEC (6mg/kg)
     - Or ivermectin (0.3 mg/kg) — As single dose — Then continued once a year for 5–6 yrs

(Continued)

71.2 ALBENDAZOLE, PYRANTEL PAMOATE, PIPERAZINE CITRATE (Continued)

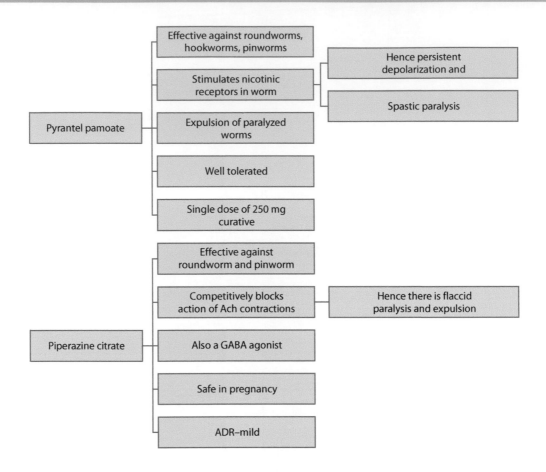

Pyrantel pamoate
- Effective against roundworms, hookworms, pinworms
- Stimulates nicotinic receptors in worm → Hence persistent depolarization and → Spastic paralysis
- Expulsion of paralyzed worms
- Well tolerated
- Single dose of 250 mg curative

Piperazine citrate
- Effective against roundworm and pinworm
- Competitively blocks action of Ach contractions → Hence there is flaccid paralysis and expulsion
- Also a GABA agonist
- Safe in pregnancy
- ADR–mild

71.3 PRAZIQUANTEL

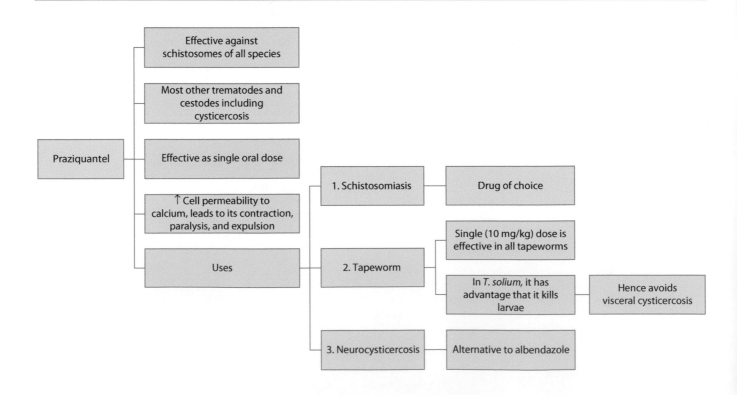

Praziquantel
- Effective against schistosomes of all species
- Most other trematodes and cestodes including cysticercosis
- Effective as single oral dose
- ↑ Cell permeability to calcium, leads to its contraction, paralysis, and expulsion
- Uses
  1. Schistosomiasis → Drug of choice
  2. Tapeworm
     - Single (10 mg/kg) dose is effective in all tapeworms
     - In *T. solium,* it has advantage that it kills larvae → Hence avoids visceral cysticercosis
  3. Neurocysticercosis → Alternative to albendazole

71.4 LEVAMISOLE AND NICLOSAMIDE

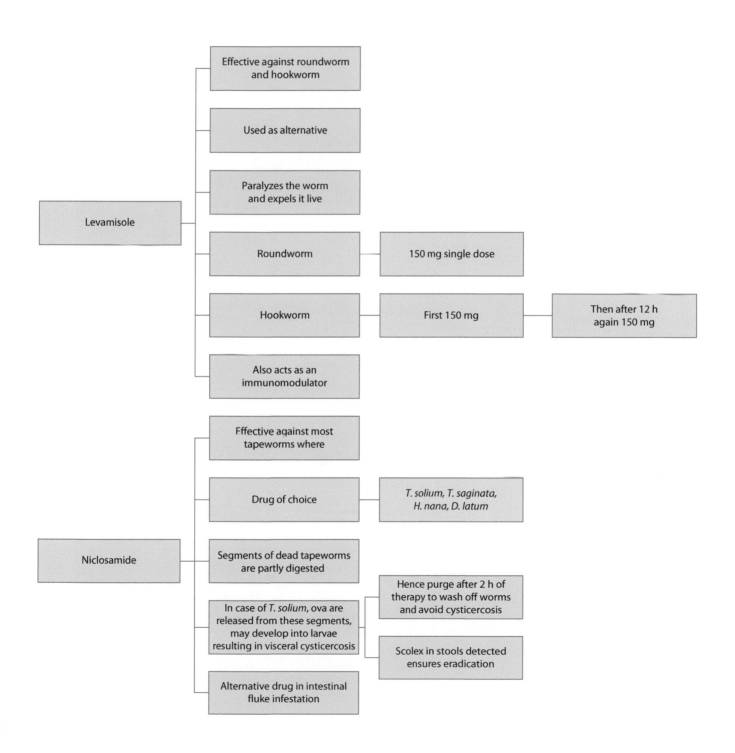

71.5 DIETHYLCARBAMAZINE (DEC)

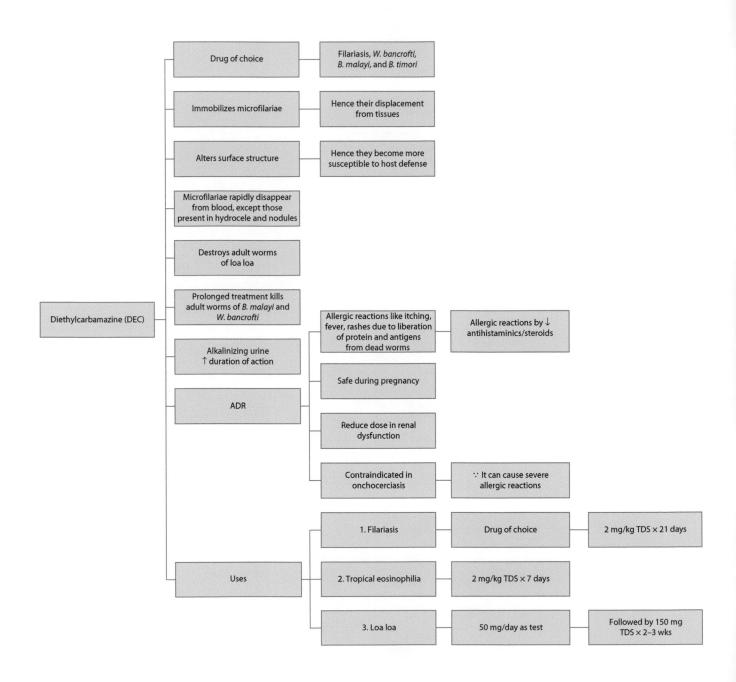

71.6 IVERMECTIN

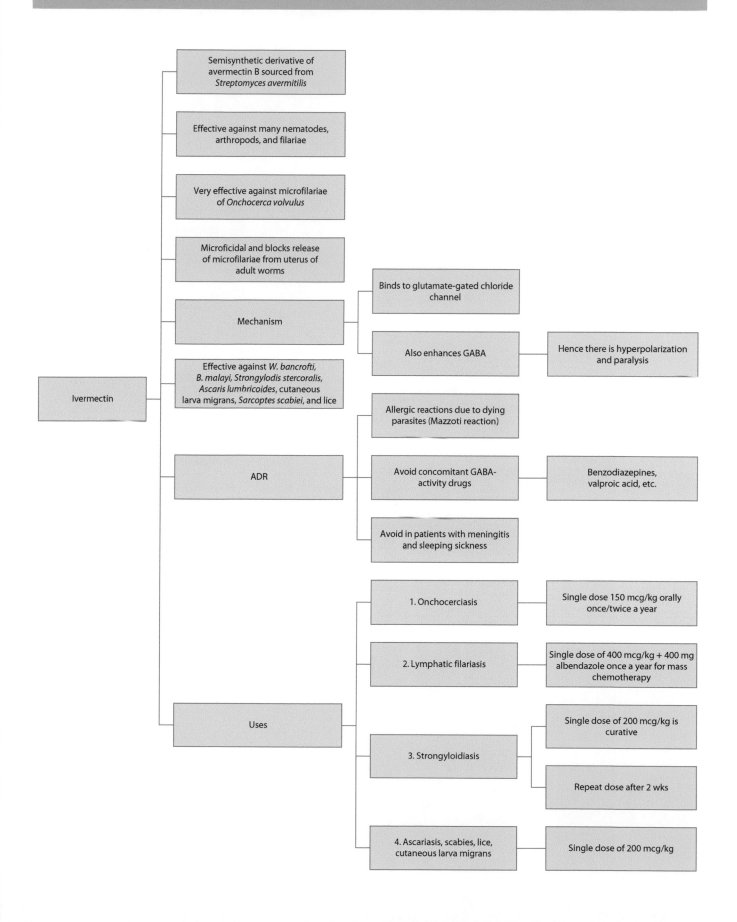

Ivermectin

- Semisynthetic derivative of avermectin B sourced from *Streptomyces avermitilis*
- Effective against many nematodes, arthropods, and filariae
- Very effective against microfilariae of *Onchocerca volvulus*
- Microficidal and blocks release of microfilariae from uterus of adult worms
- **Mechanism**
  - Binds to glutamate-gated chloride channel
  - Also enhances GABA → Hence there is hyperpolarization and paralysis
- Effective against *W. bancrofti*, *B. malayi*, *Strongylodis stercoralis*, *Ascaris lumbricoides*, cutaneous larva migrans, *Sarcoptes scabiei*, and lice
- **ADR**
  - Allergic reactions due to dying parasites (Mazzoti reaction)
  - Avoid concomitant GABA-activity drugs → Benzodiazepines, valproic acid, etc.
  - Avoid in patients with meningitis and sleeping sickness
- **Uses**
  1. Onchocerciasis → Single dose 150 mcg/kg orally once/twice a year
  2. Lymphatic filariasis → Single dose of 400 mcg/kg + 400 mg albendazole once a year for mass chemotherapy
  3. Strongyloidiasis → Single dose of 200 mcg/kg is curative; Repeat dose after 2 wks
  4. Ascariasis, scabies, lice, cutaneous larva migrans → Single dose of 200 mcg/kg

71.7 MISCELLANEOUS

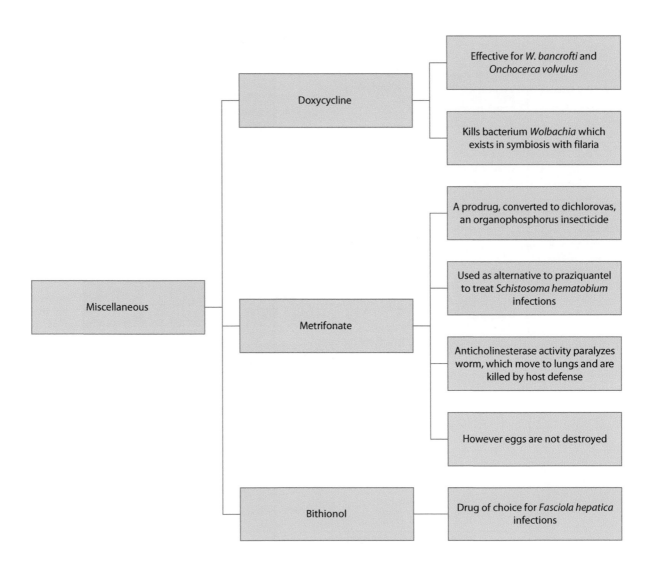

71.8 PREFERRED DRUGS FOR HELMINTIC INFESTATIONS

Worm	Drugs of choice	Alternative
1. *Ascaris lumbricoides* (roundworm)	Mebendazole (M)/albendazole (A) piperazine (Pp)	Pyrantel (P)
2. *Ankylostoma duodenale* (hookworm) *Necator americanus*	M/A	Pyrantel (P)
3. *Enterobius vermicularis* (pinworm)	M/A/P	Pp
4. *Trichuris trichura* (whipworm)	M	A
5. *Strongyloides stercoralis*	A	Thiabendazole
6. *Dracunculus medinensis* (guineaworm)	Metronidazole	M
7. *Neurocysticercosis* (tapeworms)	Niclosamide/praziquantel A A	Praziquantel
8. Hydatid disease	A	M
9. Filaria	DEC + A	Ivermectin + A
10. Schistosomes	Praziquantel	–
11. *Onchocerca volvulus*	Ivermectin	–
12. *Fasciola hepatica* (sheep liver fluke)	Bithionol	–

71.9 DRUGS FOR SCABIES AND TREATMENT OF PEDICULOSIS

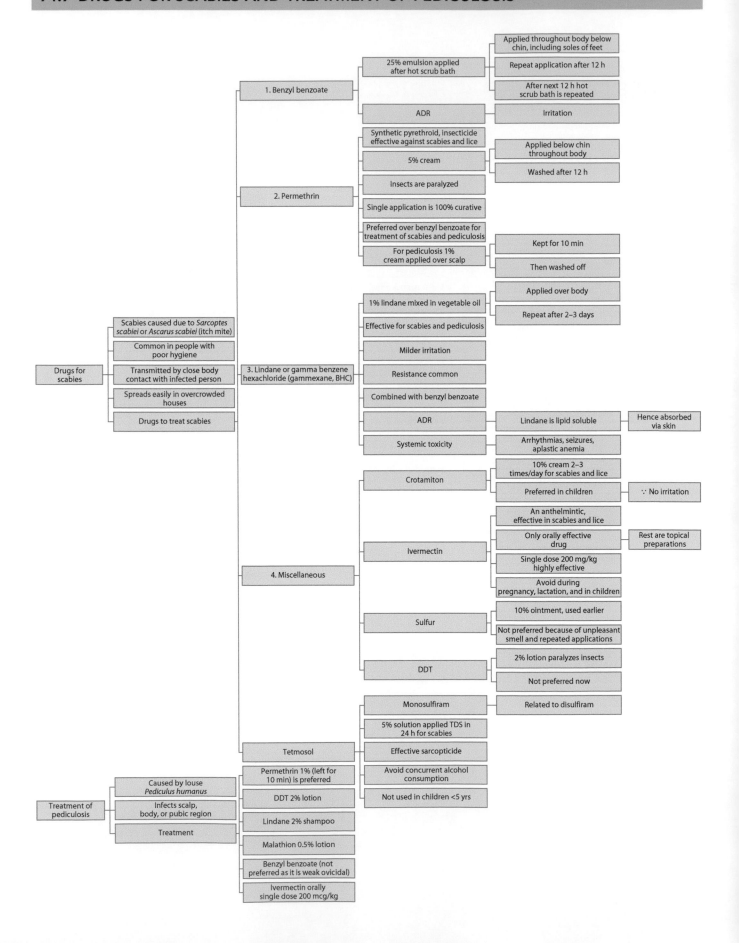

Drugs for scabies
- Scabies caused due to *Sarcoptes scabiei* or *Ascarus scabiei* (itch mite)
- Common in people with poor hygiene
- Transmitted by close body contact with infected person
- Spreads easily in overcrowded houses
- Drugs to treat scabies

1. Benzyl benzoate
- 25% emulsion applied after hot scrub bath
  - Applied throughout body below chin, including soles of feet
  - Repeat application after 12 h
  - After next 12 h hot scrub bath is repeated
- ADR
  - Irritation

2. Permethrin
- Synthetic pyrethroid, insecticide effective against scabies and lice
- 5% cream
  - Applied below chin throughout body
  - Washed after 12 h
- Insects are paralyzed
- Single application is 100% curative
- Preferred over benzyl benzoate for treatment of scabies and pediculosis
- For pediculosis 1% cream applied over scalp
  - Kept for 10 min
  - Then washed off

3. Lindane or gamma benzene hexachloride (gammexane, BHC)
- 1% lindane mixed in vegetable oil
  - Applied over body
  - Repeat after 2–3 days
- Effective for scabies and pediculosis
- Milder irritation
- Resistance common
- Combined with benzyl benzoate
- ADR
  - Lindane is lipid soluble → Hence absorbed via skin
- Systemic toxicity
  - Arrhythmias, seizures, aplastic anemia

4. Miscellaneous
- Crotamiton
  - 10% cream 2–3 times/day for scabies and lice
  - Preferred in children → ∵ No irritation
- Ivermectin
  - An anthelmintic, effective in scabies and lice
  - Only orally effective drug → Rest are topical preparations
  - Single dose 200 mg/kg highly effective
  - Avoid during pregnancy, lactation, and in children
- Sulfur
  - 10% ointment, used earlier
  - Not preferred because of unpleasant smell and repeated applications
- DDT
  - 2% lotion paralyzes insects
  - Not preferred now
- Monosulfiram
  - Related to disulfiram
- Tetmosol
  - 5% solution applied TDS in 24 h for scabies
  - Effective sarcopticide
  - Avoid concurrent alcohol consumption
  - Not used in children <5 yrs

Treatment of pediculosis
- Caused by louse *Pediculus humanus*
- Infects scalp, body, or pubic region
- Treatment
  - Permethrin 1% (left for 10 min) is preferred
  - DDT 2% lotion
  - Lindane 2% shampoo
  - Malathion 0.5% lotion
  - Benzyl benzoate (not preferred as it is weak ovicidal)
  - Ivermectin orally single dose 200 mcg/kg

Antiseptics and disinfectants

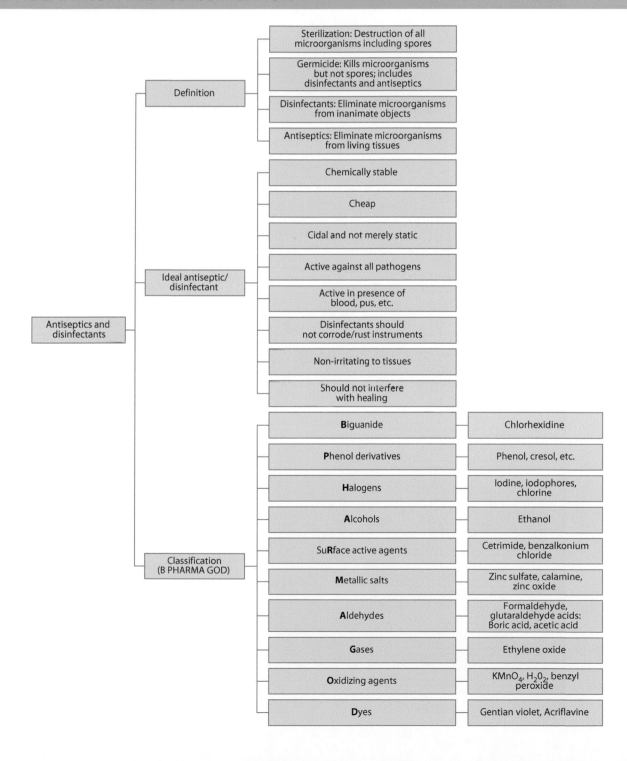

72.2 BIGUANIDES

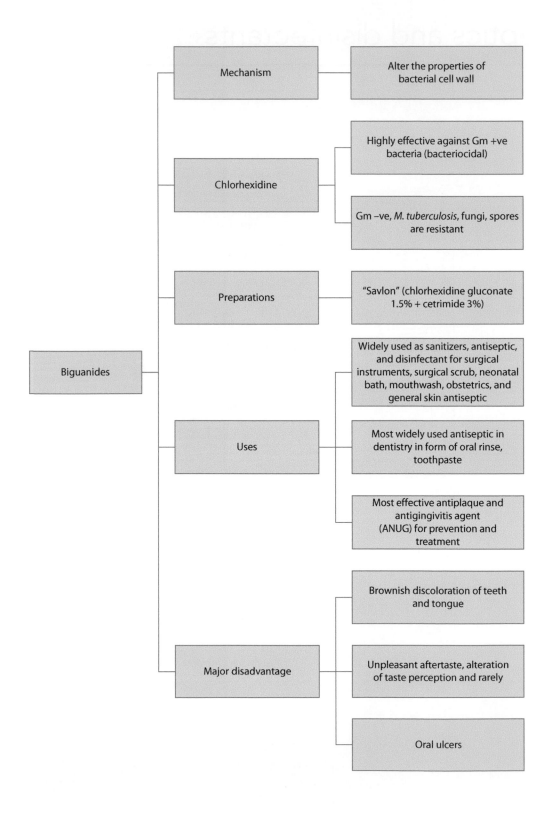

Biguanides

Mechanism — Alter the properties of bacterial cell wall

Chlorhexidine — Highly effective against Gm +ve bacteria (bacteriocidal)

— Gm –ve, *M. tuberculosis*, fungi, spores are resistant

Preparations — "Savlon" (chlorhexidine gluconate 1.5% + cetrimide 3%)

Uses — Widely used as sanitizers, antiseptic, and disinfectant for surgical instruments, surgical scrub, neonatal bath, mouthwash, obstetrics, and general skin antiseptic

— Most widely used antiseptic in dentistry in form of oral rinse, toothpaste

— Most effective antiplaque and antigingivitis agent (ANUG) for prevention and treatment

Major disadvantage — Brownish discoloration of teeth and tongue

— Unpleasant aftertaste, alteration of taste perception and rarely

— Oral ulcers

72.3 PHENOLS

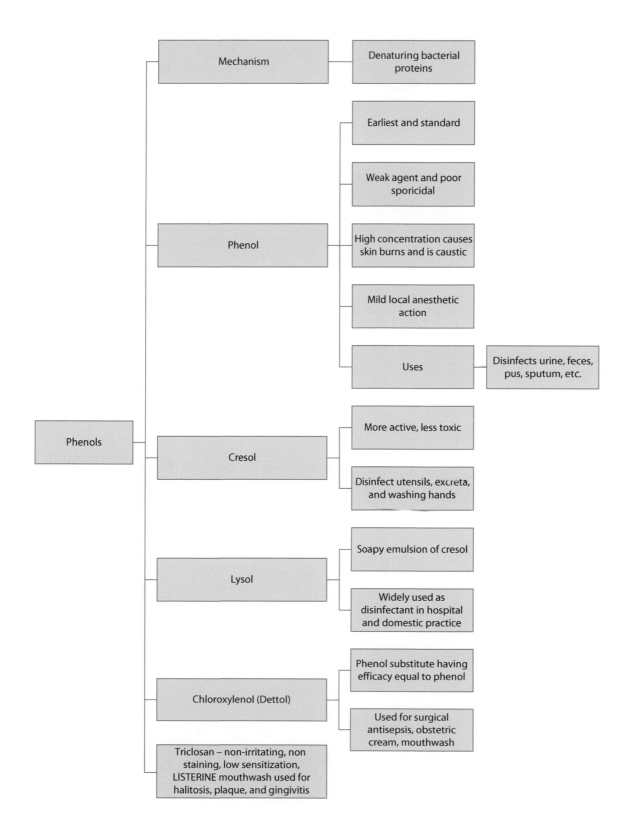

72.4 HALOGENS

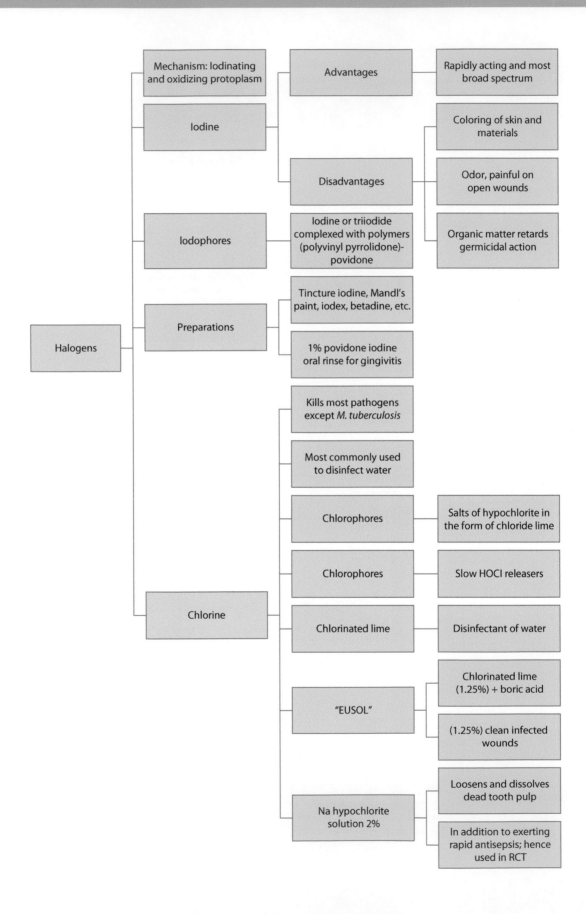

72.5 ALCOHOLS

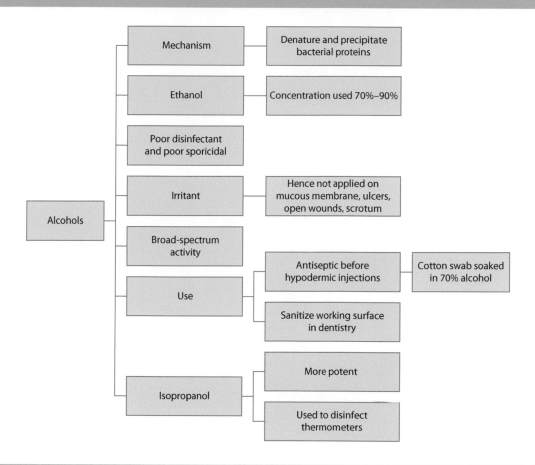

72.6 SURFACE ACTIVE AGENTS

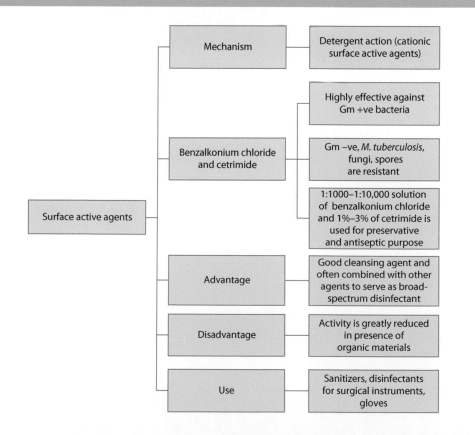

72.7 METALLIC SALTS

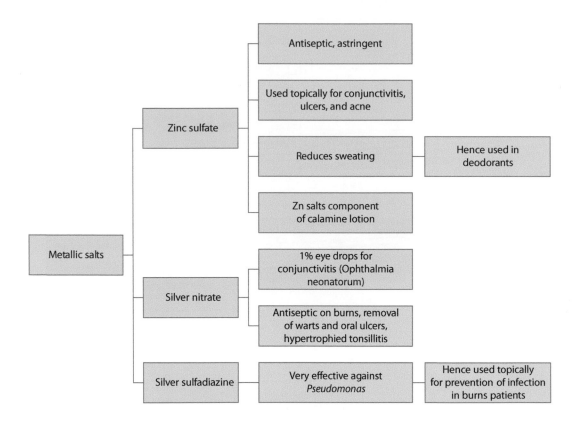

72.8 ALDEHYDES

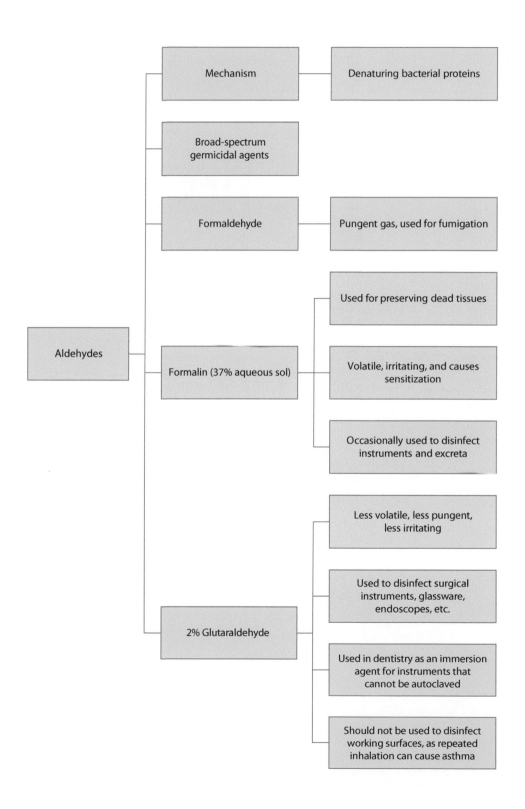

72.9 ACIDS

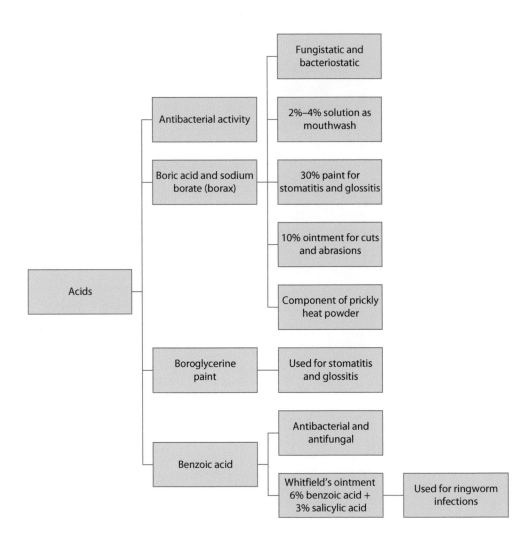

72.10 GASES

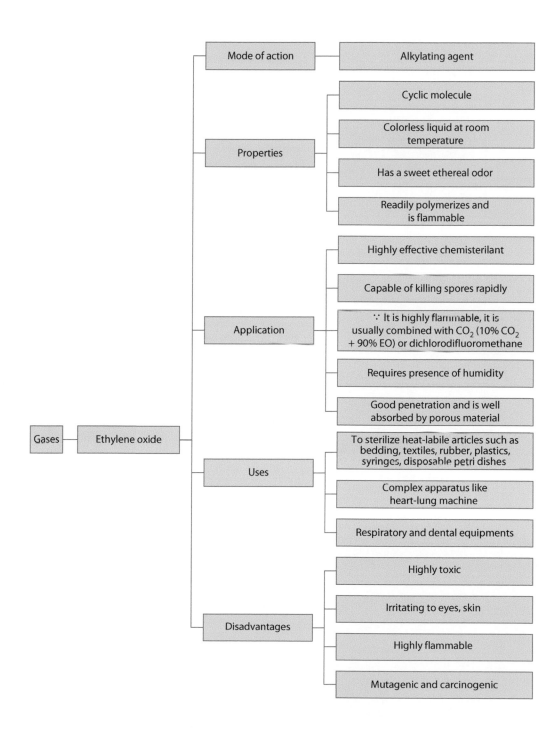

72.11 OXIDIZING AGENTS

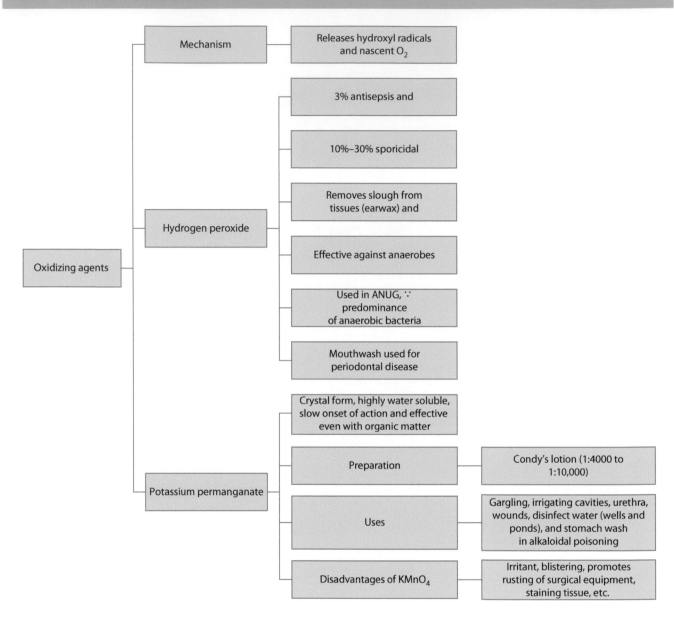

Oxidizing agents

Mechanism — Releases hydroxyl radicals and nascent O_2

Hydrogen peroxide
- 3% antisepsis and
- 10%–30% sporicidal
- Removes slough from tissues (earwax) and
- Effective against anaerobes
- Used in ANUG, ∵ predominance of anaerobic bacteria
- Mouthwash used for periodontal disease

Potassium permanganate
- Crystal form, highly water soluble, slow onset of action and effective even with organic matter
- Preparation — Condy's lotion (1:4000 to 1:10,000)
- Uses — Gargling, irrigating cavities, urethra, wounds, disinfect water (wells and ponds), and stomach wash in alkaloidal poisoning
- Disadvantages of $KMnO_4$ — Irritant, blistering, promotes rusting of surgical equipment, staining tissue, etc.

72.12 DYES

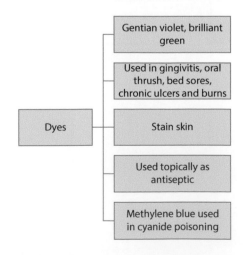

Dyes
- Gentian violet, brilliant green
- Used in gingivitis, oral thrush, bed sores, chronic ulcers and burns
- Stain skin
- Used topically as antiseptic
- Methylene blue used in cyanide poisoning

Cancer chemotherapy

73

73.1 INTRODUCTION AND PHASES OF CELL CYCLES

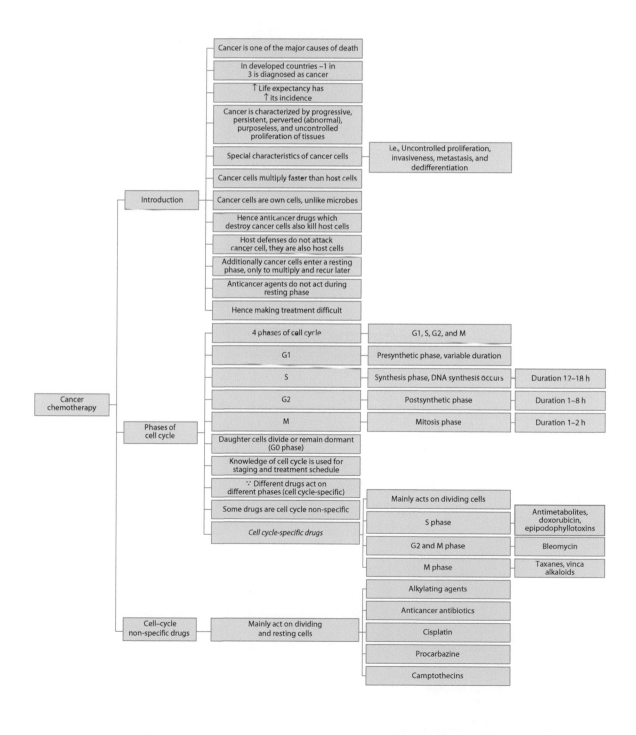

73.2 COMMON ADVERSE EFFECTS OF ANTICANCER AGENTS AND MEASURES TO PREVENT ADVERSE EFFECTS

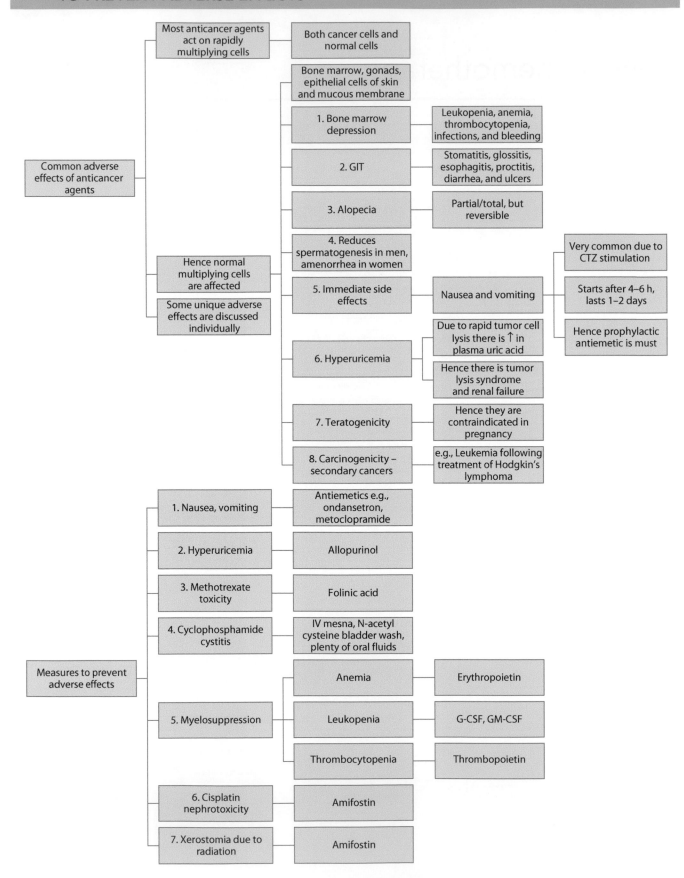

73.3 CLASSIFICATION OF ANTICANCER AGENTS

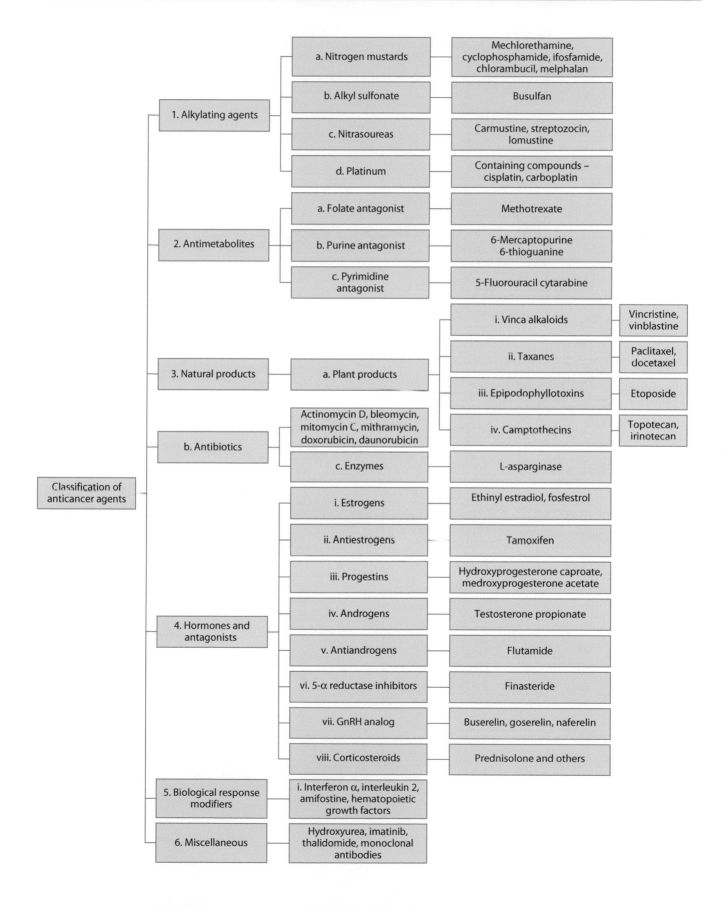

73.4 ALKYLATING AGENTS AND NITROGEN MUSTARDS

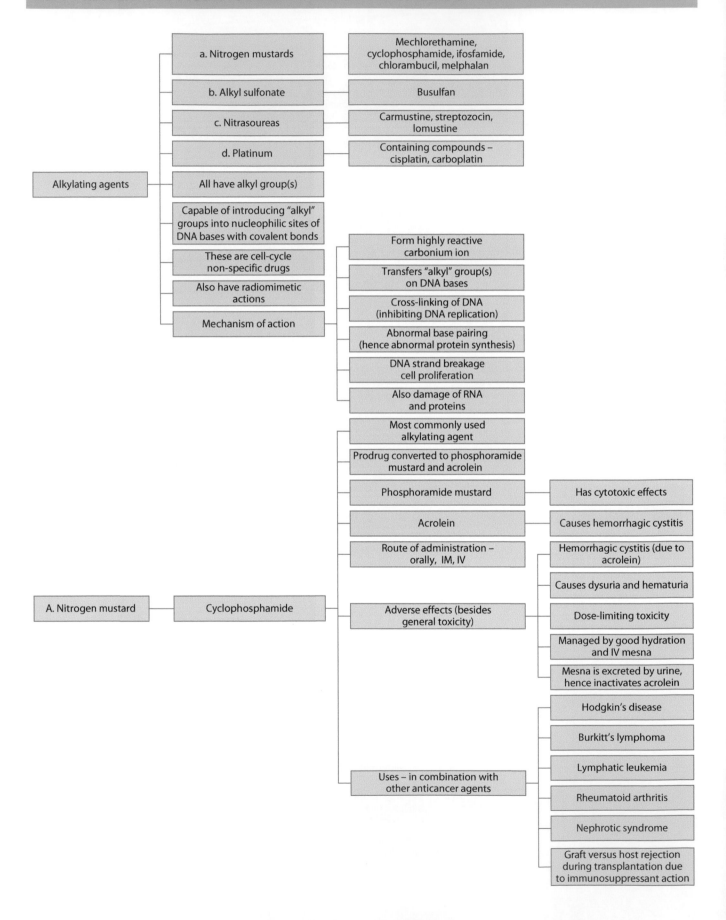

73.5 OTHER ALKYLATING AGENTS, ALKYL SULFONES, AND NITROSUREAS

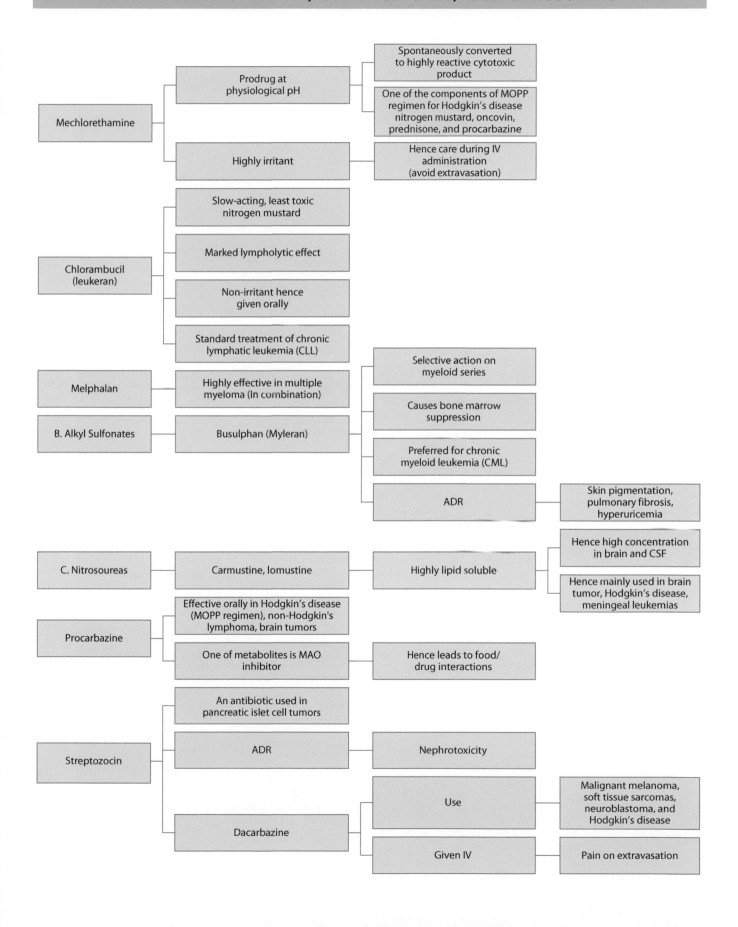

73.6 PLATINUM-CONTAINING COMPOUNDS

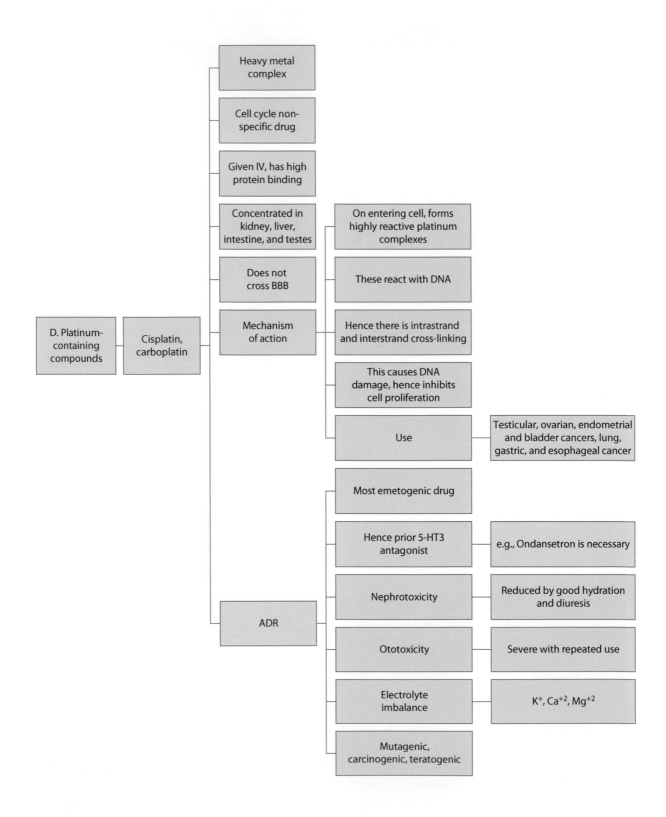

73.7 ANTIMETABOLITES – FOLATE ANTAGONISTS – METHOTREXATE (MTX)

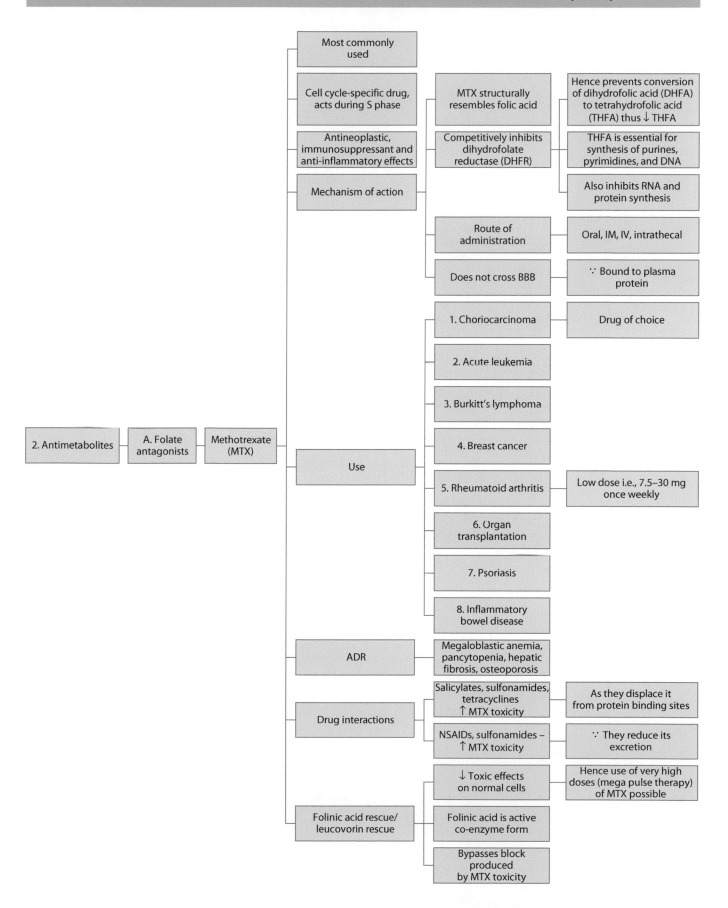

73.8 PURINE – ANTAGONISTS AND PYRIMIDINE ANTAGONIST

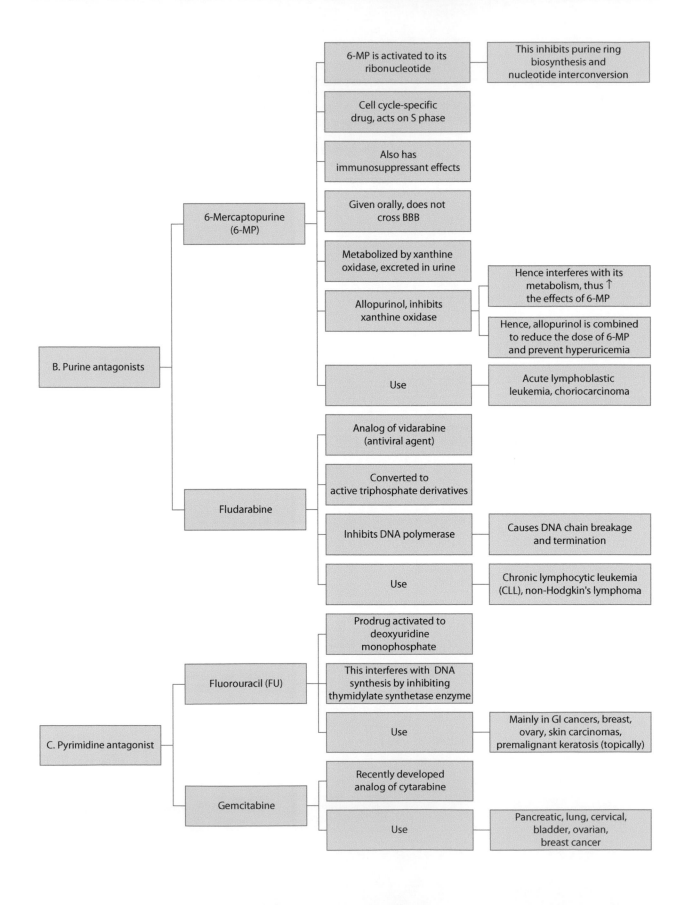

73.9 NATURAL PRODUCTS – PLANT PRODUCTS: VINCA ALKALOIDS

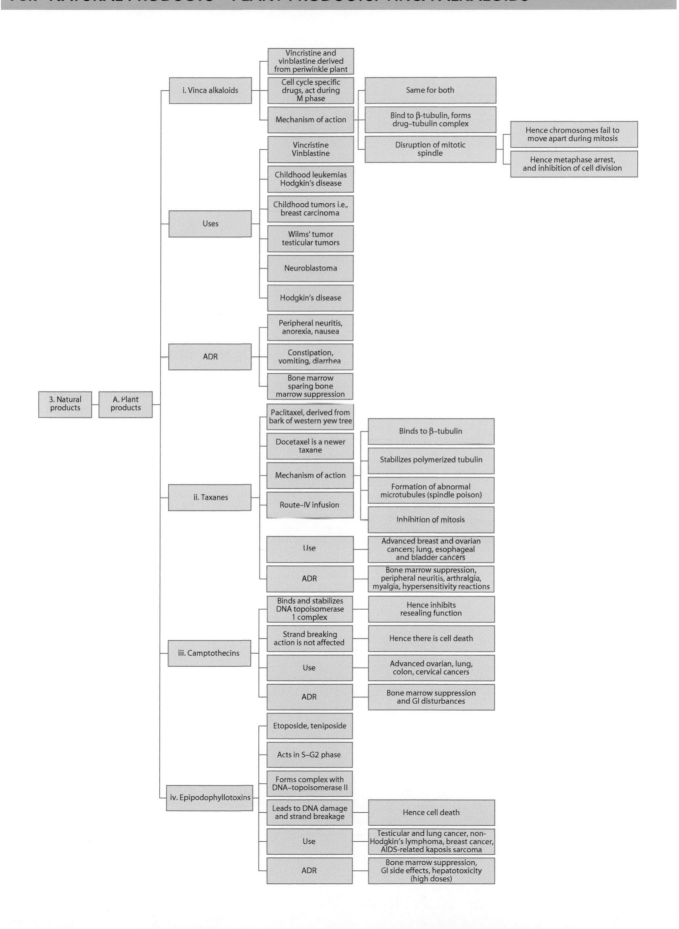

73.10 ANTICANCER ANTIBIOTICS

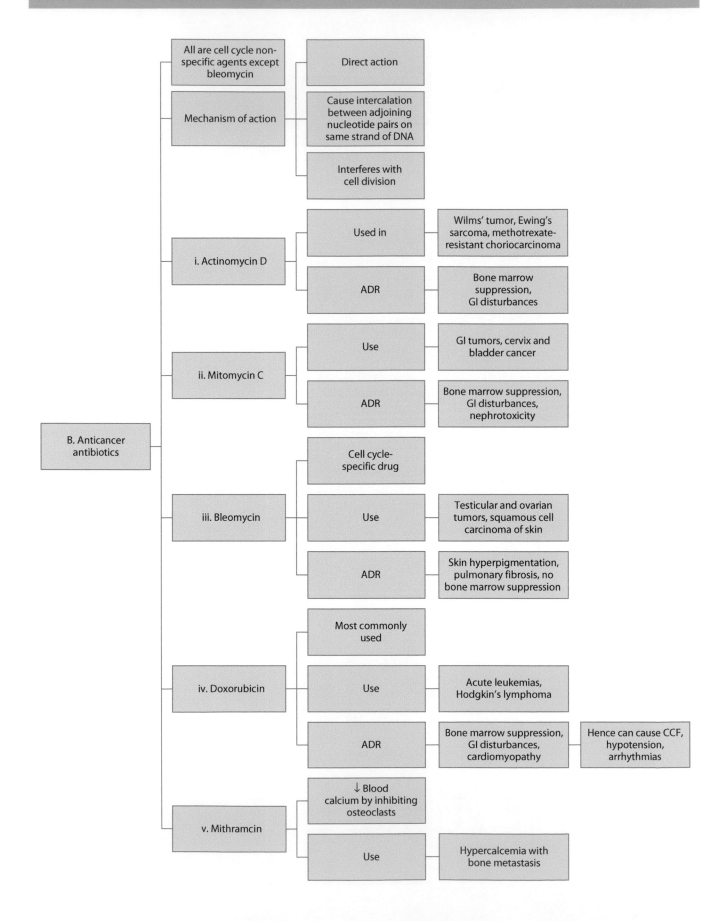

73.11 ENZYMES

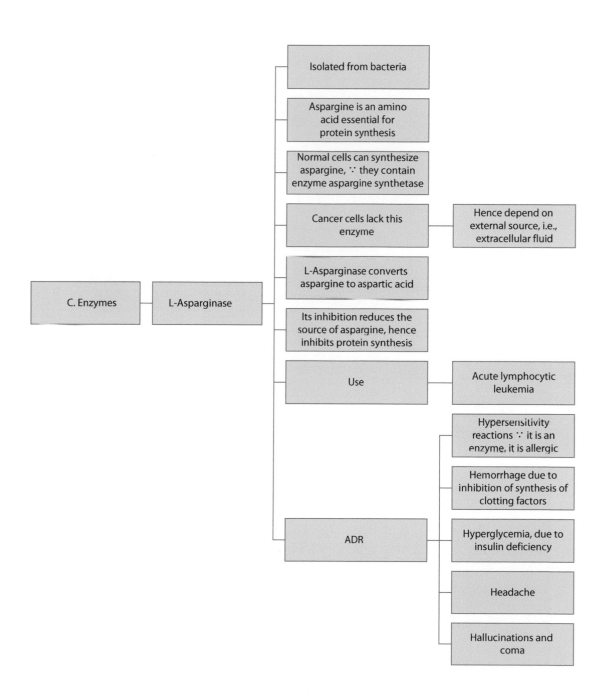

73.12 HORMONAL AGENTS

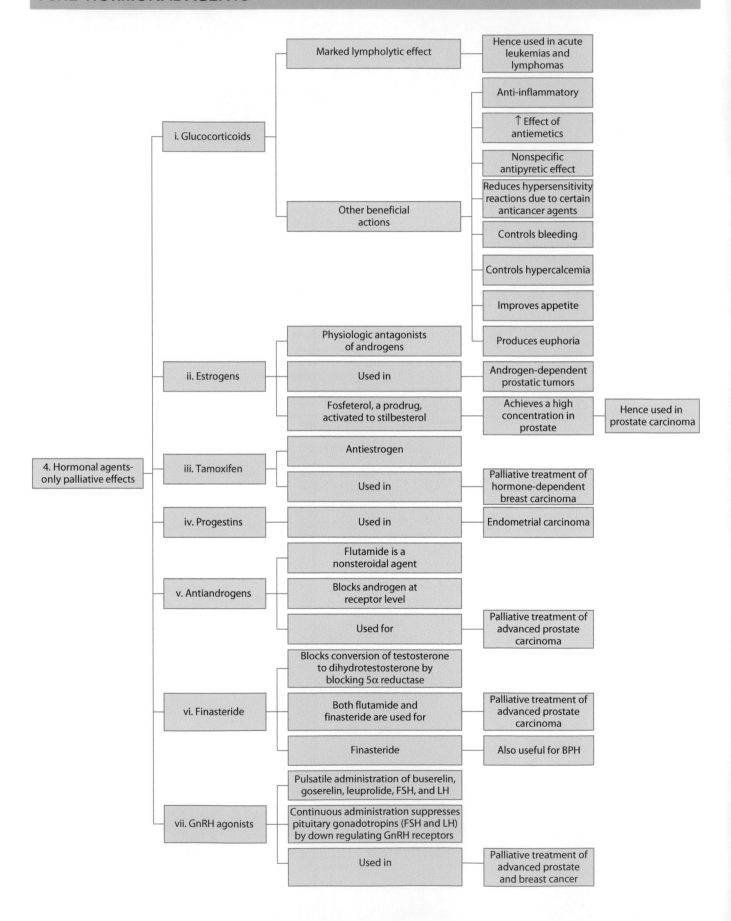

73.13 BIOLOGICAL RESPONSE MODIFIERS

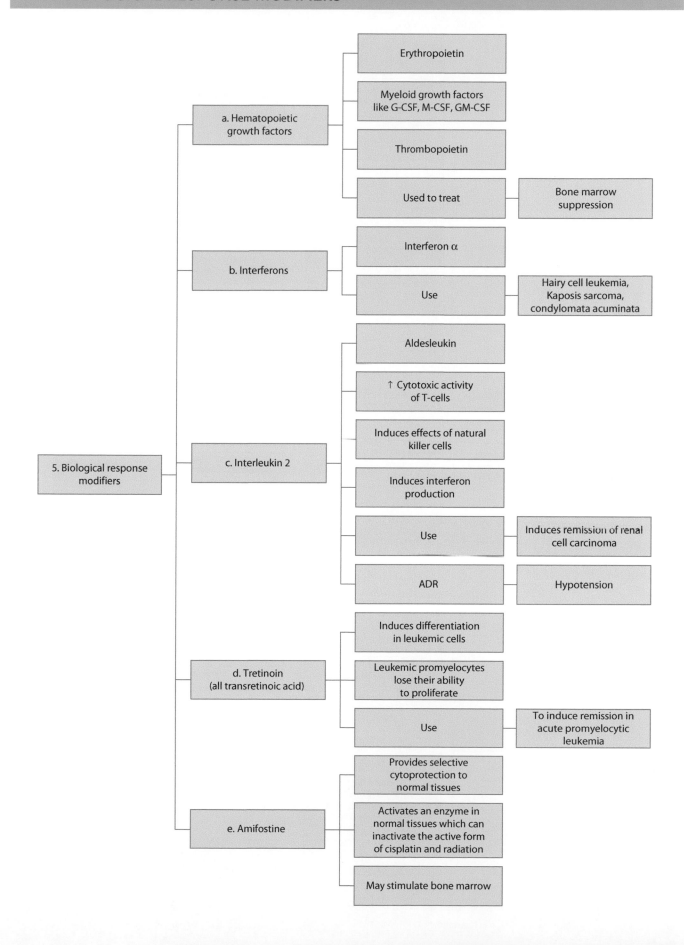

73.14 MISCELLANEOUS

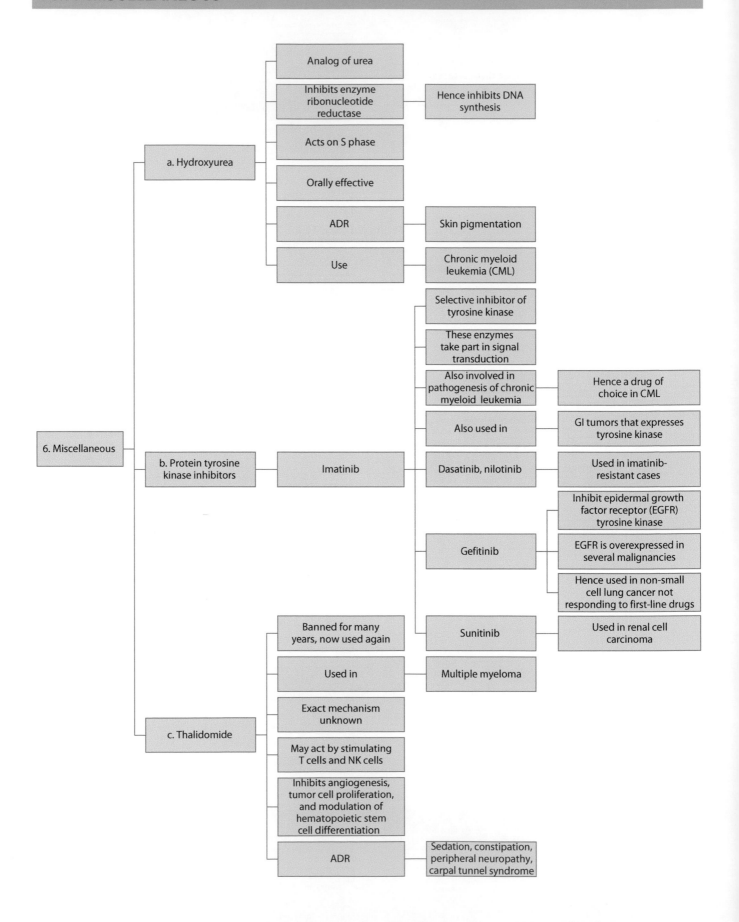

73.15 MONOCLONAL ANTIBODIES AND RADIOACTIVE ISOTOPES

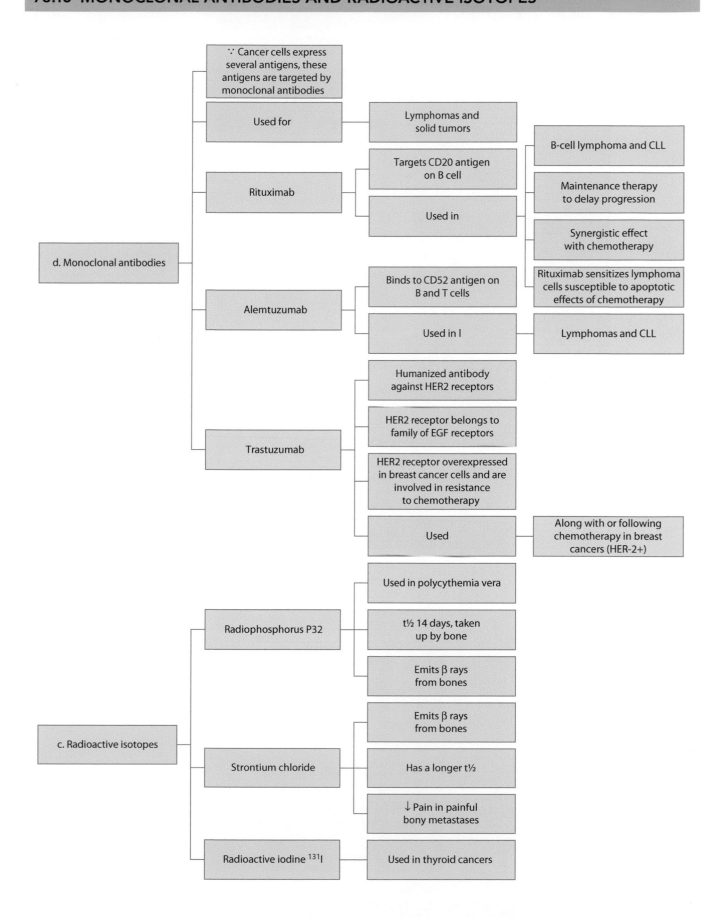

73.16 RESISTANCE TO ANTICANCER DRUGS AND GENERAL PRINCIPLES OF CANCER TREATMENT

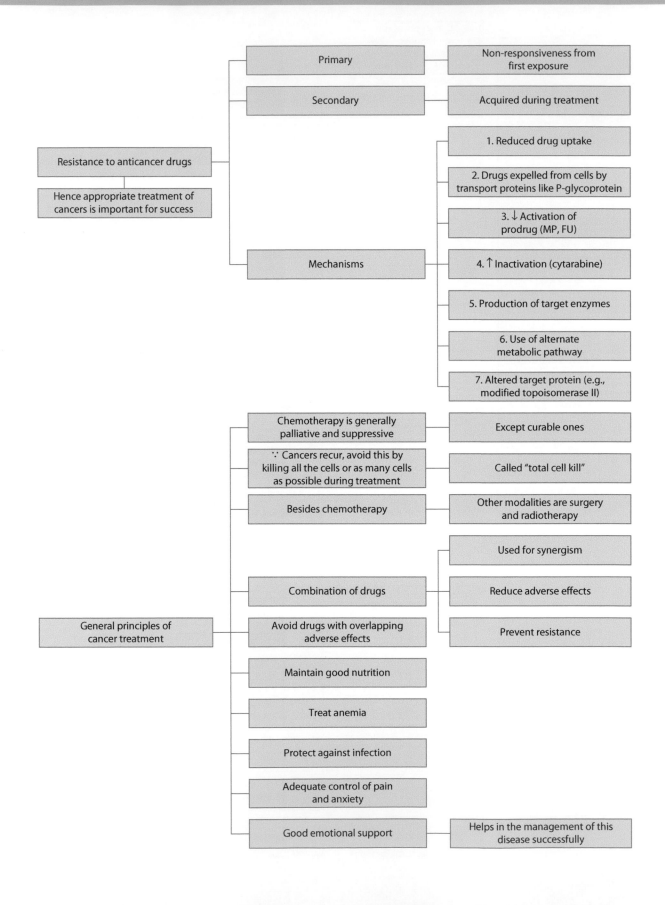

Miscellaneous

Chelating agents

74.1 CHELATING AGENTS

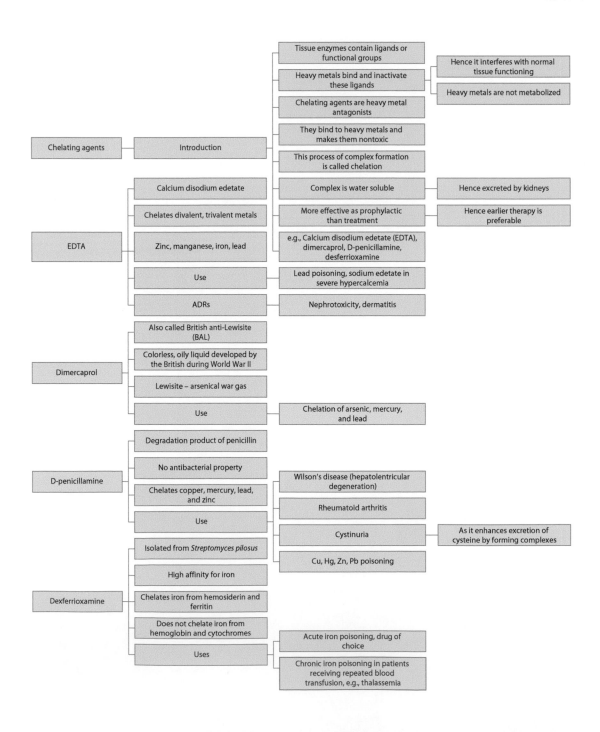

Immunosuppressants and immunostimulants

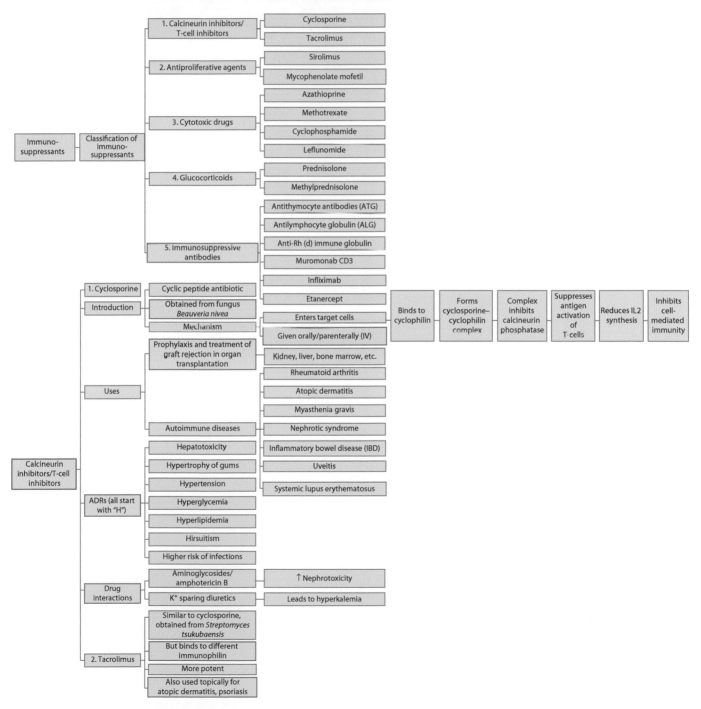

75.2 ANTIPROLIFERATIVE AGENTS

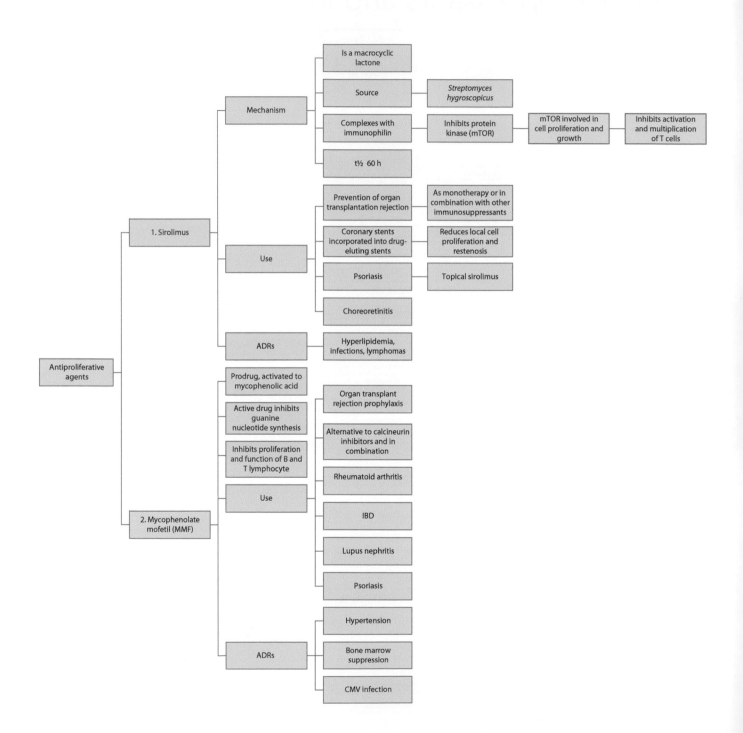

75.3 CYTOTOXIC AGENTS AND GLUCOCORTICOIDS

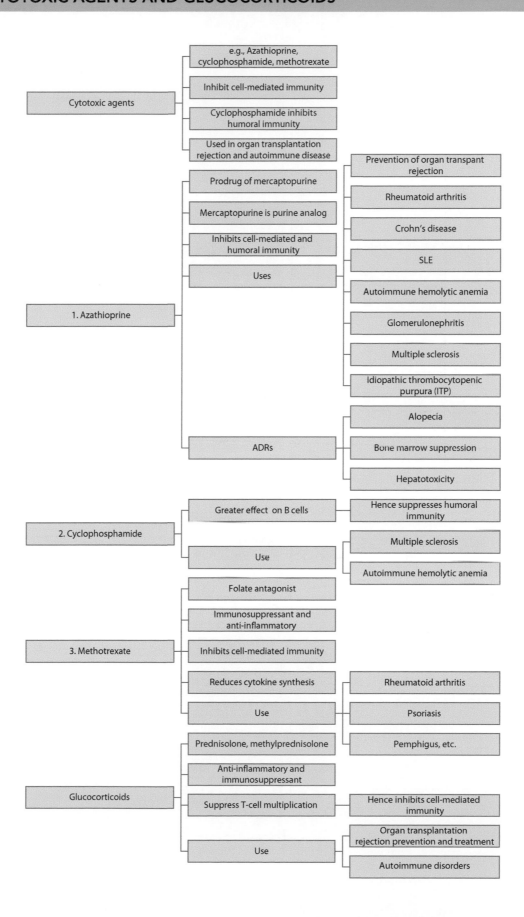

75.4 IMMUNOSUPPRESSIVE ANTIBODIES

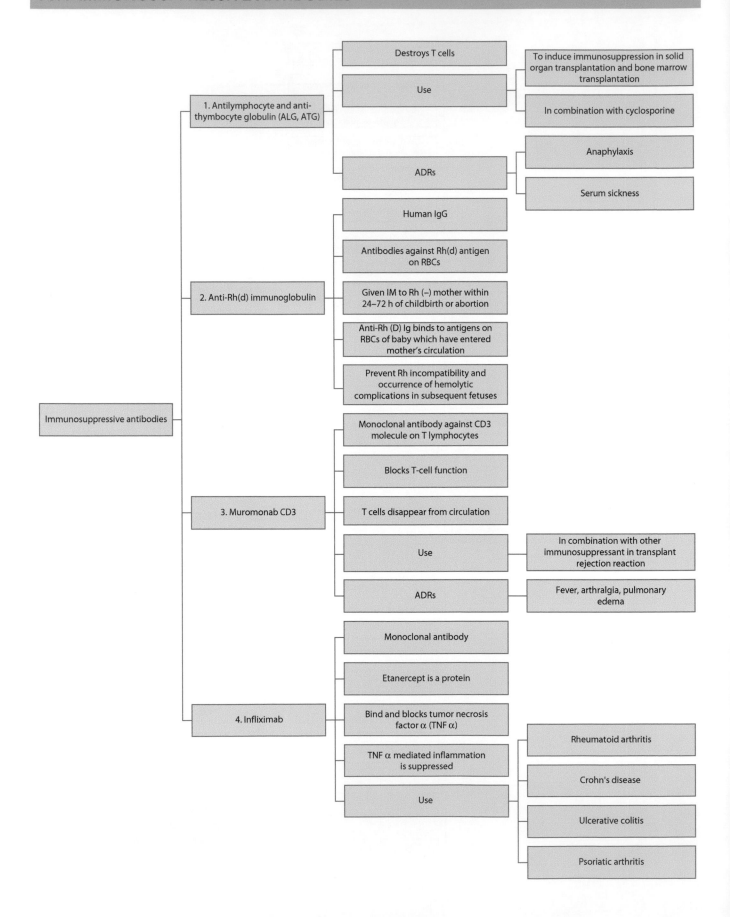

75.5 IMMUNOSTIMULANTS

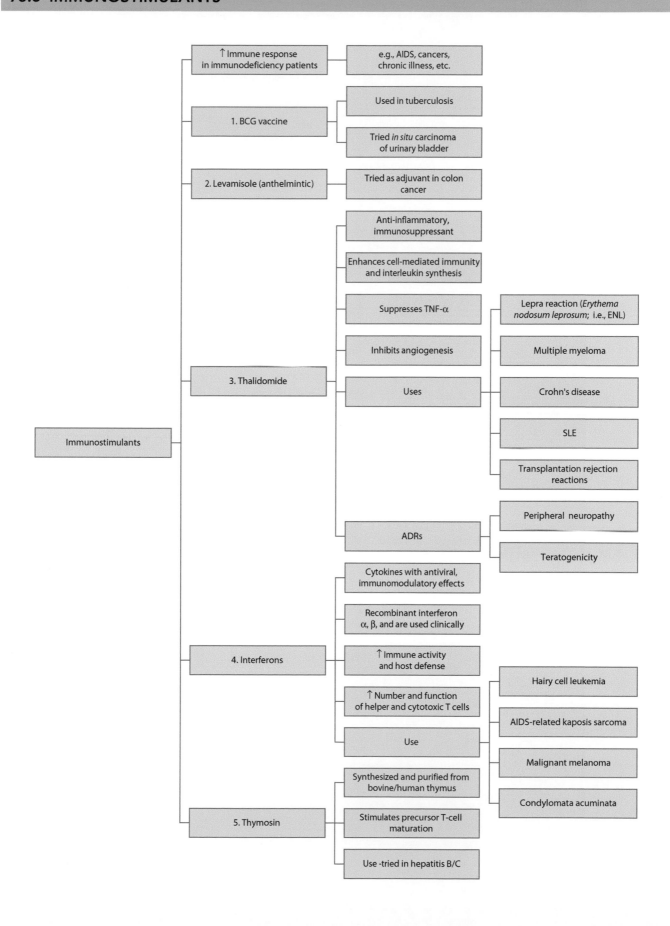

Index